THE ROUTLEDGE INTERNATIONAL HANDBOOK OF COMMUNITY PSYCHOLOGY

This handbook offers a unique critical and cross-disciplinary approach to the study of Community Psychology, showing how it can address the systemic challenges arising from multiple crises facing people across the world.

Addressing some of the most pressing issues of our times, the text shows how Community Psychology can contribute to principled social change, giving voice, enabling civic participation and supporting the realignment of social and economic power within planetary boundaries. Featuring a collaboration of contributions from world-leading academics, early career researchers and community leaders, each chapter gives theory and context with practical examples of working with those living in precarious situations, on matters that concern them most, and highlights positive ways to contribute to progressive change. The editors examine economic, ecological, demographic, gender, violence, energy, social and cultural, and political crises in relation to psychological theories, as well as public policy and lived experiences, presenting an approach situated at the intersection of public policy and lived experiences. Viewed through four different perspectives or lenses: a critical lens; a praxis lens; an ecological lens and a reflective lens, this compendium of critical explorations into Community Psychology shows how it can contribute to a fairer, more just, resilient and sustainable world.

Also examining the lessons learnt from the COVID-19 pandemic about the pervading nature of social inequality, and the potential of solidarity movements ranging from local to international levels, this is ideal reading for undergraduate and postgraduate students and scholars in Community Psychology and related areas, including social psychology, clinical psychology and applied psychology.

Carolyn Kagan is Professor Emerita of Community Social Psychology at Manchester Metropolitan University, UK. She is retired and is now a scholar-activist, involved with projects that connect localism, environmental and social justice, and community resilience.

Jacqueline Akhurst is a Professor Emerita of Rhodes University, South Africa. Her community-based research utilises Action Research or Activity Theory. Her recent focus has been on community-based service learning in higher education.

Jaime Alfaro is Professor and researcher at the Center of Studies of Well-Being and Social Coexistence, Universidad del Desarrollo, Chile. He has a PhD in social science, University of Girona, Spain.

Rebecca Lawthom is Professor of Community Psychology and Head of the School of Education at the University of Sheffield, UK. She works with others in participatory and collaborative ways to achieve valued change. Her research interests cohere around marginalisation and she writes within the fields of disability, ageing and methods.

Michael Richards is a critical community psychologist who is deputy programme leader of a child and adolescent mental health programme and deputy director of the Arts and Wellbeing Research Centre at Edge Hill University, UK.

Alba Zambrano is an academic of the Department of Psychology Universidad de La Frontera, Chile, in the field of Community Psychology. Research interests include community strengthening processes, prevention of psychosocial problems based on evidence and socio-community inclusion. She is director of the Life Skills Program UFRO JUNAEB agreement.

The Routledge International Handbook Series

The Routledge Handbook of Smart Technologies
An Economic and Social Perspective
Edited by Heinz D. Kurz, Marlies Schütz, Rita Strohmaier and Stella S. Zilian

Routledge International Handbook of Diaspora Diplomacy
Edited by Liam Kennedy

The Routledge Handbook of European Integrations
Edited by Thomas Hoerber, Gabriel Weber and Ignazio Cabras

The Routledge Handbook of Global Development
Edited by Kearrin Sims, Nicola Banks, Susan Engel, Paul Hodge, Jonathan Makuwira, Naohiro Nakamura, Jonathan Rigg, Albert Salamanca and Pichamon Yeophantong

Handbook of Urban Mobilities
Edited by Ole B. Jensen, Claus Lassen, Vincent Kaufmann, Malene Freudendal-Pedersen and Ida Sofie Gøtzsche Lange

The Routledge Handbook of Sport and Sustainable Development
Edited by Brian P. McCullough, Timothy Kellison and E. Nicole Melton

The Routledge International Handbook of Therapeutic Stories and Storytelling
Edited by Clive Holmwood, Sue Jennings and Sharon Jacksties

The Routledge Handbook of Environmental Movements
Edited by Maria Grasso and Marco Giugni

The Routledge International Handbook of Indigenous Resilience
Edited by Hilary N. Weaver

The Routledge International Handbook of Practice-Based Research
Edited by Craig Vear

THE ROUTLEDGE INTERNATIONAL HANDBOOK OF COMMUNITY PSYCHOLOGY

Facing Global Crises with Hope

Edited by
Carolyn Kagan, Jacqueline Akhurst, Jaime Alfaro,
Rebecca Lawthom, Michael Richards
and Alba Zambrano

Routledge
Taylor & Francis Group

LONDON AND NEW YORK

Cover Image: © Getty Images

First published 2022
by Routledge
4 Park Square, Milton Park, Abingdon, Oxon OX14 4RN

and by Routledge
605 Third Avenue, New York, NY 10158

Routledge is an imprint of the Taylor & Francis Group, an informa business

British Library Cataloguing-in-Publication Data
A catalogue record for this book is available from the British Library

Library of Congress Cataloging-in-Publication Data
Names: Kagan, Carolyn, editor.
Title: The Routledge international handbook of community psychology:
facing global crises with hope / edited by Carolyn Kagan, Jacqueline Akhurst,
Jaime Alfaro, Rebecca Lawthom, Michael Richards, Alba Zambrano.
Description: Milton Park, Abingdon, Oxon; New York, NY: Routledge, 2022. |
Series: Routledge international handbooks | Includes bibliographical references and index. |
Identifiers: LCCN 2021031683 (print) | LCCN 2021031684 (ebook) |
ISBN 9780367344153 (hardback) | ISBN 9781032160917 (paperback) |
ISBN 9780429325663 (ebook)
Subjects: LCSH: Community psychology–Handbooks, manuals, etc.
Classification: LCC RA790.55 .R68 2022 (print) |
LCC RA790.55 (ebook) | DDC 362.2/2–dc23
LC record available at https://lccn.loc.gov/2021031683
LC ebook record available at https://lccn.loc.gov/2021031684

ISBN: 978-0-367-34415-3 (hbk)
ISBN: 978-1-032-16091-7 (pbk)
ISBN: 978-0-429-32566-3 (ebk)

DOI: 10.4324/9780429325663

Typeset in Bembo
by Newgen Publishing UK

"It is certain, in any case, that ignorance, allied with power, is the most ferocious enemy justice can have."
James Baldwin, No Name in the Street, 1972.

We dedicate this book to all those who struggle with injustice across our divided globe. We celebrate, accept and recognise the need to remain unified and knowledgeable about the crises that face us. This book is dedicated to continued joint action for and with justice in mind.

CONTENTS

FIGURES

TABLES

NOTES ON CONTRIBUTORS

Jacqueline Akhurst is a Rhodes University Professor Emerita. Her community-based research utilises action research or activity theory. Recently her focus has been community-based service learning in higher education. https://orcid.org/0000-0003-1566-9092

Cinzia Albanesi is full Professor of Community Psychology, University of Bologna and president of the European Association of Community Psychology. Her research interests focus on community development, community partnership and participatory processes, service-learning and school-based intervention to promote well-being and civic competences. https://orcid.org/0000-0001-8240-6159

Jaime Alfaro has a PhD in social science, University of Girona. He is Professor and researcher at the Center of Studies of Well-being and Social Coexistence, Universidad del Desarrollo, Chile. https://orcid.org/0000-0003-0397-3716

Caterina Arcidiacono is a psychologist, Jungian psychoanalyst and Full Professor in Community Psychology, at the University of Naples Federico II. She is currently a member of the European Federation of Psychologists' Associations standing Committee on Community Psychology, vice president of the Associazione Italiana di Psicologia and past president of both the ECPA (European Community Psychology Association) and SIPCO (Italian Society of Community Psychology). https://orcid.org/0000-0003-3699-6981

Paola Balla, PhD, is a Wemba-Wemba and Gunditjmara woman who lectures with Moondani Balluk Indigenous Academic Centre, Victoria University. She utilises art as sovereign act, in both process and outcome for expressing Black matriarchy and First Nations ways of "being, knowing and doing". https://orcid.org/0000-0002-1321-1363

B. Mackenzie Barnett is a master's student in clinical psychology fascinated by the study of human growth and development within the broader systems they interact with. Born and raised in Canada, she has spent time living in Europe and Asia.

Garret Barnwell is a South African clinical psychologist, writing and practising mostly from critical and Community Psychology perspectives stemming from the South. This focus includes ecopsychosocial dimensions of decoloniality, climate and environmental justice. https://orcid.org/0000-0002-9414-2776

M. Isidora Bilbao-Nieva is a doctoral candidate in Ecological-Community Psychology at Michigan State University. https://orcid.org/0000-0003-0957-0723

Sally Birdsall lectures in science and sustainability education at undergraduate and postgraduate levels. Her current research explores pedagogies that can help people cope with contentious issues such as the climate emergency, focusing on the interrelationship between emotions, world views and agency. https://orcid.org/0000-0002-8348-7605

Gay Bradshaw holds doctorates in ecology and psychology. She is founder and director of The Kerulos Center for Nonviolence and The Tortoise and the Hare Sanctuary located in southern Oregon, USA.

Mark H. Burton is an independent scholar-activist, involved with a number of campaigns that connect economy, environment and social justice in Greater Manchester. He was formerly a psychologist and manager of health and social care services. https://orcid.org/0000-0001-8327-5533

Marcelo Calegare is Professor at the Faculty of Psychology and the postgraduate programme in psychology at the Federal University of Amazonas, Brazil. He is a member of the Community Psychology Working Group of the National Association for Research and Graduate Studies in Psychology. https://orcid.org/0000-0001-6814-5300

Bernice Calmes is the director at Art.1 Middle Netherlands, the provincial registry for discrimination incidents. She works on this project with a team of trainers headed by Niki Eleveld, coordinator of Education, and Mustapha Bah, coordinator of Innovation.

María Antonieta Campos Melo has a degree in psychology from the Universidad de la Frontera and is a student in the Community Psychology master programme at the Universidad de La Frontera. She is a researcher in community leadership and gender issues. She is also a professional with experience in linking with the environment of higher education institutions and community work from a Latin American approach. https://orcid.org/0000-0003-4257-0565

Moisés Carmona Monferrer is an associate professor in the social psychology and quantitative psychology department at the University of Barcelona. He has been a community psychologist for over 20 years in the city of Barcelona where he has developed interventions and research projects. https://orcid.org/0000-0002-4259-6434

Sergio Chacón Armijo has a master's degree in social and Community Psychology and is Professor in the psychology department of the Catholic University of Temuco. He is director of the LATAM Nucleus of the Global Implementation Society, head of Development at Fundación Mujer Levántate and invited expert on the stigma commission of the Iberoamerican network of NGOs working on drug addictions. https://orcid.org/0000-0001-7442-1754

Elvira Cicognani is Full Professor of Community Psychology and currently head of the Department of Psychology at the University of Bologna. Her research interests focus on civic and political engagement among youth, active citizenship interventions, health behaviours and community health promotion. https://orcid.org/0000-0002-8653-290X

Jenna Condie is a senior lecturer in digital society at Western Sydney University. Her interdisciplinary research traverses critical psychology, geography and technology studies. Her work is orientated towards enabling equitable mobilities, just places, safe spaces and emancipatory technologies. https://orcid.org/0000-0002-0811-0517

Immacolata Di Napoli, PhD, is a community psychologist and researcher at the University of Naples Federico II. Her principal research area is community trust. She has developed a scale for community trust and has taken part in action research projects in local contexts. https://orcid.org/0000-0002-7255-7735

Pierce S. Docena is a founding member of the LGBT Psychology Special Interest Group of the Psychological Association of the Philippines. He is currently an assistant professor at the University of the Philippines Visayas Tacloban College. https://orcid.org/0000-0002-3913-8782

Paul Duckett has been researching and teaching in Critical Community Psychology since the late 1990s. His work focuses on the cultural and political factors that impact understandings of disability and mental health, and impact on teaching practices in university settings. https://orcid.org/0000-0002-7340-1054

Andrea Ellwood is a mum, first and last.

Ciro Esposito is a psychologist and PhD student in mind, gender and language at the University of Naples Federico II. His main research topics are individual, relational and community well-being, social justice and gender issues, addressed from the perspective of Community Psychology. https://orcid.org/0000-0003-2440-4336

Rubén David Fernández Carrasco is researcher and associated teacher at the University of Barcelona. He is a consultant in participatory and community-based actions, and researcher and facilitator in applied drama in pursuit of social change and liberation. https://orcid.org/0000-0003-4772-7533

Isabel Fernandes de Oliveira has a PhD in clinical psychology from the University of São Paulo, Brazil. She is currently a Professor and researcher at the Federal University of Rio Grande do Norte, Brazil. She works with Community Psychology, Marxian social theory, social policy and psychologist practice. https://orcid.org/0000-0002-2153-762X

Jorge Mario Flores Osorio has worked for more than 30 years in excluded and impoverished communities with an emphasis on Mayan communities in Guatemala and Chiapas. His work has led to the development of a community research strategy called Research-Reflection-Action. https://orcid.org/0000-0002-1024-1081

Kerry Fox graduated with an MA in fine art in 2019: her work explores her journey as a mother carer. Combining art with activism, she explores how the process of making and materials give agency to strength, fragility and liminality

Antonella Guarino is post-doctoral research fellow at the Department of Psychology of the University of Bologna. Her research interests include promotion of active citizenship in schools and communities, service-learning, mental health promotion and participatory processes. https://orcid.org/0000-0003-3742-5574

Takehito Hagiwara is a specially appointed professor of the University of Human Arts and Sciences. He graduated from Keio University and earned his master of social sciences (2000) under the supervision of Professor Kazuo Yamamoto. His research interests include Community Psychology, school counselling and crisis intervention. https://orcid.org/0000-0002-5383-2818

Niki Harré is a Professor in the School of Psychology at the University of Auckland. Her research addresses issues of environmental sustainability, values, religion, political activism and how to inspire action for the common good. https://orcid.org/0000-0001-6378-324X

Daniel Hikuroa uses earth systems science and environmental humanities approaches and methods, and is based in Te Wānanga o Waipapa, at the University of Auckland.

Carolyn Kagan is Professor of Emerita Community Social Psychology at Manchester Metropolitan University. She is retired and is a scholar-activist, involved with projects that connect localism, environmental and social justice, and community resilience. https://orcid.org/0000-0001-6015-6179

Daniel Kelly is a Pākehā writer of Irish ancestry, sent south by the combination of colonisation, enclosure and hunger that informs his research today. He is a PhD candidate at the University of Auckland and a keen community gardener. https://orcid.org/0000-0003-2391-4422

Fernando Lacerda Júnior is Associate Professor at the Federal University of Goiás/Brazil. He is a member of the Critique, Insurgency, Subjectivity, and Emancipation Research Group. https://orcid.org/0000-0002-0486-5162

Rebecca Lawthom is Professor of Community Psychology and head of the School of Education at the University of Sheffield. She works with others in participatory and collaborative ways to achieve valued change. Her research interests cohere around marginalisation and she writes within fields of disability, ageing and methods. https://orcid.org/0000-0003-2625-3463

Charles Z. Levkoe is Canada Research Chair in Equitable and Sustainable Food Systems and Associate Professor at Lakehead University. His community-engaged research uses a food systems lens to explore the connections between justice, ecological regeneration, regional economies and active democratic engagement. https://foodsystems.lakeheadu.ca/ https://orcid.org/0000-0003-4950-2186

Nosipho Faith Makhakhe, PhD, is lecturer in health promotion and postdoctoral fellow at the University of KwaZulu-Natal. Her research interests include HIV prevention among high-risk populations, as well as participatory action research methods that incorporate intervention mapping and design.

Nick Malherbe is a researcher at the Institute for Social and Health Sciences, University of South Africa and South African Medical Research Council–University of South Africa Masculinity and Health Research Unit. His research interests include community-building, culture and violence. https://orcid.org/0000-0002-4968-4058

Eric Julian Manalastas was the founding coordinator of the LGBT Psychology Special Interest Group of the Psychological Association of the Philippines. He recently finished his PhD in social psychology at the University of Sheffield, UK. https://orcid.org/0000-0002-6907-4302

Nqobile Msomi is an early career lecturer at Rhodes University and counselling psychologist, registered with the Health Professions Council of South Africa. She coordinates Rhodes University's Psychology Clinic, a community-based training institution for counselling and clinical psychologists. https://orcid.org/0000-0002-9232-2028.

Laura Muñoz Restrepo is a graduate student of psychology and sociology from the Pontificia Universidad Javeriana of Bogotá, Colombia, and has worked with the research group Social Bonds and Peace Cultures. Laura has experience in the psychosocial accompaniment of rural community organisations. https://orcid.org/0000-0001-6667-0697

Moniq M. Muyargas is a member of the LGBT Psychology Special Interest Group of the Psychological Association of the Philippines. She is currently an assistant professor at the University of the Philippines Iloilo. https://orcid.org/0000-0003-1092-3231

Karen Nairn's current research is with young activists working for social change in Aotearoa, which builds on earlier research with young people who grew up during New Zealand's neoliberal reforms, as reported in *Children of Rogernomics: A Neoliberal Generation Leaves School.* https://orcid.org/0000-0002-0855-8434

Sipho Ngcongo is a master's student in health promotion, School of Psychology at the University KwaZulu-Natal. Sipho is a critical reflexive scholar with a keen interest in Community Psychology and sexual consent-related research.

Alejandra Olivera-Méndez has a PhD in rural social development from the University of Reading, England. She is a professor in the programme Innovation in Natural Resources Management at the Postgraduate College, San Luis Potosí Campus, Mexico. She is also coordinator of the Rural Psychology Latin American Network. https://orcid.org/0000-0002-3144-6553

Fortuna Procentese, PhD, is Professor of Community Psychology at the University of Naples Federico II, director of the postgraduate course in Emergency Psychology (development path for resilient communities), president of the Italian Society of Community Psychology (SIPCO), and member of the European Community Psychology Association (ECPA) board. https://orcid.org/0000-0002-1617-0165

Amy F. Quayle, PhD, is a lecturer in psychology at Victoria University, Melbourne, Australia. She has examined the experience of racialised oppression and implications for identities, communities and possibilities created through community arts practice for individual, community and social change. https://orcid.org/0000-0003-3824-1056

Kai Reimer-Watts is a PhD student in Community Psychology at Wilfrid Laurier University, with a master of climate change (MCC) from the University of Waterloo. His work explores the intersections of the arts, movement-building and grassroots activism to promote a more just, safe climate future. https://orcid.org/0000-0003-0058-4539

Michael Richards is a critical community psychologist who is deputy programme leader of a child and adolescent mental health programme and deputy director of the Arts and Wellbeing Research Centre at Edge Hill University, UK. https://orcid.org/0000-0002-6857-580X

Manuel Riemer, PhD, is a professor of Community Psychology and sustainability science at Wilfrid Laurier University and director of the Viessmann Centre for Engagement and Research in Sustainability (wlu.ca/veris). His community-based action research is focused on the intersection of community, environment and justice with projects related to cultures of sustainability and sustainability justice. wlu.ca/veris https://orcid.org/0000-0001-5478-2034

Te Kerekere Roycroft is a doctoral candidate at Te Wānanga o Waipapa – The University of Auckland. Her research centres on the generationally evolving definitions of both *whakapapa*-based and adoptive *tūrangawaewae* for *whanaunga* who live at "home" and in urban environments. https://orcid.org/0000-0001-5066-9712

Katherine Runswick-Cole is Professor of Education in the School of Education at the University of Sheffield. Her background is in critical disability studies, disabled children's childhood studies and critical and Community Psychology. https://orcid.org/0000-0001-9658-9718

Sara Ryan is Professor of Social Care at Manchester Metropolitan University. A sociologist by background, her research focuses on disability studies, in particular learning disability and critical autism studies. She is a strong proponent of scholar activism. https://orcid.org/0000-0002-7406-1610

Stella Sacipa Rodríguez (MA) has retired as Professor of Peace Psychology from the Pontificia Universidad Javeriana of Bogotá, Colombia, where she led the research group Social Bonds and Peace Cultures for many years. Her work has focused on ways to support and accompany victims of war.

Herling Sanhueza Yáñez has a master's degree in Community Psychology and is an academic and coordinator of the line of community intervention, Universidad de Las Américas. She has taught in universities in Chile, at undergraduate and graduate level, both in the social-community area and clinical psychology. Her area of specialisation is: mental health problems, networks and community processes in rural and urban areas in Chile. https://orcid.org/0000-0003-2249-6599

Mohamed Seedat is the head of the Institute for Social and Health Sciences at the University of South Africa. He writes about violence, the psychologies underlying South Africa's democratic and development imaginations, and engaged approaches to research and development. https://orcid.org/0000-0001-9018-3370

Yvonne Sliep, PhD, holds an honorary position at the School of Psychology, University KwaZulu-Natal, South Africa, and is an international consultant for collective healing and peacebuilding in Africa. She specialised in narrative research and narrative theatre in community based co-created interventions.

Christopher C. Sonn, PhD, is Professor of Community Psychology at Victoria University, Melbourne, Australia. His research examines various forms of structural violence and its effects on social identities, intergroup relations and belonging. https://orcid.org/0000-0002-6175-1030

Mirella L. Stroink is Professor of Psychology and Dean of Health and Behavioural Sciences at Lakehead University in Canada. Applying complex adaptive systems theory to human cognition and behaviour, her research examines psychological resilience, systems thinking, food and well-being in the ecological and social context. https://orcid.org/0000-0002-8311-0939

Shahnaaz Suffla is Associate Professor at the Institute for Social and Health Sciences, University of South Africa. Shahnaaz's research interests are draw from the intersections of decolonial, African, community and peace psychologies, and are located within liberatory philosophies and epistemologies. https://orcid.org/0000-0002-4597-5472

Beatriz A. Torre is a founding member and current chairperson of the LGBT Psychology Special Interest Group of the Psychological Association of the Philippines. She is currently an assistant professor at the University of the Philippines Diliman. https://orcid.org/0000-0001-5269-4815

Claudia Tovar Guerra, PhD, is Professor of Psychology at the Pontificia Universidad Javeriana of Bogotá, Colombia. She is a current member of the research group Social Bonds and Peace Cultures. Her work includes working with communities on psychosocial accompaniment, cultures of peace and processes of civil resistance. https://orcid.org/0000-0003-2771-6837

Carlie D. Trott, PhD, is an assistant professor in psychology at the University of Cincinnati, whose participatory and action-oriented research aims to bring visibility to, and work against the inequitable impacts of climate change, socially and geographically. www.cdtrott.com/. https://orcid.org/0000-0002-4400-4287

Iana Tzankova is postdoctoral research fellow at the Department of Psychology of the University of Bologna. Her research interests include civic and political participation in adolescence and young adulthood, environmental behaviour and activism. https://orcid.org/0000-0001-7172-2009

Mariola Elizabeth Vicente Xiloj, Maya K'staniche' from Momostenango Totonicapán, Guatemala. Mariola is a lecturer at the University of San Carlos de Guatemala and has worked with indigenous and peasant groups in western Guatemala in the struggle for political recognition by the state.

Mary Watkins is co-founder of the community, liberation, indigenous and eco-psychologies specialisation at Pacifica Graduate Institute; author of *Mutual Accompaniment and the Creation of the Commons*; and co-author of *Toward Psychologies of Liberation* and *Up Against the Wall: Re-Imagining the U.S.-Mexico Border*.

Mari Yoshinaga is a professor of clinical-community laboratory at Showa Pharmaceutical University, Machida, Tokyo, Japan. Her research interests include children and adolescents' participation in community development and community-based participatory studies. She is also a representative of an organisation to ensure outdoor play for children. https://orcid.org/0000-0002-2618-7841

Alba Zambrano has a master's degree in applied social sciences and in educational sciences, with mention in social development. She is an academic in the Department of Psychology Universidad de La Frontera in the field of Community Psychology. Alba's research interests include community strengthening processes, prevention of psychosocial problems based on evidence and socio-community inclusion. She is director of the Life Skills Program UFRO JUNAEB agreement. https://orcid.org/0000-0002-0052-3456

Bruna Zani is Alma Mater Professor, University of Bologna, former full professor of Community Psychology. Her research interests are community mental health, risk behaviours in adolescence, social representations, service learning, civic engagement and political participation in young people, and personalised health budget. https://orcid.org/0000-0001-7358-5001

Sally Zlotowitz is a clinical and community psychologist working in the fields of mental health inequalities, innovation, and redesigning services and addressing the social determinants of psychological health in partnership with marginalised communities. She is currently CEO of the charity Art Against Knives in London. She is a co-founder of Psychologists for Social Change.

ACKNOWLEDGEMENTS

We would like to thank Eleanor Taylor and Alex Howard from Routledge for their support for the book from start to finish.

Linsey Parkinson has assisted with the administrative aspects of working with six editors and 70 authors across 25 chapters. She prepared the manuscript for submission with enthusiastic, efficient cheeriness, whilst still making substantial contributions to the resilience and cohesion of her local community. She lit up the last stages of preparation of the book.

Mark Burton, as well as contributing a co-authored chapter, helped with abstract translations and in overcoming the software difficulties we had as we shared chapters amongst the editors.

To our authors, a particular acknowledgement and thanks for working with us on the book during what, for many of us, has been the most trying of years, during the pandemic of COVID-19.

INTRODUCTION
Facing global crises

Carolyn Kagan, Jacqueline Akhurst, Jaime Alfaro,
Rebecca Lawthom, Michael Richards and Alba Zambrano

Abstract

We introduce the idea of interconnected global crises affecting the lives of peoples, including economic, sociocultural, political and ecological crises as well as the crisis of violence. They are all situated at the intersection of public policy and lived experiences, whether this is in families, communities or workplaces and influence how social institutions operate in different places. They also, paradoxically, present opportunities for resistance and hope, and it is this complexity and potential that is addressed in the handbook. We consider lessons learnt from the COVID-19 pandemic about the pervading nature of social inequality but also the potential of solidarity movements ranging from local to international levels. We overview all the chapters, viewed through four different perspectives or lenses: a critical lens; a praxis lens; an ecological lens; and a reflective lens.

Resumen

Introducimos la idea de crisis globales interconectadas que afectan a la vida de los pueblos, incluidas las crisis económica, sociocultural, política y ecológica, así como la crisis de violencia. Todos ellos se sitúan en la intersección de la política pública y las experiencias vividas, ya sea en las familias, comunidades o lugares de trabajo e influyen en el funcionamiento de las instituciones sociales en distintos lugares. También presentan oportunidades de resistencia y esperanza. Consideramos las lecciones aprendidas de la pandemia de COVID-19 sobre la omnipresencia de la desigualdad social, pero también las posibilidades de movimientos de solidaridad que van desde el nivel local hasta el internacional. Pasamos a una revisión general de los diferentes capítulos, vistos a través de cuatro perspectivas o lentes diferentes: una lente crítica; una lente de praxis; una lente ecológica; y una lente reflectante.

This handbook showcases the relevance of, and contribution made by some contemporary community psychologies in addressing various systemic challenges that arise from multiple crises facing people across the world. A crisis represents a crossroads – to carry on to disaster, or to pause, change direction and make moves towards recovery of some sort. The recovery we seek is for improved social, ecological and economic justice – a transformation in how financial, material and political resources are shared; ecological resources are protected; and

DOI: 10.4324/9780429325663-1

social resources are celebrated. In each chapter, the authors present a Community Psychology response to a crisis or interconnected crises.

Interconnected and systemic crises

The handbook focuses on community psychological responses to those social schisms created by and reflected in the different, interconnected and overlapping crises –crises which impede our progress towards a world with strong social justice, good stewardship over human and ecological resources, and lives lived in solidarity with each other, characterised by high levels of social trust and cohesion. These crises threaten not just individual and societal well-being, but the very sustainability of the planet and our lives upon it. We cannot ignore the fact that the book has been written during a crisis of a different sort – the COVID-19 pandemic – but, as we shall see, the very existence and impact of the pandemic cannot be separated from the wider web of crises (see chapters by Runswick-Cole et al.; Sliep et al.; Zambrano et al.).

There are a number of ways of characterising the crises to which we have alluded, but here we represent them as (i) an economic crisis; (ii) a sociocultural crisis; (iii) the crisis of conflict and violence; (iv) a political crisis; and perhaps most importantly, as it threatens the very future of the planet, (v) an ecological, environmental and energy crisis (Kagan and Burton, 2014; Kagan and Lewis, 2015).

Of course these crises are interconnected: conflicts are often due to economic issues and increasingly climate change; political populism and state-sponsored violence arise in times of economic uncertainty and dispossession (Forgas et al., 2021); the ecological, environmental and energy crises are fundamentally the results of the ravages of capitalism, shored up by political corruption and power grabbing, and increasingly give rise to conflict; threats to sociocultural cohesion arise as social trust and identities are fractured by the operation of power and dominance, a disrespect and refusal to see the "other" as equal, and underpin both economic marginalisation and conflicts. Running through these crises are tenacious issues of gender inequities and of demographic change, clearly identified in the United Nations' Sustainable Development Goals (SDGs) (Esquivel, 2016).

An economic crisis

The economic crisis is a slow fuse crisis, characterised by economic trends and the worldwide adoption of neoliberal economic practices and ideologies in the service of capitalism. These forces have built on and exacerbated an increase in inequalities, within and between groups and nations worldwide. In all types of economies, they threaten social justice and underpin an increase in insecure work or unemployment, long working hours, work intensification and feelings of alienation at work, which then all have knock-on effects on families and lead to greater social instability. The increase in wealth inequality within and between groups and nations throughout the world has contributed to health inequalities and the dilution of social trust, and a retreat to individualistic beliefs and ideologies. The "common sense" of the neoliberal era is beginning to fracture and movements for change are growing (see chapters by Arcidiacono et al.; Zlotowitz and Burton; Fernandes de Oliviera and Lacerda).

A social and cultural crisis

The social and cultural crisis is reflected in the erosion of human and cultural capital of our societies and in the fracturing of identities. A model of passivity-inducing consumerism displaces the humanising practices of social solidarity and cultural production common in many indigenous societies. In the Global North, this is fuelled by the enormous expansion of consumer credit and household debt (supported by governments and corporations), and time spent in alienating, precarious work (Değirmencioğlu and Walker, 2015). The recuperation of social-historical and cultural practices is needed, building on the many examples of alternative social norms, and harnessing the best of technological developments (see chapter by Condie and Richards).

There are changing demographic patterns and movements of peoples. Worldwide population growth is accompanied in many parts of the world by ageing and even dwindling populations, and missing generations in others. Population displacement and movement is greater across the globe than ever before, with estimates of more than 214 million people now living outside their country of origin in search of protection or opportunity and many more internally displaced. This movement is due to war, economic shocks and neoliberal strategies, and so-called natural disasters due to climate change. Those forced to move often live lives characterised by fear, degradation and danger, with the violence poverty or environmental degradation they seek to escape, appearing in other forms. These include in-family violence, xenophobic attacks, workplace exploitation and hostilities, and weakening of community cohesion. Such demographic changes are transforming social lives and communities, unevenly in different places (see chapters by Tovar Guerra et al.; Barnwell et al.).

We have explored these issues through looking at decolonial (and anti-colonial) approaches within Community Psychology, which include epistemic justice, accompaniment, the recuperation of historical memory and issues of inclusion and of technology (see chapters by Carmona and Fernandes; Condie and Richards; Malherbe et al.; Flores Osorio and Vicente Xiloj; Tovar Guerra et al.; Sonn et al.; Arcidiacono et al.).

A crisis of violence

The crisis of violence is long in the making. Violence is a central feature of life for many across the globe. Sometimes people are caught up in wars and large-scale conflicts; sometimes attempts to resist oppression are met with violence of a different scale; sometimes it is state-perpetuated violence through torture or via the demeaning treatment of minorities, low-paid workers and those supported by state benefits; sometimes it is violence enacted at a domestic level, affecting countless women and children across the world. Women and children are disproportionately badly affected by violence and the fear of violence – physical, sexual, psychological or state. In many places, collective responses to violence and to peace building are challenging the corporate interests underpinning conflict at different levels (see chapters by Duckett; Tovar Guerra et al.; Flores Osorio and Vicente Xiloj).

A political crisis

The political crisis is one in which there is a resurgence of authoritarian movements and regimes that assert populist, nationalistic and xenophobic politics across the globe. These movements are in grave danger of fracturing the liberal-democratic consensus that has prevailed in some parts of the world, and are thwarting aspirations for a liberal-democratic consensus in other places. As regimes seek to grab resources for their backers, we see a decrease in social equity, social trust and social cohesion, and a concentration of both power and resources in the hands of a minority, rendering the majority at risk of ill-health and a lack of autonomy. The political crisis intersects particularly with crises of the economy, population displacement and violence and climate change; and in many places social movements have emerged which seek to address the rise of nationalism, the democratic deficit and weakening social cohesion (see chapters by Arcidiacono et al.; Fernandes de Oliviera and Lacerda; Yoshinaga and Hagiwara; Zambrano et al.; Zlotowitz and Burton).

An ecological crisis

The ecological crisis includes not only the degradation of natural resources, which is a threat to well-being and essentially to human life itself, but also the reliance on fossil fuels for energy and the man-made changes to the climate that follow. With planetary boundaries being crossed, climate change is likely to lead to the collapse of support systems for human life. Greedy, economically driven activities have shaped working lives, decimated natural resources, destroyed communities and severed long-standing practices of living in harmony with nature in many parts of the world. As people's habitats are squeezed, we can expect to see more conflicts of the most basic kinds – competition for resources to sustain life.

Energy use is one of the sites that most easily reveals global injustice: the challenge is for high-energy users in the North to use less, whilst enabling progress in the South. A fundamental shift in how communities function will be needed in the Global North, which has much to learn from the Global South and from community-level responses to alternative energy sources. Whilst global warming and climate change often seem remote from the everyday challenges facing people in the Global North, they present day-to-day challenges for families and communities in the Global South. Even in the Global North, responses to the environmental challenge demonstrate the power of collectivity, solidarity and community building (see chapters by Harré et al.; Olivera-Méndez and Calegare; Stroink et al.; Watkins et al.; Yoshinaga and Hagiwara).

These various crises are interdependent and have a systemic nature – they are not easily described, not easily predicted and are complex. Indeed, they fall into the category of wicked problems, where complexity dominates. They differentially affect the poor, the majority of disempowered women, disabled people, minority and dominated ethnic groups. They are all situated at the intersection of public policy and lived experiences, whether this is in families, communities or workplaces, and influence how social institutions operate indifferent places. They also, paradoxically, present opportunities for resistance and hope, and it is this complexity and potential that we will address in the handbook.

Lived experience within families and communities, embraced by these systemic crises, is coloured by issues of power and powerlessness, which in turn intersect with beliefs, gender, age, ability and sexuality. These intersections differ with place. Gender and sexuality are intertwined and exist in complex interaction with societies in different ways. The patterns of power and powerlessness play out differently across time and place, but suffice to say there is an enduring domination of privilege afforded to able-bodied men and masculinity. Women and people identifying with a range of gender identities (LGBTQ+) and disabled people, across the globe, have unequal access to economic power, to health and to well-paid jobs, whilst their places in families and communities reflect a web of different kinds of influences and subjugations. Though in many places social norms have changed or are changing, we still see the dominance of able-bodiedness, gendered assumptions and patriarchal and masculineal attitudes and ideologies played out at every level and in just about every place, with impacts on social institutions, including work and workplaces, families and communities, mediated by social identities and access to resources (see chapters by Runswick Cole et al.; Manalastas et al.).

Feminist perspectives greatly assist in understanding and working with the intersections of power, resource allocation and social identities, and in offering new ways of understanding the possibilities for futures built on solidarity, not individual self-interest. Feminist thought must be considered relevant to each of the systemic crises addressed. There is a gap in the handbook: an absence of a chapter explicitly focusing on feminist work. Nevertheless, gender, sexuality and feminisms do thread through some of the chapters to a greater or lesser degree (see chapters by Condie and Richards; Manasalatas et al.; Yoshinaga and Hagiwara; Zambrano et al.). We are fascinated by this gap. In part it is a product of our commissioning of chapters (an author who was to write from a feminist perspective was unable to participate). But this does not explain the absence of feminist perspectives throughout the other chapters.

The voices of young people are the voices of the future and hold possibilities for shifting social power (see chapters by Alfaro and Bilbao-Nieva; Yoshinaga and Hagiwara). In this realm, work with students in higher education becomes important, both to help them see the systemic interconnectivity of the political with all other socio-economic and cultural influences, and also to offer them other alternatives that may engender activism and with it, greater hope. These young adults have the energy and technological know-how to mobilise others and through praxis, Critical Community Psychology offers them tools (see chapters by Akhurst and Msomi; Manalastas et al.; Zani et al.).

Collaboration is an important aspect of community psychological practice and most of the chapters reflect this in their co-authorship. There will be some unfamiliar names amongst the authors, which is as it should be. By and large, experienced and maybe familiar community psychologists have, as their co-authors, at least one person who is at an earlier stage of their career or is a community partner. This is a deliberate and small step to disrupting the hegemony of the production of community psychological work and of its rewards. The chapters are all the better for this. It is reminiscent of the "crisis" in social psychology of the 1970s, during which postgraduates challenged the eminent social psychologists present at a conference, most of whom were editors of social psychology journals, saying something to the tune of "if you want to change the discipline, put postgraduates in charge of the Journals" (Strickland et al., 1976). We do, however, recognise the additional work this collaboration has meant for authors, sometimes with mentoring and support as well as writing.

The handbook is, therefore, about how Critical Community Psychology theory and practice can contribute to principled social change, with researchers working on some of the most pressing issues of our times, in ways that give others voice, enable civic participation and support the realignment of social and economic power within planetary boundaries. The pandemic features explicitly in some chapters (see chapters by Runswick-Cole et al.; Sliep et al.; Zambrano et al.), but others address underlying issues and the challenges facing Community Psychology.

The COVID-19 pandemic

Almost as soon as we had commissioned chapters for the handbook, the COVID-9 pandemic spread across the world. Whilst this is undoubtedly a health crisis of enormous magnitude, what it has also done is to expose so many ways in which the social, economic and environmental arrangements of the twenty-first century are not well designed to preserve and sustain human life itself. Many of these arrangements are, indeed, at crisis point.

The pandemic has exposed social ruptures that determine many people's lived experiences. It has revealed the precarity in which many people live their lives; social inequalities in terms of exposure to and impact of the virus, as well as access to medical treatment; the ideological bases of different political systems; and the inadequacy of health and social safety nets in very many places.

It has also exposed the strength of women – not only those female political leaders who had the convictions and skills to prioritise people's health and survival over the relentless pursuit of profits for the few; but also those many women in low-paid health, care and cleaning work who ensured the safety of thousands; as well as those many women who led community responses to the pandemic, whilst also carrying the bulk of the additional load of caring and schooling and frequently experiencing even greater domestic abuse than usual.

The pandemic has shown the cruelty of those political systems that embrace capitalism in its foulest neoliberal forms, which sought to preserve corporations over lives. It has shown us how the most wealthy have got even wealthier, whilst many others have lost their homes and livelihoods.

It has given new meanings to the idea of marginalisation: those living at the margins of their homelands, fleeing conflict, in refugee camps or in overcrowded areas in the cities were often invisible and unheard in their struggles; they have been rendered particularly vulnerable to the pandemic due to crowded living conditions. Indigenous communities in some parts of the world have been devastated by the virus. In the Global North in particular, the pandemic has revealed the fragility of the ways in which older people are cared for, as those in care homes were not only at risk of premature death, but also cruelly isolated and separated from their families and friends. Healthcare decisions around treatment, resuscitation and vaccination have made more prominent the valuing of some lives over others (for example, non-disabled over disabled – see chapter by Runswick-Cole et al.). We recognise that COVID-19 exacerbates inequality and impacts upon personal arenas of family and public, shared communities and workspaces (Fisher et al., 2020).

However, the pandemic has also revealed the strong social value placed on care and caring, often not reflected in political and organisational values – and certainly not in the recognition given to those workers. It has demonstrated that when social trust is low, politicians are disbelieved and rules to reduce viral transmission are broken; but at the same time it has shown that people can understand risk, take responsibility and follow rules if it is made easy for them to do so. It has also demonstrated that when pushed, people in the Global North can reduce unnecessary consumption and begin to recognise what is important in life – social connection rather than material goods. It has shown the extent to which a collective purpose can override personal interests, as people did what they could to help and support others and to protect them from viral infection. It has shown how people's physical health can improve in those cities where vehicle emissions were reduced during lockdowns, but that mental health is put under great strain through the loss of social contacts and continuing states of fear and uncertainty.

Community psychologists have risen to the challenge of working together internationally to witness, respond to and share some of the positive community responses to COVID-19 that resonate with their own value-based and principled practices. These are practices that seek, as much as anything else, to work with people to achieve change through struggle, organisation, alliances and hope. (An example is the *New Bank of Community Ideas*, a joint initiative between the US-based Society for Community Research and Action (SCRA) and the European Community Psychology Association (ECPA), designed to capture small-scale, inspiring stories of resilience, solidarity and community building from around the world. Another, of longer standing, is the Global Knowledge Exchange, building connections between emerging and leading regions of Critical Community Psychology, including South Africa, Indonesia, Aotearoa New Zealand Australia, Chile, Canada and the USA.) In the UK, a community action and resilience workstream was set up within the professional body the British Psychological Society, in response to COVID-19. The Build Back Better movement aims to strengthen communities using participative processes (BPS, 2021).

Fundamentally, the pandemic has revealed the long-standing failure of good stewardship of our environments. Factory farming, the degradation of the environment and reduced biodiversity have led to increased chances of zoonotic transmission, as habitats are eroded and (particularly small) mammals come ever more closely into contact with humans.

COVID-19 has exposed, therefore, what we, as community psychologists know full well about social injustices and inequities and the fragility of social protection measures. It has also, perhaps, held a mirror up to us and our discipline, forcing us to examine further the adequacy of our praxis – showing the potential for greater international collaboration within and beyond the discipline.

The pandemic has enabled us to see more clearly the political, economic, social and ecological systems in which we are immersed and how we might "build back better". We have also seen communities' resilience and the power of the collective in maintaining support and solidarity. Resilience is, on the one hand, a deeply personal ability to bounce back from adversity; on the other hand, it is a thoroughly collective ability to not only respond to adversity but also to change – even transform – the sources of that adversity that affects people unequally (Hart et al., 2016). The sources of adversity during the pandemic, but also those that people face more generally, are closely linked to societal organisation at macrolevels – the economic, political, social and ecological realms with their interconnections. These in turn are linked to the systemic crises that we currently face.

A period of unprecedented social solidarity

Whilst the world has cowered in the face of COVID-19, there have been some recent and concurrent widespread collective acts of resistance. We have seen unprecedented forms of social solidarity, taking different forms in different places. For example, we have seen, born from a crisis of a different sort, the crisis reached by realisations of the longer-term impact of slavery and colonialism, the Black Lives Matter and anti-racist protests, mostly in the Global North, with white people joining the demonstrations for the first time in substantial numbers. These have burgeoned into more than local demonstrations of protest and solidarity, to become a worldwide movement drawing attention to the brutal colonial legacies and the continued economic marginalisation that has resulted for many.

Greta Thunberg has motivated young and old to take action on climate change – Fridays for the Future and Extinction Rebellion both preceded the pandemic. These movements have galvanised masses of people in lots of different places. Declarations of climate emergencies by major cities and even some governments have mobilised people who had hitherto been politically inactive. Similarly, the surge of protest with the #MeToo movement and other more local demonstrations against sexual and physical violence towards women, has also mobilised some people to take action for the first time.

In recent years, pro-democracy and anti-corruption street protests, born of failing governments and economies, and weak public services, have risen, largely against authoritarian governments, in places as far apart as Hong Kong, Myanmar, Chile, Tunisia, Iraq, Lebanon, Ecuador, Tunisia, Uganda and Belarus. Street protests have arisen in different places, including Hong Kong and Chile (see chapter by Zambrano et al.). Put these progressive movements alongside the growth in populism we have seen particularly in countries of the Global North, and we have a picture of social unrest and resistance, independent of the pandemic.

These demonstrations of social solidarity have taken place at the intersections of those systemic global crises, outlined above, which have strongly influenced people's experiences of, and impact of the pandemic.

Overview of the book

There is a loose structure to the book, moving from some of the grounding theoretical ideas, addressing each of the systemic crises, through praxis to reflection. However, it is best thought of as a collection of themes and variations (to borrow a musical metaphor), in which issues come and go; practice takes different forms and all culminate in greater hope and the possibility of a more just, liveable world, and a more relevant, decolonial or even anti-colonial, transformative praxis. The place-based nature of the work is an important feature of community psychological praxis; place matters and is therefore theorised alongside and within the praxis.

The stance taken throughout the book is a political one: one that makes explicit the values and principles of not only prevailing systems of knowledge and practice but also of the imagined futures of societies transformed, societies, that is, with a shift in power and resources away from corporations and the wealthy minority, in favour of the most poor, marginalised and dispossessed, and in favour of the environment. These are lofty aims and we are aware of the dangers of overclaiming our impact. We must be realistic about the contribution of Community Psychology to the shifts in power needed in order to progress: it is only through being clear about our own praxis and making links and forming alliances with others working to the same ends that we can consider ourselves part of a social movement for societal transformation – or at least attempt to prefigure a better world in which to live (Cornish et al., 2016).

As we strive to work with communities to maintain their acts of support and solidarity in a post-COVID-19 future, and to work for social transformation in other ways, we still find ourselves embroiled in a web of systemic crises. Whilst for some these do not pose immediate threat to life, for others they certainly underpin the destruction of lives and livelihoods and any possibility of human and non-human flourishing.

We have organised the book as if we were looking at Community Psychology from four different viewpoints or through four different lenses: a critical lens; a praxis lens; an ecological lens; and a reflective lens. There are linkages and overlaps between the different lenses, but the metaphor of a lens permits us to focus in, or magnify, key elements of that viewpoint. A lens is different from a gaze: a gaze invites outsiders to look in, whereas a lens is implicitly embodied so the writers and the readers become immersed in the subject matter. Lens remind us that no view can come from nowhere and the lens and shaping is an important funnel of knowledge production.

Within each lens are themes and variations and a focus on one or more of the systemic crises.

The critical lens

The five chapters viewed through a critical lens provide some foundational ideas and key groundings that are picked up in the following chapters. Chapters in this section address the sociocultural crisis, the economic crisis, the ecological crisis, the political crisis and the crisis of violence. The authors, coming as they do from different regions in the world, each in different ways reveal limitations in hegemonic community psychological work and ways forward to remediate these.

Malherbe et al. give both a rationale for and examples of how knowledge is central to the coloniality and of the need for an epistemo-political decolonisation of Community Psychology, moving beyond the dominant cultural ideologies and practices of the colonisers. Drawing on work with a low-income community in South Africa, they illustrate some of the ways in which epistemic freedom can be sought, whilst at the same time resisting epistemicide. The chapter concludes with a consideration of what epistemic freedom could mean for a truly decolonising Community Psychology.

Fernandes de Oliviera and Lacerdo take us to Brazil and an exploration of the challenges faced by the grassroots Community Psychology that emerged from the favelas in achieving lasting social change. They argue that this is, in part, due to an abandonment of radical theoretical knowledge to guide praxis, and argue a return to Marxism as a means to fully understand social dynamics as a contradictory, processual, material and historical totality. Marxism, they suggest, can help Community Psychology address, in part, the political crisis, through an understanding and articulation of the possibilities for social change under contemporary capitalism. In particular, it can allow us to see ways in which the grip of private property and elites in a class society can be weakened.

Marxist theory is a theory of political economy, and Zlotowitz and Burton draw our attention to ways in which political economy is central to community psychological endeavours, with an emphasis on the ways the economic crisis is characterised by the economic system and how its power relations structure the lives of people in their communities. They give examples from the diverse fields of mobilising against austerity in the UK and working in alliance with others in the Degrowth and economic localism movements, to show both the importance of, and ways of, integrating political economy into community psychological work.

Picking up on the ecological crisis alluded to in the previous chapter, Barnwell et al. invite us to think about the role that ecopsychosocial accompaniment can play in a Community Psychology that rejects the separation of humans from the rest of the natural world, which is at the core of the ecological crisis. They present examples of ecopsychosocial accompaniment with animals, with the rest of the natural world and with people in forced migration.

Population displacement, including forced migration is frequently a result of conflict and violence. The final chapter, viewed through the critical lens, is by Duckett, who reveals yet another lacuna in much of community psychological work, namely war and violence more generally. He urges us to move beyond thinking of violence as an interpersonal activity, to understanding violence as structural and experienced by people who lack social power. He argues that academic institutions are marked by the features of structural violence and that this might underpin Community Psychology's silence on structural violence as a result. Duckett moves beyond knowledge structures to recommend a Community Psychology focusing on social institutions, hierarchies of social power and on ways in which understanding how social policies enact social sanctions against socio-economically distressed and disadvantaged people.

Viewing Community Psychology through a critical lens requires us to confront themes of coloniality, hegemonic practices and social structures and embrace new ways of thinking about and doing Community Psychology, not just theoretically but also in praxis, in pursuit of liberation and emancipation – themes to be explored next, as we view Community Psychology through a praxis lens.

The praxis lens

Community Psychology is but one liberatory praxis, working with those oppressed, marginalised and excluded from access to social resources, power and ways to live fulfilling lives (Kagan et al., 2020). It does, though, have a unique way of combining not just psychological but also other social theories with practice – and the integration of theory and practice is its praxis. Chapters viewed through the praxis lens reveal a range of different methods and community alliances and partnerships, enacted in different places. Work in neighbourhoods, with oppressed groups, with indigenous communities and across social strata are included, all with a critical use of theory and reflection.

We open the section with a contribution from Zambrano et al., who highlight some of the ways in which the various crises – political, sociocultural and the pandemic – have served to both mobilise and silence popular protest in Chile. They examine some of the various community psychological strategies for building on popular resistance that in turn have been, and can contribute to responses to the pandemic. Through this discussion they uncover some of the characteristics of a particular, Latin American Community Psychology.

Community psychological tactics for change are taken up by Manalastas and his colleagues, as they illustrate some of the work undertaken in the course of advocating for LGBT+ rights in the Philippines. They show how advocacy for LBGT+ rights can be enacted through curriculum development; through organising within the professional body; and through collaborating with LBGT+ activists and communities beyond the academy, in policy formulation. Through doing LBGT+ and being LGBT+ they stand in solidarity with LBGT+ communities in pursuit of social change.

A different form of solidarity is offered by Tovar Guerra et al., who open our eyes to ways in which accompaniment can be an essential tool for change, in their case with communities displaced by conflict in one of the most violent countries of the world, Colombia. Through the psychological familiarisation and recovery work that features in the accompaniment process, they are able to show the psychological consequences of forced displacement and argue for a shift in focus to a preventative approach.

The following chapter, by Arcidiacono et al., draws on work in neighbourhoods in Italy to reconceptualise the notion of community trust to embrace place-based considerations. Employing a community-based participatory research process, they highlight how networking with and between extant community groups and associations can lead to an increased awareness of the role of trust, enabling this to become the "glue" that underpins active citizen participation, a strong shared sense of purpose, place and citizen well-being.

Still centred on Europe, Carmona and Fernándes also focus on neighbourhood work, this time on two neighbourhoods in Spain. They make a persuasive argument for going beyond those groups who usually participate, to involving sectors of the community who usually do not. They suggest detailed steps and skills needed to achieve more inclusive participation, with deep reflection and systematisation at different stages of the process.

"Going beyond the usual" is also a feature of Condie and Richards' chapter about another gap in Community Psychology, as they draw attention to the disconnect between digital technologies, social media and Community Psychology praxis. Using an autoethnographic method, they draw attention to new, interdisciplinary concepts concerning the digitalisation and datafication of society and its institutions. The ideas are brought to life for a new Digital Community Psychology with reference to work in housing.

The exclusion of certain sectors and the homogenisation of the concept of well-being is problematised by Alfaro and Bilboa-Nieva in relation to their work on the well-being of children and young people in Chile. They demonstrate how working at the intersection of Community Psychology and the new sociology of childhood creates a new framework for research. They argue that well-being must analyse the dynamics of power distribution, the social construction of childhood and conditions that affect young people's quality of life, but most importantly place children and young people at the heart of this research.

Yoshinaga and Hagawari respond to the challenge of research that exposes the role that young people can play through their work in the wake of the 2011 Great Japanese Earthquake, which enabled young people to participate in disaster management and in the recovery process.

The case studies they present reveal the range of creative methods they used to empower young people, primarily through increasing self-efficacy and enabling their participation in disaster management.

Creative methods and the use of the arts feature centrally in the chapter by Sonn et al. Their concern is to use arts and cultural practices to foster voice, a sense of community and place identity, and social justice consciousness, for Aboriginal self-determination and decolonial justice in Australia. They draw on liberation, indigenous and critical psychologies in their work and illustrate with examples of decolonial arts praxis.

Through the praxis lens we can see different ways of working in different cultural contexts, but all with critical reflection on those theoretical and practical resources available, with a view to ensuring that more people are enabled to participate in change processes. They all assume a strong partnership with community groups and organisations, and move on from work that situates the community psychologist as an outside expert. This combining of expert and popular knowledge also features in the praxis we will view, specifically, through an ecological lens.

The ecological lens

Those chapters viewed through the ecological lens illustrate some of the ways in which Community Psychology is beginning to rise to the enormity and complexity of the ecological crisis. All four chapters stress what can be learnt from indigenous peoples, and the strength gained by "seeing with two eyes" or combining inside indigenous knowledge with outside expert knowledge.

Trott et al., working in the southern part of Canada, argue strongly for more community psychological work to address climate justice. They draw on systems theory to describe ways in which their work, using creative arts, seeks to work *against* and *beyond* the inequitable distribution of climate-related risks and vulnerabilities, while addressing the socio-economic inequities and colonial legacies that are their root. They argue that Community Psychology is well placed to contribute to the scale of transformative change that the ecological crisis requires.

The advantages of interdisciplinary and intercultural perspectives, including Māori perspectives on aspects of the ecological crisis in New Zealand, are central to the chapter by Harré et al. They offer four vignettes from those different perspectives of place-based work, food production, school and young people's climate action. These are followed by a synthesis across perspectives that highlights both the emotionality of the work and also the dialectic of human relationships being needed for effective action *and at the same time* that action for the environment builds relationships.

Food production and distribution are aspects of the ecological crisis, but Stroink et al. argue that it is food security (not just distribution) that is an essential part of climate justice. They draw on their work with indigenous people in Northwestern Ontario, Canada, to demonstrate how both conceptualising change and working for change at the ecotone between the ecosystems of Community Psychology (including systems thinking) and critical food studies is a fruitful site for local community action. Their work seeks to prefigure alternative futures, whilst they work in partnership to examine and reimagine contemporary food systems and through this, address psychological, social and ecological health.

All of these chapters seek, in part, to protect the natural world. Olivera-Méndez and Calegare discuss the role that Critical Community Psychology might play in conservation efforts and biodiversity loss in the Brazilian Amazon and in Mexico. Their participatory action research extended to environmental protection and species protection and was underpinned by explicit community psychological work with local communities.

11

By looking through the ecological lens, we can see that counter-hegemonic world views are necessary to understand and for Community Psychology to embrace not only anti- and decolonial ways of working but non-anthropocentric understanding and practices. Working to avert or mitigate the ecological crisis requires recognising the limitations, but also the value of community psychological concepts and methods which must be combined with other kinds of knowledges and practices.

The learning and reflective lens

Whilst several chapters talk about the reflexive nature of Community Psychology, this is writ large in this section on learning and reflection. The experiences of novices to Community Psychology are important in designing curricular and pedagogical relevance to students. But learning and reflection are not just for students, nor are they end points to an action process – they are essential throughout. The chapters in this section move from a starting point of an anti-colonial stance, through the development of critical thinking in students, to where we started – with deep reflection about being community psychologists during the pandemic.

Flores Osorio and Vicente Xiloj use the device of a dialogue of knowledge in order to challenge Euro-American-centric Community Psychology from an understanding of the reality of exclusion-pauperisation suffered by First Nations in Guatemala. The two participants postulated a way of redefining the work of Community Psychology that is coherent with those anti-colonial struggles and territorial defences carried out by the Maya-Kiche' First Nation.

Deep insider perspectives also appear in the chapter by Runswick-Cole et al. They discuss, together, forms of activism and advocacy on behalf of, and with, disabled sons and daughters in the UK, and the tensions this activism holds for work in the academy, which has traditionally held activism at a distance from scholarship or at best blurred the relationship between scholarship and activism. Through their form of scholar activism, they remind us to recognise those activisms of marginalised and minoritised groups that have, thus far, been overlooked as sites for the emergence of radical social movements.

Akhurst and Msomi, working in the Eastern Cape, South Africa, discuss how the incorporation of community-based service learning into postgraduate psychology training fits with both university community engagement priorities and synergies with courses in Community Psychology, particularly as these courses help students acquire the capability to work in decolonial ways. They argue that this form of learning results in partners and trainees collaborating to address the influences of systemic crises on well-being, notably those related to poverty and inequality.

The reflective process of service learning, in pursuit of critical consciousness, is picked up by Zani et al. in the work they discuss with Italian university students. The students broaden their ambition through exploring the development of critical consciousness with younger pupils, using a process of youth participatory action research. Through discussion of these case studies the authors argue that these kinds of actions have led not only to critical consciousness, beyond participants' immediate experiences, but to competencies needed to become engaged citizens.

The final chapter, by Sliep et al., describes the creation of a dialogic space, in the year of the pandemic, through which students were supported in using narratives of life experiences to connect theory with the complex context of South Africa. With insights from both students and facilitators, they argue that when critical consciousness is "embedded in action" through a reflexive process, it signifies a shift or movement, a change in the status quo. In this way, reflexivity becomes a tool for interrogation, change and transformation.

These chapters regarding learning and reflection all draw on the importance of critical thinking and critical consciousness as part of the curriculum, and highlight different ways in which this can be achieved in universities and beyond. This critical consciousness is an essential component of decolonial approaches to community psychological work, and underpins much of the work covered in previous sections.

The endnote of the book, written by the editors, revisits the ecological crisis as an example of the emergence of new forms of social organisation and struggle. Most importantly, it highlights how Community Psychology as a discipline, hand in hand with other social movements, has some of the tools, reflected in the rest of the book, to enable hope not only to become practical but also to be restored and maintained.

References

BPS. (2021). Community action and resilience. www.bps.org.uk/coronavirus-resources/community-action

Cornish, F., Haaken, J., Moskovitz, L., & Jackson, S. (2016). Rethinking prefigurative politics: introduction to the special thematic section. *Journal of Social and Political Psychology, 4*(1), 114–27.

Değirmencioğlu, S.M., & Walker, C. (2015). *Social and psychological dimensions of personal debt and the debt industry*. Palgrave.

Esquivel, V. (2016). Power and the Sustainable Development Goals: a feminist analysis. *Gender & Development, 24*(1), 9–23. https://doi.org/10.1080/13552074.2016.1147872

Fisher, J., Languilaire, J.C., Lawthom,, R., Nieuwenhuis, R., Petts, R.J., Runswick-Cole, K., & Yerkes, M.A. (2020). Community, work, and family in times of COVID-19. *Community, Work & Family, 23*(3), 247–52. https://doi.org/10.1080/13668803.2020.1756568

Forgas, J. P., Crano, W. D., & Fiedler, K. (Eds.). (2021). *The psychology of populism: The tribal challenge to liberal democracy*. Routledge.

Hart, A., Gagnon, E., Eryigit-Madzwamuse, S., Cameron, J., Aranda, K., Rathbone, A., & Heaver, B. (2016). Uniting resilience research and practice with an inequalities approach. *SAGE Open, 6*(4), 215824401668247. https://doi.org/10.1177/2158244016682477

Kagan, C., Burton, M., Duckett, P., Lawthom, R., & Siddiquee, A. (2020). *Critical community psychology: critical action and social change*. Routledge.

Kagan, C., & Lewis, S. (2015) Community, work and family and the metamorphosis of social change. Invited keynote paper presented to the *Community Work Family Conference*, Malmo, 2015. Available from http://eprints.mdx.ac.uk/17580/1/malmo_Cwf_paper.pdf

Kagan, C.M., & Burton, M.H. (2014) Culture, identity and alternatives to the consumer culture. *Educarem Revista*, Curitiba, Brasil, n. 53, 75–89 (Dossier: Educação, Cotidiano e Participação: desafios e contribuições para a formação). http://ojs.c3sl.ufpr.br/ojs/index.php/educar/article/view/36583

Strickland, L.H., Aboud, F.E., & Gergen, K.J. (1976). *Social psychology in transition*. Plenum.

PART I

Community Psychology through a critical lens

1

EPISTEMICIDE AND EPISTEMIC FREEDOM

Reflections for a decolonising Community Psychology

Nick Malherbe, Shahnaaz Suffla and Mohamed Seedat

Abstract

Community Psychology has, in the main, contributed to different modes of epistemicide, that is, the destruction, distortion, marginalisation and silencing of other-than-Northern knowledges and ways of knowing. Increasingly, however, decolonising enactments of Community Psychology have resisted the discipline's complicity in entrenching unequal knowledge hierarchies that depend on epistemicide. (Re)inspired by the latest iterations of the decolonial turn, which have sought to mobilise epistemologies of the South in an attempt to advance epistemic freedom, we critically appraise some of the epistemologically just praxes and the intellectual and political struggles intrinsic to a liberatory knowledge-making project. We then reflect on our own Community Psychology work. Specifically, we recount how re-membering conflict, struggle and everyday care within a low-income South African community with whom we collaborate has been able to cherish epistemic freedom, while guarding against epistemicide. In this, we offer a critical consideration of the messiness, hybridity and contradictions, as well as the radical solidarities and agency that accompany work of this sort. We conclude by reflecting on what epistemic freedom, and its associated challenges, could mean for a decolonising Community Psychology that seeks to resist the coloniality of knowledge.

Resumen

La psicología comunitaria ha contribuido, principalmente, a diferentes modos de epistemicidio, es decir, a la destrucción, distorsión, marginación y silenciamiento de conocimientos y formas de conocimiento que no son del Norte. Sin embargo, cada vez más, las representaciones descolonizadoras de la psicología comunitaria han resistido la complicidad de la disciplina en fortalecer las jerarquías desiguales de conocimiento que dependen del epistemicidio. (Re) inspirados por las últimas iteraciones del giro descolonial, que han intendado movilizar las epistemologías del Sur por promover la libertad epistémica, evaluamos críticamente algunas de las praxis epistemológicamente justas y las luchas intelectuales y políticas intrínsecas a un

DOI: 10.4324/9780429325663-3

proyecto por la construcción de conocimiento libertador. Luego reflexionamos sobre nuestro propio trabajo en la psicología comunitaria. Específicamente, contamos cómo recordar el conflicto, la lucha y el cuidado diario, dentro de una comunidad sudafricana de bajos ingresos con la que colaboramos, ha sido capaz de apreciar la libertad epistémica, mientras evitando al epistemicidio. En esto, ofrecemos una consideración crítica del desorden, la hibridación y las contradicciones, así como las solidaridades radicales y la agencia que acompañan a este tipo de trabajo. Concluimos reflexionando sobre lo que la libertad epistémica y sus desafíos asociados podrían significar para una psicología comunitaria descolonizadora que busca resistir la colonialidad del conocimiento.

Introduction

If we understand power as constituted along colonial cartographies, then it follows that colonial centres hold immense influence over which knowledges are made to seem legitimate, coherent and rational, and which are not (see Masaka, 2018; Poks, 2015). In considering the nuances of colonialism and knowledge production, it is perhaps insufficient to conceptualise power and knowledge as merely representing a single hybridised entity à la Foucault (1980). It may be more useful to explore how contemporary colonial power structures (i.e. coloniality) not only shape the creation of knowledge systems (i.e. epistemologies), but in fact depend on the destruction of other-than-Northern knowledges and ways of knowing. Indeed, if coloniality is to secure ideological hegemony as well as lay claim to what comprises the human, it must work to deny the intellectual life of the colonised by destroying their knowledge systems (de Sousa Santos, 2016). This process of imposing colonial epistemologies onto – and *almost* destroying – knowledges generated within colonial territories is known as epistemicide (Masaka, 2018).

Despite community psychologists becoming increasingly concerned with the coloniality of knowledge (Seedat & Suffla, 2017), and epistemic violence (Malherbe et al., 2017), few Community Psychology engagements have focused on epistemicide as such. Relatedly, there is little work that has sought to understand how community psychologists concerned with epistemic justice are able to support grassroots community-led initiatives in their efforts to resist epistemicide. Nonetheless, and as we demonstrate in this chapter, there is a growing body of Critical Community Psychology that addresses itself to epistemic freedom (e.g. Ali-Faisal, 2020; Carolissen & Duckett, 2018; Kessi, 2017; Reyes Cruz & Sonn 2010; Suffla & Seedat, 2017). Situated within this critical tradition, we draw on our own work, in a South African community, to illustrate some of the complexities, challenges and limitations that community psychologists face when attempting to resist epistemicide.

Epistemicide, coloniality and knowledge production

Coloniality represents the structures of power that were established during the era of so-called classic colonialism in the late fifteenth century, but that survive today in dominant cultures, labour relations, intersubjective interactions, social systems, institutions and knowledge-making practices (see Maldonado-Torres, 2007). Thus, in addition to addressing itself to power and being, coloniality is also concerned with knowledge (see Maldonado-Torres, 2016), which is to say that coloniality seeks to ensure that all models of thinking, seeing and interpreting – no matter how alienating – cohere with the rules and norms of a supposedly universal Western modernity (Mignolo, 2007).

How does epistemicide fit into coloniality's broader matrices of social domination? In his pioneering work on this topic, de Sousa Santos (2005, 2016) argues that modern science, as it has been conceived in the colonial centres, has always sought legitimacy through the destruction of those knowledges produced in the Global South. Certainly, much scientific "progress" is premised on the regulation, control and sometimes destruction of colonised peoples and their knowledge systems, all while staking claim to the values of impartiality, objectivity and Truth (Bennett, 2007; Teo, 2019). In undermining, asphyxiating and destroying indigenous knowledges, epistemicide looks to neutralise, invisibilise and efface the people to whom these knowledges belong (see Masaka, 2018). Once knowledges of the colonised are erased, the coloniser is able to assume a benevolent, paternal role either in imparting knowledge or as the sole bearer of "valid" knowledge (Bennett, 2007; Mills & Lefrançois, 2018). The notion of epistemicide helps us understand how epistemology connects with coloniality, that is, how the destruction of indigenous knowledges relates to the cheapening of the lives of those who created these knowledges (de Sousa Santos, 2016; Mignolo & Walsh, 2018). It is apparent, then, that we cannot consider epistemicide and coloniality separately.

De Sousa Santos (2016) has argued that when knowledge creation relies on epistemicide, what emerges is abyssal thinking, where that which is deemed legitimate is infused with an imperial modality of reason that reduces colonised peoples to the status of sub-human. Sub-human colonial subjects are effectively constructed as irrational, incompetent non-knowledge holders who are underdeveloped, undeveloped and/or developed wrongly, and therefore must have their interests determined through "superior" colonial knowledges (Mills & Lefrançois, 2018; Ngũgĩ wa Thiong'o, 2009). As such, and because being makes possible knowing, epistemicide is enacted with a view towards erasing the ontological density of colonised peoples (Mignolo & Walsh, 2018), thereby relegating these peoples to a zone of non-being wherein their humanity is refused (see Fanon, 1967). In this sense, coloniality operates at intrapsychic and structural levels, where colonised people may act to silence their own knowledges in order to receive the kinds of recognition necessary to survive within systems of coloniality (Bennett, 2007).

There is, of course, a bitter irony to epistemicide. Colonial powers always depend upon the indigenous knowledges that they denigrate and destroy (see Masaka 2018). How, for instance, could settler colonialists survive in unfamiliar conditions without drawing from local knowledges? Herein lies one of the central contradictions of epistemicide, and indeed coloniality more broadly. It is also important to note that epistemicide usually fails in its mission to destroy indigenous knowledge forms in toto (Masaka, 2018). This failure signifies that epistemicide is always met with insurgent decolonial resistance (Ndlovu-Gatsheni, 2018, 2021), much of which challenges the inherent contradictions of coloniality. Thus, we do not adequately consider coloniality and epistemicide if we do not also synchronously and actively engage with the pursuit of decolonisation and epistemic freedom.

Epistemic freedom

To resist epistemicide is to struggle for what Ndlovu-Gatsheni (2018) calls epistemic freedom. He maintains that epistemic freedom differs from academic freedom in that it is not about proclaiming whatever one wishes, and has little to do with institutional autonomy. Rather, epistemic freedom insists on both the right to interpret the world from one's locus of enunciation – which sits at the intersection of knowledge and the politics of place (Mignolo, 1999) – and to use methodologies that actively oppose coloniality. Epistemic freedom seeks to liberate reason from coloniality (see Ndlovu-Gatsheni, 2018) through an epistemic delinking from the logic of modernity and its naturalised assumptions (Poks, 2015). Therefore, struggles for epistemic freedom may entail working outside of the kinds of narrative linearity and supposed rationality that have, in large part, been favoured by Western modernity since the Enlightenment

(Poks, 2015; Teo, 2019). In this way, we can reclaim suppressed knowledges from Otherness (see Gqola, 2010), and build pluriversal futures that, in rejecting coloniality's partialised humanism, stress the fullness of humanity (see Fanon, 1967). The privileging of indigenous knowledges may then not only open up pathways for decolonisation, but also reveal how dominant knowledges – far from de facto universal – are, in fact, indigenous to their own contexts (Teo, 2019).

The centuries of violence enacted in the name of coloniality's cognitive empire, Ndlovu-Gatsheni (2021) argues, indicate the imperative of epistemic freedom. Yet, if it is to serve as an opening into other freedoms, epistemic freedom cannot constitute an end in and of itself (Ndlovu-Gatsheni 2018). Epistemic freedom is a deeply personal project that entails learning to unlearn, and then relearning in order to create and build (Tlostanova, 2015; Tlostanova & Mignolo, 2012). It requires the cultivation of a decolonial attitude on the part of knowledge-making subjects, as well as a conviction that everyone is a legitimate knower and producer of knowledge (Maldonado-Torres, 2016; Ndlovu-Gatsheni, 2018). This decolonial attitude entails an openness to knowledges that exist outside of the European and North American canons (Tlostanova & Mignolo, 2012), as well as a commitment to working across and beyond epistemic borders (Mignolo, 2007). In considering these twinned pillars of the decolonial knowledge-making attitude, Anzaldúa's (1987) concept of border thinking is useful. Border thinking entails a literal "thinking from the borders", or learning to know with and through knowledges that are not necessarily recognised under coloniality's cognitive empire. Through border thinking, we can begin to deconstruct and look beyond the artificial borders by which coloniality entraps knowledges (Poks, 2015). Border thinking allows us to approach that which has not always been understood as knowledge – or whose status as knowledge has been muted through epistemicide (e.g. affects, spirituality, quotidian practices and movement) – as legitimate ways of knowing. To think on, with, beyond and through borders is to engage theories of lived knowledge that are created beyond the colonial matrix of power, and to facilitate the creation of an "epistemology of the exteriority; that is, of the outside created from the inside" (Mignolo & Tlostanova, 2006, p. 206).

Refuting epistemicide in the name of epistemic freedom can feel like an abstract and enormously ambitious task. However, it is important to note that struggling for epistemic freedom does not stand outside of history. There is a long tradition of movements for epistemic freedom from which to draw inspiration, build upon and critically engage. In demanding epistemic justice and participation, these movements have sought to advance counter-hegemonic knowledges – or what de Sousa Santos (2016) calls insurgent cosmopolitanism – in an attempt to refuse colonial ways of knowing and break with that which coloniality deems commonsensical (see Bennett, 2007). For instance, in slavocratic South Africa, much of the country's Muslim population immersed themselves in Islamic knowledge traditions as a way of subverting a Dutch/English Christian colonial order that denied the interiority of colonial subjects (Gqola, 2010). Today, we see the continuation of such decolonial epistemic struggles in indigenous ecological activism in Canada (Lowan-Trudeau, 2017), efforts to resist the neoliberalisation of local knowledges in Ecuador (Laurie et al., 2005), attempts to incorporate indigenous knowledges into university curricula in Australia (Sonn et al., 2000), labours to integrate indigenous knowledge systems into higher education systems in South Africa (Kaya & Seleti, 2014), and many other movements for epistemic freedom that are taking place all over the world (see de Sousa Santos, 2005). The flourishing of these different struggles does not, however, point to the profusion of epistemic freedom. To the contrary, they indicate the pervasiveness of epistemicide (Ndlovu-Gatsheni, 2021). Notwithstanding, these struggles demonstrate that while coloniality can erase people, it never successfully kills ideas (Mignolo & Walsh, 2018), and that although subaltern knowledges are subjugated by coloniality, they are never completely erased (Ndlovu-Gatsheni, 2021).

Community Psychology, epistemicide and epistemic freedom

Within the discipline of psychology, the notion of epistemicide is rarely afforded significant attention. There is, however, an increasing number of critical psychologists who are concerned with epistemic violence (Teo, 2019). Epistemic violence is enacted whenever dominant groups represent marginalised groups in inaccurate, essentialised and/or harmful ways (see Spivak, 1988). Thus, where epistemic violence signifies a mode of oppressive representation, epistemicide represents the destruction of the knowledge-making resources and traditions of meaning-making. When epistemic violence is prolonged and systematised, it tends to lead to epistemicide.

Mainstream psychology's tendency towards epistemic violence, by ignoring the psychological knowledges of Othered peoples, has over time resulted in epistemicide. We see the co-constituent effects of epistemicide and epistemic violence in psychology's long history of aligning with colonialism and coloniality (see Teo, 2019). Examples include: attempts by psychologists to render the colonised – especially resisting colonial subjects – mentally ill (Mills & Lefrançois, 2018); the Eurocentric training that many psychologists in the Global South continue to receive (Capella Palacios & Jadhav, 2020); the ways by which psychology cohered with the colonial project in India (see Hartnack, 1987); the individualising and Eurocentric approaches assumed by many mental health NGOs in Palestine (Makkawi, 2009); the intersection of psychology with apartheid ideology in South Africa (Kessi, 2017); and how, in the mid-nineteenth century, escaped African slaves in the Americas were diagnosed with "drapetomania", a bogus mental disorder that was said to have compelled slaves to run away from slaveowners (Gould, 1981). In each of these instances, colonial schemas of human psychology are drawn upon to impose colonial knowledge forms with a view towards destroying indigenous knowledges along with the people to whom these knowledges belong.

Although much of Community Psychology has perhaps not been as directly implicated in practices of epistemicide and epistemic violence as many mainstream iterations of psychology have, much mainstream Community Psychology remains tethered to psychology's Euro-American-centric epistemological impulses (see Seedat & Suffla, 2017). We saw this in Community Psychology's early, United Statesian conceptions, many of which were ambivalent towards the decolonising social movements of the day (Gokani & Walsh, 2017), while remaining committed to epistemes that relied on an ahistorical, liberal individualism (Malherbe & Dlamini, 2020). Today, well-funded Community Psychology initiatives are oftentimes unconcerned with issues of coloniality and epistemicide.

Yet, there are, just as there have always been, progressive iterations of Community Psychology all over the world that are committed to enhancing epistemic freedom (see Reich et al., 2007). Seedat and Suffla (2017), for instance, have sought to retrieve African knowledge archives which stretch Community Psychology's disciplinary boundaries. In a similar vein, Ali-Faisal (2020) has proposed an Islamic anti-patriarchal liberation psychology framework that endeavours to recover Islamic histories, centralise a range of Muslim voices and reject colonial representations of Islam (also see Seedat, 2021). Speaking to community-engaged praxes, Reyes Cruz and Sonn (2011) have stressed how an intercultural perspective is able to contribute to a decolonising standpoint that understands community engagement through a given community's cultural knowledges. Kessi (2017) similarly emphasises that if we are to orient Community Psychology research towards epistemic justice, links must be fostered between researchers, participants and communities more broadly. Sonn et al. (2017), in emphasis, insist that community psychologists should commit themselves to epistemic freedom in their engagements with social movements, the ways by which they build alliances with these movements, and in the manner by which they work with communities to reclaim subaltern ways of knowing.

Epistemic freedom has, in recent years, also been taken up as a pedagogical imperative by a number of community psychologists. Exemplary here is the special issue of the *American Journal of Community Psychology* on "Teaching Toward Decoloniality in Community Psychology and Allied Disciplines", edited by Carolissen and Duckett (2018). Together, the articles in this special issue capture how teaching decolonial Community Psychology is central to advancing epistemic freedom (also see Kessi, 2017; Reyes Cruz & Sonn, 2011). Building on this work, Malherbe and Dlamini (2020) have called for an ethic of discomfort that strives to unsettle Community Psychology teaching curricula and will the discipline towards epistemic freedom. In applying notions of epistemic freedom to pedagogy, Malherbe and colleagues (2017) sought to disrupt their university's knowledge-making conventions by facilitating a space wherein groups of young people from six African countries were able to teach university staff about their experiences with, and involvement in, community-engaged projects on youth safety.

It would seem, then, that while much of Community Psychology, just like mainstream psychology, has cohered with or been complicit in epistemicide (Seedat & Suffla, 2017), there is a rich body of work that has sought to purpose the discipline for epistemic freedom and justice, particularly in the spheres of community praxis, pedagogy and community engagement. Almost all of this work, however, is concerned with epistemic violence, rather than the more radical and longitudinal notion of epistemicide. In what follows, we consider this latter concern in our own work.

Community Psychology, epistemicide and epistemic freedom: some reflections from South Africa

Community context

Established during the 1980s in apartheid South Africa, the community of Thembelihle, located in the south-west of Johannesburg, initially served as an informal settlement for brickmakers working at a nearby factory. Over the years, Thembelihle has grown considerably and is, according to the most recent census data, home to a population of over 21,000 people (ISHS, 2018; Statistics South Africa 2011). Just under half of this population faces unemployment, with crime rates climbing each year (ISHS, 2018). Since 2001, community activist groups have been locked into tense relations with government authorities over a number of issues, including a lack of social services, land contestations and forced removals related to the contested presence of dolomitic rock in the community (Cornell et al., 2020).

The University of South Africa's Institute for Social and Health Sciences, the institution with which we are affiliated, has – for over 30 years – partnered with residents of Thembelihle on a number of community-engaged projects. This work has sought to harness the knowledges of local activists, teachers, (re)productive workers, cultural workers, care workers, community leaders and youth groups to form political coalitions, articulate and enact psychosocial justice and, ultimately, advance epistemic freedom. Undergirded by a collaborative and critical participatory ethic, these community projects endeavour to address a multifaceted conception of violence (i.e. violence as direct, epistemic and structural). In doing so, such community-engaged work comprises multiple components which are geared towards intra- and inter-community cohesion and solidarity as well as strengthening service delivery systems in the community.

Like all community–university partnerships, our work is structured by unequal dynamics of power. Our reflexive engagement with this work entails continuously evaluating the ways by which we move towards decoloniality and even, unwittingly, regress towards coloniality. We are made to negotiate the uneven (de)colonising potentialities inherent to our institutional embeddedness (see Suffla et al., 2020), and remain alert to the imperative to connect the knowledges produced within the community partnership to community members' ontological and material realities (i.e. how these knowledges can assist people in their daily lives and struggles for psychosocial justice).

In what follows, we speak to the notion of re-membering, and how this informs our community-engaged work in Thembelihle, after which we reflect on three community-engaged projects that have harnessed different modes of re-membering towards epistemic freedom. Together, these three projects demonstrate the challenges, limitations and hope inherent to decolonising Community Psychology engagements that strive to contribute to struggles for epistemic freedom.

Advancing epistemic freedom through re-membering

Epistemic freedom addresses epistemicide not through a mythological return to an idealised pre-colonial past, nor by looking to a future that takes little heed of the conditions of the present. Instead, epistemic freedom requires that we recognise the dynamism, historicity, decolonial potential and insurgent capacities of the knowledges of colonised peoples (Masaka, 2018). Accordingly, Ndlovu-Gatsheni (2018) argues that epistemic freedom demands that efforts are made to: (1) return to the centre of enunciation; (2) shift the centre of knowledge; (3) decolonise normative foundations of critical theory; (4) rethink how we think; and (5) learn to unlearn so that we may relearn (also see Mignolo, 1999; Mignolo & Walsh, 2018; Ndlovu-Gatsheni, 2021; Tlostanova & Mignolo, 2012).

Following the above, we have sought to advance epistemic freedom within our community-engaged work through the notion of re-membering, which represents one of a number of framing devices within our work. Although a complex concept, re-membering, in essence, represents an attempt to reckon with and reconstruct a past that is mired in colonial trauma. Indeed, as Ngũgĩ wa Thiong'o (2009) argues, coloniality has dismembered colonised peoples from their pasts, and therefore also from their identities, ways of knowing and sense of being (also see Malherbe, 2020a). The lived and felt memories of colonialism have, in this way, been disavowed by coloniality (Gqola, 2010). Re-membering looks to retrieve, recover and (re)construct the pasts and knowledge formations that coloniality has (almost, but not completely) severed (see Malherbe, 2020a). In other words, if we acknowledge that a "community is formed and re-formed every time its history is told" (see Poks, 2015, p. 66), the process of re-membering can facilitate the retrieval of the pluriversal epistemologies – and related subjectivities – that coloniality has sought to destroy. However, because memories of colonial trauma have been suppressed and devalued, they cannot always be directly re-membered, and may need to be recalled and invoked through alternative methodologies and border thinking (Gqola, 2010; Teo, 2019). Thus, to re-member is not only to retrieve the knowledges that coloniality has sought to destroy, but equally to constitute these knowledges within a decolonising vision of epistemic freedom.

Re-membering community conflict

When working in structurally violent settings marked by coloniality, community psychologists risk engaging in epistemicide in two respects. Firstly, there is the risk of reproducing the neo-colonial logic of the liberal peace that seeks to absolve violences through top-down, statist structures which are removed from people's realities on the ground (see Suffla et al., 2020). In the case of Thembelihle, we see evocations of the liberal peace in news reports that, for the most part, construct the community as a monolithic entity whose grievances derive primarily from its refusal to adhere to a state-centric liberal social order (Malherbe et al., 2021). Secondly, even when community psychologists working in structurally violent settings reject liberal notions of peace, it is possible to adhere to mythologised understandings of community cohesiveness that ignore knowledge histories mired in disunity, contradiction and intra-community conflict. As Cornell and her colleagues (2020) write, in Thembelihle, as with many other communities, attempts at solidarity-making and coalition-building will always rub against the community's long history of factional social movements and oppositional struggles. Therefore, if we are to guard against epistemicide and take on a decolonising approach to practicing Community Psychology, we should not look to understand violence through a linear or monolithic hermeneutic that mutes the various – often incompatible – community-based understandings of violence, nor should we ascribe to individualist and state-centric conceptions of liberal peace. Promoting epistemic freedom within violent settings demands that community knowledge systems and antagonistic subject positions are taken into account within the decolonising political agenda (see Malherbe & Dlamini, 2020). When community psychologists embrace, rather than ignore or paper over contradiction or tensions in this way, they can begin to return to the centre of enunciation (see Ndlovu-Gatsheni, 2018).

To re-member community conflict requires not only that community psychologists take seriously the various conflicting knowledges that comprise any community, but also that people articulate these knowledges in ways they deem appropriate, rather than through means that cohere with a predetermined research agenda. In our work, we have sought to understand historical knowledges of community conflict and tension in Thembelihle by collaborating with different community members to construct an oral history of the state-directed relocations, or forced removals, that took place in the community in the early 2000s (see Cornell et al., 2020). While memories of the relocations are, by definition, unstable (see Gqola, 2010), they are nonetheless able to offer us insights into how power has been distributed, contested, reformulated, won and lost in Thembelihle (see Wale, 2016). To re-member such community histories in a manner that is suitably convergent, complex, nuanced and multifaceted can serve to resist the liberal peace as well as the temptation to discount community tensions with evocations to an idealised notion of cohesion. We anticipated that the politics of these historical knowledges could illuminate the existing politics and practices of coloniality and decoloniality in Thembelihle.

Despite taking place in the post-apartheid era, Thembelihle's relocations strike an uncanny resemblance to colonial and apartheid racist social logic, and therefore represent a site of trauma for many residents (Cornell et al., 2020). However, this was not the case for all residents. Relocations in the community were re-membered in different, and oftentimes oppositional ways. In interviewing some of the community members and government officials who had been involved in the relocations, we found that many in the community had resisted the removals. As one community member noted, "No one wanted to relocate, but because of the inferiorities that were instilled in the people, some ended up moving out of fear and fled. But we stood our ground." Others, however, endorsed the relations, with one community member describing this process as just, voluntary and fair by proclaiming that "We started by identifying the beneficiaries and those beneficiaries were sent to the housing department for [a] screening […] then they came back [and stated that] this can qualify, this cannot qualify […] everybody went voluntarily." There were also a number of violent conflicts between these different parties. A community member recalled:

> When I came back the second day from work [assisting with the relocation process],
> I found about ten men with guns in the garden [...] and then they told me "no, it's
> security, to protect you". "Me? For what?" "Because of the protests in Thembelihle."

Such conflict was downplayed by state representatives ("Thousands of families were moved from Thembelihle, moved to fully-fledged houses") who, for their part, attributed the tensions surrounding the relocations to noncompliant community members (see Cornell et al., 2020).

We need not understand the divergent historical knowledges of Thembelihle as antithetical to a coherent decolonising agenda. Instead, they indicate the range of experiences and desires which can be taken up by those striving for decoloniality. Developing insurgent cosmopolitanism in Thembelihle therefore entails heeding various community knowledges and drawing out the common elements of these knowledges (e.g. a desire for secure living conditions; respect for histories of struggle; autonomy) in an attempt to enunciate a broader decolonising vision (see de Sousa Santos, 2016). In holding historical contradictions within a decolonising agenda, community members draw on the tenets of epistemic freedom to enhance and strengthen such an agenda. While an individual subject may not see their way of knowing reflected in any precise way in community struggles for justice, these struggles can work to honour a common set of political and social desires that cut across different community knowledges. At the same time, however, care must be taken not to entrench antagonistic subject positions beyond reproach. We may, in this way, work to centre local knowledges and reject abyssal thinking by shifting the normative foundations for understanding community conflict (de Sousa Santos, 2016; Ndlovu-Gatsheni, 2018).

Re-membering community conflict through divergent oral histories is not without its challenges. This was made clear to us in an early attempt to work with residents of Thembelihle to construct a timeline of the relocation events. We soon realised that such a knowledge form prioritises linearity over epistemic freedom, and thus necessitates some form of epistemicide. Yet, even when constructing nonlinear oral histories, honouring epistemic freedom presents several challenges. There were, for instance, cases where the politics embodied by a particular episteme contrasted with our own political standpoints. Similarly, the oral histories were, in the end, defined in large part by the most dominant community voices (e.g. one interview took place over two days, while another lasted only a few minutes). Yet, in working with residents of Thembelihle to outline their community's histories – most of which are ignored by mainstream knowledge practices (see Malherbe et al., 2021) – we did not attempt to *know* Thembelihle in any definitive way. Rather, by using oral history to re-member the historical trajectories of power in the community, we sought to understand how such knowledges of power could be drawn on for purposes of decolonisation. Epistemic freedom can, in this way, connect decoloniality to an expansive conception of community-building that is sensitive to multiple ways of knowing and, therefore, being.

Re-membering community struggle

Lau and Seedat (2015) argue that within Community Psychology storytelling can function to recover the values, beliefs and practices inherent to indigenous knowledges. However, because stories may represent subjective interpretations, fictionalised and/or semi-fictionalised accounts that are only dubiously verifiable, they tend to be considered as adjacent and subordinate to "legitimate" knowledge rather than representing knowledge as such. Yet, one comes to know community life – and indeed lives within communities – through stories. Community-engaged social justice efforts similarly draw inspiration and learn from stories of resistance and struggle.

Thus, where the denigration of the story as a form of knowledge may be considered a mode of epistemicide, engaging storytelling as a legitimate knowledge form can allow us to rethink thinking itself (see Ndlovu-Gatsheni, 2018).

There are, of course, many different ways by which to tell community stories, but if these stories are not – in some way – privileged, their decolonising potential is likely to fall away through systemic degradation. In our community-engaged work in Thembelihle, we have attempted to flesh out the visceral nature of storytelling by engaging with high school students, community leaders and activists, schoolteachers, foreign nationals and cultural workers to produce digital stories on community struggle. Digital stories, which are short audiovisual vignettes wherein a spoken narrative is accompanied by a series of photographs, are able to bridge different knowledge paradigms (Lau et al., 2017). In this respect, the epistemic freedom that is afforded by digital storytelling gives way to a kind of border thinking that, in moving through different knowledge forms (Lau & Seedat, 2015), is rooted in a fundamental humanism (see Anzaldúa, 1987).

With one participant commenting that "In politics there can't be unity", it was clear that a single digital story could not capture the range of knowledges that construct a particular struggle narrative. Yet, within a system of coloniality that disinvests from, and systemically degrades the lives of poor Black people, the community members were able to quilt together a set of common struggles (e.g. struggles around employment, affordable education, and resourced learning and working environments). As one elderly community member proclaimed:

> It's to combine all these struggles and make it one struggle, the struggle of saying we don't want to see our kids moving in the same direction, we don't want to see the youth, the women in Thembelihle suffering the way we have suffered.

Therefore, in creating their digital stories, participants were able to witness and relate to one another, themselves and their community in new ways (Lau & Seedat, 2015). In this, participants utilised the digital stories to construct the world from their loci of enunciation ("You can listen at someone else when he's narrating, where he *is* from and how does that person *experience* the life in Thembelihle"), and in this regard the participants advanced a modality of epistemic freedom.

Synthesising individual voices into a single story allowed for the creation of different knowledge forms that exceeded the sum of their parts. In this, the digital stories differed from the oral histories in that the groups were encouraged to forge new, coherent knowledges out of those which they were re-membering, rather than produce a set of diffracted historical knowledges. Forging singular knowledges out of the group voice could, in this way, foster a sense of solidarity and commitment to a range of struggles, illustrated by a community member's insistence that "We are a community and we take ourselves as such, you understand?" This was certainly challenging, as participants, who would oftentimes occupy contesting politics and positionalities, were required to construct a story. Nonetheless, at public screening events audiences made connections between the different digital stories. For instance, when viewed alongside one another, it became clear that the struggles for material justice (e.g. electricity, clean water and safe infrastructure for all), on which the activists focused in their digital story, were imbricated in the psychosocial struggles of the community, articulated by a storyteller as the "fight against conditions of unemployment, condition of poverty, condition of mental slavery". Audience members practiced epistemic freedom at the screening events by offering different ways of knowing Thembelihle as well as mobilising and making connections between these knowledges.

There were a number of challenges in our attempts to advance epistemic freedom through the different digital stories. Although digital stories facilitate the kind of multimodal communication that is able to centre the emotionality of respective knowledge forms, the relatively short duration of a given digital story (in our case, none exceeded five minutes), along with the kind of narrative linearity that digital stories demand, meant that some knowledges – or ways of knowing community struggle – were lost. This was, in part, due to the process itself, whereby participants worked to construct a single story, despite occupying contesting subject positions. Thus, unlike the oral histories, not all of those who produced digital stories could re-member in as expansive a way as they might have wished. Indeed, for the digital story to create knowledges that are useful, communicability must be prioritised. Yet, this inherent restriction of the digital story need not represent an unsurpassable limitation of the methodology. Epistemic freedom is always hindered by the limitations inherent to one's medium of expression. Therefore, when considering the coherence of digital stories alongside the narrative expansiveness of oral histories, we are confronted with how critical community psychologists are able to approach epistemic freedom through a range of methodologies, each of which embodies its own set of communicative advantages and constraints.

Each digital story sought to reconstitute stories of struggle (which are, by definition, rooted in the past) for the decolonial requirements of the present conjuncture. However, the social changes that resulted from the digital stories were, at first glance, uneven. Although all of the digital stories were screened in public places within and beyond Thembelihle (e.g. sports fields, central business districts, community halls and markets), it was the story produced by the community leaders and activists that resulted in the most tangible social change. Their digital story featured in what became a successful campaign for electrification in Thembelihle (see Suffla et al., 2020). Yet, epistemic freedom cannot only be assessed against such instrumental metrics. We also need to understand epistemic freedom as a force that enables different knowledges to travel, and assists us in knowing the world in new, potentially rehumanising, ways. For example, many of those who watched the schoolteachers' digital story expressed feeling moved. This story was also useful in setting up solidarity networks between different teachers in the community. Therefore, while not every digital story resulted in material change, each worked to formalise community-oriented ways of knowing that, under systems of coloniality, have been denigrated, asphyxiated and/or ignored.

Re-membering everyday community care

Although a complex and, at times, poorly defined concept, the everyday refers to those aspects of our lives that are familiar and habitual, but nonetheless dynamic and in flux (Harrison, 2000). Embedded within the everyday are knowledges that, because of their seemingly instinctual and unexceptional nature, tend to go unarticulated. At different moments, the everyday offers to us banal, oppressive and subversive knowledges. It is also within the everyday that we can locate decolonial imaginaries which are not always recognised as such. Community psychologists are thus challenged to work with people to articulate these different everyday knowledges and to harness their decolonising potentialities (Suffla et al., 2020).

Coloniality seeks to render the individual, European, white, heterosexual, able-bodied male subject paramount to understandings of the human condition. Knowledges of connectedness, mutuality and community are, by this abyssal logic, severed or made to seem superfluous (see Maldonado-Torres, 2016). In our work, we sought to examine how, and if, residents of Thembelihle resisted coloniality's individualising and Eurocentric hermeneutic within everyday life. Accordingly, we worked with a number of community members, as well as a film production company, to produce a documentary film entitled *Thembelihle: Place of Hope* (see Suffla et al., 2020). Although the documentary was broad in its focus, for the purpose of this chapter, we will consider how it depicted everyday community care in Thembelihle. A stark instance of such care was observed in the documentary's representation of a local brick-making collective which distributed profits equally among its workers rather than along hierarchal capitalist structures (i.e. workers having to sell their labour to bosses, who then retain the surplus value produced by the workers). The bricks themselves were used largely for community development initiatives. Similarly, instead of relying on competitive pricing, a small-scale farmer working in Thembelihle distributed his produce in accordance with people's needs, sometimes giving away for free that which he had cultivated. In another example, teachers and nurses in the community incorporated into their work an activist component, fighting for legislative reforms that would benefit learners and patients (Malherbe, 2020b). Together, each of these caring knowledge-actions served as a humanising counter-narrative to the dominant depictions of Thembelihle that tend to focus on little more than violence (see Malherbe et al., 2021). This was reflected by the farmer in his assertion that "As a matter of fact, this garden reflects the people of Thembelihle." Within these everyday enactments of community care, lay knowledges of decolonial resistance – as well as prefigurative visions of a decolonised future – were captured by one participant's proclamation that "we do have a vision of a better future and, as voting citizens, we deserve a better future".

At public screenings of the documentary, epistemicide's near evisceration of caring community knowledges in Thembelihle was made apparent to those in attendance. The raising of critical consciousness through the documentary screenings was powerfully encapsulated by an audience member in her proclamation, "Don't say 'no' I'm fine. I'm not poor. I'm not sick. I'm not hungry. You must be conscious!" Almost all audience members noted that they were unaware of the different ways by which care was being enacted, on a daily basis, within this relatively small community. Several local business owners who watched the documentary were excited to see the brickmakers' workers' cooperative. Other audience members claimed to feel considerable pride at seeing how residents were resisting coloniality through everyday protest action, while others were outraged at the extent of the impoverished conditions facing different community members. Several activists in the community went on to use the documentary to garner government support for some of their demands, and to promote a sense of pride for the political victories that they had achieved in Thembelihle over two decades of organised activism. These activists also used the documentary to communicate with and create coalitions between other community-based movements. In short, the documentary served as a means by which to transfer and build upon everyday community knowledges. The point of the documentary screenings, like those of the digital stories, was therefore not simply to valourise the manner by which caring knowledges persist against coloniality's systemically uncaring nature (Malherbe, 2020b). Rather, audience members engaged with one another to unlearn the individualising modes of care that are rewarded by coloniality, and relearn and re-member what it means to perform care at a community level (see Tlostanova & Mignolo, 2012; Ndlovu-Gatsheni, 2018).

Coloniality's emphasis on the individual segregates caring knowledges from one another, effectively preventing the transferability and expansion of these knowledges. Thus, everyday care, as a kind of knowledge-action, dissipates when it does not receive structural support. Although the documentary was used in campaigns to garner state support for various caring initiatives in Thembelihle (e.g. those of teachers and the demands of activists), such support was not always realised. Under South Africa's dire economic conditions (which have been exacerbated by the COVID-19 pandemic), many of the community members who had participated in the documentary struggled to sustain community care interventions (Malherbe,

2020b). The brickmakers, for instance, could not maintain their egalitarian business model, and have had to seek work elsewhere. Activists faced comparable challenges with respect to their political organising. For those decolonising Community Psychology engagements that look to work with people to advance epistemic freedom, it is essential that such work is connected to collective efforts that seek to garner structural and material support for these freedoms. If we do not attempt to sustain different community knowledges in a structural fashion, we risk not only being complicit in epistemicide but also destroying the kinds of hope and decolonial imaginings which so often accompany such knowledge forms. As recounted by a nurse who featured in the documentary, "The spirit is there in Thembelihle. People want to see themselves living like people in other communities where there is everything. People are not just sitting back. They're fighting for what they want."

Conclusion

In this chapter, we reflect on how re-membering tensions and conflict, stories of struggle and everyday care in a community context has, and has not, been able to speak to epistemic freedom as a decolonial imperative. This work remains challenging. It is, for instance, difficult to harness knowledges towards action under social conditions that denigrate forms of knowing that do not cohere with coloniality's dehumanising and exploitative mandates. Traditional knowledge platforms, mired in coloniality's individualising hermeneutic logic, are likely to be hostile to knowledges which align with a decolonising vision. Nonetheless, these tensions and contradictions also point community psychologists towards praxes founded on nuanced and contextually embedded approaches to knowledge-making that explicitly pursue epistemic freedom.

We conclude by reflecting on two salient implications for decolonising praxes that our work highlights. First, epistemic freedom may be bolstered through solidarity work with social movements and through structural change. Epistemic freedom is comprehended as more than the mere rejection of conditions of epistemicide. The enactments of a decolonising Community Psychology that constitutes the work of epistemic freedom in solidarity with social movements is about embedding praxes within the various knowledge practices, histories and ways of knowing – explicit and hidden – that characterise a given community. Epistemic freedom assumes the support of social movements to engage in praxes that facilitate shifts in the centre of enunciation, alter normative logics and challenge abyssal thinking. By taking seriously people's lived and felt knowledge systems in this way, decolonising community praxes engage in the rethinking of thought (see de Sousa Santos, 2016; Ndlovu-Gatsheni, 2018). Second, decolonising Community Psychology is about building the capacities and practices of collective and individual patience, fortitude and tenacity to transform the difficulties which accompany efforts to privilege knowledges that are incompatible with dominant knowledge forms. In this, decolonising praxes denote living with struggle and engaging in emotionally charged work that is geared towards an uncompromised vision of psychosocial liberation.

References

Ali-Faisal, S.F. (2020). Islamic anti-patriarchal liberation psychology: A framework to decolonize psychology for Muslims. *Feminism & Psychology, 30*(3), 343–62.

Anzaldúa, G. (1987) *Borderlands/La Frontera: The new Mestiza.* Aunt Lute Book Company.

Bennett, K. (2007). Epistemicide! The tale of a predatory discourse. *The Translator, 13*(2), 151–69.

Capella Palacios, M., & Jadhav, S. (2020). How coloniality shapes the making of Latin American psychologists: Ethnographic evidence from Ecuador. *International Review of Psychiatry, 32*(4), 348–58.

Carolissen, R., & Duckett, P. (Eds.). (2018). Teaching toward decoloniality in community psychology and allied disciplines [Special issue]. *American Journal of Community Psychology*, *62*, 241–9. https://doi.org/10.1002/ajcp.12297

Cornell, J., Seedat, M., Malherbe, N., & Suffla, S. (2020). Splintered politics of memory and community resistance. *Journal of Community Psychology*, *48*(5), 1677–95.

de Sousa Santos, B. (Ed.). (2005). *Democratizing democracy: Beyond the liberal democratic canon.* Verso.

de Sousa Santos, B. (2016). *Epistemologies of the South. Justice against epistemicide.* Routledge.

Fanon, F. (1967). *Black skin, white masks.* Grove Press.

Foucault, M. (1980). *Power/knowledge: Selected interviews and other writings, 1972–1977.* Pantheon.

Gokani, R., & Walsh, R.T. (2017). On the historical and conceptual foundations of a community psychology of social transformation. *American Journal of Community Psychology*, *59*(3–4), 284–94.

Gould, S.J. (1981). *The mismeasure of man.* Norton.

Gqola, P.D. (2010). *What is slavery to me?* Wits University Press.

Harrison, P. (2000). Making sense: Embodiment and the sensibilities of the everyday. *Environment and Planning D: Society and Space*, *18*(4), 497–517.

Hartnack, C. (1987). British psychoanalysts in colonial India. In M. Ash & W. Woodward (Eds.), *Psychology in twentieth-century thought and society* (pp. 233–52). Cambridge University Press.

Institute for Social and Health Sciences (ISHS). (2018). *Report: 2013–2018* (Unpublished report). Institute for Social and Health Sciences, University of South Africa.

Kaya, H.O., & Seleti, Y.N. (2014). African Indigenous knowledge systems and relevance of higher education in South Africa. *International Education Journal: Comparative Perspectives*, *12*(1), 30–44.

Kessi, S. (2017). Community social psychologies for decoloniality: An African perspective on epistemic justice in higher education. *South African Journal of Psychology*, *47*(4), 506–16.

Lau, U., & Seedat, M. (2015). The community story, relationality and process: Bridging tools for researching local knowledge in a peri-urban township. *Journal of Community & Applied Social Psychology*, *25*(5), 369–83.

Lau, U., Suffla, S., & Kgatitswe, L.B. (2017). Catalysing transformation through stories: Building peace in recognition, struggle and dialogue. In M. Seedat, S. Suffla, & D. J. Christie (Eds.), *Emancipatory and participatory methodologies in peace, critical, and community psychology* (pp. 147–64). Springer.

Laurie, N., Andolina, R., & Radcliffe, S. (2005). Ethnodevelopment: Social movements, creating experts and professionalising Indigenous knowledge in Ecuador. *Antipode*, *37*(3), 470–96.

Lowan-Trudeau, G. (2017). Gateway to understanding: Indigenous ecological activism and education in urban, rural, and remote contexts. *Cultural Studies of Science Education*, *12*(1), 119–28.

Makkawi, I. (2009). Towards an emerging paradigm of critical community psychology in Palestine. *The Journal of Critical Psychology, Counselling and Psychotherapy*, *9*(2), 75–86.

Maldonado-Torres, N. (2007). On the coloniality of being: Contributions to the development of a concept. *Cultural Studies*, *21*(2–3), 240–70.

Maldonado-Torres, N. (2016). Outline of ten theses on coloniality and decoloniality. *Fondation Frantz Fanon.* http://frantzfanonfoundation-fondationfrantzfanon.com/IMG/pdf/maldonado-torres_outline_of_ten_theses-10.23.16.pdf

Malherbe, N. (2020a). Articulating liberation psychologies of culture. *Journal of Theoretical and Philosophical Psychology*, *40*(4), 203–18.

Malherbe, N. (2020b). Community psychology and the crisis of care. *Journal of Community Psychology*, *48*(7), 2131–7.

Malherbe, N., & Dlamini, S. (2020). Troubling history and diversity: Disciplinary decadence in community psychology. *Community Psychology in Global Perspective*, *6*(2/1), 144–57.

Malherbe, N., Seedat, M., & Suffla, S. (2021). Analyzing discursive constructions of community in newspaper articles. American Journal of Community Psychology, 67(3–4), 433–46.

Malherbe, N., Suffla, S., Seedat, M., & Bawa, U. (2017). Photovoice as liberatory enactment: The case of youth as epistemic agents. In M. Seedat, S. Suffla, & D.J. Christie (Eds.), *Emancipatory and participatory methodologies in peace, critical, and community psychology* (pp. 165–78). Springer.

Masaka, D. (2018). The prospects of ending epistemicide in Africa: Some thoughts. *Journal of Black Studies*, *49*(3), 284–301.

Mignolo, W.D. (1999). I am where I think: Epistemology and the colonial difference. *Journal of Latin American Cultural Studies*, *8*(2), 235–45.

Mignolo, W.D. (2007). Delinking: The rhetoric of modernity, the logic of coloniality and the grammar of de-coloniality. *Cultural Studies*, *21*(2–3), 449–514.

Mignolo, W.D. & Tlostanova, M.V. (2006). Theorizing from the borders: Shifting to geo- and body-politics of knowledge. *European Journal of Social Theory, 9*(2), 205–21.

Mignolo, W.D., & Walsh, C.E. (2018). *On decoloniality: Concepts, analytics, praxis.* Duke University Press.

Mills, C., & Lefrançois, B.A. (2018). Child as metaphor: Colonialism, psy-governance, and epistemicide. *World Futures, 74*(7–8), 503–24.

Ndlovu-Gatsheni, S.J. (2018). The dynamics of epistemological decolonisation in the 21st century: Towards epistemic freedom. *Strategic Review for Southern Africa, 40*(1), 16–45.

Ndlovu-Gatsheni, S.J. (2021). The cognitive empire, politics of knowledge and African intellectual productions: Reflections on struggles for epistemic freedom and resurgence of decolonisation in the twenty-first century. *Third World Quarterly, 42*(5), 882–901.

Ngũgĩ wa, Thiong'o (2009). *Re-membering Africa.* East African Educational Publishers.

Poks, M. (2015). Epistemic disobedience and decolonial healing in Norma Elía Cantú's Canícula. *Studia Anglica Posnaniensia, 50*(2–3), 63–80.

Reich, S., Riemer, M., Prilleltensky, I., & Montero, M. (Eds.). (2007). *International community psychology: History and theories.* Springer.

Reyes Cruz, M., & Sonn, C.C. (2011). (De)colonizing culture in community psychology: Reflections from critical social science. *American Journal of Community Psychology, 47*(1–2), 203–14.

Seedat, M. (2021). Signifying Islamic psychology as a paradigm: A decolonial move. *European Psychologist, 26*(2), 131–41.

Seedat, M., & Suffla, S. (2017). Community psychology and its (dis)contents, archival legacies and decolonisation. *South African Journal of Psychology, 47*(4), 421–31.

Sonn, C.C., Arcidiacono, C., Dutta, U., Kiguwa, P., Kloos, B., & Maldonado-Torres, N. (2017). Beyond disciplinary boundaries: Speaking back to critical knowledges, liberation, and community. *South African Journal of Psychology, 47*(4), 448–58.

Sonn, C.C., Garvey, D.C., Bishop, B.J., & Smith, L.M. (2000). Incorporating Indigenous and crosscultural issues into an undergraduate psychology course: Experience at Curtin University of Technology. *Australian Psychologist, 35*(2), 143–9.

Spivak, G.C. (1988). Can the subaltern speak? In L. Grossberg & C. Nelson (Eds.), *Marxism and the interpretation of culture* (pp. 271–313). University of Illinois Press.

Statistics South Africa. (2011). Community profile databases: Thembelihle. In *Census.* https://census2011.adrianfrith.com/

Suffla, S., Malherbe, N., & Seedat, M. (2020). Recovering the everyday within and for decolonial peacebuilding through politico-affective space. In Y.G. Acar, S.M. Moss, & O.M. Uluğ (Eds.), *Researching peace, conflict, and power in the field: Methodological challenges and opportunities* (pp. 343–64). Springer.

Teo, T. (2019). Academic subjectivity, idols, and the vicissitudes of virtues in science: Epistemic modesty versus epistemic grandiosity. In K. O'Doherty, L. Osbeck, E. Schraube, & J. Yen (Eds.), *Psychological studies of science and technology* (pp. 31–48). Palgrave Macmillan.

Tlostanova, M. (2015). Can the post-Soviet think?. *Intersections: East European Journal of Society and Politics, 1*(2), 38–58.

Tlostanova, M.V. & Mignolo, W.D. (2012). *Learning to unlearn: Decolonial reflections from Eurasia and the Americas.* The Ohio State University Press.

Wale, K. (2016). *South Africa's struggle to remember: Contested memories of squatter resistance in the Western Cape.* Routledge.

2

CONTRIBUTIONS OF MARXISM TO COMMUNITY PSYCHOLOGY

Emancipation in debate

Isabel Fernandes de Oliveira and Fernando Lacerda Júnior

Abstract

Brazilian Community Psychology emerged as a synthesis of the attempts to theorise the social practices developed by psychologists in favelas, social movements or poor neighbourhoods. It is possible to identify activities linked to social struggles for political and/or human emancipation. Community Psychology needs Marxism in order to promote liberation. Marxism understands social dynamics as a contradictory, processual, material and historical totality. Our analysis highlights two contributions. First, Marxian debates on political emancipation and human emancipation can be helpful to Community Psychology in understanding what kind of social change is possible within capitalism and what kind of social change requires the suppression of private property and class society. Second, Marxism is crucial to understand the social and historical context in which psychological-community work is inserted: an increasingly barbaric stage of capitalism.

Resumen

La Psicología Comunitaria en Brasil surgió como una síntesis de los esfuerzos de teorizar las prácticas sociales desarrolladas por psicólogas y psicólogos insertados en favelas, movimientos sociales o barrios pobres. Es posible identificar actividades vinculadas a las luchas sociales por emancipación política y/o humana. Psicología Comunitaria necesita recurrir al marxismo para contribuir hacia la liberación. El marxismo entiende la sociedad como una totalidad contradictoria, procesual, material e histórica. Nuestro análisis destaca dos aportaciones. Primero, los debates marxistas sobre la emancipación política y la emancipación humana y su aporte para que la Psicología Comunitaria comprenda qué tipo de cambio social es posible dentro del capitalismo y qué tipo de cambio social requiere la superación de la propiedad privada y de la sociedad de clases. En segundo lugar, el marxismo es crucial para comprender el contexto social y histórico en que se inserta el trabajo comunitario de la psicología: una etapa cada vez más bárbara del capitalismo.

 DOI: 10.4324/9780429325663-4

Introduction

In this chapter, we argue that Marxist foundations can be useful to a Community Psychology (CP) that seeks to be transformative, emancipatory and revolutionary. We will highlight the contribution of Marxism to CP as an integral set of theoretical foundations for the critique of social life under capitalism and a perspective that guides psychologists who struggle for human emancipation. We think that the main contribution of Marxism to CP is not to offer a set of specific pragmatic tools, techniques or methods. Certain "methods" or "theses" may be appropriate to understand or change certain objects, while they cannot help to understand or change other objects. For example, a group of radical behaviourists in Brazil found that behaviourism could not be merely "applied" by CP in order to develop conscientisation, but instead, it needed to be reframed (see Castro & Lacerda Jr., 2014).

The chapter begins offering a brief history of CP in Brazil. Then, we highlight two contributions of Marxism to CP. (1) Radical critique of capitalism in which social life is considered as a processual, contradictory, material and historical totality. Marxist social theory addresses essential elements for understanding the genesis, dynamics and the need to overcome the capitalist mode of production. (2) Understanding social change as a struggle for human emancipation. The perspective of human emancipation makes it possible to assess the degree to which techniques, methods or practices promote liberation in specific contexts.

Community Psychology in Brazil: a brief history

In order to introduce the history of Brazilian CP, we present the following timeline, which does not express every trend, but serves as a useful overview of how the field developed (Baima, 2019; Freitas, 1996, 2005; Góis, 2003, 2005; Lacerda Jr., 2010; Lane, 1996). Starting in the 1970s, Brazilian psychologists offered free psychological services in favelas, poor communities and rural territories. From the late1970s psychologists (some with personal experiences of Freirean conscientisation) engaged in struggles for democracy and social change through alliances with social movements, trade unions or political parties. They began problematising practices of mainstream psychology, to create alternative social practices to help oppressed groups develop critical consciousness and transformative praxis. In the late 1980s, efforts were made to theorise the above-mentioned experiences, in journal or book publications – enabling professionals to be identified as community psychologists. With the diffusion and institutionalisation of CP, in the 1990s, some community psychologists were employed in public services or by NGOs. Meanwhile, critical community psychologists criticised the institutionalisation of trends within CP that reproduce techniques from mainstream psychology, not always looking for social changes or alliances with social movements. In the 2000s, thousands of jobs were created for community psychologists in public services. CP became seen as a synonym for psychology focused on social welfare and poverty reduction. Direct experiences with social movements or inside working-class communities outside the state apparatus became increasingly rare with the result that during the first part of 2010s, conservative and individualistic trends of mainstream psychology become more widespread within CP. On the margins, critical community psychologists problematised institutionalisation, arguing for the recovery of Brazilian CP's historical memory, especially actions in alliance with social movements struggling for liberation.

Social struggles for democracy and self-criticism of psychology

This history of CP in Brazil requires the consideration of: (1) the 1964 military coup and the struggles for re-democratisation, 1979–1985; (2) the emergence of critical and theoretical trends within Brazilian psychology, from the late 1970s.

The 1964 coup that put the military in power was a response by the big bourgeoisie, rural landowners and imperialism to a reformist movement that mobilised the working class. Its function was to sustain the dependence of the Brazilian social formation on US imperialist interests and exclude working-class participation in defining its political course. The resultant autocratic political regime began to collapse in 1979, when a resumption of the working class's struggles and organisations gave vital energy to the struggles of other sectors of civil society for democracy (Antunes, 2011; Netto, 2014).

Psychology was forced to confront two tasks in the post-coup context: to present itself as a socially relevant profession and demonstrate that it was not a threat to the political regime. Psychologists in this period – especially the representatives of professional bodies (Hur, 2012) – were characterised as "guardians of the order" (Coimbra, 1995) due to the hegemony of ideas and practices that essentially served the needs of capitalism, especially within clinical psychology, industrial psychology, and educational psychology (see: Lacerda Jr., 2013; Yamamoto, 1987).

However, individualistic and instrumental practices and ideas for the reproduction of capitalism were challenged by intellectuals and professionals "caught up" by the struggles for social transformation that marked the transition from the period of bourgeois autocracy to bourgeois democracy between 1979 and 1985 (Lacerda Jr., 2013). Almost immediately after the coup of 1964, some psychologists got involved with urban and rural guerrilla organisations that saw in armed struggle the only way to face state terror: all of them died as victims of state terrorism (Souza & Jacó-Vilela, 2017). During the struggles for democracy that increased massively since 1979, we saw the direct involvement of dozens of psychologists. Some of them were survivors of torture practices by the state, like Coimbra (1995); others were directly involved in grassroots movements for human rights or democracy (see Hur, 2012). Some of the pioneers of Brazilian CP, like Andery (2001) or Góis (2003), were directly involved with these struggles, and their proposals for creating new practices in Brazilian psychology cannot be understood apart from their alliances with struggles for democracy (Baima, 2019).

In different fields of Brazilian psychology, multiple "alternative" theories and practices emerged, questioning the "social function" of psychology (Yamamoto, 1987). The emergence of CP in Brazil is only understandable when considering psychologists' engagement with social struggles for democracy and better living conditions for the working class, characterising the social conflicts since 1979. The relationship with social movements was remarkable in the activities of CP pioneers in Brazil (such as Andery, 2001; Góis, 2003; Machado, 1988; Vasconcellos, 1985).

The first experiences were rarely called "Community Psychology", but rather the "social approach" (Caniato, 1988), "psychology for the people" (Góis, 2003), or "psychology in favelas" (Gonçalves, 2019). The term CP appeared later, mainly through the efforts of psychologists who founded the Brazilian Association of Social Psychology (ABRAPSO) – a space that allowed debates and theorising of the practices developed in communities.

As in other proposals of "alternative psychologies" that appeared during the first years of the 1980s, it is possible to find in the first CP experiences: (1) a critical stance towards psychology (in particular, its elitism); (2) efforts to learn from other fields; (3) creative activities in order to develop new practices that contribute to transforming living conditions of the working class, especially where most precarious. The first experiences were deeply influenced by the winds of "re-democratisation" that marked the end of the business–military dictatorship (Freitas, 1996; Lacerda Jr., 2010, 2013).

Dissatisfaction with mainstream psychology and indignation over social inequalities were common features that led professionals to CP (Freitas, 1996). For example, Góis (2003), directly influenced by Paulo Freire, describing his first experiences (in the early 1980s), highlights how class struggles create situations in which psychologists need to understand personal suffering as the result of ideology and alienation. Thus, psychologists who want to work side by side with oppressed groups need to understand that their professional activities will only promote liberation if they also are concerned with the organisation of grassroots groups and movements struggling politically against the state (Góis 2003, p. 47).

Learning from Freire, Góis (2003) developed a very ambitious project in a poor working-class neighbourhood of Fortaleza (the capital of the state of Ceará), affecting more than 13,000 people. Resultant CP activities covered social practices aimed at: (a) the healing of personal value and power of oppressed people; (b) opposition, critique and the overcoming of "ideology of submission" and "oppressed character"; (c) promotion of community organisation and vindicatory popular struggle.

In these experiences described by Góis (2003), community psychologists developed three very different kinds of activities: (1) free psychological services for workers, like individual and group psychotherapy – these activities were coordinated only by psychologists; (2) cooperation with other professionals, like educators or social workers, developing activities of "political education" or even literacy groups; (3) support, assistance or consultancy to activities (creation of a local newspaper or community garden, organisation of a women's group to tackle oppression and so on) through self-determined activity of local social movements or specific groups. The activities developed by psychologists thus went beyond particular professional frontiers and were defined according to demands of the community workers.

Furthermore, Andery (1984) used experiences of community organisation from liberation theology and popular education (Freire, 1982) to create a method for psychologists to approach poor workers through dialogue. Firstly, psychologists need to research the history and culture of communities and subsequently to open dialogues, to problematise social issues and define plans of intervention, through conscientisation.

These first CP practices were usually guided by cooperation between psychologists and working-class movements, characterised by dialogue with different fields of knowledge and practice, going beyond psychology (such as popular education, participatory research, liberation theology, public health). Unlike other regions of the world, the main interest informing many experiences was "liberation". Baima's (2019) historical synthesis of the period points out that, during the 1980s, the great majority of CP practices adopted a standpoint favouring social transformation, through challenging the dictatorial state and capitalism, aiming to create another system of social relations.

The above were all influenced by concepts originating from Marxism, especially class struggles, class consciousness and concepts of human as a social-historical being (Machado & Lacerda Jr., in press). It is important to note that CP was preceded by social practices that were the result of the militant or voluntary activity by psychologists concerned with social inequalities and with building democracy and structural changes in Brazilian society. These experiences were later defined as CP.

Institutionalisation of Community Psychology: political and theoretical setbacks

The "democratic transition" from the military dictatorship ended with the promulgation of the 1988 Federal Constitution, which asserted social rights and democratic freedoms. However, it was an incomplete transition. The new democratic–bourgeois society inherited several institutions created by the military dictatorship, such as the military police forces that remain today. The economic model kept intact the privileges of the bourgeoisie and the big landowners. This prevented the realisation of rights, which often existed only on paper. Great pressure was needed from organised groups in order for the rights recognised by the constitutions to be respected. Thus, the transition took place: "without breaking the existing state system, without substantive change in the class nature of political power and by compromises resulting from agreements 'from above'" (Netto, 2014, p. 257).

The "democratic transition" was accompanied by the intensification of the bourgeois ideological offensive that was expressed by the implementation of neoliberal programmes of economic "opening" and "adjustment". For this reason, the establishment of public services in different areas such as social assistance, health and education took place only partially and precariously (Behring & Boschetti, 2009).

All of this affected psychology as a profession. In the year in which psychology legally became a profession, 1962, the size of middle classes and elites enabled it to exist as a liberal profession, especially in the form of clinical psychologists in private practice. However, with the worsening economic conditions (shrinking the middle class), combined with the exponential growth in the number of professional psychologists that took place during the 1980s and 1990s, it became impossible for every psychologist to work only for the minority of the Brazilian population (i.e. middle and upper classes). So, although partial and precarious, the expansion of public services in the welfare sector made it possible for psychologists to work in "new fields", as waged workers (Oliveira & Paiva, 2016; Yamamoto & Oliveira, 2014). It was this conjuncture of partial realisation of social rights, a result of the social struggles of the working class, and the shrinking of professional space for a liberal modality that created the conditions for CP to occupy academic spaces or professional activities employed by the state.

The growth of ABRAPSO and the creation of spaces in universities made it possible for the first theoretical elaborations on the practices carried out in the previous period to spread within mainstream psychology during the 1990s (Freitas, 1996; Góis, 2003; Lane, 1996). Throughout the 2000s, theoretical development has continued, with many arguing for the specific nature of CP (Góis, 2005; Nepomuceno et al., 2008). However, others criticised how some practices of CP were becoming a tool for neoliberal austerity policies. For example, the emphasis on "autonomous communities" could be very useful in the dismantling of universal social rights (Freitas, 2005; Lacerda Jr., 2010; Zonta, 2010).

Another significant change was the emergence of spaces for professional work. The decisive consolidation in 2004 of the National Social Assistance Policy enabled thousands of psychologists to enter public social assistance facilities to work with the working class's most precarious sectors (Oliveira & Paiva, 2016). Psychology in the field of social assistance was not always practiced by professionals guided by CP. However, a close relationship has been established between social assistance and CP, in official guidance documents for professional practice (CREPOP, 2007) and theoretical reflections (Costa & Cardoso, 2010; Ximenes, Paula, & Barros, 2009).

The institutionalisation of CP had two problematic results: (1) the creation of a new specialism, justified more by its theories and methods than by its relationship with the working class or social transformation (Gonçalves, 2019); (2) the displacement of anti-capitalist projects of social change by more moderate political ideals focusing on partnership between grassroots social movements and state apparatuses or NGOs. Sometimes this meant the co-option of combative social movements through funding social programmes focused on very specific social groups, usually at the expense of dismantling services offered to the public (Baima, 2019).

Increasingly, individualistic and technicist trends, such as Positive Psychology, criticised in the early years of CP in Brazil, have gained some terrain (e.g. Yunes et al., 2016). In addition, there are criticisms of CP as moving away from experiences built directly through cooperation with grassroots movements (Zonta, 2010), increasingly uncritical stances towards the state organisations, and the abandonment of political projects that seek to go beyond capitalism (Baima, 2019; Lacerda Jr., 2010, 2013).

In summary, the institutionalisation of CP had contradictory results. On the one hand, it contributed to the consolidated efforts of different theorists and professionals concerned with poverty reduction, the transformation of oppressive processes or the overcoming of social inequality. On the other, it opened up space for the return of concepts of "community", "individual" and "intervention" that had been severely criticised in the 1980s.

It is in this context that we are concerned with the recovery of the historical memory of Brazilian CP, especially the creative role played by psychologists alongside working-class people in favelas, communities and social movements. Since Marxism is a revolutionary theory, elaborated from a working-class perspective and focused on human emancipation (Löwy, 1989), it could strengthen currents within the contradictory field of CP that aim for the social and structural transformation of capitalism.

Marxist contributions for Community Psychology

Insofar as it was the existence of ethical–political projects aimed at liberation that enabled the emergence of critical conceptions of CP (Gonçalves, 2019; Freitas, 2005; Kagan et al., 2011), it can be argued that the Marxist societal project in defending human emancipation is fertile ground for the renewal of insurgent practices in CP. The revolutionary conception of social transformation through the construction of Communism proposed by Marx expresses a more precise and coherent definition of social change than other proposals in the field (see Baima, 2019). It is important to acknowledge that Communism as Marx understands it is something totally different from the experiences of "really existing communism" that permeated the history of 20th century, despite its use of Marxism as official state ideology. Marx (1975) understands Communism as a social system organised around the freedom of individual personalities and the disappearance of labour exploitation and state repression. None of these existed in the USSR and do not exist in China today.

However, the Marxian conception of human emancipation is inseparable from certain other dimensions of Marx's theory, namely: (1) an analysis of work and its contribution to the process of producing social life; (2) a dialectical conception that includes historicity in contradictory and permanent motion; (3) a societal collective project aimed at social revolution and human emancipation. Suppression of any one of these makes it impossible to understand the complexity of Marx's thought (Netto, 2011).

A careful reading of Marx's work enables an understanding of reality in its complexity and historicity. Marx starts from explaining how a given society, in this case, capitalist society, organises itself to produce the goods and means necessary for its maintenance and reproduction. Consequently, macrostructural dynamics is its primary concern. However, Marx did not ignore or underestimate the role of the individual in history. He unveils capitalist sociability through his ontology of the social being, having as the fundamental category of the human world, work – an activity in which the individual and his or her consciousness are decisive (Teixeira, 1999).

Social life is founded through and crossed by an immanent dialectic between subjectivity and objectivity in which, on the one hand, there is the sphere of individuality, consciousness and the intentional projects of individuals who seek to satisfy their needs, and, on the other hand, there is the sphere of society, of objective processes that are set in motion by human activity (Lukács, 1976/2008; Marx, 1844b/1975; Teixeira, 1999).

There have been several attempts to adapt Marxian ideas to create a Marxist psychology or to conceptualise the received "subject matter" of psychology (Oliveira & Amorim, 2012). However, this is *not* Marxist psychology. The artificial separation of knowledge into disciplines cannot be solved through adding adjectives (e.g. Marxist sociology, Marxist political science). The method of Marxism does not support disciplinary divisions that do not explain social reality as a totality. Nevertheless, it is possible to start from its assumptions and categories to develop a psychology that is critical of social classes, exploitation, social inequalities, race and gender oppressions, alienation and other social processes that emanate from capitalist modes of production.

As previously discussed, the rich and diverse mosaic of knowledge grouped within the notion of "CP" did not produce consistent and conscious analyses of what social change really means. Does it involve the annihilation of class society? How might new social practices and societal structures be created? If CP wants to promote social changes in order to satisfy working-class needs, it is necessary to explain how these needs were created and which kind of struggles might overcome capitalist society's contradictions. Marx's theory may be of further use to CP by highlighting some more categories: private property, exploitation, the state and emancipation.

Private property and exploitation at the heart of capitalism

From his youth, Marx widely questioned private property as the foundation of the modern state. He demonstrated how the existence of private property produced a split between private interests and the general will or public needs (Marx, 1842/1975; Vieira, 2019). Capitalist dynamics are based on private property, particularly the ownership of the means of production. This creates social conditions that coerce workers to sell their labour power in order to receive wages and acquire personal products necessary to their personal fulfilment. In this sense, when Marx criticises private property, he is not against personal property per se, but is referring to everything (buildings, machines, advanced technologies, land) that is necessary to produce commodities and wealth through labour exploitation. Marx argues that private property assumes a particular form that is possible only through a specific system of social relations. On the one hand, there are those who only have their labour power by which to earn their living; and, on the other, there are those who have money, means of production and subsistence, who seek to realise the value of the wealth they have through the purchase of the labour power of others, thereby establishing a workforce (Marx, 1867/1996).

In other words, private property in capitalism allows a social division of labour in which the product objectified by work (time, labour) is expropriated from the worker. The labour force becomes a commodity that is bought by those who have the fundamental means of production and reproduction of life (Marx, 1844b/1975; 1867/1996). This separation, of the worker, from the objects produced, which are now seen as private property, is, according to Marx, estranged or alienated work. Alienated labour and private property "are but different expressions of one and the same relationship" (Marx, 1844b/1975, p. 281). Without the latter, there would be no split between product owners and direct producers who cannot appropriate what they produce immediately nor the heritage historically accumulated by humanity, as in this statement:

> The process [...] takes away from the labourer the possession of his means of production; a process that transforms, on the one hand, the social means of subsistence and of production into capital, on the other, the immediate producers into wage labourers.
>
> *(Marx, 1867/1996, p. 705)*

The development of the two ontologically fundamental classes that characterise capitalism is expressed in the ideology of bourgeois society. According to the ideals of freedom, equality and fraternity propagated during the first victorious bourgeois revolution (Declaração dos Direitos do Homem e do Cidadão, 1789), human beings are born free and equal. However, the bourgeoisie, as a ruling class, structured a political system of power that favoured coercion, social inequality and political domination (Tonet, 1989).

In theory, capitalist economy favours competition between free subjects living under mutual and impersonal social relations in which anyone can buy and sell commodities. However, this is not real equality. In the capitalist market, structural inequalities intervene as social constraints that impose on the great majority only one alternative: to sell their own creative forces, that is, to convert their bodies and abilities into commodities. The subjugation of workers is thus a primary and essential feature of capitalism. According to Marx (1867/1996, p. 705), for capital to exist:

> two very different kinds of commodity possessors must come face to face and into contact; on the one hand, the owners of money, means of production, means of subsistence, who are eager to increase the sum of values they possess, by buying other people's labour power; on the other hand, free labourers, the sellers of their labour power, and therefore the sellers of labour.

The capitalist mode of production operates to obtain increasing value through the subjugation of workers. Wage labour institutionalises the labour force's exploitation via a relationship in which the worker produces more goods in a given time than is received in wages (surplus value). Technology in the production process can accelerate exploitation, increasing the number of goods produced in a period. This is exacerbated over time by another parasitic system (distribution and exchange) that enables the circulation of goods and the realisation of their value as money. This constitutes what Marx calls the capital–labour contradiction, perpetuating the growing exploitation, inequalities and poverty in capitalism.

In the beginning, the basis for the incorporation of workers into the wage-labour system, was their expulsion from the land (Marx, 1867/1996). Today, however, it is impossible in any way to conceive of a life that is not mediated by labour force exploitation. Furthermore, the forms of exploitation have intensified: informal and precarious work, without any social protection, represent strategies to increasingly exploit the workforce and increase social inequality (Antunes, 2011).

So, to think about a psychological praxis directed at the working class, demands a recognition that private property is the basis of the capital–labour contradiction. It is a question of continually contesting the condition of the labour force as a commodity. If CP abandons criticism of political economy, it cannot present any historically feasible proposal for emancipatory social transformation (see Ratner, 2019). The logic of exploitation is indestructible within the framework of capitalism, and its limits are the need for survival and the reproduction of the workforce. Thus, the fundamental strategy of change that operates in the tension between classes is "politics", which does not exist without the state (Abranches, 1985). It is, therefore, necessary to understand the state, in order to promote transformational change.

Social change beyond the state

Marx understands the state as a management committee for the interests of the bourgeoisie that introduces organised violence and promotes the ideological hegemony of the ruling class into everyday life. The state operates in order to maintain private property and the exploitation of many human beings by just a few. Historically, it is possible to identify its role as mediator of the relations between the bourgeoisie and the proletariat, civil society and the market, government and governed. However, the state under capitalism exists in order to maintain the capitalist dynamics that underlie it. Marx (1843a/1975) affirms that civil society (which includes the economy) generates the state and, therefore, defines its origin and finitude.

The state is a product, a consequence, and emerges from production relations; it expresses the class structure's interests inherent in the social relations of production (Engels, 1880/1989, 1884/1990).

Thus, a political state is necessary in the absence of a "General Will" within society. The state is not neutral; it always operates in favour of the dominant class, because real political power is never equally distributed between citizens. The bourgeois class (the owners of the means of production) has the power over the way society is organised to guarantee the reproduction of material life, and it directs the work processes (of exploitation in particular). Therefore it extends its power, as the dominant class, to the state, to represent its interests (Montaño & Durigetto, 2010).

The state acts as an element of domination, organised violence and coercion of civil society, since a gap is created between the people and their representation. Hence, the state becomes as a material force that emanates from civil society, but works under the appearance of being an independent entity, separated from society.

Gramsci (1971) exposes the complex relations between state and civil society in times of monopoly capitalism. Gramsci unveils how the development of capitalism also produces diverse social and political organisations that can represent workers or capitalists (unions, political parties, professional movements). Civil society comprises organisations that are permeable to distinct class interests. This means that structural changes cannot take place without the occupation of social organisations that become tools to attain political hegemony – something necessary to social change (Montaño & Durigetto, 2010). Far from reducing the role of the productive and economic sphere, Gramsci emphasises "how the economic sphere determines the production and reproduction of the superstructure in the historical context in which the State became complex" (Montaño & Durigetto, 2010, p. 44).

If the state is the mediator of relations between classes and is a tool for attaining ideological hegemony, then the working class is always at a disadvantage in political disputes, even within democratic legislative apparatuses that cannot dissolve the social antagonism between classes.

In order to assure the maintenance of private property, every state establishes individual freedom as the first fundamental right that also asserts political freedoms. It was only as the result of working-class social struggles that labour laws were promulgated to assure social rights and tackle social issues like mass unemployment and precarious working conditions. When this happened – for example, in some countries the emergence of the welfare state focused on the social needs of workers alongside the economic interests of capital – the state, apparently, acted as a sphere of conciliation. However, this does not convert the state into a political entity capable of solving class conflicts: these can be overcome only through the entire transformation of society.

Our main conclusions are that there is no human emancipation without superseding the state. Democracy within capitalist (or bourgeois) society (in Marx's words: political emancipation) creates political changes (e.g. concession of social rights, more space for political representation within the state apparatus), but it does not go beyond the existence of social classes, exploitation and private property. Democracy can improve the life of the working class, but does not go beyond a society that is founded on alienated labour and private property. With political emancipation, human rights exist only as citizen rights granted by a political community at the state level. Marx (1843b/1975) asserts that human subjects under capitalism are those represented by their selfish self, separate from their social self as citizens. The existence of such a split is, in itself, an alienation that characterises everyday life. These rights, as in Article 2 of the Declaration of the Rights of Man (sic) and the Citizen, following the French Revolution of 1789, are freedom, property, security and resistance to oppression. Freedom, or liberty, consists of the right to do everything that does not harm others. It is about freedom as an isolated human, separate from another. According to Marx (1843b/1975), this freedom translates into property rights of every citizen to enjoy and dispose of goods, income, the fruit of work and industry. However, since the workers' only property is their labour power, this freedom, ideologically presented as political emancipation, represents the freedom to enter, unequally, into contracts of employment.

In the same vein, the principle of equality is little more than the freedom of private property. Equality is one in which the law is the same for everyone, whether protecting or punishing. We know it as legal equality. It is associated with security, represented by protection within private property. Security is the supreme social concept of bourgeois society, manifested in the institutional form of the police. It is the apogee of individualism. Therefore, so-called human rights do not transcend the bourgeois logic whose support is the state.

Human emancipation is a change that goes beyond private property and requires social revolution. Marx (1844a/1975, p. 205) asserts that

> it represents a protest by man against a dehumanised life, because it proceeds from the point of view of the particular, real individual, because the community against whose separation from himself the individual is reacting, is the *true* community of man, *human* nature. (emphasis in original)

Human emancipation requires overcoming social barriers to the free development of the individual who consciously relates to humanity, private property, alienated labour and the state (Löwy, 1989). Without considering the conditions for the possibility of overcoming bourgeois society, any process of human emancipation does not go beyond the condition of mere utopia.

Liberation beyond the state, private property and alienated labour

According to the timeline presented in the beginning of this chapter, we see that, despite the existence of many theoretical and political trends in Brazilian Community Psychology, there is a dominant development. While, in its origins, there was a predominance of practices (often clandestine) in cooperation with social movements and working-class organisations against private property and the capitalist state, the field came to be dominated, especially in the last 20 years, by practices and knowledges that focus on partnership with the state and restricted to advocating poverty reduction. In short, the horizon of Community Psychology has shifted from the perspective of human emancipation to the perspective of political emancipation. This development can be understood as an adaptation to the status quo. From the Marxist criticisms above, the state is not and cannot be a partner of the working class. The most basic issues facing the oppressed can only be overcome with the suppression of private property and alienated labour. For this reason, we presented Marxist theses to alert psychologists to the social barriers that limit programmes in partnership with or within the state.

We want to be clear: there is no "liberation" when we focus only on poverty reduction through state programmes. If this is the future of Brazilian Community Psychology, it is not going to help liberatory efforts. "Liberation" was the keyword that differentiated "critical community psychology" (Kagan et al., 2011) and "social community psychology" (Freitas, 2005; Lacerda Jr., 2010) from the most naive trends of CP. However, Martín-Baró (1987/1996) warned about the impossibility of producing liberation without working-class political organisation and without revolutionary changes in the capitalist social order:

> Only revolutionary practice will enable Latin American peoples to break the inflexibility of social structures that rigidly serve the interests of the few; only then will it be possible to overcome the "one hundred years of solitude" that keeps them on the sidelines of history, yoked to a predetermined fate.
>
> *(p. 220)*

It is precisely the centrality of the revolutionary struggle against capitalism for the whole liberation process that makes Marxism an important source to enrich CP. If we do not consider Martín-Baró's warning, efforts in favour of CP's institutionalisation may engender social transformation that does not require anti-capitalist activities. In other words, by mere specific professional practices, psychologists cannot contribute to the social transformation of capitalist dynamics. Such an ideological thesis undermines the political engagement of professionals building alliances with social movements. This warning was issued many years ago by Cuban psychologists (de la Torre, 1995): CP can become a conservative ideology when seeking "social change" without "social revolution".

Current trends of Brazilian CP are primarily focused on the execution of public social policies created to ease social tensions. While we recognise some open spaces within social policies and many benefits of policies that assure minimum guarantees of living conditions for the working class, it is also important to highlight that a more democratic capitalist society does not break with the class and unequal structural basis of capitalism. That is why we need Marxism, inspiring ideas and practices within CP, especially if we want "liberation" or "human emancipation".

Learning from Marxism, Freire's (1982) concept of conscientisation, and criticising liberal proposals of CP, Zonta (2010) proposes a model of CP that is coherent with human emancipation. CP always has to recognise its activity as: therapeutic in the sense that there are individual mechanisms that block the critical understanding of social reality; pedagogic in the sense that conscientisation always means learning and appropriation of knowledge; political in the sense that social change demands social struggle.

Still according to Zonta (2010), individual and group activities vary according to the social issues facing specific social groups. However, every intervention of CP for human emancipation needs to consider three instances of conscientisation: (a) to **see** – that is, to learn to observe critically the group's own experience and the social reality in which it develops; (b) to **judge** – to decode what is observed through critical interpretation of experience as a problem to be solved; (c) to **act** – there is no conscientisation without action, through organised, collective and transformative practice. This means that not every action can be understood as praxis. Group activities developed by community psychologists related to action have always to consider three questions (Zonta, 2010): What is to be done? How? What are the specific tasks needed? These three questions always consider both objective (what are the material needs or the accumulated force of a social group) and subjective processes. He proposes this framework because:

> "To work within a community, does not mean that one is doing Community Psychology. It is necessary to build a Psychology with a theory and a method absolutely identified with working classes and engaged with a project of social change towards an equal and, because of that, just society."
>
> *(Zonta, 2010, p. 116)*

The different proposals of Brazilian CP that seek human emancipation resonate with these words. To lose of sight the struggle for an equal society – that is, socialism –relates to the problems facing Brazilian CP (Lacerda Jr., 2014). In other words: although bourgeois democracy devises a very favourable scenario for the working class to carry out struggles for its objective interests, its mere existence does not guarantee the overcoming of capitalism and, therefore, effective human emancipation. This requires the superseding of the state, alienated labour and private property.

In recovering the foundations of Marxian thought, we try to answer some of the main challenges faced by CP in Brazil: the capitalist state is not a partner and must be overcome; the formal guarantee of citizenship does not guarantee the real overcoming of social inequality. Without overcoming alienated work and establishing cooperative forms of work, there is no possibility of eliminating poverty; and, finally, only the organised political action of the working class (and not of a professional category, such as psychology) can transform the structural bases of capitalist society.

Without overcoming capitalism, the dream that seeks to move between denouncing its fundamental contradictions and announcing a new possible world is just an impossible dream (Freire, 1982). We are proposing possible dreams that come from the materialistic analysis of reality and strive to carry out emancipatory societal projects. This is what the Psychology of Liberation of Martín-Baró (1986/1996) proposes; this is the main lesson of Marxism for CP.

References

Abranches, S.H. (1985). *Os despossuídos: crescimento e pobreza no País do Milagre* (2ª ed.). Jorge Zahar.

Andery, A.A. (2001). Psicologia na comunidade. Em S.T.M. Lane and W. Codo (Eds.), *Psicologia social: O homem em movimento* (pp. 203–20). Brasiliense.

Andery, A.A. (1984). Trabalhos em comunidade: seu significado para a produção de novos conhecimentos científicos. *Psicologia: Ciência e Profissão, 4*(1), 30–4.

Antunes, R. (2011). *O continente do labor*. Boitempo.

Baima, L.S. (2019). *Psicologia e Luta de classes no Brasil: uma análise histórica da inflexão política da Psicologia Comunitária* (Tese de Doutorado) Faculdade de Psicologia, Pontifícia Universidade Católica de Campinas, São Paulo.

Behring, E.R. & Boschetti, I. (2009). *Política social: fundamentos e história* (6ª ed.). Cortez.

Caniato, A. (1988). Implicações do enfoque social na prática do psicólogo em saúde mental. *Psicologia & Sociedade, 4*, 178–88.

Castro, T.C. & Lacerda Jr., F. (2014). A relação Psicologia Comunitária e Behaviorismo: das críticas às propostas de diálogo. *Estudos e Pesquisas em Psicologia, 14*(3), 732–55.

Coimbra, C. (1995). *Guardiães da ordem: Uma viagem pelas práticas psi no Brasil do "Milagre"*. Oficina do Autor.

Costa, A.F.S. & Cardoso, C.L. (2010). Inserção do psicólogo em Centros de Referência de Assistência Social – CRAS. *Gerais: Revista Interinstitucional de Psicologia, 3*(2), 223–9.

CREPOP. (2007). *Referências técnicas para atuação do(a) psicólogo(a) no CRAS/SUAS*. Conselho Federal de Psicologia.

Declaração dos Direitos do Homem e do Cidadão. (1789). Accessed November 2020, https://bit.ly/36LYPgd

de la Torre, C. (1995). *Psicología latinoamericana: Entre la dependencia y la identidad*. Publicaciones Puertorriqueñas. [also, Havana: Editorial Felix Varela; reprinted, 2010, Buenos Aires: Paidós].

Engels, F. (1884/1990). The origin of the family, private property and the state: in the light of the researches by Lewis H. Morgan. In K. Marx & F. Engels, *Collected works* (Vol. 26, pp. 129–276). International Publishers.

Engels, F. (1880/1989). Socialism: Utopian and scientific. In K. Marx and F. Engels, *Collected works* (Vol. 24, pp. 285–325). International Publishers.

Freire, P. (1982). Educação: o sonho possível. In C.R. Brandão (Org.). *O educador: vida e morte* (pp. 91–101). Graal.

Freitas, M. de F. Q. de (2005). (In)Coerências entre práticas psicossociais em comunidade e projetos de transformação social: Aproximações entre as psicologias sociais da libertação e comunitária. *Psico, 36*(1), 47–54.

Freitas, M. de F.Q. de. (1996). Psicologia na comunidade, psicologia da comunidade e psicologia (social) comunitária: Práticas da psicologia em comunidade nas décadas de 60 a 90. In R.H. de F. Campos (Ed.). *Psicologia social comunitária: Da solidariedade à autonomia* (pp. 54–80). Vozes.

Góis, C.W.L. (2003). *Psicologia comunitária no Ceará*. Instituto Paulo Freire de Estudos Psicossociais.

Góis, C.W.L. (2005). *Psicologia comunitária: Atividade e consciência*. Publicações Instituto Paulo Freire de Estudos Psicossociais.

Gonçalves, M.A. (2019). *Psicologia favelada: Ensaios sobre a construção de uma perspectiva popular em psicologia*. Mórula.

Gramsci, A. (1971). *Selections from the prison notebooks*. Lawrence and Wishart.

Hur, D.U. (2012). Políticas da psicologia: Histórias e práticas das associações profissionais (CRP e SPESP) de São Paulo, entre a ditadura e a redemocratização do país. *Psicologia USP, 23*(1), 69–90.

Kagan, C., Burton, M., Duckett, P., Lawthom, R., & Siddiquee, A. (2011). *Critical community psychology*. Blackwell BPS Textbooks.

Lacerda, F. Jr. (2014). Socialism. In T. Teo (Ed.). *Encyclopedia of critical psychology* (1815–1820). Springer.

Lacerda, F. Jr. (2013). Critical psychology in Brazil: A sketch of its history between the end of the 20th century and the early 21st century. *Annual Review of Critical Psychology, 10*, 110–48.

Lacerda, F. Jr. (2010). Notas sobre o desenvolvimento da psicologia social comunitária. In F. Lacerda Jr. & R.S.L. Guzzo (Orgs.).*Psicologia e sociedade: Interfaces no debate sobre a questão social* (pp. 19–41). Alínea.

Lane, S.T.M. (1996). Histórico e fundamentos da psicologia comunitária no Brasil. In R.H. de F. Campos (Org.). *Psicologia social comunitária: Da solidariedade à autonomia* (pp. 17–34). Vozes.

Löwy, M. (1989). *Método dialético e teoria política*. Paz e Terra.

Lukács, G. (1976/2008). *Para uma ontologia do ser social I* (Trad. C.N. Coutinho, M. Duayer, & N. Schneider). Boitempo.

Machado, M.N.M. (1988). Mudança em comunidades: pesquisa e intervenção. *Psicologia & Sociedade, 4*, 36–40.

Machado, G.P. & Lacerda, F. Jr. (in press). Marxismo e psicologia comunitária: uma relação presente na psicologia brasileira? *ArquivosBrasileiros de Psicologia*.

Martín-Baró, I. (1987/1996). The lazy Latino: The ideological nature of Latin American fatalism (P. Berryman, Trad.). In A. Aron & S. Corne (Eds.), *Writings for a liberation psychology* (2nd ed., pp. 198–220). Harvard University Press.

Martín-Baró, I. (1986/1996). Toward a liberation psychology (A. Aron, Trad.). In A. Aron & S. Corne (Eds.), *Writings for a liberation psychology* (2nd ed., pp. 17–32). Harvard University Press. (Reprinted from *Boletín de Psicología, 5*(22), pp. 219–31, 1986).

Marx, K. (1842/1975). Debates on the law on thefts of wood (C. Dutt, Trans.). In K. Marx & F. Engels, *Collected works* (Vol. 1, pp. 224–63). International Publishers.

Marx, K. (1843a/1975). Contribution to the critique of Hegel's *Philosophy of Law* (M. Milligan and B. Ruhemann, Trans.). In K. Marx & F. Engels, *Collected works* (Vol. 3, pp. 5–129). International Publishers.

Marx. K. (1843b/1975). On the Jewish question (C. Dutt, Trans.). In K. Marx & F. Engels, *Collected works* (Vol. 3, pp. 146–74). International Publishers.

Marx, K. (1844a/1975). Critical marginal notes on the article "The king of Prussia and social reform" by a Prussian (C. Dutt, Trans.). In K. Marx & F. Engels, *Collected works* (Vol. 3, pp. 189–206). International Publishers. Online version: www.marxists.org/archive/marx/works/1844/08/07.htm

Marx, K. (1844b/1975). Economic and philosophic manuscripts of 1844 (M. Milligan and D.J. Struik, Trans.). In K. Marx & F. Engels, *Collected works* (Vol. 3, pp. 229–346). International Publishers.

Marx, K. (1867/1996). Capital: A critique of political economy (Book 1; S. Moore and E. Aveling, trans). In K. Marx and F. Engels, *Collected works* (Vol. 35). Lawrence & Wishart.

Montaño, C., & Duriguetto, M. L. (2010). *Estado, classe e movimento social*. Cortez.

Nepomuceno, L.B., Ximenes, V.M., Cidade, E.C., Mendonça, F.W.O., & Soares, C.A. (2008). Por uma psicologia comunitária como práxis de libertação. *Psico, 39*(4), 456–64.

Netto, J.P. (2014). *Pequena história da ditadura brasileira (1964–1985)*. Cortez.

Netto, J.P. (2011). *Introdução ao estudo do método de Marx*. Expressão Popular.

Oliveira, I.F., & Amorim, K.M.O. (2012). Psicologia e Política Social: o trato à pobreza como "sujeito psicológico". *Psicologia Argumento, 30*, 567–73.

Oliveira, I.F. & Paiva, I.L. (2016). Atuação do psicólogo no campo das políticas sociais: mudanças e permanências. In D.U. Hur & F. Lacerda Jr. (Orgs.). *Psicologia, políticas e movimentos sociais* (pp. 142–56). Petrópolis: Vozes.

Ratner, C. (2019). *Psychology's contribution to socio-cultural, political, and individual emancipation*. Palgrave Macmillan.

Souza, J.A.M. de, & Jacó-Vilela, A.M. (2017). Luta Armada na Psicologia: Prática de Classe contra o Terrorismo de Estado. *Psicologia: Ciência e Profissão, 37*(spe), 44–56.

Teixeira, P.T.F. (1999). A individualidade humana na obra marxiana de 1843 a 1848. *Ensaios Ad Hominem, 1*, 175–246.

Tonet, I. (1989). Liberdade, igualdade, fraternidade: De 1789 a 1989. *Ensaio, 17/18*, 307–14.

Vasconcelos, E.M. (1985). *O que é psicologia comunitária?* Brasiliense.

Vieira, J.L. (2019). O problema da propriedade privada para o jovem Marx. *Transf/Form/Ação, 42*(2), 123–50.

Ximenes, V.M., Paula, L.R.C. de, &Barros, J.P.P. (2009). Psicologia comunitária e política de assistência social: diálogos sobre atuações em comunidades. *Psicologia: Ciência e Profissão, 29*(4), 686–99.

Yamamoto, O.H. (1987). *A crise e as alternativas da psicologia*. EDICON.

Yamamoto, O.H., &Oliveira, I.F. (2014). Definindo o campo de estudo: as políticas sociais brasileiras. In I.F. Oliveira & O.H. Yamamoto (Orgs.).*Psicologia e políticas sociais: temas em debate* (pp. 21–45). EDUFPA.

Yunes, A.M., Garcia, N.M., &Juliano, M.C.C. (2016). O desafio de construir políticas públicas de atenção às famílias a partir de tecnologias sociais e com foco na promoção de resiliência comunitária. In V.M. Ximenes, J.C. Sarriera, Z.A.C. Bomfim, & J. Alfaro (Orgs.). *Psicologia Comunitária no mundo atual: desafios, limites e fazeres* (pp. 49–72). Expressão Gráfica e Editora.

Zonta, C. (2010). Aspectos educativos envolvidos no processo de apropriação do conhecimento e desenvolvimento da consciência nas práticas comunitárias. In F. Lacerda Jr. &R.S.L. Guzzo (Orgs.). *Psicologia e sociedade: Interfaces no debate sobre a questão social* (pp. 99–117). Alínea.

3

COMMUNITY PSYCHOLOGY AND POLITICAL ECONOMY

Sally Zlotowitz and Mark H. Burton

Abstract

We explore a number of ways in which Community Psychology can become more attuned to political economy. Firstly we identify the paradigmatic connections between mainstream economics and psychology. Then we explore political economy as the context for practising Community Psychology, with emphasis on the ways in which the economic system and its power relations structure the lives of people in their communities. We examine potential cross-fertilisations between political economy and Community Psychology and then give examples from our own work of community psychological practice within counter-hegemonic economic practice and movements. The examples are community wealth building, degrowth and psychologists organising against austerity policies in the UK movement Psychologists Against Austerity/Psychologists for Social Change. We conclude that community psychologists can do more to integrate a political–economic dimension into their work.

Resumen

Exploramos varias maneras para que la psicología comunitaria pudiera sintonizar más con la economía política. Primero identificamos las conexiones paradigmáticas entre la disciplina económica dominante y la psicología. Luego exploramos la economía política como el contexto para la práctica de la psicología comunitaria, con énfasis en las formas en que el sistema económico y sus relaciones de poder estructuran la vida cotidiana de las personas en sus comunidades. Examinamos potenciales fertilizaciones cruzadas entre la economía política y la psicología comunitaria y luego ofrecemos ejemplos desde nuestro propio trabajo de la práctica psicológica comunitaria dentro de la práctica y los movimientos económicos contrahegemónicos. Los ejemplos son la Construcción Comunitaria de la Riqueza, el decrecimiento y los psicólogos que se organizan contra las políticas de austeridad en el movimiento del Reino Unido, Psychologists Against Austerity/Psychologists for Social Change (Psicólogos Contra la Austeridad / Psicólogos para el Cambio Social). Concluimos que los psicólogos comunitarios pueden hacer más para colocar e integrar una dimensión político-económica en su trabajo.

DOI: 10.4324/9780429325663-5

Introduction

One way of thinking about Community Psychology is as an alternative, non-individualist psychology. As an alternative, critical, psychology, it explores relationships between the macro, meso and micro scales of human activity and being (Kagan et al., 2019). This is more than a theoretical exploration, since Community Psychology works with people in their lived contexts to support their self-liberation from oppression and their maximisation of well-being. Dimensions of those lived contexts, at all three scales, include the state, civil society and communities, and economic forces and relationships. The first two dimensions have been much discussed in Community Psychology. The state (including national and local government and state-structured institutions) has always been a concern for the discipline, and a specific focus on public policy has emerged with vigour in the last decade (see, for example, the collection introduced by Maton, 2013). Civil society and community have long been central preoccupations. The economy, however, has been largely neglected by the discipline, although as we will see there are some exceptions.

Nevertheless, economic forces and relations strongly influence communities, their creation and evolution, their structure and functioning, and their relations with institutions of both state and civil society. Moreover, the economy is a major influence on the lived experience of communities and their members, determining resource levels and structuring the pattern of life (Leonard, 1984). "Community psychology goes beyond an individual focus and integrates social, cultural, economic, political, environmental, and international influences to promote positive change, health, and empowerment at individual and systemic levels" (Society for Community Research and Action, n.d.).

Despite its relevance, the economic sphere has received little attention in the published literature of Community Psychology. A literature search using the keywords "Community Psychology", "Economy" and "Economic" resulted in only a handful of published outputs, some of them our own. This absence seems strange and probably reflects both the individualistic bias of most psychology together with a reluctance to cross the academic barrier between psychology and economics.

Our concern in this chapter is more with political economy than economics as such; that is, the way in which economic relations are intimately connected to the power structures and relations in society, with a particular emphasis on the role of dominant groups and classes in an unequal accumulation of resources through expropriation and exploitation, using the full political resources of state and civil society to that end. For instance, the United Kingdom is deeply divided economically:

> the UK is the fifth most unequal country in the world, according to the OECD. Financial wealth is held by a small minority, 44% of the UK's wealth owned by just 10% of the population, five times the total wealth held by the poorest half. More than a fifth of the population live on incomes below the poverty line despite the majority of these households being in work.
>
> *(CLES, n.d.)*

Proponents of the current political economic system in the UK have told their own story of human psychology, notably viewing this economic inequality "as beneficial, because it creates psychological inducements for greater productivity, innovation, and wealth creation" (Beattie, 2019 p. 8); or as B. Johnson, now the UK prime minister once put it (2013), "some measure of inequality is essential for the spirit of envy and keeping up with the Joneses that is, like greed, a valuable spur to economic activity".

This has become the dominant view of human nature in the Global North, that we are essentially greedy, competitive and self-serving and that this is also the key to so-called progress. This redefines the very story of who we are as social beings. As community psychologists who often witness the cooperative, generous, resilient, resistant, collective and altruistic acts of those most disadvantaged by current economic policies, we have a different story to tell about human psychology. It embeds the understanding of our behaviour in social structures, power differentials and context. As two community psychologists working in the UK, we have come together as authors to make the case for more psychologists to be active in the wider movement transforming the political economy and to offer some suggestions for this, with an emphasis on the overlaps with a Critical Community Psychology agenda.

Background

The similarities between the orthodox, dominant disciplines of economics and psychology

Despite the relative lack of connection between psychology and economics, the two disciplines share some basic assumptions. Arnsperger and Varoufakis (2006) identified three assumptions of the now dominant neoclassical economics, what they call "(methodological) individualism, instrumentalism and equilibration". That is, socio-economic explanation must start at the level of the individual agent (hence "methodological"), in terms of their action, or agency. Individuals act to maximise their self-interest and do so within a system that tends to equilibrium. Burton (2015) noted that this broadly corresponds to the core assumptions of mainstream psychology, especially that which developed in the English-speaking world from the early 20th century (Danziger, 1990). The two fields do come together in the interdiscipline of behavioural economics. What has been termed "heterodox" economics, where other assumptions and traditions, for example ecological, feminist, Marxist and Keynesian currents make contributions (Calderón et al., 2017; Chang, 2014; Jo et al., 2019), has been largely absent from the mainstream discipline of economics as well as the interdiscipline. Taken together, the schools of heterodox economics offer ways of thinking that chime more with the critical perspective in Community Psychology.

Synthesising the various approaches (Chang, 2014; SSM, 2016) would suggest the following assumptions. The economy is made up of interest groups including classes, institutions and individuals, in their ecological and social contexts. People are rational and irrational, selfless and selfish, depending on their context. The world is a complex web of nested, interconnected systems, of which the economy is one, characterised by uncertainty despite its regularities. The economy involves the transformation of materials and energy into objects and services used by people, largely commodified and monetised at present. Economies change through the combination of exploitation and accumulation, interaction with social and ecological boundaries, influence, struggle, deliberation and accident. Moreover, economies are reproduced through human action, yet in constant flux. Yet economies can be changed through concerted and principled human action.

Political economy: context for Community Psychology

The economic realm is a significant context for the concerns of Community Psychology, as well as its practice. Community Psychology always emphasised preventing psychological and other social problems rather than merely treating them once they appeared. It has been well documented that economic factors affect various dimensions of well-being, including health (Carlisle, 2001). Yet, too often is "the economy" seen as a structural issue that is not considered a site of intervention for applied psychologists, or is so only indirectly, through supporting people back into education or work.

Since 1970, there have been six global recessions, depending on the definition used, causing increases in poverty and weakening of the social safety net. In 2007–8 the global economy was hit by an interconnected series of shocks. Analyses differ as to the primary causes, but the immediate impact was the bailout of large financial institutions by governments and central banks and the consequent imposition of austerity, the reduction of government spending in the attempt to recoup the money from the public. While in most places there was no net loss of employment, millions ended up in lower-paid and more insecure jobs, with poorer conditions, often casualised via "zero-hour contracts" and the "gig economy". This phenomenon has been called the "emergence of the Precariat class" (Standing, 2014, p. 10). People have lost income, whether from employment or cuts in welfare payments, while personal and household debt has risen in most economies (Walker et al., 2014). They have lost roles, self-esteem and purpose as well as social contacts and networks. Physical and mental health has suffered.

All these things have not happened to all those hurt by societal economic changes, but one or more have affected them all (Barr et al., 2015; Psychologists Against Austerity, 2015; Sage, 2018). As economic inequalities have risen, evidence shows the negative implications for everyone's health and well-being, as social problems such as crime rise (Wilkinson & Pickett, 2009). However, it is those already affected by wider structural inequalities who are likely to have been most affected.

The focus of Community Psychology is the community itself, and these large-scale economic shocks affect the very contexts in which Community Psychology is practised. In the UK, for example, the deindustrialisation of the 1980s, particularly in communities that grew up around coal mines or heavy industries, has led to outmigration in search of work and an ageing of the population in those settlements. It has also led to a weakening of the largely work-based collective support systems (union branches, social clubs). For those who remained, the pattern of work in often low-paid, casualised and non-unionised sectors, has changed the patterns of everyday life and the pattern of ties and identifications in those communities. More recently, we have seen the closing down of public services and community spaces as a result of austerity, leading to a further breakdown of community ties and resources (West, 2016).

Even if recessions, inherent in the crisis-prone capitalist economy, cannot be prevented without fundamental political change (the end of capitalism?), there are multiple points at which the impact of these changes can be lessened. For example, community psychologists can ally with others to challenge and change social policy on job creation and social security. They can work with groups of people affected by these changes to increase their ability to collectively withstand the mediated impact of these changes. We will explore some examples below of these ways of working.

Cross-fertilisations between political economy and Community Psychology

How might political economy inform the theory and practice of Community Psychology and how might Community Psychology inform political economy? We will consider each in turn.

Our argument is that community psychological problem definition and action requires an understanding of the ways that economic relations structure and affect the social spaces in which we operate, and also of the beliefs, concepts and actions of the members of the community and others with whom they interact.. To take one example, communities are often beset by what are actually conflicts over distribution: who gets what and who deserves what. Suppose some residents from a neighbourhood want to restrict traffic through their streets. What is the terrain in which they do this? Firstly, it is underinvestment in public transport and the privileging of the private motor car that makes this necessary in the first place. Competition among motor manufacturers has led to inducements to buy the latest models and these have been getting ever bigger and heavier in recent years. The overall growth of motor traffic makes roads congested and drivers, often guided by "satnavs", take shortcuts through residential neighbourhoods. Some residents have come to see their identity as enhanced by their possession of a car, and they are resistant to restrictions, even though they and their children would benefit. In the neighbourhood in question, the residents are organised and understand how to make bids for funding. In another nearby neighbourhood, fewer residents have cars, housing is more dense, there are more children, and pollution levels and traffic volumes are higher. But there the residents are not well organised. The disadvantage of that second neighbourhood is the result of the political economy of industry and hence employment, refracted through social class to give us two communities with a similar interest in traffic restriction, but with unequal scope to make it happen. The very problem, the dominance of the profitable motoring-petrochemical industrial complex is also an economic reality, little mitigated politically since so many citizens rely on those sectors for their livelihoods, and, as we saw, to some degree their sense of self-worth.

The above example suggests some limits to a Community Psychology that only focuses on the neighbourhood level in isolation from the political economy. It also suggests that an adequate critical community psychological practice would connect the disparate communities in a common struggle and make visible the wider economic system context that influences behaviour and decisions. That involves both making demands and enacting changes on the ground, while also addressing the policy and political level, locally and nationally. Although more difficult than a locality orientated approach, this would tend to conscientise the citizens involved, as they "read the world", that is, the system of political and economic forces that underpin lived reality, making those invisible forces more visible.

That concept of "reading the world" comes from the work of Paulo Freire (e.g. 1972) and others who have combined an analysis of consciousness (in the sense of social and political awareness) with the theory of ideology, rooted in materialist political economic analysis. Much of Freire's work has been available in English since the 1970s, yet it is still relatively unknown among English-speaking psychologists (but not among other community practitioners). It is, however, one of the pillars of Critical Community Psychology and liberation psychology (Burton & Guzzo, 2020; Montero et al., 2016).

Something like this can be seen in action in radical housing movements in Spain and the UK. A number of social movement organisations combine direct action to protect people from evictions and against rent hikes, whether by private landlords, supposedly "social" landlords, or lenders of housing capital. This is combined with elucidation of housing policy, its sources and determinants, and political mobilisation to confront it. Examples are the Plataforma de Afectados por la Hipoteca (PAH: Platform for People Affected by Mortgages) in Barcelona, one of the roots of Barcelona en Común, the political movement now running the city council; and the Acorn union of renters in the UK, as well as more local groups such as Focus E15 in London (e.g. Carey et al., 2018).

The so-called neoliberal phase of capitalist political economy allows people to have little sense of ownership or participation in decisions that are made: "the market knows best". As Guinan & O'Neill (2019, p. 384) argue, people often feel, rightly, that they lack meaningful influence over the places where they live and work, instead having the sense that they and their communities are being buffeted by powerful external forces – often economic in nature – over which they have little or no collective control.

A Community Psychology that neglects this level of analysis will underestimate both the alienation people can feel in their everyday lives and their investment in the status quo. It would therefore be impaired in supporting the participation of oppressed and marginalised groups in decision-making, policymaking and democracy.

By understanding the impact of political–economic forces and decisions on people at a concrete, lived level; how consciousness can be raised, through popular education and struggle; and how common pitfalls in the micro-politics of groups can be avoided, maybe Community Psychology, as a kind of "under-labourer" (one who does relatively menial work for another worker, cf. Locke, 1690/1997, who suggested philosophy's subordinate role to that of science), could offer a helpful service to social and political movements working for liberation and transformation.

Examples of community psychological political economy

Community wealth building and other new economic initiatives

Community wealth building (CWB) is a systemic approach to inclusive local economic development that challenges traditional economic systems. Its purpose is to ensure that "wealth" is kept and built within local communities, for the benefit of local people, rather than being extracted by "outside" firms or individuals (CLES, 2020), which often makes a wealthy elite still wealthier while wealth fails to "trickle down". CWB draws upon developments in cities in the USA, such as Portland, Oregon, and Cleveland, Ohio, and on earlier work on "local economic multipliers" by the New Economics Foundation (NEF consulting, n.d.). Pioneers of solidarity finance, including community-owned banks supporting local economies, are also found in Brazil (Jayo et al., 2009). It has been pioneered by The Democracy Collaborative (USA), the Centre for Local Economic Strategies (CLES) (UK) and others. It is based on a series of principles that aim to democratise the economy. CLES describes five core principles for CWB in the UK:

1. Plural ownership of the economy
2. Making financial power work for local places
3. Fair employment and just labour markets
4. Progressive procurement of goods and services
5. Socially productive use of land and property

In 2020, CWB was gradually gaining ground in the UK as part of a broader movement of new economic policies and practices, despite the mainstream economic paradigm. Its successful implementation in the small city of Preston in the north of England, has become well known in the UK and internationally. The CWB movement in the UK is generally being led by local government, especially those local authorities with an overall Labour Party (the centre-left party in power in many British cities) majority. Local governments in London, Scotland and the north of England responded to the COVID-19 pandemic by deciding to deepen and speed up CWB as a means of recovering from the economic crisis now facing the country (CLES, 2020; McKinley, Brett, & Lawrence, 2020).

For local government, the starting point for the application of these principles is to identify the institutions, mostly public sector institutions, that are "anchored" to a place (i.e. not going to leave to chase greater profits). These "anchor institutions" include hospitals, museums, universities and councils (elected municipal bodies managing a variety of services and policies). One of the core strategies is to ensure the maximum local impact of anchor organisations' economic footprints, for example through their spending, investment and employment practices, to support locally based and new forms of democratic businesses, such as workers' cooperatives, community-owned businesses and/or the local community and voluntary sector. Other interventions include the development of community land trusts for local housing or community-owned regional banks.

In Preston, six anchor institutions were involved, including the Police and Crime Commissioner's Office, the University and both the county and town councils. These local anchor institutions worked primarily to shift procurement towards local suppliers and those benefiting local citizens in other ways.

The University supported the development of the cooperative sector in the city by supporting the creation of the Preston Co-operative Development Network, to help establish 10 new worker co-ops, each receiving start-up advice and business support, for instance a local food cooperative to supply catering for the local authorities. Other strategies implemented in Preston included maximising the social return on the councils' pension fund, allocating £200m for investment in Lancashire; the development of a community bank; ensuring new housing developments include jobs and opportunities for local people; and implementing a living wage, benefiting 4,000 employees.

These interventions resulted in the anchor institutions increasing the money that they spent locally in Preston from 5% to 18% and within the county of Lancashire from 39% to 79%, which equated to £200 million pounds for the local economy. In 2018, due to the combined impacts on employment and well-being, Preston was declared the "Most Improved City in the UK" (CLES, 2019).

In Cleveland, USA, similar CWB strategies have meant cooperatives beginning to deliver laundry, energy and catering services for a number of anchor institutions, including universities and hospitals, with one construction programme emphasising the development of minority and female-owned businesses and cooperatives (Kelly et al., 2016).

Strategies for CWB differ according to the local context and resources, but they all emphasise local asset ownership, local jobs and resources, the co-production of local public services and local democratic control. Consequently, while being essentially a top-down intervention, CWB is also part of a broader social movement towards progressive "localisation", which includes a shift towards citizens growing and supplying food (and other essential goods) locally, and reducing the demand on global supply chains (see www.localfutures.org/).

What role in CWB for Critical Community Psychology?

Community (and other applied) psychologists could take up a number of roles in response to, and to help strengthen, the growing new economies movement in the UK (Zlotowitz & Lloyd, 2019), assuming that "under-labourer" role described above.

Firstly, there is a need to ensure that these new economic approaches, including CWB, are decolonised (Bola, 2019), that is, to acknowledge the history and contribution of European colonisation to the metropolitan concentration of wealth and power. Slavery, the colonisation of the Americas and other regions, and the genocide of indigenous people are at the root of the capitalist system (Blackburn, 1998; Federici, 2004; Horne, 2020). That exploitation of the

Global South, and its diaspora, continues and the current economic system continues to hurt most harshly the Black and indigenous majority communities and those affected by intersecting circuits of oppression. In the UK, this has been starkly revealed by the impact of the austerity regime implemented after the Great Financial Crisis (Hall et al., 2017); and also, by the disproportionate effects of the COVID-19 pandemic on Black and ethnic minority people and communities, a consequence of structural inequalities. In the US, Movement Generation and Cooperative Jackson are leaders in prefiguring such decolonised new economies and a "just transition" to those new economic models (Bola, 2019).

Cooperation Jackson (n.d.) is a place-based project, "building a solidarity economy in Jackson, Mississippi, anchored by a network of cooperatives and worker-owned, democratically self-managed enterprises". By organising with marginalised workers and communities, it is bringing to life an alternative local solidarity economy "built on equity, cooperation, worker democracy, and environmental sustainability to provide meaningful living wage jobs, reduce racial inequities, and build community wealth". As community psychologists we can look for opportunities to collaborate with marginalised communities in building similar initiatives.

Connected to these local economy initiatives, and to CWB principles, is the often hidden question of land ownership. In England alone, a mere 1% of the population owns more than 50% of the land, with 30% of land still in the hands of the aristocracy and gentry (Shrubsole & Powell-Smith, n.d.). While this is in large part attributable to the peculiar history of Britain, where the aristocracy and rising bourgeoisie interassimilated (Anderson, 1992; Nairn, 1977), racial injustice is deeply connected to land in terms of ownership and access to green space and is currently being challenged by groups such as Land in Our Names in the UK, who are actively addressing land and racial justice issues. Land is an underexplored dimension, not just in conventional economics but, so far, in Community Psychology itself. As a place-based approach, CWB aims for socially productive use of land and property. Options such as community-led housing, community land trusts and the transfer of community assets to community ownership could be fertile areas for a community social psychological approach.

The first author of this chapter (SZ) has been working with others as part of the London charity MAC-UK, to begin to connect the principles of CWB with MAC-UK's work to redesign services with, by and for the most marginalised young people and their communities (MAC-UK, n.d.; Zlotowitz et al., 2016). For instance, as several local London boroughs are implementing a local inclusive economy strategy to their recovery from COVID-19 (e.g. Newham, Hackney), we want to make the case that excluded young people should be shaping this approach within these places. Young people who experience poverty, inequality and violence in their communities can attest to the importance of how their lives and futures are shaped by these basic elements of political economy. These young people are often alienated by and/or resistant to local political systems and sometimes earn a livelihood outside the formal economy. As community psychologists, we can help by publicising the relationship between these experiences and psychological health and well-being for those who are working more formally in the new economies movement, adding weight to its advocacy work (Zlotowitz, 2020). "Community health building" needs to become an important part of the case for the approach.

At MAC-UK, in addition to supporting young people into employment and directly employing young people, we are considering if and how, as part of our new strategy, we can catalyse community self-determination through the development of youth-led workers' cooperatives and other social enterprises. Workers' cooperatives emerged in the 1800s as sites of resistance to exploitative capitalism and can be understood as emancipatory working-class praxis (Dhillon, 2016). Indeed, this democratisation of the economy through such organisations that allow young people to play meaningful roles, receive meaningful support and connections, gain access to social networks and implement community action, can have positive psychological outcomes, and such participation is core to Community Psychology's theories of change (Christens, 2012; Peterson & Zimmerman, 2004). Our practice to date has repeatedly demonstrated that marginalised young people value autonomy and opportunities to contribute to and improve their communities and the experiences of their younger peers rather than just gaining a livelihood. This is work we mean to build on at MAC-UK, so that excluded young people can participate in and benefit from workers' cooperatives and other forms of community-owned businesses.

Other practices familiar to community psychologists, such as participatory action research (PAR) (Fals Borda & Rahman, 1991), might serve the CWB movement. In partnership with marginalised communities, PAR could offer structured aid to community-led reflection and action, embedded in local knowledge, context and relationships in the places which are implementing CWB.

The degrowth movement, beyond the economy

Implicit in much of what we've discussed so far has been a critique not just of mainstream psychology but also of dominant economic theory and policy. Like psychology, political economy, as a body of theory, meta-theory, values, practices, findings and policy prescriptions, is a contested terrain. While that contestation reaches into the heart of the mainstream discipline of economics, currently dominated by neoclassical theory, it also applies to the assumptions and policies of most economists and political actors about what the economy should be like. In most of the schools of economics, just as in the world of economic policy, there is a set of interlocking normative assumptions that are deeply problematic from the standpoints of social justice and ecological safety. Central to this broad consensus is the assumption, and prescription, that the economy should continue to expand: economic growth is almost universally seen as a desirable thing, bringing employment and prosperity while ensuring the continued viability of the economic system. It is even seen as essential in order to address the dis-economics of growth, the increase in inequality, scarcity of physical resources and damage to ecological and planetary systems. Approaches that emphasise local economies and ecological safety, such as CWB and the Green New Deal (popular in a variety of progressive circles, Dale, 2019), do not escape this assumption that "growth is good". Indeed CWB, in its core practice of retaining monetary flows locally, is more accurately understood as Community Wealth Capture, where that wealth (or strictly speaking, value) is produced in the first place by a productive economy that is hardly challenged in terms of its central motor of accumulation.

Yet, it does not take much specialist knowledge to understand that continued expansion, if that means a continued expansion of material and energy throughput, cannot continue for ever. This has been understood at least since the 1970s (Meadows et al., 1974). Indeed, it could be said that the fundamental problem threatening human life on this planet is the ever-increasing flow of materials, both renewable and non-renewable, via the activities of extraction, production, distribution and use, to eventual disposal or dispersal, into the "sinks" in the planet's air, soil and water. These flows are linked to what is measured as economic activity, for example via gross domestic product (GDP). While, in principle, economic activity can diverge from material flows, in practice, such decoupling is at best only relative: the two things are linked and they mostly vary together (Parrique et al., 2019). GDP growth is a key statistic that governments and central banks use to monitor their macroeconomic policies. When it falters, panic sets in.

Opposition to the growth doctrine has come from a number of sources, paradigmatically, the development of alternative approaches to economics, and normatively, as alternative goals for political economic policy and practice. In the first category is the discipline of ecological economics, in several variants, which situates the economy within the natural world. Instead of a circular model wherein money and goods flow between households, firms and the state, it emphasises the importance of the sources of natural resources (both finite and renewable) and of the ecological sinks where the waste from the economic system ends up. Ecological economics emphasises the importance of the flows of materials and energy into and out of the human economy.

Some writers on political economy have developed a counter-paradigmatic, and normative, approach known as degrowth. The term was popularised, as *decroissance*, by the French economist Serge Latouche (2010, 2012a, 2012b), although it seems to have first been used by the post-Marxist theorist André Gorz. The title of one of Gorz's books, *Critique of Economic Reason* (2010), gives a clue as to why this is a counter-paradigmatic approach, since it attacks the idea that decisions about society and human well-being can be reduced to an economic calculus. Latouche (2012) similarly uses the metaphor of "escaping from the economy". Over the last decade or so the degrowth movement has grown, initially in Continental Europe but also finding common cause with post-development theorists and activists from the Global South and sections of the ecological economics community (Muraca, 2013). It integrates intellectuals and activists working at various levels, from practical projects building alternatives, to social and political movements for societal-level transformation, to an ecological economy and society.

There has been little exploration of the potential connection between degrowth and (Critical) Community Psychology, although one article has attempted this. Natale et al. (2016) suggest that there is a natural alliance between degrowth and Critical Community Psychology since both assume the need to challenge the status quo, while being critically vigilant for the professional and theoretical assumptions inherent in narrowly defined disciplinary practices. They see both frameworks as working to understand individual and social phenomena from a multilevel and ecological perspective, with Critical Community Psychology having at its disposal a variety of techniques and good practices for building community, together with empowerment, care and support for activists. The general social and economic theory of degrowth would add to the micro- and meso-level emphases of Community Psychology. Both frameworks also prioritise more cooperative, community-based and participatory ways of living. Finally, degrowth emphasises revisiting the foundations of the current system, while Critical Community Psychology advocates aim for transformative, strategic interventions for promoting well-being.

Many of the practices of the degrowth movement appear to have a family resemblance to much of Critical Community Psychology. Drawing on a participative methodology with degrowth scholar-activists, Brossman and Islar (2020) organised the lived practices of the degrowth movement under five headings: 1) rethinking society (imagining and constructing alternatives); 2) acting politically (advocating, resisting, organising); 3) creating alternatives (practices of consuming consciously and less, sharing in manifold ways, alternative mobility patterns, sourcing and consuming food ethically, doing things yourself and producing cooperatively as practices that create alternative lifestyles and structures); 4) fostering connections (emphasising the nurturance of relationships and the building of diverse yet supportive community); and 5) in a departure from the themes covered in most of the degrowth literature, "unveiling the self" ("being self-aware and fostering well-being, being mindful, practising arts and enjoying the body, showing vulnerability, rejecting self-promotion and facing conflicts"

p. 926). The multiple points of connection with Critical Community Psychology should be obvious.

The second author of this chapter is a founder and collective member of a degrowth organisation in the Greater Manchester region of the UK. Steady State Manchester explores and promotes an alternative approach to economic development in the city and region, essential if all shall live well and within planetary limits. It encourages organisations to actively pursue the "Viable Economy and Society" (Burton, 2020) for a safe and good future for all citizens in the region and worldwide. Two of the collective members (Mark Burton and Carolyn Kagan) are advocates of Critical Community Psychology, and the work of the collective draws on that perspective. For example, workshops have explored alternative approaches to social, economic and spatial transformation in Greater Manchester via a variety of participative methods such as World Café, Ketso and back-casting (literally working back from a desirable end point to establish a plan of action). The Viable Economy and Society revision was based on an open collective process of reading, discussion and review. Intersectoral edges (Kagan et al., 2019, pp. 222–9) are sought and created to enable the small collective to have an influence beyond its size, while helping allies to develop their ideas and practices. Examples of this have included joint campaigns on fossil fuel divestment, public transport, urban and peri-urban planning, and the construction of alternative exchange systems. So, while Community Psychology is not prominent in the degrowth movement, its ways of working do have a relevance and could make a significant contribution to both the movement's concepts and its effectiveness.

Psychologists for Social Change

Another way of engaging with political economy is through an active network of psychologists and others campaigning together for principled social change. Originally set up as Psychologists Against Austerity (PAA) in 2014, the network has been an active voice in making the connection between growing economic hardship and inequalities and poor psychological health, especially for the most marginalised (Psychologists Against Austerity, 2015). The aim of the PAA campaign was to mobilise psychologists and others, and psychological knowledge, to demonstrate the impact of economic ideology on the increasing prevalence of psychological distress. With a strapline "equality is the best therapy", the network campaigned before the 2015 UK General Election as part of the wider anti-austerity movement. Equipped with a briefing paper, *The Psychological Impact of Austerity* (Psychologists Against Austerity, 2015), which describes five psychological "ailments" that increased as a consequence of austerity policies, the network took part in political debates, lobbied parliamentary representatives and drew on professional roles to appear in the media. Examples in the briefing paper included how cuts to domestic abuse services led to more women being trapped in abusive relationships, how the increasing use of foodbanks perpetuated family shame and humiliation, and how reactionary welfare reform created more insecurity.

In 2016, the network became Psychologists for Social Change and is now a strong national and international network of local groups made up of applied psychologists, academics, students, therapists, psychology graduates, those with lived experience of structural inequalities or formal services, related applied occupations (such as social workers), and many others who are interested in a broad range of social and political action directed towards creating a psychologically healthy society. The aim is to encourage more psychologists to use their roles, their knowledge, skills and relatively privileged positions, drawing on shared experience and knowledge, to foment social, economic and political action that helps shape public, political and policy debates towards a more just, equitable and sustainable world.

Caring for political-economic activists

Running across all the above areas of intervention, we are very aware of the need to ensure that those working to shift the economic paradigm, in whatever capacity, are emotionally supported, and Community Psychology too recognises the importance of support for activists. This is especially true for those activists from marginalised communities who may be at risk of facing more harmful responses from those defending their stake in the status quo. Battling against conventional economic systemic pressures, whether working and struggling inside or outside the public sector, requires resistance, resilience, persistence and creativity. To enable this amongst activists, community psychologists can offer support with reflection, facilitation of peer support, interpersonal and group communications and empathic listening, though it might also be necessary to help actors see the need for such "psychological" support.

Conclusions

The above discussion indicates some of the ways in which the political economy of communities influences the terrain in which Community Psychology is practised. It also indicates some of the ways that community psychologists might both take these factors into account, and more than that, to influence them in a politically and economically engaged praxis. The examples are not to be taken as prescriptions or models for imitation but rather as one exploration of some of the possibilities for such work. We anticipate that in the coming years, community psychologists will respond to the challenge of integrating a political-economic-ecological dimension into their work, thereby continuing to overcome the disciplinary narrowness still too common in the parent discipline.

References

Anderson, P. (1992). *English questions*. Verso.

Arnsperger, C., &Varoufakis, Y. (2006). What Is neoclassical economics? The three axioms responsible for its theoretical oeuvre, practical irrelevance and, thus, discursive power. *Real World Economics Review, 38.* www.paecon.net/PAEReview/issue38/ArnspergerVaroufakis38.htm

Barr, B., Kinderman, P., &Whitehead, M. (2015). Trends in mental health inequalities in England during a period of recession, austerity and welfare reform 2004 to 2013. *Social Science & Medicine, 147,* 324–31. https://doi.org/10.1016/j.socscimed.2015.11.009

Beattie, P. (2019). The road to psychopathology: Neoliberalism and the human mind. *Journal of Social Issues, 75*(1), 1–24.

Blackburn, R. (1998). *The making of New World slavery: From the Baroque to the Creole*. Verso.

Bola, G. (2019). Why we must decolonize economics. *New Economics Foundation Magazine, 1,* 22–23.

Brossmann, J., & Islar, M. (2020). Living degrowth? Investigating degrowth practices through performative methods. *Sustainability Science, 15*(3), 917–30. https://doi.org/10.1007/s11625-019-00756-y

Burtòn, M. (2015). Economy and planet: A blind spot for community psychology? *Universitas Psychologica, 14*(4), 15–21. https://doi.org/10.11144/Javeriana.upsy14-4.epbs

Burton, M. (2020). *The viable economy … and society* (revision of 2014 "The Viable Economy"). Steady State Manchester. https://steadystatemanchester.files.wordpress.com/2014/11/the-viable-economy-master-document-v4-final.pdf

Burton, M., & Guzzo, R. (2020). Liberation psychology: Origins and development. In L. Comas-Días & E. Torres Rivera (Eds.), *Liberation psychology: Theory, method, practice, and social justice* (pp. 17–40). American Psychological Association. http://dx.doi.org/10.1037/0000198-002

Calderón, A.A., Simarro, R.M., Jiménez, A.B., & Erades, C.M. (Eds.). (2017). *Hacia una Economía Más Justa: Manual de corrientes económicas heterodoxas*. Economistas sin Fronteras.

Carey, N., James, S., Dennis, A., Zlotowitz, S., Gillespie, T., & Hardy, K. (2018). Building alliances with marginalised communities to challenge London's unjust and distressing housing system. *Clinical Psychology Forum, 309,* 34–8.

Carlisle, S. (2001). Inequalities in health: Contested explanations, shifting discourses and ambiguous policies. *Critical Public Health*, *11*(3), 267–81.

Centre for Local Economic Strategies (CLES). (n.d.). *How to build community wealth.* https://cles.org.uk/community-wealth-building/how-to-build-community-wealth/

Centre for Local Economic Strategies (CLES). (2019). Community wealth building 2019: Theory, practice and next steps. (p. 30). https://cles.org.uk/wp-content/uploads/2019/09/CWB2019FINAL-web.pdf

Centre for Local Economic Strategies (CLES). (2020). *Own the future: A guide for new local economies.* https://cles.org.uk/wp-content/uploads/2020/07/Own-the-future-revised-mutuals-copy.pdf

Chang, H. (2014). *Economics: The user's guide: a Pelican introduction.* Pelican Books.

Christens, B.D. (2012). Targeting empowerment in community development: A community psychology approach to enhancing local power and well-being. *Community Development Journal*, *47*(4), 538–54.

Cooperation Jackson. (n.d.). *Cooperation Jackson.* Cooperation Jackson. https://cooperationjackson.org

Dale, G. (2019, October 28). Degrowth and the Green New Deal. *The Ecologist*, web edition. https://theecologist.org/2019/oct/28/degrowth-and-green-new-deal

Danziger, K. (1990). *Constructing the subject: Historical origins of psychological research.* Cambridge University Press.

Dhillon, G.S. (2016). *Social justice and worker cooperatives* [Wilfrid Laurier University]. https://scholars.wlu.ca/etd/1799

Fals Borda, O., & Rahman, M.A. (1991). *Action and knowledge: Breaking the monopoly of power with participatory action-research.* Intermediate Technology Publications and Apex Press.

Federici, S. (2004). *Caliban and the witch: Women, the body, and primitive accumulation.* Autonomedia; Pluto.

Freire, P. (1972). *Pedagogy of the oppressed.* Penguin.

Gorz, A. (2010). *Critique of economic reason.* Verso.

Guinan, J., & O'Neill, M. (2019). From community wealth-building to system change. *IPPR Progressive Review*, *25*(4), 382–92.

Hall, S., McIntosh, K., Neitzert, E., Pottinger, L., Sandhu, K., Stephenson, M., Reed, H., & Taylor, L. (2017). *Intersecting inequalities: The impact of austerity on Black and Minority Ethnic women in the UK.* Runnymede Trust.

Horne, G. (2020). *The dawning of the apocalypse: The roots of slavery, white supremacy, settler colonialism, and capitalism in the long sixteenth century.* Monthly Review Press.

Jayo, M., Pozzebon, M., & Diniz, E.H. (2009). Microcredit and innovative local development in Fortaleza, Brazil: The case of Banco Palmas. *Canadian Journal of Regional Science*, *32*(1), 115–128.

Jo, T.-H., Chester, L., & D'Ippoliti, C. (Eds.). (2019). *Routledge handbook of heterodox economics: Theorizing, analyzing, and transforming capitalism.* Routledge.

Johnson, B. (2013). *The third Margaret Thatcher lecture.* Centre for Policy Studies. www.cps.org.uk/files/factsheets/original/131128144200-Thatcherlecturev2.pdf

Kagan, C., Burton, M., Duckett, P., Lawthom, R., & Siddiquee, A. (2019). *Critical community psychology: Critical action and social change* (2nd ed.). Routledge.

Kelly, M., McKinley, S., & Duncan, V. (2016). Community wealth building: America's emerging asset-based approach to city economic development. *Renewal*, *24*(2), 51–68. www.lwbooks.co.uk/renewal/24-2/community-wealth-building

Latouche, S. (2010). *Farewell to growth* (David Macey, Trans.). Polity Press.

Latouche, S. (2012a). *La sociedad de la abundancia frugal: Contrasentidos y controversias del decrecimiento.* Icaria.

Latouche, S. (2012b). *Salir de la sociedad de consumo: Voces y vías del decrecimiento* (1st Spanish ed.). Ocataedro.

Leonard, P. (1984). *Personality and ideology: Towards a materialist understanding of the individual.* Macmillan.

Locke, J. (1690/1997). *An essay concerning human understanding.* Penguin Books.

MAC-UK. (n.d.). *Transforming the health, social and economic inequalities of excluded groups.* https://mac-uk.org/

Maton, K. (2013). Community psychologists in the policy arena: Perspectives from four continents. *Global Journal of Community Psychology Practice*, *4*(2), 2–4.

McKinley, S., Brett, M., &Lawrence, M. (2020). Democratic by design: A new community wealth building vision for the British economy after Covid-19. Common Wealth & The Democracy Collaborative. https://uploads-ssl.webflow.com/5e2191f00f868d778b89ff85/5f7d93ca26285b806fefc970_Democratic%20by%20Design.pdf

Meadows, D.H., Meadows, D.L., Randers, J., & Behrens, W.W. (1974). *The limits to growth: A report for the Club of Rome's project on the predicament of mankind.* Pan Books. www.donellameadows.org/wp-content/userfiles/Limits-to-Growth-digital-scan-version.pdf

Montero, M., Sonn, C., & Burton, M. (2016). Community psychology and liberation psychology: Creative synergy for ethical and transformative praxis. In M.A. Bond, I. García de Serrano, & C. Keys (Eds.), *APA handbook of community psychology* (1st ed.; Vol. 1) (pp. 149–167). American Psychological Association.

Muraca, B. (2013). Decroissance: A project for a radical transformation of society. *Environmental Values*, *22*(2), 147–69. https://doi.org/10.3197/096327113X13581561725112

Nairn, T. (1977). The twilight of the British state. *New Left Review*, January–April (101–102), 3–61. https://newleftreview.org/issues/I101/articles/tom-nairn-the-twilight-of-the-british-state

Natale, A., Di Martino, S., Procentese, F., & Arcidiacono, C. (2016). De-growth and critical community psychology: Contributions towards individual and social well-being. *Futures*, *78–79*, 47–56. http://eprints.leedsbeckett.ac.uk/3008/1/De-growth%20and%20critical%20community%20psychology.pdf

NEF Consulting. (n.d.). *Local Multiplier 3 (LM3)*. www.nefconsulting.com/our-services/evaluation-impact-assessment/local-multiplier-3/

Parrique, T., Barth, J., Briens, F., Kraus-Polk, A., Spangenberg, S.H., & Kerschner, C. (2019). *Decoupling debunked: Evidence and arguments against green growth as a sole strategy for sustainability*. European Environmental Bureau. http://eeb.org/library/decoupling-debunked

Peterson, N.A., & Zimmerman, M.A. (2004). Beyond the individual: Toward a nomological network of organizational empowerment. *American Journal of Community Psychology*, *34*(1/2), 129–45.

Psychologists against Austerity. (2015). *The psychological impact of austerity: A briefing paper*. Psychologists Against Austerity/Psychologists for Social Change. www.psychchange.org/psychologists-against-austerity.html

Psychologists for Social Change. (n.d.). www.psychchange.org/

Sage, D. (2018). Reversing the negative experience of unemployment: A mediating role for social policies? *Social Policy & Administration*, *52*(5), 1043–59. https://doi.org/10.1111/spol.12333

Shrubsole, G., & Powell-Smith, A. (n.d.). Who owns England? https://whoownsengland.org/

Society for Community Research and Action (SCRA). (n.d.). *What is community psychology?* www.scra27.org/what-we-do/what-community-psychology/

Standing, G. (2014). The precariat. *Contexts*, *13*(4), 10–12.

Steady State Manchester (SSM). (2016). A comparison table of 9 schools of economics by Ha-Joon Chang with a further school, ecological economics, added by Mark Burton. https://steadystatemanchester.files.wordpress.com/2012/07/assumptions-of-ecological-economics-mb.pdf

Walker, C., Burton, M., Akhurst, J., & Degirmencioglu, S.M. (2014). Locked into the system? Critical community psychology approaches to personal debt in the context of crises of capital accumulation. *Journal of Community & Applied Social Psychology*. https://doi.org/10.1002/casp.2209

West, L. (2016) *Distress in the city: Racism, fundamentalism and democratic education*. Trentham.

Wilkinson, R., &Pickett, K. (2009). *The spirit level: Why more equal societies almost always do better*. Penguin.

Zlotowitz, S. (2020). It's not just all in your head. *New Economics Foundation Magazine*, *2*, 22.

Zlotowitz, S., Barker, C., Moloney, O., & Howard, C. (2016). Service users as the key to service change? The development of an innovative intervention for excluded young people. *Child and Adolescent Mental Health*, *21*(2), 102–8.

Zlotowitz, S., & Lloyd, J. (2019, August 11). Beyond the individual in mental health and wellbeing. *Stir to Action Magazine*, *26*. www.stirtoaction.com/blog-posts/beyond-the-individual-in-mental-health-wellbeing

4

GROUNDING COMMUNITY PSYCHOLOGY IN PRACTICES OF ECOPSYCHOSOCIAL ACCOMPANIMENT

Garret Barnwell, Gay Bradshaw and Mary Watkins

Abstract

Ecopsychosocial accompaniment is a practice that has the potential of repositioning community psychologists from a place of elevated expertise to a horizontal position on more equal footing from which solidarity can emerge. It requires radical availability; steadfast witnessing; self-reflexivity; attunement to the knowledge, needs and desires of others; and committed response-ability. Accompaniment can be engaged in with a person, a human community, other-than-human animal(s), a mountain or a river. Accompaniment is at the heart of building inclusive spaces graced by efforts to build justice and mutual security, trust and respect. Such spaces pre-empt violence by cultivating dignified and equitable conditions where life can thrive sustainably. Ecopsychosocial accompaniers are students of the historical context of the situation in which accompaniment is taking place. They work alongside others to transform sociocultural contexts which have generated pervasive social and ecological misery through ongoing coloniality, rapacious capitalism and racism. The authors use forced migration – an outcome of all the interdependent crises articulated in the Introduction – to explore ecopsychosocial accompaniment as an essential practice in Community Psychology.

Resumen

El acompañamiento ecopsicosocial es una práctica que tiene la potencial de reasignar a los psicólogos de la comunidad desde una posición de experto elevado a una posición horizontal en una base de mayor igualdad en la cual puede emerger la solidaridad. Esto requiere de una disponibilidad radical y de atestiguarse; autorreflexión; ajustarse al conocimiento, necesidades y deseos de los otros; y compromiso a una responsabilidad. El acompañamiento puede comprometerse con una persona, una comunidad humana, con el mundo aparte de humanos, animales, una montaña o un río. El acompañamiento es el corazón de la construcción de espacios inclusivos honrados por los esfuerzos para construir justicia y seguridad común, verdad y respeto. Tales espacios previenen la violencia, cultivando condiciones dignas e igualitarias donde la vida puede desarrollarse sosteniblemente. Los acompañantes ecopsicosociales son

DOI: 10.4324/9780429325663-6

estudiantes del contexto histórico de la situación en la cual el acompañamiento esta ocurriendo. Trabajan junto con otros para transformar contextos socioculturales que han generado miseria social y ecológica generalizada a través del continuo colonialismo, el insaciable capitalismo y el racismo. Los autores usan la migración forzada – resultado de las crisis interdependientes articuladas en la Introducción – para explorar el acompañamiento ecopsicosocial como práctica esencial de la Psicología de la Comunidad.

Ecopsychosocial accompaniment

The Western professionalisation of psychosocial understandings has created unintended consequences, too often disempowering community members whom it seeks to serve, neglecting the knowledge indigenous to a group and usurping leadership. The shadow of acquiring an expert status through the academy can be unacknowledged hubris, born of coloniality. Critical Community Psychology is concerned with the decolonisation of oppressive social systems that reproduce themselves within Community Psychology and invade psychological space (Kagan, Burton, Duckett, Lawthom, & Siddiquee, 2019). As community psychologists try to struggle free of colonial ways of seeing and being, the practice and ethics of ecopsychosocial accompaniment, with roots in liberation movements, liberation theology and liberation psychology, help provide a potential pathway to solidarity (Kagan et al., 2019; Watkins, 2015; Watkins, 2019; Watkins & Shulman, 2008). We seek to lift up the practice of ecopsychosocial accompaniment so that it can orient relationship building in Community Psychology and disable power structures of oppression as we join *with* others to strengthen and build beloved communities where justice, dynamic peace and ecological well-being can co-flourish.

We, the authors, are intergenerational and binational (US and S. Africa), with multidisciplinary backgrounds (ecology, conflict transformation and management, humanitarian assistance, clinical and liberation psychologies). We have converged around the practice of mutual accompaniment from varied community practice contexts: forced migration, other-than-human animal collective trauma and environmental justice.

Paul Farmer (2013), a co-founder of Partners in Health, describes what it means to accompany someone:

> [It] is to go somewhere with him or her, to break bread together, to be present on a journey with a beginning and an end. There's an element of mystery, of openness, of trust, in accompaniment. The companion, the accompagnateur, says: "I'll go with you and support you on your journey wherever it leads. I'll share your fate for a while" – and by "a while", I don't mean a little while. Accompaniment is about sticking with a task until it's deemed completed –not by the accompagnateur, but by the person being accompanied.
>
> *(p. 234)*

The root of *acompañamiento* is *compañero* or friend. It draws from the Latin *ad cum panis*, to break bread with one another.

In contradistinction to a relationship skewed and dominated by one partner with expert status and higher social privilege intervening from above, accompaniers desire horizontal and mutual relationships where multiple voices can come forward and through their dialogue discern a path of action together. Like musical accompanists, they try to attune themselves to how to support the best efforts of others. Kagan et al. (2019) explains that accompaniment is an "active process of being in the presence of another person and journeying with her or him"

(p. 231). In this practiced and intentional humility lie the seeds for deep listening, learning from others' knowledge and life experiences, bearing witness and working in solidarity. This is not a question of uncritical deference, offers activist-accompanier Staughton Lynd (2010), but of equality.

Beyond critical psychology, "accompaniment" is a term used in arenas as diverse as social medicine, peace activism, human rights, pastoral support, social psychology, animal rights and liberation psychology. The concept is used when speaking of accompanying the ill who are also poor (Farmer, 2011), those caught in prison and detention systems, political dissidents, refugees, those suffering under occupation, those with intellectual disabilities, victims of torture and other forms of violence, those forcibly displaced, those suffering violations of human rights, and those attempting to live peacefully in the face of paramilitary and military violence, as in the peace communities in Colombia. In countless other situations of human and environmental duress, what we are describing as accompaniment is engaged in without recourse to the term. In Latin America, "psychosocial accompaniment" has arisen as a role that is distinct from that of psychotherapist or psychological researcher, though it may include elements of each. Colombian community psychologist Stella Sacipa-Rodriguez (in Sacipa-Rodriguez & Montero, 2014, p. 67) describes it as the creation of psychosocial spaces for compassionate listening and witnessing, where mutual respect and acknowledgement can be engendered so that social bonds and support can be established and then strengthened.

The adjective "psychosocial" emerged as a corrective to psychological understandings that neglected the importance of social context due to an underlying individualistically oriented paradigm. It is past time for us to combine "eco" with "psychosocial" to correct psychology's failure to focus on the environmental and place-based context of the human being. While Community Psychology has pursued "ecological" approaches that restore the connections between the individual and the social, "eco-" has not referred specifically to built and natural environments. Psychosocial well-being is not independent of ecological or environmental well-being. Ecopsychosocial accompaniment requires radical availability, steadfast witnessing, self-reflexivity, attunement to others' needs and desires, and committed response-ability. Accompaniment can be engaged in with a person, a human community, other-than-human animal(s), a mountain or a river. It can be accomplished at various levels of organisation, from grassroots relationships to policy creation and implementation, to create deep structural change. Accompaniment is at the heart of building inclusive spaces graced by efforts to build security, trust and mutual respect. These pre-empt or redress violence by cultivating dignified and equitable conditions where life can thrive sustainably. For critical psychologists, this mutual accompaniment includes supporting decolonial struggles, partnering to assist marginalised groups to reclaim identities and represent their own social worlds (Kagan et al., 2019). Accompaniers – inside and beyond Community Psychology – seek to transform the legacies of sociocultural and historical contexts which have generated pervasive social and ecological misery, opening spaces that struggle to be free of coloniality, rapacious capitalism and racism.

Accompaniers work within their own community or they may be "outside accompaniers" (2021), invited to participate. Rather than positioning themselves as "allies", outside critical psychologists can seek to "accomplice" (Indigenous Action Media), shouldering the risks facing community members. Outside accompanists may have more privilege than community members they work alongside. If so, care needs to be taken to track and be responsible for the effects of this privilege and to be open to critique and counsel concerning them. For instance, peace accompaniers in conflict situations – who live with a community that is less likely to be attacked if there are international accompanists present – may desire a world without privileging whiteness, even as they use their whiteness in an effort to protect communities of colour who are building peace (Mahrouse, 2014).

Community psychologists need to become students of the situation in which they plan to accept requests for accompaniment, learning about the history behind the present moment and the structural pillars that sustain social and ecological misery. This assists them to be accompaniers across levels of organisation, working not only to ameliorate suffering but to work together to transform its generation. To illustrate the principles, practices and ethics of ecopsychosocial accompaniment, we will address forced migration – an outcome of all of the interdependent crises articulated in the Introduction, and one we are each intimately involved in from different vantage points: in the accompaniment of migrants (Watkins), trans-species accompaniment (Bradshaw), and earth accompaniment (Barnwell).

Ecopsychosocial accompaniment of forced migrants in the U.S.

According to the United Nations (UN) Refugee Agency, conflict and climate change forced 79.5 million people to flee their homes in 2019. One percent of humanity, one in 97 people, is currently displaced. Right-leaning, xenophobic and racist governments have built walls around the world to deter forced migrants from entering their countries, as well as gulags of detention prisons to contain them. Often having suffered persecution, torture, violence, and/or the destruction of their homes and livelihood, far too many forced migrants find themselves stranded at militarised borders and jailed in detention prisons, in need of accompaniment. Too often, they are met with disdain, death-dealing neglect and even hatred, rather than the welcome they so desperately need.

Many individuals and groups have mobilised to accompany migrants from the inception of their journeys through the point of their establishing a secure home in another place. Accompanying migrant caravans, providing human rights and asylum process training, visiting detainees in immigration prisons, accompanying migrants to immigration court, offering support to their families if they are deported and extending a hand in finding housing, employment and healthcare are some of the work of accompanists. Community psychologists in solidarity with migrants and the groups that support them can provide targeted assistance, deploying their skills and learning new ones.

Activist-accompanier, historian and lawyer Staughton Lynd advocated for "reciprocal accompaniment", and urged would-be accompaniers to find skills that could be of use in a given situation.

> "Accompaniment" is simply the idea of walking side by side with another on a common journey. The idea is that when a university-trained person undertakes to walk beside someone rich in experience but lacking formal skills, each contributes something vital to the process.
>
> *(Lynd & Grubacic, 2010, p. 20)*

Community psychologists have learned new skills to meet the particular needs of those they are accompanying. For instance, the Colombian social psychologists at The Social Bonds and Cultures of Peace research group devote themselves to accompanying victims of violence who were displaced from the countryside by armed conflict. Through their listening and witnessing, they became aware that many of the displaced families wanted it to be clear in public records that their loved ones were falsely assumed to be guerrillas. They also wanted to know where their loved ones' remains are so that proper burials could be conducted. Honouring these deep desires, the psychologists needed to become knowledgeable about and effective in interfacing with relevant judicial and public authorities and processes (Sacipa et al., 2007).

Psychologists team up with immigration lawyers to offer forensic evaluations of asylum seekers, helping document and explain to the immigration judge the kinds of traumas a person has undergone, the effects of these on their mental health and testimony, and the probable psychological consequences of being deported. This form of accompaniment provides an opportunity for forced migrants to convey their life story to someone who can witness not only their challenges, but their strengths, courage and resilience (Gangsei & Deutsch, 2007). Their stories retain the social, ecological, economic and political contexts which are too often lost in clinical encounters narrowly focused on post-traumatic stress disorder symptomology.

Community psychologists Regina Langhout and Sylvane Vaccarino-Ruiz (2021) have studied the deleterious health effects of deportation raids on children and adults in their community of Santa Cruz, California. They have accompanied 9-to 12-year-old immigrant youth and helped them claim their experience of these raids in the face of the wider community's efforts to disappear them, denying their destructive impact on the whole community. Their work, along with others, was used to develop a Society for Community Research and Action (2021) policy brief that offered national and judicial policy recommendations, local jurisdiction policy recommendations and policy recommendations for neighbourhoods and institutions.

I, Mary Watkins, accompanied young adults to create an oral history of their families' forced migration and their experiences living in Santa Barbara, California, without immigration documents (Immigration Rights Committee, 2008). The youth used these stories to educate and dialogue with the Anglo community. They hoped to shift destructive narratives about their community, to engender empathic understanding and to mobilise their citizen neighbours to work in solidarity with them to promote supportive legislation and to combat harmful practices of the police.

Sadly, the challenges of many migrants without documents also include forced deportation, negating the value of the deep sacrifices that were already suffered to make the journey. Through the Post-Deportation Human Rights Project (PDHRP), liberation and community psychologist Brinton Lykes has been collaborating with human rights lawyers, immigrant community groups in the US, deportees and families without immigration documents to explore the effects of current US detention and deportation policies on Salvadoran and Guatemalan families residing in the Northeast US. Brabeck, Lykes, and Hershberg (2011) describe how through their accompaniment of family members who have suffered deportation directly or indirectly, they learn from the experiential knowledge of community members. This enables them to discuss the relevant issues with fellow citizens, in hopes of bridging the growing chasm between citizens and non-citizens and to construct a shared understanding of and response to injustices that immigrant families (many of whom include US-born citizen children) face.

Accompaniment can also be expressed through immigration prison abolition efforts, as well as advocacy for non-punitive paths to citizenship. Accompanists can work against the criminalisation of forced migrants, shining light on the destructive functions of such derisive and false narratives. They are critical for anti-racist work that is essential to the dismantling of immigration prisons and harshly restrictive "walls" of governmental policies.

These kinds of accompaniment are antidotes to the walls that have been built and the restrictive and punitive laws that have been passed to stem the flow of migration; they are, as well, an affective antidote to the hatred, disdain and disregard that flow from racist xenophobic orientations (Casey & Watkins, 2014). Community psychologists can be of help in accompanying immigrants throughout their struggle to find a safe home, leveraging their institutional and cultural resources to support migrants and the organisations that support them (Fernández, 2020).

Accompanists need to continuously engage in reflexivity, acknowledging and reflecting upon the potential ill-effects of their privilege on those they are working with – be it professional, class, race or citizenship privilege. They need to take care to divest themselves of habits – including those born of white privilege – that can thwart and even unintentionally insult grassroots leadership. In addition, they need to critically address and replace narratives of "giving aid" and "helping" that fail to recognise the reciprocal and mutual nature of accompaniment. Jonathan Weigel of Partners-in-Health differentiates aid from accompaniment. He describes "aid" as a short-term, one-way encounter where one person helps and another is helped.

> Accompaniment seeks to abandon the temporal and directional nature of aid; it implies an open-ended commitment to another, a partnership in the deepest sense of the word […] To replace the hubris of traditional frozen assistance with humility, trust, patience, and constancy – to replace aid with accompaniment. This is not an easy approach. It entails radical availability.
>
> *(Weigel, 2013, pp. xxv–xxvi)*

Standing with the wild

The "community" that most Community Psychology addresses is far too limited. It is ironic that while Community Psychology uses the term "ecological", it is not addressing what Quechuans call the *ayllu* (Mendoza and Zerda, 2011). A schoolteacher, Justo Oxa, describes the unbroken wholeness of a Quechuan way of being in community where non-human life is an integrated substrate of everyday life and values:

> The community, the ayllu, is not only a territory where a group of people live; it is more than that. It is a dynamic space where the whole community of beings that exist in the world lives; this includes humans, plants, Animals, the mountains, the rivers, the rain, etc. All are related like a family. It is important to remember that this place, the community, is not where we are from, it is who we are. I am not from Huantura, I am Huantura.
>
> *(Oxa, quoted in de la Cadena, 2015, p. 239)*

While the Quechuan concept of a trans-species community, interwoven in, not separate from the rest of Nature may seem radical relative to present, modern-day living, relative to the anthropological record, colonialism's mandate of domination of Nature is anomalous, representing 1% of the entire human species (Narvaez, 2013). Many traditional indigenous peoples exemplify ontologies of oneness where human lives and identities are patterned with those of other beings (Deloria, 2006). John Fadden, Mohawk (Ganienkehaka) Iroquois, similarly speaks of his people's land ethics:

> The Haudenosaunee (People of the Longhouse) view everything as a circle with everything more or less equal. We're all related. In a sense, we are related to all things of reality. The earth is our mother. The moon is our grandmother. The sun is our

elder brother. That view, also, reflects the Haudenosaunee land ethic [...] On my mother's side we've been here thousands of years. It's a nice feeling to know that part of my genetic makeup has been here for that long period of time. We are a part of this place.

(Fadden, 2020)

A parallel, positive convergence has developed in Western science (Low et al., 2012; Bradshaw, 2017). Instead of viewing the Earth through the kaleidoscope of reductionism, parsing every millimetre of life into smaller and smaller shards, science has joined non-dual indigenous and spiritual traditions where it is understood that life-form diversity springs from the substrate of one (Kimmerer, 2013; Francis, 2015). Gaia is sentient with each of her family, a unique thread in the seamless tapestry of life.

The need for reparation of Nature is vital. Every continent, every ocean and the sky has been denuded. Grief pours from emptied canyons, forests and waters once bursting with the calls and cries of arcing Eagles, proud Pumas, scarlet Salmon and uncountable other species. Climate change and human appropriation of diverse ecosystems have forced innumerable, diverse species ranging from Frogs to Polar Bears to migrate far and wide from their native habitats in search of food, water and shelter (Abate, 2019). The Wild has become a refugee in its own home. Centring the *ayllu* in Community Psychology opens accompaniment to include trans-species relations.

While aid is given to endangered species through conservation, it has not reversed the growing list of extinctions. Something more is needed: profound transformation of the human psyche and culture – something that dissolves human privilege and undertakes a profound relational transformation.

In the Canticle of the Creatures Francis looks to nature for guidance on how we are to model our relationships [...] We are co-responsible with and for one another, especially for the poor and excluded. We are co-responsible for the life of the natural environment, showing gratitude and respecting nature's proper limits.

(Perry, 2020)

It is a challenging task. Nature accompaniment asks the accompanier to disable the psychological, social and cultural struts which hold humans aloof and above other creatures, and to literally stand on equal footing. In so doing, human accompaniers begin their own profound healing from the ravages of colonialism. Accompaniment's horizontality unleashes the psychological imprisonment rendered by human privilege and the primacy of the human-human contract. John Muir writes of this liberation:

We are now in the mountains and they are in us, kindling enthusiasm, making every nerve quiver, filling every pore and cell of us. Our flesh-and-bone tabernacle seems transparent as glass to the beauty about us, as if truly an inseparable part of it, thrilling with the air and trees, streams and rocks, in the waves of the sun, – a part of all nature, neither old nor young, sick nor well, but immortal. Just now I can hardly conceive of any bodily condition dependent on food or breath any more than the ground or the sky. How glorious a conversion, so complete and wholesome it is, scarce memory enough of old bondage days left as a standpoint to view it from! In this newness of life we seem to have been so always!

(Muir, 1911, p. 10)

It is in this shared, unimpeded relational space, outside the walls, exits and retreats afforded by modernity's synthetic world, where accompaniers learn to occupy their Homo sapiens form, and bring the resources and abilities that such membership bestows, while simultaneously journeying in solidarity with Animal kin.

There is often a feeling of unguarded nakedness, vulnerability and disorientation in the early stages of this metamorphic transformation from encasement to radical availability. Yet, in the presence of the wild, colonial-wired reactions soon discharge and the accompanier is embraced by a "glorious [...] conversion, so complete and wholesome" (Muir, 1911, p. 10).

By dropping the shield of privilege and control, senses long suppressed awaken and their ancient intelligence revitalises. This is the point where deep listening begins. This is the space to hear the voice and needs of the accompanied: the old growth forest threatened by rapacious industry; the Orca torn from his family, condemned to live and die in a cement tank, the Wolves hiding by day and hunting by night to flee the hunter's gun; and the Hummingbirds, desperate for succour, traditional migration paths dried up by climate change and smothered by expanding roads and houses, that must fly hundreds of off-track miles to find flowers. An indicator of the impact of human-forced Wildlife migration is the spate of unprecedented sightings. Lions and Cougars venture into empty city streets; absent for two centuries, a Northern Gray Whale swims in waters off Israel; North Atlantic Gannets appear in California's coastal waters, while Pacific Auks have been forced to the Atlantic. While this has brought Animals and humans into closer contact, no corresponding ethic and practice of mutual accompaniment and inclusivity have followed. Cougars and Bears found near humans are viewed as dangerous interlopers and are summarily shot or trapped and killed.

A global movement has begun to stand with these individuals and their societies to forge a communal ethic. The work of Canadian naturalist Charlie Russell provides details of how mutual accompaniment to foster a trans-species community readily evolves.

Charlie lived around Grizzly Bears his entire life, from 1941 to 2018, in the rugged mountains of Alberta's Front Range, British Columbia and Alaska. He spent nearly every day in the mountains with the purpose of understanding Grizzly Bears and supporting their right for self-determination.

> I've never wanted to know about bears, I've only wanted to understand them. As a result, my questions aren't the same as what biologists want to know [...] People say in order to understand someone you have to love them – I think that's probably why I can understand bears a little, because I love them. Understanding someone means you care about them. Learning becomes something that isn't just about you, collecting facts for your own purpose. It's about seeing the world through their eyes and getting to know what is important to them.
>
> *(Bradshaw, 2020, p. 20)*

In 1996, during his sojourn in Russia, Charlie plumbed the depths of accompaniment to radical availability. The purpose of his stay in the Kamchatka wilderness was to show, and test for himself, that humans could live peacefully with Brown Bears, (Eurasia's counterpart to the North American Grizzly) absent the constant threat of persecution and death.

Shortly after his arrival, Charlie was asked to rescue, rear and reintroduce orphaned Brown Bear cubs whose mothers had been slaughtered illegally for their body parts. Charlie built a cabin under the spectacular volcano near the sparkling Kambolnoye Lake and began his education to become a mother Bear. Typically, cubs stay with their mother for three to four years, spending not only spring and summer, but denning with her through the winter. Despite his intimate experience with Grizzlies, Charlie needed to cultivate the sense and sensibilities of a mother Brown Bear. "Knowing about bears was all well and good, but these weren't 'any old bears'. All ten cubs were completely unique. You have to pay attention to the bear right in front of you" (Bradshaw, 2020, p. 38).

There were intrinsic obstacles to overcome in the process of mother-bearing. Charlie had to stand at the razor's edge of life's paradox – the simultaneous existence of separation and union. On the outside, he inhabited a human form. On the inside, he had to be Bear-like. To think and make decisions like a mother Bear, Charlie needed to become one from the inside out, and that began with learning how to think like a Bear. He existed as a human, but to accompany the cubs, and his neighbouring Bear community, Charlie had to become part of the Brown Bear world of experience, their Umwelt, and exquisitely attune to the needs and desires of the Bears.

This involved letting go of human identity by dissolving internalised beliefs in and attitudes towards human-constructed reality which walls off our species from the rest of Nature. Charlie did not consider himself a Bear, but he relinquished any vestige of privilege and ways of being that were not congruent with those of Nature.

Such species-pluralistic ethic and culture, wherein humans and Bears are guided by shared values and precepts, is reflective of how all Wildlife lives. While each individual Animal is constrained by his particular physiology and form, he is connected and guided by the vast, unbroken intelligence underlying all life. Charlie followed these rules and as a result, in addition to rearing his own cubs, was invited by a wild mother Brown Bear, whom he called Brandy, to watch over her precious children. Over those 10 years, Brandy and Charlie lived in mutual accompaniment. She taught him Bear ways, and he learned through giving care to her cubs.

In Charlie's eyes, being open to Bears meant moving in synchrony with Nature's pulse, unhampered by strictures of human domination. He understood that the bodies we occupy are secondary to the being who lies within. The mutuality of such accompaniment was clear to Charlie: "If you are completely open and honest and love someone and you are with them, no one and nothing else matters. That's how you begin to learn who they are and they learn who you are".

Charlie was responsible for the cubs until they were able to live on their own. He stayed until three sets of cubs successfully grew into adults and joined wild Brown Bear society to raise families of their own. He stayed with his task to accompany Brandy and the cubs until they deemed it complete, at which point, Charlie left for Canada. He may have returned home, but he was forever changed.

Russell's story is replayed again and again as rescue and sanctuary movements attempt to respond to the massive displacements of not only humans but other-than-human Animals impacted by human appropriation and destruction of their habitats. To care for the billions of Snakes, Parrots, Tortoises and the multitude of Animals who have been displaced and harmed, individuals and groups are changing the fundaments of their lives and social patterns to be able to provide for these refugees. Were Community Psychology to reframe "community" as "*ayllu*", such trans-species accompaniment would need to be included.

From separation towards mutual restoration through earth accompaniment

Colonialism and neoliberal capitalism have unravelled ecologies at an unprecedented rate (Moore, 2016). More than three-quarters of the earth's land surface has been dramatically altered, according to the Intergovernmental Science-Policy Platform on Biodiversity and Ecosystem Services (Díaz, Settele, Brondízio, Ngo, Guèze, Agard, … & Zayas, 2019). For cap-italism, a river, a forest, or a mountain is often worth more diverted, cut down or mined out than if they were left to be – having the right to flow, flourish and exist. Today, the world faces a dangerous triad of land degradation, biodiversity loss and climate change. The ramifications of these crises are astronomical. By 2050, deteriorating ecological conditions owing to the climate and environmental crisis are expected to produce between 25 million and one billion internal and cross-border migrants.

From climate justice to environmental racism, community psychologists are presented with many opportunities to work towards solidarity with the earth and those resisting neoliberal capitalism. Earth accompaniment – as Watkins (2019) has termed the process of standing in solidarity with earth and the life that lives upon her – demands critical reflection on how we reached this point and emancipatory action rooted in compassion for all life.

Vandana Shiva (2015) has pointed out this absurdity that real life is diminished and corporations are bolstered for the purpose of mass extraction and the accumulation of wealth. Shiva calls for an alternative earth democracy that recognises that all life has intrinsic worth and that its diversity should be defended and allowed to flourish. In all its forms, this approach of accompanying the more-than-human world takes on a position of "nonviolence and compassion, diversity and pluralism, equality and justice, and respect for life in all its diversity" (Shiva, 2015, p. 6). In practice, it calls for policies to promote local solutions, community rights and ecological sovereignty (Shiva, 2020).

Accompaniment presents community psychologists with opportunities to play a meaningful role in grassroots community struggles. For instance, one author of this chapter, Garret Barnwell, has accompanied the grassroots community organisation Dzomo La Mupo (DLM) – meaning "the voice of creation" in the local Tshivenda language – through documentation and advocacy. DLM was established by community members to restore indigenous forests, protect indigenous seeds and sacred natural sites, and revive traditional knowledge systems after years of apartheid-era violence in Vhembe district in South Africa. I came to this work with DLM after getting to know individual members by participating in a community-based ecotherapy project. When hearing that I was working on the psychological impacts of environmental degradation, it was suggested by the project's coordinator and members that I focus on the area. This relationship soon evolved beyond research, however.

Apartheid, which means "separate" in Afrikaans, one of South Africa's 11 official languages, institutionalised segregation and white supremacy. Early in its claim to power, the apartheid government saw strategic economic value in the soil created by the dense Afromontane forests in Vhembe to establish exotic pine plantations. Underpinning the environmental racism of apartheid was the view that Black South Africans could be objectified and eliminated, and that the world they lived in could be commodified and treated as an open-access system through which initially the colonisers and now the corporate elite accumulate wealth. These processes were often characterised by violence, displacement and ecocide.

Today, DLM's actions are rooted in traditional views – *Mupo* – that embodies all life as sacred and interconnected. This way of being is in stark contrast to apartheid violence that took place in the late 1940s onward in the area. Through the interactions that I have had with DLM members, they've explained that bulldozers tore through ancestral lands, decimating 22 square miles of life, in and around some of the most sacred places where people had lived, farmed and performed essential rituals for generations.

As part of my research that documented these processes, a community member described his experiences as a child: "*I used to live here with my father and the family, but we were chased away so that they could plant the pine tree [...] This used to be a beautiful place*".

Today, he explained: "*Most rivers have dried up or have been contaminated by chemicals used on the plantations*".

"We tried to remove the pines but we couldn't". He continued: *"All the people were chased away and their homes were destroyed [...] The animals that were [...] here didn't have homes. There were lots of wild animals, but people started pouching [...] They [the white man] could even kill six or seven impalas [deer] per day"*.

People were removed from their land so that apartheid-era government-owned corporations could establish large-scale pine plantations. During this ecocide, entire communities were internally displaced.

A traditional leader explained to me: *"There was a lot of emotional strain on the community because it [forced displacement and removals] immediately breaks families. It breaks communities. It breaks their well-being"*.

After the fall of apartheid, community members gathered in dialogue to remember the rivers, villages and other vital places in what DLM refers to as ecological dialogues. These inclusive community processes were recollective and ignited a struggle to reconnect, restore and protect ancestral land and these sacred natural sites – known as *Zwifho* in the local Tshivenda language. *"These sacred places are the roots of our clan"*, another participant reported. Communities have conducted rituals in these sacred spaces – forests, mountains or rivers – for generations, bringing community, ancestors and other-than-human communities together. For DLM members, these spaces were said to have motivated their struggle and are central to healing. However, they are contentious spaces that are threatened by ongoing environmental and land injustices.

Today, pine and tea plantations surround the sacred sites. DLM's ecological dialogues are a form of what liberation psychologist Ignacio Martín-Baró (1994) referred to as *conscientización* (conscientisation). Through gradually uncovering not only the mechanisms of oppression but also the relationship with the *Zwifho* within a group process, new possibilities for action were imagined. DLM has around 200 members who participate in different forms of earth accompaniment. For instance, DLM members have started a project of rewilding. Trees have been planted around the community, along eroding riverbanks and around the sacred natural sites to reforest communities. A member of DLM reflected on the rewilding action that emerged through ecological dialogues: *"It is healing to me. I feel happy when I am planting them [the seeds and trees]. My heart is filled with joy. When I see other villages looking for trees and planting them wherever they have shortage of trees, it gives me strength"*.

DLM also engages directly with the government to decolonise traditional ideas about heritage, which in South Africa may open communities to extractive forms of tourism owing to the National Heritage Act not recognising the sovereignty and sanctity of these spaces. These approaches resist top-down policies and motivate for community-based governance, as do similar struggles emerging around the world (Shiva, 2020). As a part of these processes, through community dialogues, DLM has established principles to safeguard the *Zwifho*. These principles state that sacred sites are not for entertainment, tourism or the dumping of waste. Nothing from the *Zwifho* should be removed, and any activity that contributes to deforestation or harm of the *Zwifho* is prohibited. DLM are guardians of the sacred natural sites and work with traditional leadership and governance structures. Shiva explains: "The recognition of sovereignty and Indigenous knowledge create a major shift in the political context of the ownership, use, and control of generic resources" (Shiva, 2020, p. 79). Around the world, accompanists may align themselves with initiatives that counter extractive practices by assisting in restorative justice and promoting community sovereignty.

Despite spurious protections – such as heritage status – many of these sites are still unprotected. As a form of ecopsychosocial accompaniment, Barnwell has assisted the DLM members in the witnessing that ongoing barriers to access, lack of protection and land injustices place stress on communities and affirms restorative justice. The findings of multiple individual and group dialogues have translated into ecopsychosocial reports that are being used by DLM to complement movements towards community protections for three sacred sites. The research and reports produced have been used in lobbying the South African Heritage Resource Agency whose mandate is being challenged to protect these sites in a way that does not lead to their commodification, which is sometimes that case for heritage status.

The documentation of the psychosocial impacts of environmental degradation is not unique. For instance, James Thornton, founding CEO of Client Earth, an environmental legal organisation that uses the law to bring about climate and ecological justice, noted already in the 1990s that psychology could be used to enable effective environmental policies. Thornton (1997, p. 3) stated: "if they (psycho-legal arguments) can be based on a clear showing of negative impact on humans, there is a much better chance of success [in the courts]". In his seminal book, *A New Species of Trouble*, Kai Erickson (1996) has practically demonstrated how psychosocial case studies can be a form of ecopsychosocial accompaniment, supporting communities in the documentation of the impact of human-made environmental disasters for reparations.

However, earth accompaniment is not only focused on ecological harms, such as pollution, ecocide and the reparation thereof, but is also grounded in concern for and the promotion of ecological goods. In his work, I have tracked the sociopolitical histories and how the intergenerational relationships with the more-than-human world shape and mutually create community life. The reports do not only bear witness to collective trauma, but also the meaning of *Zwifho* and the affective bonds that individual community members have to these sacred spaces. These ecopsychosocial reports can then complement broader community land restitution processes. This affirming stance requires epistemic disobedience to mainstream psychology's framing, which tends to de-politicise psychological distress and de-animate people's relationship with the other-than-human life. Thus, earth accompaniment is centred on community and ecological strengths and refrains from damage-centred narratives that have historically harmed communities (Tuck, 2009).

A challenge for earth accompanists is to articulate the intergenerational bond between communities and places to allow for the voice of place to be present in whatever action is taken. Schlosberg (2009, p. 188) explains: "to attain both environmental and ecological justice, we must be sure that views from the margins, the remote, and the natural world are recognized and represented, either directly or through proxies". Testimonies were taken at *Zwifho* for the ecopsychosocial reports, and public dialogue between the government and community members convened by DLM were held at the sacred sites. Community custodians are considered proxies – not only representing the community interests but also the inherent rights and responsibilities towards Mupo (creation). Thus, earth accompaniment requires community psychologists to move towards the margins to find practical ways in which the earth's voice may be seen, acknowledged and adequately represented. From data collection to practical acts of solidarity, the accompanist relies on deep listening that may challenge traditional ways of knowing, which may demand non-local or non-indigenous accompanists to move into the role of the learner and/or co-creator.

To meaningfully work with the wounds of what Rob Nixon (2011) terms "slow violence" – the insidious environmental injustices that creep across boundaries and evade temporality – requires accompanists to follow a community's pace. The accompanist may add reflexivity but responds to what the accompanied views as being needed at the time. In terms of Barnwell's reports, the recommendations were related to safeguarding the *Zwifho* and addressing historical injustices, such as access issues that perpetuate dialogical distress. These reports form one minor piece in what has been an intergenerational struggle that will surely continue for generations.

Accompanists are mutually transformed through this life-affirming praxis. Conscientisation is an ongoing process with no end state (Freire, 1996), and I have been confronting my history of being a white male in South Africa who was privileged owing to the brutality of apartheid. Through the process of earth accompaniment, I have not only been able to work within a more extensive process of transitional justice in South Africa, which has assisted in confronting and reconciling my heritage, but I am slowly uncovering a deeper understanding of the more-than-human world and, in so doing, realising my responsibilities. This liberatory process has only been possible through my relationships with DLM members and people like Mphatheleni Makaulule.

Many forms of earth accompaniment are emerging at a rapid pace. A recent special issue in *Community Psychology in Global Perspective* draws attention to the possibilities for accompanying communities in resistance to climate and environmental injustices (Fernandes-Jesus, Barnes, & Diniz, 2020). Psychologists are creating supportive spaces to work through the complicated feelings that are associated with the climate crises (see Climate Psychology Alliance, 2021) and are actively participating in non-violent movements, such as Extinction Rebellion (XR Psychologists) and Fridays for the Future (Francescato, 2020).

Conclusion

Martín-Baró (1994) asserted that the choice for psychologists is "between accompanying or not accompanying the oppressed majorities". He said it is

> not a question of whether to abandon psychology; it is a question of whether psychological knowledge will be placed in the service of constructing a society where the welfare of the few is not built on the wretchedness of the many, where the fulfilment of some does not require that others be deprived, where the interests of the minority do not demand the dehumanization of all.
>
> *(p. 46)*

As we claim our place in the *ayllu* – those webs of life that include humans, other-than-human animals, soil, water, trees and air – community psychologists will be better able to grasp the interdependence of the well-being of all community members. Forced displacement and migration are symptoms of *ayllu* that have been exploited, becoming zones of abandonment. Ecopsychosocial accompaniment can occur at the original sites of displacement, along the paths to new destinations, and at the places of resettlement. Relationships of mutual accompaniment lay the foundation for understanding how to redress conditions that have become unliveable, as well as how to create places of sanctuary and renewal where life can regain conviviality. Mutual accompaniment welcomes the interchange of knowledges, visions and actions for the sake of not only healing, but the bodying forth of vibrant and just relationships of solidarity.

References

Abate, R.S. (2019). *Climate change and the voiceless: Protecting future generations, wildlife, and natural resources.* Cambridge University Press.

Brabeck, K., Lykes, M. B. & Hershberg, R. (2011). Framing immigration to and deportation from the United States: Guatemalan and Salvadoran families make meaning of their experiences, *Community, Work, and Family, 14*(3), 275–296. http://doi.org/10.1080/13668803.2010.520840

Bradshaw, G.A. (2017). *Carnivore minds: Who these fearsome animals really are*. Yale University Press.

Bradshaw, G.A. (2020). *Talking with bears: Conversations with Charlie Russell*. Rocky Mountain Books.

Casey, E., & Watkins, M. (2014). *Up against the wall: Re-imagining the U.S.-Mexico border*. University of Texas Press.

Climate Psychology Alliance. (2021). https://bit.ly/3iUMI5b

de la Cadena, M. (2015). *Earth beings: Ecologies of practice across Andean worlds*. Duke University Press.

Deloria, V. Jr. (2006). *The world we used to live in: Remembering the powers of the medicine men*. Fulcrum Press.

Díaz, S., Settele, J., Brondízio, E. S., Ngo, H. T., Guèze, M., Agard, J., ... & Zayas, C. (2019). Summary for policymakers of the global assessment report on biodiversity and ecosystem services of the Intergovernmental Science-Policy Platform on Biodiversity and Ecosystem Services. *Intergovernmental Science-Policy Platform on Biodiversity and Ecosystem Services*. https://doi.org/10.5281/zenodo.3553579

Erikson, K. (1996). *A new species of trouble: The human experience of modern disasters*. W.W. Norton.

Fadden, J. (2020). Community voices: John Fadden carries on Mohawk traditions. *Northern Woodlands*. https://bit.ly/36Z4zE4

Farmer, P. (2011). *Re-imagining accompaniment: Global health and liberation theology. Conversation between Paul Farmer and Father Gustavo Gutiérrez*. Ford Family Seminar Series, Notre Dame University, South Bend, IN.

Farmer, P. (2013). *To repair the world: Paul Farmer speaks to the next generation*. University of California Press.

Fernandes-Jesus, M., Barnes, B., & Diniz, R. F. (2020). Communities reclaiming power and social justice in the face of climate change. *Community Psychology in Global Perspective, 6*(2/2), 1–21. https://doi.org/ft8f

Fernandez, J. (2020). Liberation psychology of and for transformative justice: Centering *acompañamiento* in participatory action research. In L. Comas-Díaz & E. T. Rivera (Eds.), *Liberation psychology: Theory, method, practice, and social justice* (pp. 91–110). American Psychological Association.

Francescato, D. (2020). Why we need to build a planetary sense of community. *Community Psychology in Global Perspective, 6*(2/2), 140–64. https://doi.org/fvc4

Francis, P. (2015). On care for our common home: Laudatosi. Encyclical Delivered on May 24.

Freire, P. (1996). *Pedagogy of the oppressed*. Continuum.

Gangsei, D., & Deutsch, A. (2007). Psychological evaluation of asylum seekers. *Torture, 17*(2), 79–87.

Immigration Rights Committee (2008). *In the shadows of paradise: The experiences of the undocumented community in Santa Barbara*. PUEBLO Education Fund.

Indigenous Action Media. Accomplices not allies: Abolishing the ally industrial complex. https://bit.ly/371JkS9

Kagan, C., Burton, M., Duckett, P., Lawthom, R., & Siddiquee, A. (2019). *What is critical community psychology? Critical community psychology: Critical action and social change*. Routledge.

Kimmerer, R.W. (2013). *Braiding sweetgrass: Indigenous wisdom, scientific knowledge and the teachings of plants*. Milkweed Editions.

Koopman, S. (2014). Making space for peace: International accompaniment in Colombia. In F. McConnell, N. Megoron, & P. Williams (Eds.), *The geographies of peace: New approaches to boundaries, diplomacy and conflict* (pp. 109–30). I. B. Tauris.

Langhout, R.D., & Vaccarino-Ruiz, S.S. (2021). "Did I see what I really saw?" Violence, percepticide, and dangerous seeing after an Immigration and Customs Enforcement raid. *Journal of Community Psychology, 49*, 927–46.

Low, P. et al. (2012). *The Cambridge declaration on consciousness*. http://fcmconference.org/img/

Lynd, S., & Grubacic, A. (2010). *From here to there: The Staughton Lynd reader*. PM Press.

Mendoza, J., & Zerda, M. (2011). Psicología comunitaria social en Bolivia. In M. Montero & I. Serrano García (Eds.), *Historias de la psicología en América Latina: Participación y transformación* (pp. 65–90). Paidós.

Muir, J. (1911). *My first summer in the Sierras*. The Riverside Press.

Mahrouse, G. (2014). *Conflicted commitments: Race, privilege, and power in solidarity activism*. McGill-Queens University Press.

Martín-Baró, I. (1994). *Writings for a liberation psychology*. Harvard University Press.

Moore, J. (2016). The rise of cheap nature. In J. Moore (Ed.), *Antropocene or capitalocene? Nature, history, and the crisis of capitalism* (pp. 78–115). Kairos Books.

Narvaez, D. (2013). The 99 percent – Development and socialization within an evolutionary context: Growing up to become "a good and useful human being". In D. Fry (Ed.), *War, peace and human nature: The convergence of evolutionary and cultural views* (pp. 341–57). Oxford University Press.

Nixon, R. (2011). *Slow violence and the environmentalism of the poor.* Harvard University Press. http://doi.org/gfv5mq

Perry, M. (2020). Homily for the Feast of the Pardon of Assisi (August 2). https://bit.ly/2Z2HOed

Sacipa-Rodriguez, S., & Montero, M. (Eds.). (2014). *Psychosocial approaches to peace-building in Colombia.* Springer International.

Sacipa, S., Vidales, R., Galindo, L., & Tovar, C.P. (2007). Psychosocial accompaniment to liberate the suffering associated with the experience of forced displacement. *Universitas Psychologica, 6,* 589–600.

Schlosberg, D. (2009). *Defining environmental justice: Theories, movements, and nature.* Oxford University Press.

Shiva, V. (2015). *Earth democracy: Justice, sustainability and peace.* Zed Books.

Shiva, V. (2020). *Reclaiming the commons: Biodiversity, Indigenous knowledge, and the rights of Mother Earth.* Synergetic Press.

Society for Community Research and Action (2021). The effects of deportation on families and communities. A policy statement by the Society for Community Research and Action. www.scra27.org/what-we-do/policy/policy-position-statements/effects-deportation-families/

Thornton, J. (1997). Wild Nature, sanity, and the law. *The Trumpeter, 14*(3). https://bit.ly/2Y6nOXQ

Tuck, E. (2009). Suspending damage: A letter to communities. *Harvard Educational Review, 79*(3), 409–28. http://doi.org/gdrb3g

Watkins, M. (2015). Psychosocial accompaniment. *Journal of Social and Political Psychology, 3,* 324–41.

Watkins, M. (2019). *Mutual accompaniment and the creation of the commons.* Yale University Press.

Watkins, M. (2021). Toward a decolonial approach to accompaniment from the "outside". In G. Stevens & C. Sonn (Eds.), *Decoloniality, knowledge production and epistemic justice in contemporary community psychology* (pp. 101–120). Springer.

Watkins, M., & Shulman, H. (2008). *Toward psychologies of liberation.* Palgrave Macmillan.

Weigel, J., Basilico, M. & Farmer, P. (2013). Taking stock of foreign aid. In P. Farmer, A. Kleinman, J. Kim & M. Basilico (Eds.), *Reimagining global health: An introduction* (pp. 287–301). University of California Press.

XR Psychologists. https://bit.ly/3jw6Hrg

5

COMMUNITY PSYCHOLOGY AND WAR

Structural violence and institutional silence

Paul Duckett

Abstract

This chapter begins and ends with a reflection on a moment when I anxiously presented a keynote presentation to a Community Psychology conference on the topic of violence and war. I asked the discipline whether it had a serious problem in dealing with violence. In this chapter I unpack that moment by first considering how violence is defined and how Community Psychology has typically focused on interpersonal violence. I then describe structural violence to more fully capture the nature of violence experienced by people who lack social power and how a fuller understanding of the violence of war could benefit Community Psychology. I then consider how academic institutions are marked by the features of structural violence and consider whether Community Psychology has been compromised into silence on structural violence as a result. I conclude by offering a way forward for Community Psychology that is underpinned by a more consistent focus on social institutions, hierarchies of social power and on understanding social policies as forms of social sanction that are enacted against socio-economically distressed and disadvantaged people.

Resumen

Este capítulo comienza y termina con una reflexión sobre un momento en el que presenté, con ansiedad, una presentación principal en una conferencia de la psicología comunitaria sobre el tema de la violencia y la guerra. Le pregunté a la disciplina situviera un problema serio al tratar de la violencia. En este capítulo, analizo ese momento considerando primero cómo se define la violencia y cómo la psicología comunitaria se ha enfocado principalmente en la violencia interpersonal. Luego describo la violencia estructural para captar más plenamente la naturaleza de la violencia experimentada por las personas que carecen del poder social y cómo una comprensión más completa de la violencia de la guerra podría beneficiar a la psicología comunitaria. Luego considero cómo las instituciones académicas están marcadas por las características de la violencia estructural y considero si, como resultado, la psicología comunitaria ha sido apresionada al silencio sobre la violencia estructural. Concluyo ofreciendo un camino a seguir por la psicología comunitaria que se sustenta en un enfoque más consistente en las instituciones sociales, las jerarquías del poder social y en la comprensión de las políticas

DOI: 10.4324/9780429325663-7

sociales como formas de sanción social que se promulgan contra las personas desfavorecidas con dificultades socio-económicas.

Anxiously, in 2004 I got up on stage at the International Conference of European Community Psychology ready to give my first keynote presentation. This was early in my career and I was about to tell the conference that Community Psychology had a major problem in relation to how it dealt with the topic of violence. Before I reflect on my conference presentation and what happened after it and what violence I was referring to, I first define the ways violence is defined.

Defining violence

The definition of violence cited in the World Health Organization's seminal *World Report on Violence and Health* (WHO, 2002), and subsequently reinscribed in its recent global campaigns for violence prevention (the Violence Prevention Alliance), focuses mainly on interpersonal violence with some mention of the relational, community and societal factors that lead to and help reduce it. The main focus is on violence as perpetrated by an individual against another individual. For Community Psychology, this individualistic focus might be considered problematic. However, community psychological research on violence largely focuses on interpersonal violence as does such work in mainstream psychology (Salazar & Cook, 2002). Though Community Psychology does recognise the gendered nature of violence (e.g. Banyard, Plante, & Moynihan, 2004), it does not consistently focus on forms of structural violence. Structural violence is a term often ascribed to Galtung (1969), who defined it as violence cause by a social structure or a social institution preventing people from meeting their basic needs such that it causes morbidity and premature death. Such violence emerges from hierarchies of power where those at the top have the power of sanction over those at the bottom, and where that sanction is used against people based on their age, ethnicity, impairment, geographic location, gender, political orientation, religion, social class and so on. It is referred to as violence rather than "social inequality" or "social discrimination" as it is harm caused by human action (Lee, 2019), and the term "violence" foregrounds the nature of that harm.

The work of community activist Cathy McCormack is a particularly impressive documentation of structural violence. She coined the phrase "the war without bullets" to capture her experience of living and working in one of the most socially and economically disadvantaged communities in Europe – Easterhouse in Glasgow. The phrase captures how social policies enacted by both governments, and the industrial and commercial activity of corporations were waging a war of socio-structural, political, ideological and psychological violence against poor people – a type of "class war". Policies that were manufacturing unemployment, inequality and material poverty created a system of socio-economic apartheid that was causing mass casualties (Fryer & McCormack, 2012). The violence here was in the maintenance of social conditions of extreme economic hardship and the deliberate ramping up of social inequalities that, combined, created highly toxic social environments. The effect of that violence is shown in the statistics on mortality for that population. In 2002, Easterhouse residents were almost five times more likely to die as a result of an "accident", six times more likely to die as a result of ischaemic heart disease, three times more likely to die as a result of lung cancer and 13 times more likely to die as a result of a stroke than those living in nearby more affluent areas (MacLean, 2003). In 2002, the life expectancy of residents in Easterhouse was 10 years lower than that for the rest of the UK. An understanding of structural violence helps to pull us away from definitions of violence that largely focus on the interpersonal level and to draw attention to the broader causes and effects of violence. McCormack uses war as a metaphor to describe the violence enacted against the people of Easterhouse. But war itself can also be defined as a form of structural violence (Lee, 2019).

The violence of war

War is an obvious form of violence, but the violent impact of war is not often fully considered. War does more than kill people in combat. War forces whole communities to live for years in fear and hunger. War fractures the infrastructure of roads; water supplies and sanitation; food production, distribution and security; electricity; social, educational and health services; law and order; housing and environmental services; and broader social support structures. All of this causes significant risks to public health. Here we find morbidities and mortalities due to: infectious diseases; injuries from post-conflict ordinance (such as landmines); poisonings and burns from discarded munitions; increased vector-borne diseases due to disruptions to sanitation and clean water supplies and overcrowded, poor living conditions caused by displacement; problems with reproductive health including an increased number of birthing complications; impact of food insecurity (such as malnutrition); mental health problems; and long-term genetic impacts of exposure to chemicals and radiation (such as those from depleted munitions). It is once the indirect violence of war is understood that we get more of a sense of the nature of that violence. And, that violence is structural because it is targeted against people based on their geographical location, nationality, ethnicity, political beliefs or religion. It is also particularly targeted against women and children – they are the ones who are more likely to be displaced, disinherited and impoverished and make up most of the population of war refugees.

There is another problem of how the violence of war is tallied – there is an almost exclusive focus on episodic violence. Mainstream understandings of violence typically assume violence comes in the form of a discrete event that disrupts an otherwise violence-free life. An understanding of violence more apposite for many people's lives is of an ongoing, cumulative experience of violence that is not just lifelong but intergenerational (Myers et al., 2015). This is what is captured by the notion of structural violence. These structural causes of violence are often ones that have been instigated for generations – such as violence against Black people and violence against women. Such violence is a banal, punishing, ongoing grind that wears people down physically, psychologically and spiritually, and from which there is little or no respite. This is also the grinding violence of industrialisation that subjects millions of workers to toxic and dangerous working conditions, causing injury and premature death as well as psychological injuries resulting from excessive workplace pressures and devaluing, demeaning, poorly paying and insecure jobs (Fryer & Fagan, 2003). And this is the grinding violence that results from the multifaceted and long-lasting impacts of war.

Has Community Psychology focused enough on war to open a critical discussion on violence that would provide a means to more fully engage in the topic of structural violence and to understand the limits of focusing on its interpersonal and episodic manifestations? Well, war became of particular and troubling relevance to Community Psychology in 2003.

Is Community Psychology troubled by war?

Mainstream psychology has worked closely, since its inception, with the military-industrial complex and has profited from war as a result. This was well documented in the *Hoffman Report* (Hoffman et al., 2015), which brought that working relationship to the public's attention when it reported on the context to the collusion between the American Psychological Association (APA) and the US Department of Defense during the "war on terror" (Duckett & Değirmencioğlu,

2017). At the same time, some sections of psychology have stood against war, such as the peace psychology groups within psychology's professional bodies across Asia, Australasia, Europe and the US as well as independent groups such as Psychologists for Social Responsibility, the Radical Psychology Network, and Counselors for Social Justice. In 2003, these groups were notably active in taking a public stance against the Iraq war (Editor, IBPP, 2003). The Iraq war also preoccupied networks of political and critical psychologists. For example, it was explicitly identified in the conference theme of the International Society of Political Psychology in July 2004. In contrast, during 2002 and 2003 Iraq was not noticeably a topic of discussion for Community Psychology networks. But it became a discussion point in 2003 when a small group of community psychologists from Waikato University, Aotearoa/New Zealand, decided to boycott that year's US Society for Community Research and Action (SCRA) biennial conference. The group sent a letter to the SCRA email LISTSERV explaining that they had decided not to attend the conference because of the US administration's instigation of the Iraq war. They asked for their letter to be read out at the conference so that other delegates would understand why they were not there but also in the expectation that it would help facilitate some discussion at the conference on the war in Iraq (see Mulvey, Guzman, & Ayala-Alacantar, 2003 for a copy of the letter). However, the letter was not read out to the conference. Indeed, conference organisers actively prevented the letter from being discussed by the conference (Duckett, 2004). This was the moment that led me and others to conclude that Community Psychology had a major problem when it came to the topic of violence (see Değirmencioğlu, 2003; Duckett, 2005; Lykes, 2003). And this is what led to my keynote presentation at the European Community Psychology Network Conference in 2004 (Duckett, 2004).

I used my presentation to ask whether community psychologists were surprised at how mute the public positioning of Community Psychology appeared to have been on the war in Iraq, and the refusal to engage in discussion on the topic at the SCRA conference. I used my keynote to ask why, at the very moment when community psychologists might have been expected to be discussing the topic of war, they appeared to be not only collectively silent but actively resistant to having such a discussion. As I stood there anxiously at the podium raising that issue with conference delegates, I did not know what to expect.

I was under no illusion that my presentation would be a catalyst for change, and I was right. Very little since 2004 appears to have changed. There remains little published on either war or structural violence in Community Psychology journals, though some community psychologists have published important work on structural violence outside of Community Psychology journals (e.g. Burton & Kagan, 2007). So, a colleague and I had another go at breaking the silence and in 2017 we edited a special issue on war of the *Journal of Community and Applied Social Psychology* (Duckett & Değirmencioğlu, 2017). In preparation, we undertook a review of the Community Psychology literature published since 2003 and we found that war remained of marginal concern for the discipline. We found that when war was mentioned, it mostly appeared as context rather than as a central topic of interest. So, for example, war was mentioned in work involving First Nations peoples (Halloran, 2007) but only in relation to setting out the historical context of injustices experienced rather than as a prelude to a discussion about structural violence. In other papers, war featured as a form of a marginal independent variable when measuring other phenomena of interest, such as a factor impacting attitudes towards refugees (Hanson-Easey & Moloney, 2009). War was also a key element to the paper by Paaskesen (2013) on formerly abducted youth in Uganda, but again war was brought in as background context rather than foregrounded in a discussion of the nature of violence. As of early 2021, Community Psychology's focus on violence remained largely on interpersonal violence and there remained relatively little published on structural violence in

Community Psychology journals and even less of an indication of the discipline taking anything approaching a position on war. But that is not to say that there are not some signs that things could be changing.

How things might be changing for Community Psychology's focus on violence

Though few and far between, those occasions where work on structural violence is published are certainly noteworthy. For example, community psychological work coming from the occupied territories of Palestine has been challenging the individualised, depoliticised notions of violence and victimhood (e.g. Meari, 2015) and recentring on structural forms of violence (e.g. Makkawi, 2014; Hammad & Tribe, 2020). Makkawi makes a call for a "critical community psychology" in Palestine, pointing to his disappointment with mainstream Community Psychology in terms of its lack of relevance to the struggle of the Palestinian people. He states that a new type of Community Psychology is required if it is to be relevant and progressive for people who have been colonised and subject to the state-sponsored violence of war. The linkage to structural violence was also evident in the programme of the International Conference of Community Psychology in 2020. Neither violence or structural violence was mentioned in the conference themes and its appearance was patchy. But from the 52 abstracts published in the conference programme, three were focused on such violence – one on epistemic violence (Ellison et al., 2020), one on the violence of capitalism (Fryer et al., 2020), and one on structural violence more generally (Bailey et al., 2020). Common to these three conference abstracts was a focus on either postcolonial theory or critical theory. Structural violence was also explicitly referred to in a conference webinar entitled *Critical Transnational Conversations on Structural Violence and Radical Possibilities* (Balla, Fernández, & Fine, 2020). In that webinar, the link to structural violence was made, as with Makkawi's paper, through connecting to the notion of Critical Community Psychology.

Back in 2004, Critical Community Psychology was not a "thing" in the sense that it was not a commonly cited term, but it was beginning to be mentioned in some publications (e.g. Fryer & Fagan, 2003), and it had prominence in the Monterey Declaration of Critical Community Psychology (Angelique & Kyle, 2002). The use of the term signified a belief that Community Psychology had failed to be a socially progressive alternative to mainstream psychology (Evans, Duckett, Lawthom, & Kivell, 2016) and had failed to give psychological work a political or ideological steer (Duckett, 2009). The key concepts that sat at the core of the discipline, such as empowerment, valuing diversity, and primary prevention, were all sufficiently pliable to be deployed by the political right as much as by the political left (Duckett, 2009). For example, by the 1990s the notion of empowerment had become a vehicle by which the state transferred responsibility onto the private citizen and as a rationale for the contraction of state-based services and a ballooning of the private sector. Celebrating diversity became a vehicle for corporations to identify new, niche consumer markets and for governments and corporations combined to re-render social inequalities as of cultural rather than political interest (Klein, 1999). And prevention became appropriated as a method of social control (e.g. crime prevention) and became weaponised for use in the arena of geopolitics (e.g. "pre-emptive" military incursions).

Critical psychology and critical theory have been prominent in many of the critiques of Community Psychology's lack of political direction. As international Community Psychology networks developed in the late 1990s (e.g. Marsella, 1998), connections formed between community psychologists across Europe whose work was informed by, inter alia, German critical psychology, British Marxism and French poststructuralism. Connections were also strengthened among those whose approach was informed by liberation psychology (particularly in Central and South America), postcolonial theory (particularly in Australasia, Asia and South Africa), and critical race theory (particularly in the US). Since 2000, critical psychological approaches have been conspicuously feeding into the discipline (e.g. Fryer & Duckett, 2014; Fryer & Fox, 2015; Fryer & Laing, 2008; Kagan & Burton, 2001; Kagan et al., 2011; Painter, Terre Blanche, & Henderson, 2006; Prilleltensky & Nelson, 2002, 2009). The lack of a clear political steer in Community Psychology essentially helped give space for such work to develop and it has been in that space that the promising signs of Community Psychology engagement with the notion of structural violence have appeared. However, given that much of the material brought in from critical psychology has been quite negative and somewhat disparaging about Community Psychology, there have been signs of a bifurcation occurring in the discipline – a critical version splitting from the mainstream version. So, though there are some signs of a shift occurring that might create more room for Community Psychology to have a greater focus on structural violence and to be less absorbed by interpersonal violence, it remains too early to tell how much will shift, what the nature of that shift might be and where that shift might lead the discipline.

But there is a final issue related to structural violence and Community Psychology, and that is a particular type of violence that occurs in a particular type of social institution that Community Psychology, even in its critical iteration, appears to be particularly blinkered towards. And it is this that might ultimately hold things back. And this is pointed to in my experience of delivering a keynote presentation to a Community Psychology conference.

The structural violence in higher education

The conference at which I gave my keynote was held in an academic setting and I was speaking to an audience of mostly academics. This was 2004 and higher education had been through major reforms across Europe including a dramatic increase in student enrolments, increased inter-institutional competition for funding and an increased casualisation of the workforce (Gill & Gill, 2000). These changes were pushing through organisational reforms that were rapidly turning academia into a profession of high workloads, insecure contracts, role uncertainty and low morale (Bett, 1999; Fisher, 1992), to the point that stress levels among academics were becoming among the highest of any occupation (Fisher, 1992; Winefield, 2003). This was most true for those in lower-grade jobs who soon became an academic underclass that has been growing ever since (UCU, 2019, 2020). Women, in particular, have become overrepresented in that academic underclass (Lafferty & Fleming, 2000; Reay, 2000). Pay inequalities also grew considerably, making universities increasingly unequal places with, for example, the pay of vice chancellors ballooning from 2.9 times the pay of regular lecturers in the mid-1980s to around 16 times by 2005 (Rolands & Boden, 2020). All of this was occurring at the end of what Toro described as Community Psychology's "heyday" and at the start of its period of greatest growth (Toro, 2019).

Social hierarchies that grade status, prestige, wealth and power, and inscribe relationships of power and subordination among its members have long been a characteristic of higher education, but these social hierarchies steepened considerably from the 1980s onwards. In higher education this social stratification is not only a characteristic of the relationship among its members, but also inherent to the mission of the institution (Bourdieu, 1998) – the conferring of social status to its members through the awarding of educational qualifications (e.g. degrees), job status (e.g. tenure), and other titular awards (e.g. professor). And the social prestige that is conferred by the institutions to its members is generally not what could be described as promoting social mobility or tackling social inequality. Though the sector has historically engaged in philanthropic activities and does offer some opportunities to some people from disadvantaged social backgrounds (Gerber & Cheung, 2008), its overall effect is to replicate existing social inequalities. For example, students from socially and economically privileged backgrounds are more likely to gain access to the elite universities and then progress into the most prestigious jobs, while those from less privileged backgrounds continue to find themselves at non-elite institutions and progress into the less prestigious jobs (Argentin & Triventi, 2011).

With universities mostly reinforcing existing social inequalities and becoming increasingly shaped within by steeply unequal systems of distributed power, academia can be reasonably viewed as an institution prone to structural violence. Worse still, the positions of power within it can be readily abused through the inscription of poorly defined and loosely applied concepts of academic excellence to determine who receives reward and who receives sanction (Brusoni et al., 2014) and academic freedom (that regulates what is and isn't acceptable professional behaviour), and untrained, poorly prepared and conflicted leadership teams (Jenkins, 2014). So, an academic conference held at a university campus might be considered an environment where structural violence is etched into the very social fabric of the setting and where there might be insufficient safeguards to ensure that violence does not erupt. That might provoke a degree of anxiety for anyone who seeks to speak at an academic conference, particularly if they plan to speak critically about those attending.

It is uncommon to consider universities as inherently violent social institutions. Universities are mostly portrayed as places of safety and security. This might be partly a residue of how universities once operated in loco parentis – the university undertook the responsibilities of the student's parent or guardian (Fisher, 1995). Arguably, that legacy continues in the way university students are still commonly referred to by university staff as "kids" and treated as biologically mature children (Furedi, 2016). In loco parentis gave universities explicit license to under-report violence that occurred on their campuses and that under-reporting continued in many institutions long after their in loco parentis status lapsed (Pezza & Bellotti, 1995; Campbell & Bryceland, 1998), and it is only recently that the violence occurring within universities has come to the public's attention, particularly violence against women. In 2015, for example, Sydney University in Australia declared that it had been under-reporting incidents of sexual violence on campus (Munro, 2016). And in 2017, the Australian Human Rights Commission released results of a survey of Australian higher education institutions that found on average one in five students surveyed had experienced sexual harassment in a university setting, with this figure being as high as 1 in 2.6 for some universities. In that same year, the Association of American Universities published their report which estimated that almost 12% of university students had experienced sexual violence whilst at university (Cantor et al., 2017). In the UK, an investigation undertaken by the *Guardian* newspaper led to a story that ran in the newspaper with the heading "Sexual Harassment at Epidemic Levels in UK Universities" (Batty, Weale & Bannock, 2017). Most of these victims of violence have been women. The violence of the institution might also be seen in the alarming rates of poor mental health more generally among students and, in particular, the rates of student suicide (Westefeld & Furr, 1987; Westefeld, Witchard, & Range, 1990; Grayson, 1994; AUCC, 1999). In the UK in 2017, it was reported that one student committed suicide every four days (Shackle, 2019). In Australia, it was reported in 2017 that 65% of students aged 16–25 years reported high or very high psychological distress and 35.4% reported thoughts of self-harm or suicide (Headspace & National Union of Students, 2017). Such surveys break the image of universities as safe and protective environments. Rather, we see unconscionably large numbers of people at university, particularly students, at risk of considerable harm. There is every reason to consider universities as structurally violent as those people experiencing that harm are often those at the bottom of the institution's social hierarchy and who lack social power.

Research on one particular form of abuse of power, bullying, is hardly studied at all in higher education in spite of it being well studied in primary and secondary education as well as in the workplace more generally (Lund & Ross, 2016). That is not because bullying does not occur in universities, but that researchers do not often turn their attention to it (Pörhölä et al., 2020). From the studies that have been conducted, bullying at university clearly occurs (Chapell et al., 2004; Lund & Ross, 2016; Sinkkonen, Puhakka, & Meriläinen, 2014). Most recently, COVID-19 has unearthed the case of junior academic staff being bullied by their managers into face-to-face teaching during the pandemic (Fazackerley, 2020). The bullying of students by staff, particularly academic staff, is of particular concern because of those power disparities that are baked into higher education. In a study conducted in Finland, it was reported that in 44% of the cases of bullying experienced by students, the bullying was undertaken by academic staff. The problem with this research is that there is little of it. What research exists has largely focused on students who bully other students. There is less research on staff who bully students and even less research on staff who bully other staff. Of the research that has been conducted on the latter, the conclusion has been that bullying is impacted by the unequal distribution of power across the university social hierarchy (Sharma, 2017), unethical leadership (Erkutlu & Chafra, 2014), weak and destructive leadership (Björklund, Vaezb, & Jensen, 2020), and the use of the concept of "academic freedom" to defend inappropriate professional behaviours (Mahmoudi, 2020).

Fogg (2008) describes the lack of understanding of bullying in the academic workplace among academics as a type of naivete, and Sharma (2017) argues that it is this naivete that is the main camouflage that permits such bullying to take place. Academics don't often report bullying (Agervold, 2007) and when they do, their institutions do not have the capacity, where-withal or the proper policies and procedures in place to deal with it (Hollis, 2015; Salin, 2003). Higher education is a sector of the labour market that would, if only data were honestly recorded, be that in which amongst the most violence in the workplace occurs (Zapf et al., 2003). But bullying, along with many other forms of violence within the institution, are hidden so as to protect the public image of the higher education sector (Fogg, 2008; Hollis, 2015). Community Psychology is not an obvious part of the academy that is helping to reveal the violence occurring across the university sector. It is only referred to in a very limited number of papers published in Community Psychology journals (e.g. Javorka & Campbell, 2020; Schulze & Budd, 2020). One might wonder whether a focus on structural violence might provide the opportunity, and perhaps even the appetite, to reflect on Community Psychology as not only a discipline that might promote work that could counter structural violence but as a discipline that is housed in a structurally violent institution.

Conclusion

So, Community Psychology has taken on the mantle of a discipline that appears to have previously prevented discussion of the structural violence of war, remained wedded to a limited understanding of violence, and become resolute in its unwillingness to move its focus away from interpersonal violence and onto structural violence. The apparent lack of focus on structural violence, or at least the simplistic understanding of violence that is commonly operationalised in Community Psychology articles in academic journals, may be an echo of the apparent naivete or nonchalance towards the violence of the higher education sector itself. For whatever reason, Community Psychology has appeared to be denuded in its ability to meaningfully engage with the notion of structural violence. The topic of war, however, might offer a pathway for the discipline to engage more progressively with the topic of violence, and to extend its understanding of the nature of violence. War reveals issues that may previously have been rendered opaque, such as the concentration on episodic rather than generational forms of violence and trauma, and a focus on direct rather than indirect violence. It also revealed, in 2003, the reluctance of the discipline as a whole to engage in a discussion of the politics of violence, the moment it stayed silent on the war in Iraq. That silence has generally remained, though recently there have been signs that Community Psychology's orientation towards violence might be undergoing a shift towards understanding structural violence. But the signs of this transformation remain embryonic and might be little more than a pulsing through of a fragmenting force in the discipline – a splintering of the discipline into a mainstream Community Psychology and a Critical Community Psychology. The shift is appearing through the greater connections being made between violence and:

- social institutions,
- hierarchies of social power, and
- social policies as forms of social sanction against socio-economically distressed and disadvantaged people.

From the nascent activity occurring in what is coming to be known as Critical Community Psychology, the potential to bring in that focus on structural violence appears to be coming from work that is informed by such theoretical and philosophical positions as:

- critical theory
- Marxism
- poststructuralism
- liberation theology
- postcolonial theory
- critical race theory

Drawing on such positions might be sufficient to provide enough people with enough tools and enough momentum to signal a sufficient turn of focus away from interpersonal violence and on to structural violence. It might provide the means to foreground a more sophisticated and penetrating analysis of violence. This might cause ruptures in the discipline and a potential bifurcation of Community Psychology into a mainstream version and a critical version, with the latter perhaps more likely to offer something progressive, relevant and meaningful for those living through the intergenerational onslaught of structural violence. But it might also create the space needed to take a critical look at the higher education sector where community psychologists, like myself, are trained, where we teach and where we engage in research and open up a fuller discussion of how understanding of structural violence impacts on our work, on our relationships and on our discipline. After all, "If we are to envision a less violent world, we must first understand how violent the world is" (Reza, Mercy, & Krug, 2001, p. 104).

References

Agervold, M. (2007). Bullying at work: A discussion of definitions and prevalence, based on an empirical study. *Scandinavian Journal of Psychology*, *48*, 2, 161–72.

Angelique, H., & Kyle, K. (2002). Monterey declaration of critical community psychology. *Community Psychologist*, *35*, 35–6.

Argentin, G., & Triventi, M. (2011). Social inequality in higher education and labour market in a period of institutional reforms: Italy, 1992–2007. *Higher Education, 61*, 309–23.

Association for University and College Counselling. (1999). *Degree of disturbance: The new agenda – the impact of increasing levels of psychological disturbance amongst students in higher education.* British Association for Counselling.

Bailey, D.L., Cooper, D., Hansen-Rayes, N., Jimenez, T., Olson, B., & Somerville, D. (2020, November). Thinking holistically about place-based communities: exploring the spectrum of community psychologist roles. International Conference of Community Psychology. Online. www.vu.edu.au/about-vu/news-events/events/8th-international-conference-of-community-psychology-iccp-2020

Balla, P., Fernández, J., & Fine, M. (2020, July). *Critical transnational conversations on structural violence and radical possibilities.* International Conference of Community Psychology [Video] YouTube. www.youtube.com/watch?v=X1a4pHU0PjE

Banyard, V.L., Plante, E.G., & Moynihan, M.M. (2004). Bystander education: bringing a broader community perspective to sexual violence prevention. *Journal of Community Psychology, 32*(1), 61–79.

Batty, D., Weale, S., & Bannock, C. (2017, March 5). Sexual harassment "at epidemic levels" in UK universities. *The Guardian.* www.theguardian.com/education/2017/mar/05/students-staff-uk-universities-sexual-harassment-epidemic

Bett, M. (1999). *Independent Review of Higher Education Pay and Conditions.* HMSO.

Björklund, C., Vaez, M., & Jensen, I. (2020). Early work-environmental indicators of bullying in an academic setting: a longitudinal study of staff in a medical university. *Studies in Higher Education.* https://doi.org/10.1080/03075079.2020.1729114

Bourdieu, P. (1998). *State nobility: Elite schools in the field of power.* Stanford University Press.

Brusoni, M., Damian, R., Sauri, J.G., Jackson, S., Kömürcügil, H., Malmedy, M. … Zobel, L. (2014). *The concept of excellence in higher education.* European Association for Quality Assurance in Higher Education. Occasional Paper 20. www.enqa.eu/wp-content/uploads/2014/09/The-concept-of-Excellence-in-Higher-Education.pdf

Burton, M., & Kagan, C. (2007). Psychologists and torture: more than a question of interrogation. *The Psychologist, 20*(8), 484–87.

Campbell, K., & Bryceland, C. (1998). *Policing the campus: Providing a safe and secure environment.* Home Office Police Policy Directorate.

Cantor, D., Fisher, B., Chibnall, S., Townsend, R., Lee, H., Bruce, C., & Thomas, G. (2017). *Report on the AAU Campus Climate Survey on Sexual Assault and Sexual Misconduct.* www.aau.edu/sites/default/files/AAU-Files/Key-Issues/Campus-Safety/AAU-Campus-Climate-Survey-FINAL-10-20-17.pdf

Chapell, M.S., Casey, D., De la Cruz, C., Ferrell, J., Forman, J., Lipkin, R. … Whittaker, S. (2004). Bullying in college by students and teachers. *Adolescence, 39*, 53–64.

Değirmencioğlu, S.M. (2003). Action makes psychology more useful than fun. *The Community Psychologist, 36*(4), 27–9.

Duckett, P. (2009). Critical reflections on key community psychology concepts: off-setting our capitalist emissions? *Forum Gemeindepsychologie, 14*(2). www.gemeindepsychologie.de/ fg-2-2009.html

Duckett, P.S. (2004). Globalised violence, community psychology and the bombing and occupation of Afghanistan and Iraq (Keynote). *International Congress of European Community Psychology.* Berlin (Germany), September.

Duckett, P.S. (2005). Globalised violence, community psychology and the bombing and occupation of Afghanistan and Iraq. *Journal of Community and Applied Social Psychology, 15*(5), 414–23.

Duckett, P.S., & Değirmencioğlu, S. (2017). War, peace and community psychology (Special Section Editorial). *Journal of Community and Applied Social Psychology, 27*(4), 271–2.

Editor, IBPP (2003). Special article: A statement on the Iraq war from Psychologists for Social Responsibility: sense and nonsense. *International Bulletin of Political Psychology, 14*(13), Article 2. https://commons.erau.edu/ibpp/vol14/iss13/2

Ellison, E.R., Kivell, N., Madyaningrum, M.E., & Olson, B. (2020, November). Theory as revolution: building and applying critical theory(ies) for solidarity and transformation. *International Conference of Community Psychology.* Online.

Erkutlu, H., & Chafra, J. (2014). Ethical leadership and workplace bullying in higher education. *Hacettepe Üniversitesi Eğitim Fakültesi Dergisi (H. U. Journal of Education), 29*(3), 55–67.

Evans, S., Duckett, P., Lawthom, R., & Kivell, N. (2017). Positioning the critical in community psychology. In M. A. Bond, I. Serrano-Garcia, & C. B. Keys (Eds.), *APA handbook of community psychology* (vol. 1: Theoretical foundations, core concepts, and emerging challenges, pp. 107–28). American Psychological Association.

Fazackerley, A. (2020, September 25). UK universities "bullying" junior staff into face-to-face teaching. *The Guardian*. www.theguardian.com/education/2020/sep/25/uk-universities-bullying-junior-staff-into-face-to-face-teaching

Fisher, A.B. (1992). Welcome to the age of overwork. *Fortune* (November), *64*, 70–1.

Fisher, B.S. (1995). Crime and fear on campus. *Annals of the American Academy of Political and Social Science*, *539*, 85–101.

Fogg, P. (2008). Academic bullies. *Chronicle of Higher Education, 55*(3), B10.

Fryer, D., & Duckett, P. (2014). Community psychology. In T. Teo (Ed.). *Encyclopaedia of critical psychology* (pp. 284–290). Springer.

Fryer, D., & Fagan, R. (2003). Toward a critical community psychological perspective on unemployment and mental health research. *American Journal of Community Psychology*, *32*(1/2), 89–96.

Fryer, D., & Fox, R. (2015). Community psychology: Subjectivity, power, collectivity. In I. Parker (Ed.). *Handbook of critical psychology* (pp. 145–154). Routledge.

Fryer, D., & Laing, A. (2008). Community psychologies: What are they? What could they be? Why does it matter? A critical community psychology approach. *Australian Community Psychologist*, *20*, 7–15.

Fryer, D., & McCormack, C. (2012). The war without bullets: socio-structural violence from a critical standpoint. *Global Journal of Community Psychology Practice*, *3*(1), 87–92.

Fryer, D., Stevens, G., Teo, T., Regina, L., Dobles, I., & TeAkwekotuku, N. (2020, November). Fostering and sustaining anti-capitalist solidarities. *International Conference of Community Psychology*. Online.

Furedi, F. (2016). *What's happened to the university? A sociological explanation of its infantalisation*. Routledge.

Galtung, J. (1969). Violence, peace, and peace research. *Journal of Peace Research*, *6*(3) 167–91.

Gerber, T.P., & Cheung, S.Y. (2008). Horizontal stratification in postsecondary education: forms, explanations, and implications. *Annual Review of Sociology*, *34*, 299–318.

Gill, T.K., & Gill, S.S. (2000). Financial management of universities in developing countries. *Higher Education Policy*, *13*, 125–30.

Grayson, P. (1994). Campus suicide: A memoir. *Journal of College Student Psychotherapy*, *9*(1), 57–68.

Halloran, M.J. (2007). Indigenous reconciliation in Australia: Do values, identity and collective guilt matter? *Journal of Community and Applied Social Psychology*, *17*(1), 1–18.

Hammad, J., & Tribe, R. (2020). Social suffering and the psychological impact of structural violence and economic oppression in an ongoing conflict setting: the Gaza Strip. *Journal of Community Psychology*, *48*(6), 1791–810.

Hanson-Easey, S., & Moloney, G. (2009). Social representations of refugees: place of origin as a delineating resource. *Journal of Community and Applied Social Psychology*, *19*(6), 506–14.

Headspace & National Union of Students. (2017). *National tertiary student wellbeing survey 2016*. https:// headspace.org.au/assets/Uploads/headspace-NUS-Publication-Digital.pdf

Hoffman, D.H., Carter, D.J., Lopez, C.R.V., Benzmiller, H.L., Guo, A.X., Latifi, S.Y., & Craig, D.C. (2015). *Report to the Special Committee of the Board of Directors of the American Psychological Association: Independent review relating to APA Ethics Guidelines, national security interrogations, and torture*. Sidley Austin LLP. www. apa.org/independent_review/revised_report.pdf

Hollis, L.P. (2015). Bully university? The cost of workplace bullying and employee disengagement in American higher education, *SAGE Open, 5*(2), 1–11.

Javorka, M., & Campbell, R. (2020). This isn't just a police issue: tensions between criminal justice and university responses to sexual assault among college students. *American Journal of Community Psychology*, July (Early access).

Jenkins, R. (2014, August 18). Too many poor leaders. *The Chronicle of Higher Education*. www.chronicle. com/article/too-many-poor-leaders/

Kagan, C., & Burton, M. (2001). *Critical community psychology praxis for the 21st century*. Paper presented at the British Psychological Society Conference, Glasgow, Scotland.

Kagan, C., Burton, M., Duckett, P., Lawthom, R., & Siddiquee, A. (2011). *Critical community psychology* (1st ed.). Wiley-Blackwell.

Klein, N. (1999). *No logo: No space, no choice, no jobs*. Knopf Canada.

Lafferty, G., & Fleming, J. (2000). The restructuring of academic work in Australia: Power, management and gender. *British Journal of Sociology of Education*, *21*(2), 257–67.

Lee, B.X. (2019). *Violence: An interdisciplinary approach to causes, consequences, and cures*. Wiley-Blackwell.

Lund, E.M., & Ross, S.W. (2016). Bullying perpetration, victimization, and demographic differences in college students: a review of the literature. *Trauma, Violence, & Abuse, 18*, 348–60.

Lykes, M.B. (2003). Developing an activist liberatory community psychology: one step at a time. *The Community Psychologist, 36*(4), 39–42.

MacLean, C. (2003). *Greater Easterhouse: A profile of health needs.* NHS Greater Glasgow and Clyde. www.stor.scot.nhs.uk/handle/11289/579934

Mahmoudi, M. (2020, January 16). Academic bullying: desperate for data and solutions. *Science.* www.sciencemag.org/features/2020/01/academic-bullying-desperate-data-and-solutions

Makkawi, I. (2014). Community psychology enactments in Palestine: roots and current manifestations. *Journal of Community Psychology, 43*(1), 63–75.

Marsella, A. (1998). Toward a "global-community psychology": Meeting the needs of a changing world. *American Psychologist, 53*(12), 1282–91.

Meari, L. (2015). Reconsidering trauma: towards a Palestinian community psychology. *Journal of Community Psychology, 43*(1), 76–86.

Mulvey, A., Guzman, B., & Ayala-Alacantar, C. (2003). Women from the margins: challenging U.S. military aggression, policies and SCRA. *The Community Psychologist, 36*(4), 31–3.

Munro, K. (2016, May 17). Under-reporting of sexual assault a serious problem at Sydney University. *Sydney Morning Herald.* www.smh.com.au/education/underreporting-of-sexual-assault-a-serious-problem-at-sydney-university-20160517-gox0jj.html

Myers, H.F., Wyatt, G.E., Ullman, J.B., Loeb, T.B., Chin, D., Prause, N. … & Liu, H. (2015). Cumulative burden of lifetime adversities: trauma and mental health in low-SES African Americans and Latino/as. *Psychological Trauma: Theory, Research Practice and Policy, 7*(3), 243–51.

Paaskesen, L. (2013). Negotiating reintegration and meanings of space formerly abducted youth in Uganda. *Journal of Community and Applied Social Psychology, 24*(2), 139–52.

Painter, D., Terre Blanche, M., & Henderson, J. (2006). Critical psychology in South Africa: histories, themes and prospects. *Annual Review of Critical Psychology, 5*, 212–35.

Pezza, P.E., & Bellotti, A. (1995). College campus violence: Origins, impacts and responses. *Educational Psychology Review, 7*(1), 105–23.

Pörhölä, M., Cvancara, K., Kaal, E., Kunttu, K., Tampere, K., & Torres, M.B. (2020). Bullying in university between peers and by personnel: cultural variation in prevalence, forms, and gender differences in four countries. *Social Psychology of Education, 23*, 143–69.

Prilleltensky, I., & Nelson, G. (2002). *Doing psychology critically: Making a difference in diverse settings.* Palgrave Macmillan.

Prilleltensky, I., & Nelson, G. (2009). Community psychology: Advancing social justice. In D. R. Fox, I.Prilleltensky, & S. Austin (Eds.), *Critical psychology: An introduction* (2nd ed.) (pp. 126–43) . SAGE.

Reay, D. (2000). "Dim Dross": marginalised women both inside and outside the academy. *Women's Studies International Forum, 23*(1), 13–21.

Reza, A., Mercy, J. A., & Krug, E. (2001). Epidemiology of violent deaths in the world. *Injury Prevention, 7*, 104–11.

Rolands, J., & Boden, R. (2020, December 2). How Australian vice-chancellor's pay came to average $1million and why it's a problem. *The Conversation.* https://theconversation.com/how-australian-vice-chancellors-pay-came-to-average-1-million-and-why-its-a-problem-150829

Salazar, L.F., & Cook, S.L. (2002). Violence against women: is psychology part of the problem or the solution? A content analysis of psychological research from 1990 through 1999. *Journal of Community and Applied Social Psychology, 12*(6), 410–21.

Salin, D. (2003). Bullying and organisational politics in competitive and rapidly changing work environments. *International Journal of Management and Decision Making, 4*(1), 35–46.

Schulze, C., & Budd, L. (2020). Institutional commitment to combating sexual violence: the practices and policies of U.S. universities. *Journal of Community Psychology, 48*(8), 2692–701.

Shackle, S. (2019, September 27). "The way universities are run is making us ill": Inside the student mental health crisis. *The Guardian.* www.theguardian.com/society/2019/sep/27/anxiety-mental-breakdowns-depression-uk-students

Sharma, M. (2017). *Workplace bullying: An exploratory study in Australian academia* [Unpublished PhD dissertation]. Edith Cowan University.

Sinkkonen, H.M., Puhakka, H., & Meriläinen, M. (2014). Bullying at a university: students' experiences of bullying. *Studies in Higher Education, 39*, 153–65.

Toro, P. (2019). History. In L.A. Jason, O. Glantsman, J.D. O'Brien, & K.N. Ramian (Eds.), *Introduction to community psychology: Becoming an agent of change* (pp. 23–32). Rebus Press. https://press.rebus.community/introductiontocommunitypsychology/

University and College Union. (2019). *Counting the costs of casualisation in higher education.* UCU.

University and College Union. (2020). *Second class academic citizens: The dehumanising effects of casualisation in higher education.* UCU.

Westefeld, J.S., & Furr, S.R. (1987). Suicide and depression among college students. *Professional Psychology: Research and Practice, 18*, 119–23.

Westefeld, J.S., Witchard, K.A., & Range, L.M. (1990). College and university student suicide: trends and implications. *The Counseling Psychologist, 18*(3), 464–76.

Winefield, A.H. (2003). Stress in university academics. In M. Dollard, H.R. Winefield, & A.H. Winefield (Eds.), *Occupational stress in service professionals* (pp. 237–60). Taylor & Francis.

World Health Organization. (2002). *World report on violence and health.* WHO.

Zapf, D., Einarsen, S., Hoel, H., & Vartia, M.(2003). Empirical findings on bullying in the workplace. In S. Einarsen, H. Hoel, D. Zapf, & C.L. Cooper (Eds.), *Bullying and emotional abuse in the workplace. International perspectives in research and practice* (pp. 103–26). Taylor & Francis.

PART II

Community Psychology through a praxis lens

6

INTERROGATING CHILEAN COMMUNITY PSYCHOLOGY IN TIMES OF CRISIS

Alba Zambrano, Sergio Chacón Armijo,
Herling Sanhueza Yáñez and María Antonieta
Campos Melo

Abstract

The social outbreak that occurred in Chile in October 2019, added to the COVID-19 pandemic, has made visible and exacerbated inequities of all kinds in the country (health, work, housing, education etc). This has resulted in the activation of various social and community processes that try to reverse situations of injustice and also to subvert the economic and social logic that has led us to this situation. In this scenario, the question arises, what can Chilean Community Psychology contribute to this crisis? An attempt is made to answer this question in this chapter, which addresses, from an integrated perspective, the various alternatives that our discipline has to contribute to this process of social transformation.

Resumen

El estallido social que se produjo en Chile en octubre de 2019, sumado a la pandemia por COVID-19, ha hecho visibles y ha agudizado las inequidades de todo tipo en el país (salud, trabajo, vivienda, educación, etc.). Lo anterior ha tenido como consecuencia la activación de diversos procesos sociales y comunitarios que intentan, por un lado, revertir las situaciones de injusticia y, por otro, subvertir la lógica económica y social que nos ha llevado a esta situación. En este escenario surge la pregunta: ¿qué puede aportar la psicología comunitaria chilena en esta crisis? A esta interrogante se intenta dar respuesta en este capítulo que aborda desde una mirada integrada las diversas alternativas que tiene nuestra disciplina para aportar a este proceso de transformación social.

Introduction

This chapter presents a collective reflection of community psychologists who work in universities in the south of Chile. From community action, from teaching experience and from activism, they interrogate Community Psychology (CP) about its possible responses and contributions to some of the main crises that the country is facing today. We will stress the tasks

DOI: 10.4324/9780429325663-9

that correspond to CP, to rethink public services and, at the same time, contribute with non-colonial approaches, with a strong feminist and community emphasis.

We are currently facing a national situation that shows historical continuity but also accelerated change. The outburst of social protests throughout the country, and later the pandemic experience, have challenged the creativity of local communities, as well as their resilience to face adversity. In this situation, women leaders are playing a prominent role in the process.

In October 2019, a popular insurrection occurred in Chile, which triggered a number of demonstrations that extended throughout the country. October 18 of that year, after the underground train fare increased by 30 CLP, secondary students began a massive evasion of payment, bypassing security controls and starting an unprecedented national protest. On October 25, there were 1.2 million people on a peaceful protest in Santiago, the capital city of Chile, and a similar number joined the protests in the rest of the country. This popular uprising "exploded" due to the deep and suppressed discontent with the impact of a radical and exclusionary neoliberal system, which was traumatically installed during the military dictatorship in Chile (Barria-Asenjo et al., 2021). This free-market social and economic model has caused severe social inequalities and life conditions that deprive the vast majority of people of fundamental rights, thus forcing them to work on the edge to be able to have access to barely dignified conditions.

Although throughout the history of Chile there have been multiple crises that have allowed those who live in conditions of great poverty to make progress in accessing certain rights and improving some living conditions, the distance between social groups has never substantially decreased (Contardo, 2020). The most recent Gini index measurement in 2017 ranked Chile as the tenth most unequal country in the world (World Bank, 2020). Furthermore, the Organisation for Economic Cooperation and Development (OECD) reports Chile as having the second-widest income gap between the top and bottom deciles (Pérez & Sandoval, 2020). Thus, for example, the 1% with the highest income obtains 17% of the fiscal income, and the 10% with the highest income obtains more than 50% of the total income of the country (Atria et al., 2019).

The current institutional and economic model has been at the service of maintaining privilege for the elite. Wealth concentration, always present in the history of Chile, was clearly reinforced in the 17 years of dictatorship (1973–1990). During this period of time, Chile implemented a series of economic measures that laid the foundations for the deployment of the neoliberal model. Mechanisms such as privatisation, economic liberalisation, deregulation, subsidiarity of the state, openness to international competition and labour flexibility transformed the country in a radical way. The implementation of the model redrew the boundaries between the market and the state, thus generating transformations among social groups (Araujo, 2017). This led to small elite groups accumulating wealth and power and dominating politics (Contardo, 2020).

In the so-called Chilean post-dictatorship transition period, democratic governments did not significantly contribute to narrowing gaps: on the contrary, they favoured mechanisms that transformed the public sector (education, health, transportation etc) into lower-quality services for those groups that could not access the private alternatives available in the market. In this way, the weakening of the public sector and the growing urban segregation of the segments with the greatest economic hardship eventually transformed the public sector into a precarious and dangerous one (Contardo, 2020).

Since 2006, different civil society actors have mobilised in response to the scarce results of the reforms that diverse governments have implemented over the past 30 years, which have sought to make progress on social justice issues. Students, retirees, Mapuche people and workers from different segments began to mobilise, but without becoming an organic and sustained movement. However, in 2019, triggered by the reaction of secondary students, they managed to come together and demonstrate the discontent of society (Rodríguez-Mancilla, Vargas-Muñoz, Contreras-Osses, & Quiroz-Rojas, 2020).

The outburst of successive popular demonstrations throughout the country can be attributed to a general discontent that had been increasing, and that in turn was fuelled by various factors: the injustice expressed in multiple and everyday forms of discrimination, exclusion and abuse, the growing corruption in many institutions, and a culture of unbridled consumption. Citizens demanded the end of an abusive system, and progress towards a more egalitarian society.

It is worth stressing that after 28 days of massive demonstrations, the Chilean political class reached an historic agreement on one of the main popular demands: changing the constitution that was drafted during the dictatorship of Augusto Pinochet. This pact established the call for a referendum in October 2020, so that Chilean people could reply to two questions: first, whether they wanted or not a new constitution; and secondly, what type of constitutional body should draft it.

When the referendum took place in October 2020, an overwhelming majority of citizens decided to replace the constitution. Regarding the drafting body, the vast majority as well chose a constitutional convention, composed of citizens elected exclusively for this end, with gender parity. One hundred and fifty-five people, elected by popular vote on April 11, 2021, are drafting the new constitution.

However, after several months of multiple demonstrations, the social movement was abruptly halted (at least in appearance) by the health crisis generated by the COVID-19 pandemic. At first it invaded, paralysed and generated a deep uncertainty that harshly revealed the fragility of the system, in terms of the social protection of citizens, thus making the profound inequalities more evident (Barria-Asenjo, 2021). Gradually, solidarity networks and multiple experiences of community resilience emerged and were reactivated, in order to resist the adverse and often violent living conditions, which were exacerbated by the pandemic.

Chile, like other countries, is not only experiencing the violent effects of social inequality, but its citizens have also been losing much of their autonomy with respect to the powers that have defined reality and have placed it at the service of the interests of the elite (Aragonés & Sevillano, 2020). Although the state has not completely disappeared, it has been co-opted by these elites, and a significant part of its work has been delegitimised. The pandemic evidences the weakness of the care systems for citizens, particularly for those who have had to dramatically face precariousness in various spheres of their lives. Moreover, it challenges and highlights our ways of life: unbridled consumption, individualism and our predatory and irresponsible behaviour towards the planet.

It is in this context that the Chilean social movement emerges as an engine that, despite the high social and economic costs for many people, has made it possible to recover, in part, a sense of psychological control, as well as to promote the importance of the collective. In this way, community has re-emerged as a core value. In addition, at the base of this social movement, many processes have been interwoven in a complex manner, which have paved the way for interesting dynamics that recover community values and demand both citizen participation and the capacity for collective action (Zambrano et al., 2020).

We will go on to analyse and outline the fundamental contributions that CP can make to sustain and nurture the social transformation movement in Chile, as well as to contribute to collective action that can make it possible to face the impacts of the global health crisis that is challenging Chilean people, who were already going through a deep social crisis, since the "social outbreak".

Community Psychology essentials and its contribution to human development

The history of CP shows us that its development has included the redefinition of the reality (object) of study and of professional work. Its emergence has been marked by a reaction to medical conceptions and to the individualistic emphasis of traditional psychology, and also by the need to respond to social issues that had not been resolved (Musitu, 2004).

Despite the blurred boundaries with other disciplines and practices, along with the initial inaccuracies, it can be argued that CP, as a disciplinary field, has been able to generate an alternative conception so that it can have its own paradigmatic framework and, at the same time, dialogue with other disciplines respectfully. Although it is possible to detect some differences in the specific theories throughout the development of CP in different areas, with regard to fundamental aspects we can find important coincidences, which allow us to maintain that there is a clearly defined scientific community (Montero, 2004).

For CP, it is precisely the community, as a subject and horizon (as a political and value-based project), that is the main focus of its scientific and professional work. It is aimed at developing action towards the transformation of society and at promoting improvement in the quality of life of the community, focusing mainly on structural change. This includes, for example, links, representation, access to resources and the strengthening of networks.

Evidence shows that unequal relations in the distribution of, and access to, resources between people and groups affect the degrees of freedom and control that people have over their reality, which conditions the possibilities they have for human development (Vethencourt, 2018). The capability to take advantage of the opportunities in their life contexts depends directly or indirectly on how power is organised within a society (United Nations Development Program [UNDP], 2004). It is known that Latin America has had to face successive processes of colonisation, dictatorships and extensive abuse. It is a continent that is culturally and naturally rich and diverse but also has severe inequalities and poverty.

Despite various understandings of power (Zambrano, 2012; Zambrano & Henríquez, 2019), we can argue that it is directly related to control over different resources, thereby conditioning the possibilities that individuals and communities have to acquire opportunities to develop their potential, collaborate with others and forge, ultimately, their own destiny (Vethencourt, 2018). When people have power, they have the possibility to act and create changes in their environment. Social issues, therefore, are understood from this discipline as a lack of availability and of access to the resources that are necessary for the empowerment of people and communities.

Considering that these shortcomings are directly produced by the current modes of distribution and access to these resources, the solution to the social issues requires broader social change (Le Bossé & Dufort, 2002). Therefore, the emphasis of CP is placed on the study of power relations and control over life circumstances and their effects on psychosocial processes. To achieve this, priority is given to strengthening the psychosocial processes that enable the development of self-managing communities (Montero, 2009), and to the strengthening of organisations that are part of the community network. The main role of professionals in social practices, then, is to accompany and sustain change in a collaborative relationship with communities (Rappaport, 2005; Le Bossé & Dufort, 2002; Montero, 2003; Zambrano & Henríquez, 2019).

Although the theories that have influenced Latin American CP are diverse, they share a critical view of reality, placing the emphasis on social injustice, on the need to recognise the mechanisms that locate broad groups in situations of subordination, and on the lack of recognition and visibility of alternative ways of life and knowledge, different from those of the West. The "other lives", historically made invisible and despised, are located from this perspective as a valuable and essential form of knowledge and existence (De Sousa, 2017). Therefore, in addition to Marxist influences, critical theories, liberation social psychology, popular education and militant sociology, today there are also decolonial theories, feminist perspectives (particularly decolonial and community perspectives), and the now visible epistemologies of the South (De Sousa, 2009). Although each perspective has a different emphasis, they coincide in identifying conditions of oppression, and how these are articulated in complex ways for some people (particularly women). They also emphasise the need to make visible, and recognise the value of different ways of life and worldviews, particularly retrieving those that include a relational ontology. That is, the fact that human beings exist in relation to other human beings, but also in deep connection with nature and including the spiritual dimension (Kagan et al., 2020; Garcés & Zambrano, 2019).

In short, for CP, and especially for the Latin American CP, it is essential to contribute to the well-being of people, value diversity and recognise power relations as a relevant dimension to progress social justice. For this, it is of paramount importance to encourage people to achieve a balance between individual needs and the collective objectives set by the various communities that constitute a larger society. Although societies may differ in their desired features, visions of well-being all depend on the equitable distribution of resources in a society (Sen, 2002; Prilleltensky, 2008; Sánchez-Vidal, 2017; Zambrano & Henríquez, 2019).

The foregoing implies reconciling, according to Prilleltensky (2008), self-determination and collaboration. Self-determination is possible when people have opportunities to speak out, when they are in a position to form an opinion because they have the means to do so, and when they are able to participate in community life. Self-determination, therefore, consists of expressing ideas, seeing that one's opinions are respected and taken into account, exercising rights, participating in decisions that affect one's life and determining the actions to be taken (Le Bossé & Dufort, 2002).

Collaboration, for its part, consists of encouraging cooperation between individuals and communities. To do this, it is necessary to reinforce an ethic of mutual aid, of a sense of community, and of recognising, valuing and strengthening the interdependence between members of a community.

People and communities are the best suited to define their own transformations. Therefore, well-being must be defined from within a community, and not from unique and external standards or norms. This observation has numerous implications for action, as it requires respect for diversity to be maintained in change management (Le Bossé & Dufort, 2002), favouring an approach of consensual management. This becomes particularly challenging when we seek to accompany processes in indigenous communities, which have their own world view, but have suffered from diverse forms of violence throughout their history, due to the processes of colonisation (Sonn & Quayle, 2012).

Le Bossé and Dufort (2002) point out that for CP, diversity has an essentially political connotation, since it refers to the notion of power. Some social groups that have power, have privileges that allow them to impose their points of view and their ways of doing things on other social groups that in turn systematically see that their points of view are discredited, and their ability to reflect and act is restricted. Recognising diversity is, from this perspective, to acknowledge the imbalance of existing powers expressed in the different forms that social actions take.

It follows, then, that respect for diversity implies waiving privileges and redefining power relations. It requires a cessation of implicitly or explicitly imposing unique standards and norms by professionals through their actions in aid relationships (Rappaport, 1977). Contexts that facilitate respect for diversity would be characterised by the valuing of interdependence and differences, the request and consideration of opinions, and the promotion of reflection and the integration of groups (Le Bossé & Dufort, 2002). Respect for diversity takes on its true meaning when it aims at social justice through an equitable distribution of resources and obligations.

The purpose of contributing to the building of a more just society constitutes another important value that guides community psychologists in their management of change. Social justice, for CP, is understood as a relational construct that deals with the fair and equitable allocation in society of burdens, resources and powers (Miller, 1990). As we have seen, data clearly show us that some groups have more power and opportunities to meet their needs than others. A more just society is one in which social groups increase in their abilities and opportunities to meet their needs in order to advance welfare and justice for their members (Prilleltensky, 2008; Le Bossé & Dufort, 2002; Zambrano & Henríquez, 2019). This is undoubtedly a titanic task for Latin America, as it is for Chile specifically.

The aim to advance social justice goes far beyond a purely psychological and political understanding of power. It requires a synergy of both dimensions: unless social structures and cognitive and behavioural structures are affected, what is achieved is simply to maintain the status quo (Prilleltensky, 2008).

Political responsibility derived from the commitment to work around a paradigm of social transformation and cultural amplification (Zambrano, 2012) requires psychologists in this field to work from the perspective of endogenous local development. It asks them to promote change, facilitating better levels of articulation and awareness among the various actors. In Marxist language, it is about working at the level of the social structure and the superstructure (ideology), but with resources that allow the mobilisation of dialogue, conflict, consensus and the construction of articulating projects that explicitly consider the issues of welfare, justice, power, respect and the promotion of diversity. According to Prilleltensky (2008), the interventions that seek to increase, for example, self-esteem, social support or social skills, should incorporate sociopolitical development, awareness-raising and social action. Ultimately, it is about connecting the personal with the political in all spheres so that community action promotes political changes. It is within the perspective of substantial structural change that Latin American CP is placed (Wiesenfeld, 2014).

Latin American CP proposes a type of action that emphasises participation of a clearly political nature. This manifests itself when it seeks to raise awareness and increase the power of socially disadvantaged individuals, groups and communities; when it supports processes of democratisation in relationships and structures (Zambrano & Henríquez, 2019); and when it encourages mechanisms for people to make decisions. Without a doubt, all are elements that critically challenge the established order.

Politicising implies asking radical questions about what exists. These questions are related to how we want to live together, and to criticising unquestioned relationships, such as work as exploitation, the relationship between genders as inequality, predatory relationships with nature, and racism, amongst others (Fernández-Savater, 2020).

Facing the crises: communities and their responses

We would now like to focus our analysis on showing how in Chile in general, and in some southern regions in particular, relationships of profound inequality and social injustice are reproduced, and how collective action and the empowerment of communities becomes an imperative today.

In Chile, the statement "It wasn't depression, it was capitalism" became famous. With this, we do not wish to deny the alarming figures of depression present in our country, considering that, according to the latest Health Survey of the Ministry of Health of Chile (2018), 15.8% of the population might be suffering from depression and 6.2% would meet clinical criteria to confirm said diagnosis, thus placing our country above the world average (4.4%) and making it one of the countries with the highest rates of this health condition in the region (World Health Organization [WHO], 2017).

On the contrary, we would like to illustrate, based on these figures, how our forms of social, political and economic organisation have contributed to exacerbating health inequities and their impact on people's mental health. This is not a recent issue. Already in 2009 the World Health Organization (WHO) endorsed the recommendations of the Commission on Social Determinants of Health, among which the need to fight against the inequitable distribution of power, money and resources was raised (WHO, 2009). This struggle also included the call for countries to not only place special emphasis on improving the daily living conditions and well-being of people in conjunction with the various social actors, but also to contribute to the emancipation of individuals and groups, especially [of] the marginalised, and [to] take measures to improve the social conditions that affect their health (WHO, 2009).

Although the poverty rate in terms of income in Chile appears low (8.6%), many people move in and out of poverty due to the fragility of the labour market and the high cost of living. Moreover, if we consider poverty from a multidimensional perspective, the figure rises to 20.7% (Ministry of Social Development, 2018). Despite the fact that market goods have grown at an accelerated rate (López, 2020), public and social goods have seen their growth restricted. Vulnerability is especially felt when people get sick, when they begin to age or when they lose their jobs, because the state offers them nothing, since its action, such as it is, focuses on extreme poverty.

Policies focused on addressing poverty require individuals to prove that they are poor and to compete for scarce resources with other people in similar conditions. Thus, community networks, territory and social cohesion are devalued, ineffective in addressing the multidimensionality of poverty (Alfaro, Sánchez, & Zambrano, 2012). In this scenario, social policies are rather palliative and compensatory, without the transformative power that is required.

Chile is characterised by the presence of multiple natural crises (a wide range of natural disasters: earthquakes, floods, droughts, volcanic eruptions) and social crises. These, while they activate broad solidarity networks, also reveal the weaknesses of the logic and organisation of the state. This has occurred once again with the advent of the health crisis resulting from the COVID-19 pandemic.

The pandemic surprised Chile, like other countries in the world, in full social effervescence with a series of social movements that from different fronts had been demanding greater social justice, rejection of the capitalist and patriarchal system, and another series of movements linked to environmental issues.

As some studies show (Bidisha, Mahmood, & Hossain, 2021; Tavares & Betti, 2021), it is important to consider the clear distinctions in how the pandemic has affected the different social and economic classes. People who live in poverty conditions are evidently more affected than those who have economic advantages. This impact does not only mean a greater risk of disease, but it includes all the negative effects of the measures taken by the different countries to face the pandemic.

The pandemic highlights various conditions that have been denounced as limitations to social development. In Chile, during this period, the dramatic dismantling of the public sector produced by commodification and inequality has been exposed.

The omnipresent and uncertain nature of this crisis causes many aspects of what we called normality to collapse. Everyday life becomes unpredictable, unstable, and fragile, especially for those who live in the worst life conditions, in a society that lacks a comprehensive system of care. Thus, the need for public strategies for the care of life, which should be present in all policies, is made evident.

Forced lockdown highlights a set of conditions that, although they have been present, not much attention had been paid to them. We emphasise, among others, social loneliness, abandonment and the precariousness in which older people live, as well as the increased stresses of care (Scholten et al., 2020), which, being most of the time experienced by women, have strongly increased.

The pandemic has revealed the disparity in the time that men and women dedicate to care work, thus exacerbating, in some way, a crisis of care (Malherbe, 2020), which is not only operational but also ethical and political. It raises questions for CP insofar as it underpins new, community ways of approaching the care of others. The latter arises from the verification that the capitalist and patriarchal structure of relationships has imposed a mark of competition on them on the one hand, and has relegated care to the private space on the other hand (Fisher et al., 2020). This has imposed on women the obligation to both produce and reproduce, to care, transforming this intimate space into a place of exploitation for them where multiple oppressions intersect (Malherbe, 2020).

Uncertainty seems to provoke intense and instantaneous bonds, greater awareness of human vulnerability and of dependence on others. This is not planned or a deliberate strategy. For this reason, the pandemic is also an opportunity to understand that we are interconnected and that we must become part of a "we", the basis of a collective sense. Care intersects with the awareness of our interdependence, since we are part of a whole. It becomes evident, then, that it is necessary to take care of ourselves so we can take care of others, and that our personal and social survival depends on everyone.

However, until now the policies that have been implemented in Chile have emphasised a mainly vertical set of measures, not always taking into account the diverse points of view of the citizens, especially considering the cultural and geographical diversity that can be found in the country (Zambrano et al., 2020). A significant proportion of these measures are related to social control, extending the restrictive measures that were implemented for the social outbreak. There are weaknesses in the preventive strategies and in the local support networks. There is little or no space given to citizenship initiative, and not enough attention is paid to the psychosocial impacts of the pandemic (Barria-Asenjo et al., 2021).

Going beyond the crisis to build community action

By community action we mean, in a general way, those actions that are aimed at generating changes in human relations, thereby directly affecting the distribution of power. For this, it is essential that participatory processes are facilitated in order to create or strengthen social organisations, fostering a process that enriches the associative fabric, encouraging communication and collaboration among all groups to work on a "shared project" (Zambrano & Berroeta, 2012). In this perspective, below we will briefly present some experiences that illustrate expressions of the sense of "we" inherent in the notion of community, and the development of community action to collaborate with each other, as well as to demand greater social justice and modify the situations that limit development.

From the "social outbreak", as well as from the moment the pandemic was declared, several solidarity initiatives have emerged and spread, which identify organisation and the collective as main aspects. It should be noted that this social movement, which began in October, implied significant social and economic impacts for most people. In different neighbourhoods of the big cities of Chile, groups were organised whose mission was to participate in the great national movement, using different means of protest and social demonstration. Special mention should also be made of the feminist movement, which finds in the demonstration spaces a platform to denounce not only capitalism and its effects, but also patriarchal relations that are a substantial part of the relations of injustice and oppression present in the country.

Some of the collective initiatives that were activated are the following: health brigades to care for people affected by police repression; "communal pots"[1] to face the economic impact on people who lost their jobs during this period; solidarity networks to remotely support mental health; new forms of fair trade; and exchange of time and services.

In many places solidarity networks have been implemented during the pandemic, both to support neighbours with economic or health problems, and to monitor how each family is doing in this period. Although face-to-face meetings have been restricted, leaders have maintained an updated information system and have managed to organise and channel mutual support in neighbourhoods facing greater difficulties.

Once again, the role played by women is notable. It is particularly women who take a leading role in caring not only for their families, but also for the members of the community by mobilising strategies to promote mutual support. As an example of this, we present below the opinion of a female leader from a grassroots territorial organisation in a neighbourhood on the suburbs of Temuco:

> We have learned to be more supportive, caring about our neighbours [...] who are infected, who are unemployed [...] we call them by phone. We started with a "communal pot", but later it was difficult to keep doing it because we couldn't collect things for every day [...], but now we collect things and we give them to the people who need them most. We all support each other.
> *(Female leader of the San Eugenio neighbourhood in Temuco)*

Another female leader of a neighbourhood in Angol tells us:

> The authorities, the professionals of the municipality, they do not know where help is needed the most, we are in touch with people every day, and even though we can't meet face to face now, we know who are in need, because we have managed to know how people are doing...
> *(Female leader member of a Territorial Committee)*

Despite the restrictions on social contact, people in community life spaces in urban neighbourhoods have managed to sustain mechanisms of mutual aid, support and solidarity, especially to solve basic subsistence needs.

In rural areas, meanwhile, a differentiated effect of both the "social outbreak" and the pandemic can be observed. In a country with a strong centralisation of power and services, isolated areas have traditionally solved their needs in an endogenous way (sometimes with very little state support), and the impact of the social crises is faced in a particular way, sometimes as a more distant and unfamiliar experience. Problems or tensions are impervious to change, with continuing inequalities and the scarce presence of the state to improve living conditions.

In La Araucanía region, for example, the Lafkenche territory, which is part of the Puerto Saavedra municipality, is a predominantly rural area. Like all territories ancestrally inhabited by the Mapuche people, it has a long history of dispossession and colonisation that has marked the life stories of its inhabitants and has shaped a particular local history of resistance and negotiation with the Chilean state and society.

Currently, Puerto Saavedra's local government is led by a Mapuche mayor, who has promoted a management that makes visible and centrally addresses the situation of the Mapuche people in the territory and intercultural relations. This has emerged as a political commitment greatly supported by the community, which is predominantly Mapuche (at the communal level, the Mapuche indigenous population corresponds to 80.6% of the population).

This historical relationship of resistance and negotiation between the Mapuche people, through their cultural authorities, and the different local governments, representatives of the state in the territory, has been marked by the denunciation of abuses, discrimination and inequality of opportunities. During the last few years, these denunciations have been joined by the demand for greater appreciation of the contribution that the Mapuche world makes to territorial sustainability.

The Mapuche leaders of the territory have been key in the organisation of a community that is not only mobilised by demands for more resources, but also by the power to exercise their political and cultural rights as a people, in order to have greater well-being or "good living" in the territory. Thus, environmental, spiritual and identity issues, among others, have strongly emerged, demanding that community organisation and local management are pertinent to the demands of the territory. Similarly, the high presence of women leading community processes, representing different groups and organising small productive groups, is noteworthy. Female community leaders are recognised for their ability to mediate between the community and the different government agents, in addition to forming a "front line" of support for the most vulnerable people in the community. Their presence is decisive to protect life from various threats attributed to the current hegemonic system. Without female community leaders, the state's protection work would not be possible, especially in places with wide social gaps and with greater cultural complexity. Their participation, from the private level acting in cases of violence against women in the domestic context, to the public level, as defenders of life in the territory and promoters of the Lafkenche cultural identity, makes their social actions a strategic factor in the social welfare and governance of the territory.

The social struggle generated in Chile in 2019, and the evidences made manifest by the pandemic during 2020, have not changed the urgent priorities, demands and dreams of the Lafkenche territory in Puerto Saavedra, but they have indeed connected with structural imperatives at the national level.

The importance for the state to design, plan and execute public policies with an intercultural approach, at all levels, is still being stressed. The COVID-19 pandemic has demonstrated the inefficiency of a centralist state that denies the territorial and cultural diversity of its population, that is, a state that is not prepared to safeguard the lives of the Mapuche communities.

Challenges and contributions from Chilean Community Psychology

The expression of not wanting to return to normality has become widespread, since normality was precisely the problem. Not returning to "normal" is not a matter of desire; rather, it is in these circumstances an ethical-professional imperative. We cannot evade our duty to continue supporting this process of subversion, understood, like Fals Borda, as the act of revealing the contradiction of the social order with new transformative impulses and as "a right of the peoples to fight for their freedom and autonomy, assuming it as a transition period that can bring changes, developments or revolutions, depending on the commitment and constancy of the subversive elements" (Pereira, 2008, as cited in López, 2017, p. 179).

Furthermore, subversion is a necessary tool to open up paths and, above all, to resist "abusive forms of power, which create or maintain oppression or harm" (Portelli & Eizadirad, 2018, p. 53). In this way, subversion is transformed into a morally sustained way to transform abusive social relations, which are expressed in public policies that perpetuate and normalise these asymmetrical power relations (Portelli & Eizadirad, 2018).

Below we will briefly present some of the contributions from CP that would help sustain these resistances and transformations in order to make progress in relationships and conditions that allow human development in a balanced relationship with the environment and nature.

A first emphasis that we propose, from the logic of CP, is the need for a *territorial perspective on the strengthening of care systems*. Community action must be deployed in localities, in order to leverage the empowerment of communities and movements towards the necessary social transformations, in a participatory way. This includes work in specific and physically delimited localities, but is not limited to them. The COVID-19 pandemic has forced us to think that part of the challenge involves identifying forces, movements and groups that are not necessarily subject to a specific territory, but that are working for processes of social transformation. This also means we need to review the supports that have traditionally served for the formation of links and articulation of work with communities; we refer to face-to-face dialogue in specific localities. Today the question is whether, given the restrictions on physical contact, we can still advance in the construction, strengthening and emancipation of communities and groups. Although contact and communication today are mediated by digital platforms, this connection can be an effective alternative for transitory moments of distancing. Furthermore, we cannot ignore its potential in the sense of allowing ourselves to permeate physical, territorial boundaries, in order to articulate changes that make sense to large groups of people who are willing to commit to said transformations.

Likewise, the challenge is to involve, at local levels, broader networks of organisations and public policy programmes, so that they can articulate and be capable of offering more comprehensive systems of care in the various dimensions of the lives of the people of a community. But this should not happen without considering the capacities, autonomy and particularities of communities.

It is essential to continue working with and for communities and groups with the purpose of establishing forms of relationship with the state decision-makers based on horizontality, complementarity, interdependence and collaboration (Lima et al., 2020).

A second element of paramount importance is the *active accompaniment of communities and professionals linked to community action*. Today more than ever, community organisations require professional collaboration, aimed at sustaining and strengthening social organisations in a period of high complexity and overload. They require listening, dialogue and accompaniment in their daily life experiences. To do this, we must experiment with new communication formats to favour encounters, embrace emotions and reinforce measures of resistance, solidarity and creativity. This is relevant to help make visible and reinforce the assets present in organisations and the community as a whole. Sometimes it will also be appropriate to link up with other organisations or institutions to promote initiatives.

This accompaniment must be carried out from a feminist position, which allows the identification of resistance carried out by many women who play a leading role in caring for others (including the community). We must recognise their strength and contribution, but also work to problematise the overload that these tasks represent to them. This is important in order to contribute to the democratisation of various care tasks.

Likewise, it is relevant to provide support to other professionals who are doing front-line work with particularly precarious or marginalised communities (for example, homeless people, people with mental health issues, people with addiction disorders). These are people who will require emotional support and connection with more stable systems of care and prevention of burnout.

The third proposition is that *community action must be embedded in an anti-colonial Latin American perspective*. It is essential to accompany critical participatory processes that manage to connect the particular demands of the territories with the structural factors that maintain and reproduce social injustice and the inequalities that oppress life in communities. To achieve this, we should recognise "the situated" as a locus for understanding reality, from where political action and/or social intervention is possible (Montenegro & Pujol, 2003), connected with the recognition of those historical, cultural and paradigmatic factors that determine local dynamics.

Community action, then, must be accompanied by processes of political formation of leaders with the ability to question power relations rooted in structural inequalities derived from the triple system of patriarchal, colonialist and capitalist domination (De Sousa, 2009), thereby promoting social transformations that have an impact on the form of organisation of the state and on local public policies, but also that press for changes in the way we understand and conceive the "public sector", transcending the state–civil society dichotomy.

The COVID-19 pandemic has confirmed the valuable and silent work of thousands of women and their organisations in the task of protecting and defending the lives of the most excluded communities (particularly rural, indigenous). These experiences rise as resistance, and are not only a reaction to the current health crisis, but also a consolidated response to the historical relationship of colonialism (Lugones, 2003) that has been organised for generations in our continent by marginalised communities.

This implies valuing popular knowledge, not only to solve the problems of the communities from which this knowledge arises, but also to make this knowledge available to address structural issues.

For the above, there is a need for a Latin American CP capable of facilitating processes of reconstruction of the social fabric between actors not only different from each other but also contradictory or even antagonistic. The crisis has revealed the need to act on the network of social relations within which power is articulated, and to move beyond "more of the same". This is not only a matter of promoting deep changes in the state model from the social sciences, but also of rethinking and recreating the sense of the "public", connecting the individual and the collective in a continuum so that the transformations towards a dignified life are relevant to the territories and their communities.

Fourthly, we stress the importance of the *construction of knowledge and community praxis, as a dialogical processes*, built with the community to provide spaces for exchange. De Sousa (2009) argues that the use of derivative methodologies to extract information from communities without a commitment to social transformation should not be allowed. Positions of power associated with academic extractivist logics (Grosfoguel, 2016) should be renounced in favour of horizontality, openness to daily life and the appreciation of community knowledge. From an empowerment approach, a collaborative relationship is essential, where knowledge, skills and relationships are enriched, in any community action. This view of complementarity and synergy allows power to be amplified, a logic that identifies the idea of "potency power" that is present in the notion of empowerment (Zambrano, 2012).

In short, complementary roles of collaboration and intermediation as well as social advocacy (when required) should be part of this work to support community processes.

Fifthly, it is necessary to *strengthen professional and union organisation*, for example the Chilean Society of Community Psychology. The dialogue of shared knowledge and impressions in a common space allows for the crossing of tensions, epistemological adhesions that nurture and guide the practice of each participant in this organisation. The space for dialogue makes it possible to open up paths for the common construction of investigative work, as well as of spaces for expressing and denouncing situations of injustice, violence and violation of human rights. It is a space for collectivisation that allows us to strengthen bonds, to grow and to feel less alone in the face of the voracity of a social market model that encourages individualism. It is an organisation that is also a technical reference for various public policies, as well as an authorised voice for social advocacy or denunciation.

The last proposition regards the *training for psychologists*. Here, there is the opportunity or challenge to raise the idea that CP is not limited to the mere transmission of content, but extends to the need to contribute to raising awareness regarding the responsibility that falls to us as community psychologists in the processes of social transformation. This requires specific disciplinary knowledge, but above all, the development of a willingness to be actively involved in the emancipation of excluded communities and groups. The foregoing places this academic challenge on an ethical level. With regard to training for practice, it is essential to have courses in community ethics, since the deficit in this area implies ethical problems that are later noticed in professional work, for example, in the invisibility of community voices or in assuming tasks or projects for which they may not be prepared (Winkler et al., 2012). In short, we must prepare the new generations of community psychologists to continue and consolidate these processes with a clear emphasis on acting with and for the communities, assuming the link with them as partnerships and not as mere subjects of psychosocial intervention.

Finally, we would like to emphasise, as a fundamental learning process in this period of sustained crisis, that life is made possible not in isolation, but due to the entire network of relationships that form the community or communities to which we belong. We must take care of ourselves and take care of others to make life possible. We have seen that the way to sustain our existence involves building and nurturing communities from the local level to the broadest level. However, we must go further; our species must honour and cooperate with nature to sustain life.

Note

1 *Olla común* in Chile. It is an initiative of community participation that seeks to solve the basic need to eat. People cook in public and it is supplied with food donations. It is similar to a soup kitchen, although of a more self-managed and independent nature.

References

Alfaro, J., Sánchez, A., & Zambrano, A. (Eds.) (2012). *Psicología Comunitaria y Políticas Sociales: Reflexiones y Experiencias*. Paidós.

Aragonés, J., & Sevillano, V. (2020). La desigualdad ante el espejo del Covid-19. In M. Moya & G. Willis (Eds.), *La psicología social ante el Covid 19: Monográfico del Internacional Journal of Social Psychology* (pp. 71–3). Universidad de Granada.

Araujo, K. (2017). Sujeto y neoliberalismo en Chile: rechazos y apegos. *Nuevo mundo nuevos mundos*. https://doi.org/10.4000/nuevomundo.70649

Atria, J., Flores, I., Sanhueza, C., & Mayer, R. (2019). Top incomes in Chile: A historical perspective of income inequality (1964–2015). *World Inequality Database*, Working Paper N° 2018/11.

Barria-Asenjo, N., Žižek, S., Scholten, H., Salas, G., Zambrano, A., Gallo, J., Gómez, E., & Uribe, J. (2021) Deglobalizing COVID-19: The pandemic from a decentered perspective. *Revista Sociedade e Estado*, *36*(3).

Bidisha, S. H., Mahmood, T., & Hossain, M. B. (2021). Assessing food poverty, vulnerability and food consumption inequality in the context of COVID-19: A case of Bangladesh. *Social Indicators Research*. https://doi.org/10.1007/s11205-020-02596-1

Contardo, O. (2020). *Antes de quefueraoctubre*. Editorial Planeta Chilena S.A.

De Sousa, B. (2009). *Una epistemología del Sur. La reinvención del conocimiento y la emancipación social*. Siglo XXI, CLACSO.

De Sousa, B. (2017). *Democracia y transformación social*. Siglo del Hombre Editores.

Fernández-Savater, A. (2020, September 27). ¿Es la revoluciónaúndeseable? *Infolibre*. https://cutt.ly/ahPbBIk

Fisher, J., Languilaire, J., Lawthom, R., Nieuwenhuis, R., Petts, R., Runswick-Cole, K., & Yerkes, M.. (2020). Community, work, and family in times of COVID-19. *Community, Work & Family*, *23*(3), 247–52.

Garcés, G., & Zambrano, A. (2019). Significadosentorno al desarrollo del consumoproblemático y dependencia alcohólica en comunidades mapuches rurales de la región de la Araucanía, Chile, 2016–2017. *Salud Colectiva*, *15*, 1–18. https://doi.org/10.18294/sc.2019.1932

Grosfoguel, R. (2016). Del "extractivismo económico» al «extractivismo epistémico» y «extractivismo ontológico": una forma destructiva de conocer, ser y estaren el mundo. *Tabula Rasa*, *24*, 123–43. https://doi.org/10.25058/20112742.60

Kagan, C., Burton, M., Duckett, P., Lawthom, R., & Siddiquee, A. (2020). *Critical community psychology: Critical action and social change*.(2nd ed.). Routledge. https://cutt.ly/ohPcrUY

Le Bossé, Y., & Dufort, F. (2002). El empoderamiento de las personas y comunidades: otra forma de intervenir. En F. Dufort y J. Guay (comps.). *Agir au coeur des communautés. La psychologie communitaire et le changement social* (pp. 75–115). Le Presse de l'Université Laval.

Lima, M., Barros, R., Gussi, M., Milanese, M., Gussi, M. A., & Serrano, I. (Org.). (2020). *Tratamento Comunitário. Experiência de um paradigma de transformação social*. Tecknopolitik.

López, J. (2017) Orlando Fals Borda: del cientificismo a la subversión moral. Tránsitos y reconstrucciones de un pensamiento crítico. *Ciencianueva. Revista de Historia y Política*, *1*(1), 172–85.

López, R. (2020, April 5). Un país vulnerable en la hora de la verdad. CIPER. www.ciperchile.cl/2020/04/05/un-pais-vulnerable-en-la-hora-de-la-verdad/

Lugones, M. (2003). *Pilgrimages/Peregrinajes: Theorizing coalitions against multiple oppressions*. Rowman & Littlefield.

Malherbe, N. (2020). Community psychology and the crisis of care. *Journal of Community Psychology*, *48*(7), 2131–7.

Miller, D. (1999). *Principles of social justice*. Harvard University Press.

Ministerio de Desarrollo Social. (2018). *Situación de Pobreza. Síntesis de resultados*. https://cutt.ly/5hPmjjK

Ministerio de Salud de Chile. (2018). *Encuesta Nacional de Salud 2016–2017. Segunda entrega de resultados*. Departamento de Epidemiología, División de Planificación Sanitaria, Subsecretaría de Salud Pública.

Montenegro, M., & Pujol, J. (2003). Conocimiento Situado: Un Forcejeo entre el Relativismo Construccionista y la Necesidad de Fundamentar la Acción. *Revista Internacional de Psicología*, *37*(2), 295–307.

Montero, M. (2003). *Teoría y práctica de la Psicología Comunitaria: la tensión entre comunidad y sociedad*. Paidós.

Montero, M. (2004). *Introducción a la psicología comunitaria: desarrollo, conceptos y procesos*. Paidós.

Montero, M. (2009). El fortalecimiento de la comunidad, sus dificultades y alcances. *Universitas Psychologica*, *8*(3), 615–26.

Musitu, G. (2004). Surgimiento y desarrollo de la Psicología. En G. Musitu, J. Herrero, L. Cantera & M. Montenegro (Coord.). *Introducción a la Psicología Comunitaria* (pp. 3–17). UOC.

Pérez, R., & Sandoval, S. (2020, 26 de febrero). *La geografía de la desigualdad y del poder*. CIPER. www.ciperchile.cl/2020/02/26/la-geografia-de-la-desigualdad-y-del-poder/

Pereira, A. (2008). Fals Borda:la formación de un intelectual disórgano. *Anuario Colombiano de Historia Social y de la Cultura*, *35*, 375–411.

Portelli, J., & Eizadirad, A. (2018). Subversion in education: Common misunderstandings and myths. *International Journal of Critical Pedagogy*, *9*(1), 53–72.

Prilleltensky, I. (2008). The role of power in wellness, oppression, and liberation: The promise of psychopolitical validity. *Journal of Community Psychology*, *36*, 116–36. https://doi.org/10.1002/jcop.20225

Rappaport, J. (1977). *Community psychology: Values, research and action.* Holt, Rinehart and Winston.

Rappaport, J. (2005). Community psychology is (thank God) more than science. *American Journal of Community Psychology*, *35*, 231–8. https://doi.org/10.1007/s10464-005-3402-6

Rodríguez-Mancilla, M., Vargas-Muñoz, R., Contreras-Osses, P., & Quiroz-Rojas, R..(2020). Rebelión social en la ciudad Notas sobre significaciones políticas del octubre chileno. *Universitas, Revista de Ciencias Sociales y Humanas*, *33*, 201–24. https://doi.org/10.17163/uni.n33.2020.10

Sánchez-Vidal, A. (2017). Empoderamiento, liberación y desarrollo humano. *Psychosocial Intervention*, *26*(3), 155–63.

Scholtenn, H., Quezada-Scholz, V., Salas, G., Barria-Asenjo, N., Rojas-Jara, C., Molina, R., García, J., Julia, M., Marinero, A., Heredia, M., Zambrano, A., Gómez, E., Cheroni, A., Caycho-Rodríguez, T., Reyes-Gallardo, T., Pinochet, N., Binde, P., Uribe, J., Bernal, J., & Somarriva, F. (2020). Abordajepsicológico del COVID-19: Una revision narrativa de la experiencia latinoamericana. *Revista Interamericana de Psicología*, *54*(1), e1287.

Sen, A. (2002). Why health equity? *Health Economics*, *11*, 659–66. https://doi.org/10.1002/hec.762

Sonn, C. & Quayle, A. (2012). Community psychology, critical theory and community development in Indigenous empowerment. In D. Bretherton and N. Balvin (Eds.), *Peace psychology in Australia* (pp. 261–282) (Peace Psychology Book Series). https://doi.org10.1007/978-1-4614-1403-2_15

Tavares, F.F., & Betti, G. (2021).The pandemic of poverty, vulnerability, and COVID-19: Evidence from a fuzzy multidimensional analysis of deprivations in Brazil. *World Development,* 139, 105307. https://doi.org/10.1016/j.worlddev.2020.105307

United Nations Development Program. (2004). *Desarrollo Humano en Chile. El poder: ¿para qué y para quién?, 2004.* UNDP. www.undp.org/content/dam/chile/docs/desarrollohumano/undp_cl_idh_informe2004.pdf

Vethencourt, F. (2018). Capacidades, funcionamientos y agencia como eslabones de un círculo virtuoso en la concepción de desarrollo de Sen. In M., Phelan (comp.). *El círculo virtuoso de lascapacidadesen el Desarrollo humano* (pp. 11–35). Universidad Central de Venezuela, Consejo de Desarrollo Científico y Humanístico.

Wiesenfeld, Esther. (2014). Community-social psychology in Latin America: Consolidation or crisis? *Psicoperspectivas*, *13*(2), 6–18. https://dx.doi.org/10.5027/psicoperspectivas-Vol13-Issue2-fulltext-357

Winkler, M., Alvear, K., Olivares, D., & Pasmanik, D. (2012). Querer No Basta: Deberes Éticos en la Práctica, Formación e Investigaciónen Psicología Comunitaria. *PSYKHE*, *21*(1), 115–29.

World Bank. (2020). [GINI Index by country, Excel spreadsheet] [Data set]. World Bank. https://api.worldbank.org/v2/en/indicator/SI.POV.GINI?downloadformat=excel

World Health Organization. (2009). *Comisión sobre determinantes sociales en salud. Informe de Secretaría.* https://apps.who.int/gb/ebwha/pdf_files/A62/A62_9-sp.pdf

World Health Organization. (2017). *Depression and other common mental disorders: Global health estimates.* https://cutt.ly/NhPnr0b

Zambrano, A. (2012). Las diversascaras del poder: poder para el Desarrollo humano. *Revista Estudios Contemporáneos de la Subjetividad*, *2*(2), 200–14.

Zambrano, A., Arias, S., Silva, C., Bravo, J., Sanhueza, H., & Vera, A. (2020). *Aportes desde la Psicología Comunitaria al bienestar psicosocial y a la salud mental en tiempos de pandemia COVID-19.* Documento de trabajo preparado para la Mesa Redonda "Salud mental en tiempos de pandemia". Colegio de Psicólogos de Chile AG.

Zambrano, A., & Berroeta, H. (Eds.). (2012). *Teoría y práctica de la acción comunitaria.* RIL Editores.

Zambrano, A., & Henríquez, D. (2019). Trazandorutas para el empoderamiento de la comunidaden barrios de la región de La Araucanía: aportes desde la investigación acción. *Revista Interamericana de Psicología*, *53*(3), 331–44. https://doi.org/10.30849/rip/ijp.v53i3.1258

7

PSYCHOLOGISTS TAKING ACTION FOR LGBT+ RIGHTS AND WELL-BEING IN THE PHILIPPINES

Eric Julian Manalastas, Moniq M. Muyargas,
Pierce S. Docena and Beatriz A. Torre

Abstract

This chapter describes the experiences of psychologists taking action for the rights and well-being of lesbian, gay, bisexual and transgender communities in the country context of the Philippines. We reflect on our work as Filipino psychologists in various forms of advocacy and community engagement from 2010 to the present. Three case studies are presented: knowledge generation and dissemination, community organising within the psychology profession, and collaboration with LGBT+ activists towards social change. We utilise community psychological frameworks, in our particular cultural context, to highlight the value of reaching out beyond academic spaces to build community collaboration ("nothing about us without us"), *diskarte* (the Filipino concept of creative problem-solving in the face of constraints such as limited resources), and queering (the playful subversion of normative ways of thinking and doing, to uncover systems of power and achieve group goals). We suggest that by recognising and applying key principles, strategies and perspectives used by community psychologists, we can imagine – and create – social change that empowers lesbian, gay, bisexual, transgender and other gender and sexual minorities in the Philippines and beyond.

Resumen

Este capítulo describe las experiencias de los psicólogos que trabajan por los derechos y el bienestar de las comunidades lesbianas, gays, bisexuales y transgénero en el contexto de Filipinas. Reflexionamos sobre nuestro trabajo como psicólogos filipinos en diversas formas de promoción y participación comunitaria desde 2010 hasta el presente. Se presentan tres casos de estudio: generación y difusión de conocimiento, organización comunitaria dentro de la profesión de psicología y colaboración con activistas LGBT+ hacia el cambio social. Utilizamos marcos de psicología comunitaria, en nuestro contexto cultural, para destacar el valor de ir más allá de los espacios académicos para construir una colaboración comunitaria ("nada sobre nosotros sin nosotros"), diskarte (un concepto filipino de resolución creativa de problemas frente a

DOI: 10.4324/9780429325663-10

restricciones, como recursos limitados) y queering (la subversión lúdica de las formas normativas de pensar y de hacer para revelar sistemas de poder y lograr las metas colectivas). Sugerimos que al reconocer y aplicar los principios, estrategias y perspectivas utilizados por los psicólogos comunitarios, podemos imaginar – y crear – un cambio social que empodere a las personas lesbianas, gays, bisexuales, transgénero y otras minorías sexuales y de género en Filipinas y más allá.

Many of the societal challenges that are of concern to community psychologists – such as inequalities in health; experiences of discrimination and violence; poverty and economic marginalisation – are well known to be structured by gender (see Wasco & Bond, 2010). In this chapter, we extend the analysis of gender as a form of systemic crisis (Kagan & Lewis, 2015) by highlighting the less explored but related dimensions of *sexual orientation and gender identity/ expression* (SOGIE). We ground our discussion on the work and experiences of psychologists taking action for the rights and well-being of lesbian, gay, bisexual, transgender and other sexual and gender minority (LGBT+) communities in the context of the Philippines.

We reflect on our work as Filipino LGBT+ psychologists engaged in various forms of advocacy and community engagement from 2010 to the present. Our team is composed of four early-career, pre-PhD psychologists, including two gay men, one lesbian woman and one heterosexual ally, all cisgender, with formal training *not* in Community Psychology (a specialisation that does not formally exist in the Philippines; Florendo et al., 2013), but in social psychology (Eric, Bea and Pierce), the teaching of psychology (Moniq), gender and sexuality studies (Eric), and LGBT+ psychology (Bea and Eric). All four of us have published research on Filipino LGBT+ issues and have been actively involved in teaching, activism and community practice on LGBT+ rights and well-being in the Philippines.

This chapter is organised as follows. We begin with an overview of sexual orientation and gender identity/expression as dimensions of oppression, including a critical reflection on the unique role of psychology in both perpetuating and addressing anti-LGBT+ stigma and discrimination. We then briefly outline the state of LGBT+ rights in the specific context of the Philippines. We present three case studies representing our work as psychologists taking action for Filipino LGBT+ rights in the interrelated areas of public education, creating positive change within the profession of psychology, and collaboration with community activists. The chapter concludes with reflections on the cultural values and principles that have underpinned our work, as well as limitations and directions for future engagement.

From sexual orientation and gender identity/expression to anti-LGBT+ oppression

Learning "a different language" (BPS, 2018), including being attuned to idioms and core terminology, is a basic tenet for working with communities such as gender and sexual minorities. In mainstream psychology (Rothblum, 2020) as well as human rights discourse (OHCHR, 2019), the term *sexual orientation* is used to refer to an individual's physical, romantic and/or emotional attraction towards others on the basis of gender, while *gender identity* refers to the deeply felt and experienced sense of being female, male or other gender categories in one's culture, and *gender expression* is how people present gender externally in appearance, voice and behaviour. Sexual orientation and gender identity/expression, much like the concept *gender*, are not simply individual-level characteristics. These concepts form the basis for important relationships such as same-gender partnerships, civil unions and marriages (Peplau & Fingerhut, 2007), families formed and headed by LGBT+ people (Moore & Stambolis-Ruhstorfer, 2013), and broader LGBT+ communities (Formby, 2019).

The commonly used acronym LGBT+ is a shorthand way to refer to the aggregated communities of sexual minority (*lesbian, gay and bisexual*) and gender minority (*transgender*) people (Rothblum, 2020), as well as those who are queer, questioning, nonbinary, asexual and intersex. Across the world, sexual and gender minority communities may use varying terminologies; in this chapter we use the term *LGBT+* for pragmatic communicative purposes, acknowledging that this term carries a particular social and political history that can both hinder as well as facilitate community engagement (Garcia, 2013).

Within LGBT+ communities, there is much diversity (Harper & Wilson, 2017). This includes the same diversity in age, race, socioeconomic class, language, religion and ability in other communities. However, one commonality experienced through LGBT+ communities is the systemic problem of *anti-LGBT+ stigma* (Harper & Schneider, 2003; OHCHR, 2019). Despite recent progress in visibility and equal rights for sexual and gender minorities in Western democratic countries, LGBT+ people across the globe continue to collectively experience stigma, prejudice and discrimination at both structural and personal levels. A recent review provides clear evidence for this crisis, including continuing criminalisation, restriction of freedom of expression, and discrimination, torture and violence (Mendos et al., 2020).

First, in 67 of 193 United Nations (UN) member states, consensual same-sex sexual relations are criminalised. That is, in 35% of the world's countries, being lesbian, gay or bisexual is a criminal offence. In six countries, this offence calls for the death penalty. Furthermore, 51 countries currently restrict the possibility of operating charities and civil society organisations that work on SOGIE issues or serve the LGBT+ community. The justification for these restrictions is usually made on the argument that these organisations' activities are illegal, immoral or against the public interest, indicating that anti-LGBT+ structural stigma is in operation.

Second, laws that restrict the freedom of expression in relation to SOGIE exist in 42 countries. These include regulations that prohibit LGBT+-related media content and the "promotion of homosexuality" and other "non-traditional" sexual relations. This systemic condition means that activists and community psychologists face severe restrictions in knowledge-sharing, writing and speaking about LGBT+ issues.

Third, despite evidence of high global prevalence of physical and sexual violence against sexual and gender minorities, particularly transgender people (Blondeel et al., 2018), policies protecting LGBT+ people against hate crimes exist in only 48 countries. Anti-LGBT+ discrimination in education, employment and access to services like healthcare is also a concern: only 57 countries have laws that protect against discrimination on the basis of sexual orientation or gender identity/expression.

Finally, and of particular interest to community psychologists, LGBT+ people have been subject to a long history of stigmatisation by mental health professionals: "homosexuality" was long-considered a mental disorder and only removed from the International Classification of Diseases (ICD) in 1990 (Rothblum, 2020), while "gender incongruence" remains an ICD diagnostic category to this day (Dickey, 2020). This point invites psychologists to reflect on our collective role, as a profession, in the historical oppression of gender and sexual minorities, as well as our professional duty to undo these systemic harms and contribute to the liberation of LGBT+ people (Anderson & Holland, 2015).

The context of the Philippines

The oppression experienced by LGBT+ people globally can be further contextualised by examining the specific country in which they are born, grow up and live. Our particular country context is the Philippines, a Southeast Asian democracy with a long history of colonisation under Spanish and US regimes. Economically, the Philippines is classified by the World Bank (2020) as a lower-middle-income economy. A fifth (22%) of the population of 108 million Filipinos currently live below the national poverty threshold. Culturally, the Philippines has endured a double history of colonisation: first under Spanish imperialism from the 16th to the 19th century, followed by US occupation from 1902 to 1946 (Abinales & Amoroso, 2017). An enduring effect of Spanish colonisation is in religion: the Philippines is the largest majority Roman Catholic country in Asia, with 81% of Filipinos self-identifying as Roman Catholic. Despite constitutional separation of church and state, debates and policies are often highly influenced by religious fundamentalist dogma (Ruiz Austria, 2004). Same-sex marriage, gender identity recognition, abortion, pornography and sex work are all illegal. Perhaps most strikingly, divorce remains illegal in the Philippines, the only other country other than the ecclesiastical state of the Vatican where it is not legally permitted (Abalos, 2017).

Despite general sexual conservatism in Filipino culture (Widmer et al., 1998), the Philippines is often considered one of the more LGBT+-friendly countries in Southeast Asia. Same-sex sexual behaviour is not explicitly criminalised in the Philippines, unlike in neighbouring countries Malaysia and Singapore which have retained vestiges of anti-sodomy laws from British imperialism (Sanders, 2020). Similarly, there are no laws against LGBT+ -related media content. Pride events were celebrated as early as the mid-1990s, and civil society organising for LGBT+ rights and equality is alive and well (UNDP, USAID, 2014). Compared to other Southeast Asian countries, with the possible exception of Thailand, the Philippines is considered one of the more relatively LGBT+-tolerant cultures in the region (Flores, 2019).

However, the absence of explicit oppressive policies does not mean that LGBT+ people in the Philippines live equally, free from stigma, prejudice and discrimination (Yarcia et al., 2019). Anti-LGBT+ stigma continues to operate across the Philippines. Filipino public attitudes towards same-sex sexualities are, on the surface, moderately tolerant (Manalastas et al., 2017) but become highly negative when it comes to same-gender dating (Cruz & Mallari, 2007), marriage equality (Ochoa et al., 2016), and gender transitioning (Macapagal, 2013). Young LGBT+ Filipinos may avoid coming out for fears of social rejection from family and friends (Docena, 2013), while their elderly counterparts experience actual rejection from families of origin (Guevara, 2016). LGBT+ Filipinos experience discrimination, harassment and even violence in public transportation (Silan et al., 2016), religion (Evangelista et al., 2016), schools (Atadero et al., 2014), universities (Muyargas et al., 2016), disaster relief centres (McSherry et al., 2015), employment (GALANG Philippines, 2015), and housing (GALANG Philippines, 2013). Finally, despite years of lobbying efforts, draft legislation that would prohibit discrimination on the basis of sexual orientation and gender identity/expression has failed to pass into law (Calleja et al., 2020); this means that LGBT+ Filipinos can be dismissed from school, denied employment or lose their jobs simply because of being LGBT+.

LGBT+ psychology in the Philippines

Given these challenges, our work for LGBT+ rights and well-being had its origins in a critical incident in 2009 that brought the problem of anti-LGBT+ stigma to the attention of the psychological profession (Manalastas & Torre, 2016). An LGBT+ political party had filed an application to run in the national elections but was summarily denied on two grounds: that sexual and gender minorities were "immoral" and that LGBT+ groups posed "a threat to the well-being of Filipino youth" (Commission on Elections, 2009). Realising that as a profession, we were in a position to comment on the claim that LGBT+ community organising somehow had a detrimental effect on the well-being of young people, a number of us, led by Eric, petitioned the Psychological Association of the Philippines (PAP) to take formal action. Internal lobbying led to the formation of a public interest committee within the PAP in 2010, the first time a social justice arm was institutionalised in Philippine psychology's largest professional organisation. This paved the way for the approval of a landmark policy resolution by the PAP (2011) on LGBT+ non-discrimination, published in the *Philippine Journal of Psychology* (PJP), the flagship journal of the profession, in December 2011.

Since then, the four of us, along with a growing number of colleagues, have been building an LGBT+ psychology in the Philippines, with the aim of employing organised psychology as a powerful means to advance the rights and well-being of LGBT+ Filipinos (Ofreneo, 2013). In the case studies that follow, we take turns to highlight three exemplars of these collective efforts, each utilising Community Psychology tactics for change: (1) generating and sharing knowledge (written by Pierce), (2) organising and capacitating fellow psychologists (written by Bea), and (3) collaborating with activists and mobilising local LGBT+ communities towards social change (written by Moniq).

LGBT+ psychology knowledge generation and dissemination (Pierce)

Recognising the invisibility of LGBT+ themes in the curriculum, we designed and have delivered an undergraduate special topics module titled "LGBT Psychology" in three campuses of the University of the Philippines (UP). It was first offered at the Diliman campus of UP by Eric in 2010 and subsequently adopted in two other campuses: in Tacloban by Pierce in 2014 and in Iloilo by Moniq in 2015. As an elective module, LGBT+ Psychology examines contemporary theorising and empirical research in psychological science related to the lives and experiences of LGBT+ individuals, couples, families and communities in Filipino and global contexts. It is available to both psychology and non-psychology undergraduate students, who at the end of the semester are expected to: (1) define sexual orientation and gender identity/expression (SOGIE) as key psychological ideas; (2) argue how and when SOGIE function as critical factors in various domains of psychological life; (3) explain current theories, models and empirical research in LGBT+ psychology; (4) appreciate the diversity and richness of LGBT+ lives and experiences; (5) critique various claims made regarding LGBT+ and heterosexual-cisgender people in and outside psychology; and (6) demonstrate respect for the rights and well-being of LGBT+ people.

The module delivery follows four tenets that are reflective of Community Psychology principles (Kagan et al., 2020). First, we take an evidence-informed, human rights-based approach by discussing empirical studies that emphasise the rights and well-being of LGBT+ communities. Second, the module incorporates participatory, experiential learning through activities such as social experiments, guest lectures and advocacy events. Many of our class activities highlight playful, subversive ways of learning about and challenging normative notions of gender and sexuality. For example, in one popular exercise, students collectively engage in "gender trouble" (Butler, 1990) for a day, by deliberately subverting their usual gender presentation in appearance and clothing in nonconforming ways, going about their usual activities such as attending classes, taking public transportation and so on while observing their own and other people's reactions to their genderqueer persona. The students then write reflectively about their experience, which usually elicits deep realisations about the struggles of gender-nonconforming individuals and the power of queering and troubling gender. Third, the module is LGBT+ affirmative and intersectional; we teach the module using a critical stance against heteronormativity and cisgenderism. Often this is the only module in our students' academic life where the central focus is the lives and experiences of LGBT+ people. We also make an effort to amplify the voices of relatively underrepresented members within LGBT+ communities, such as bisexual and trans individuals, older LGBT+ people and those with disabilities such as Deaf LGBT+ Filipinos. Finally, the module is anchored on principles of social justice and change. The module presents LGBT+ issues as social and community issues rather than individual problems, and we critique heteronormative, cisgenderist assumptions and practices, reflect on power structures that affect LGBT+ people's lives and deconstruct the meanings attached to the identities of gender and sexual minority groups.

One of the challenges we faced early on in teaching LGBT+ Psychology was the dearth of knowledge resources on the lives and experiences of LGBT+ Filipinos. When we started teaching this module, we relied mostly on Western references. In 2013, following the adage "create the things you wish existed", we set out to build a knowledge base of Filipino LGBT+ psychology through the publication of the first special LGBT+ issue of the *Philippine Journal of Psychology* (edited by Eric), followed by a second issue in 2016 (edited by Eric, Bea, along with our colleague Mira Ofreneo). These special issues featured original studies, conducted by Filipino psychologists, about Filipino LGBT+ lives and experiences. We also addressed the issue of limited knowledge by collaborating with members from the LGBT+ community, who share their lived experiences in our classes. For example, LGBT+ individuals talk about coming out, relationships, parenting, stigma, disability, HIV, activism and transgender concerns. These are among the most engaging and memorable in-class sessions for our students, as they are able to engage with Filipino LGBT+ experiences and learn beyond what is offered by their instructors and readings. We continue this practice as a strategy to bring members of the LGBT+ community to the centre of our teaching.

In retrospect, our efforts to "give away" (Miller, 1969) LGBT+ psychology through teaching and knowledge generation served as our academic playground. The limitations we faced along the way made us appreciate the value of community collaboration and of creative problem-solving (referred to in the Filipino language as *diskarte*), allowing us to experiment with strategies to improve the teaching of the module. These same limitations gave rise to opportunities to become better teachers, researchers and advocates by building our knowledge base and collaborating with members of the Filipino LGBT+ community. More importantly, the module afforded our students a chance to engage in action beyond the classroom. Guided by Community Psychology's values of support for community, participation, social justice and respect for diversity (Kagan et al., 2020; Nelson & Prilleltensky, 2010), our teaching and research have legitimised the place of LGBT+ themes in Philippine psychology through knowledge generation and sharing.

Organising within the psychology professional community (Bea)

Another key component of our work in promoting the rights and well-being of LGBT+ Filipinos is organising a community that we ourselves belong to, the community of psychology professionals in the Philippines. Filipino psychologists have worked individually on LGBT+ issues over past decades (e.g. Go-Singco Holmes, 1993), but as the number of Filipino psychologists interested in LGBT+ issues grew, we started to form an informal collective of colleagues who could reach out to each other for collaboration and support. This collective of psychologists and allied mental health professionals with shared advocacies for LGBT+ rights and well-being included Eric, Pierce and Bea, with Moniq eventually joining the group. From 2010, we organised dedicated LGBT+ programming in the annual conferences of two national psychology organisations, the PAP and the Pambansang Samahan sa Sikolohiyang Pilipino

(National Association for Filipino Psychology, PSSP). This contributed towards a gradual increase in the visibility of LGBT+ perspectives in Philippine psychology.

Despite these gains, critical incidents in broader Philippine society led us to seek more institutional ways to engage with issues that affect LGBT+ Filipinos. In February 2013, a national newspaper published an article on gay children in which a clinical psychologist advised parents to "arrest the situation" and warn their children that being gay is "wrong" (Bersola-Babao, 2013). The PAP quickly responded with a statement affirming the profession's position that being gay is non-pathological (PAP, 2013). While our informal collective celebrated the PAP's timely response, we wondered whether there was a need for a dedicated structure within the association to engage with fellow psychologists as well as external stakeholders like the media on LGBT+-related concerns. We dreamt of forming a nationwide network of Filipino psychologists with the capacities, skills and dedication for sustained work on LGBT+ issues.

In January 2014, the PAP officially approved our application for the LGBT Psychology Special Interest Group (PAP LGBT SIG), a formal collective of psychologists working towards LGBT+ rights and well-being. This group, led by Eric and Bea, was the first of its kind in Asia, coordinating activities among Filipino psychologists and external stakeholders such as the media, the LGBT+ activist community and policymakers, with the aim of promoting the rights and well-being of LGBT+ individuals and communities. Official recognition as part of the PAP's organisational structure paved the way for us to pursue this mission through various activities, which have largely focused on capacity building of Filipino psychologists and allied professionals to engage in research, education, advocacy and practice affirmative of LGBT+ identities and experiences. We organised and conducted a series of training workshops that aimed to equip psychologists with the knowledge, skills and efficacy to run what we called "LGBT Psych 101" sessions, public education sessions introducing LGBT+ psychology concepts and principles. Workshop participants went on to conduct LGBT Psych 101 sessions for various audiences within and outside the psychological community, including LGBT+ youth, educators, police officials and the private sector. We also conducted writing workshops for researchers doing empirical studies on Filipino LGBT+ experiences, many of whom later published their work in two LGBT+ issues of the *Philippine Journal of Psychology*. As described in the previous section, these publications addressed gaps in knowledge on LGBT+ issues in the Philippines.

Since 2014, we have been building a critical mass of members of LGBT+ psychologists. The number of PAP LGBT SIG members has continued to increase. This growth is in part due to shared goals such as social justice and inclusion, goals which resonate with some of the central values that guide community psychologists (Kagan et al., 2020; Nelson & Prilleltensky, 2010). Many of our activities have been guided by the principle of "nothing about us without us" (Charlton, 1998) through the involvement of speakers from grassroots LGBT+ organisations beyond the psychology community. For psychologists who participated in these activities, hearing personal LGBT+ Filipino accounts helped deepen their understanding of how inequality and exclusion impact well-being, and strengthen their commitment to social change.

In addition, a sense of queer playfulness and irreverent humour interwoven into many of our activities have fostered a sense of community among our group's members, many of whom identify as LGBT+. These include: encouraging members to explore drag and genderqueer identities during strategic planning workshops (fondly called "strut planning" sessions), facilitating a "pansexual speed dating"-style activity during meetings to encourage newer and older members to mingle with each other, and marching together during Pride Marches whilst carrying signs that say "Gay kids need your love, not our counselling", "Gay or straight, happiness will find you", and "Out, proud, and single psychologist. Call me!" These strategies are some ways we subvert the conventional formality of organised psychology and forge a group grounded not just in our professional identities but in our personal and political ones as well.

Success in organising notwithstanding, one challenge we have faced is working with clinical and counselling practitioners to ensure the provision of LGBT+ affirmative services. Despite well-received capacity-building efforts in this area, we continue to receive informal reports of non-affirmative practice. This may reflect gaps in training in the Philippines. As Salvador (2016) points out, there is a lack of LGBT+ affirmative training in Philippine clinical and counselling psychology. At a deeper level, this may also be grounded in a disconnect between the dominant, individually focused approaches in clinical/counselling psychology versus those emphasised in LGBT+ rights and well-being work which, similar to Community Psychology, takes a systems-oriented perspective that focuses on challenging and changing social structures towards social justice (Nelson & Prilleltensky, 2010). Recently, in order to introduce an LGBT+-inclusive perspective across practice areas, we have collaborated with colleagues from the PAP's clinical and counselling psychology divisions to conduct workshops on LGBT+ affirmative psychosocial support practice. Similar training sessions on incorporating LGBT+ experiences in the teaching of psychology and on parenting LGBT+ youth have also been made possible by collaborations with other groups within and outside the PAP. These experiences provide promising examples of how collaboration across subdisciplines can strengthen our ability to address issues at multiple levels (Kloos, 2016).

Despite challenges we continue to face, our work within organised psychology has led to significant gains in empowering Filipino psychologists to engage in education, research, practice and advocacy for LGBT+ rights and well-being. Using strategies informed by Community Psychology principles of social justice, inclusion and collaboration, we have found ways to work as "agents for social change" in our roles as insiders in an organisation (Nelson & Prilleltensky, 2010).

Collaborating with LGBT+ activists and communities (Moniq)

Apart from knowledge generation and professional community development, a third exemplar of our work is direct collaboration with local LGBT+ activist groups to mobilise for LGBT+ rights, in situations where there are limited resources, calling upon the need for *diskarte* (creative problem-solving), often in playful, unconventional ways.

In Tacloban, for example, community activities such as LGBT+ Pride were not commonplace in the city. In March 2016, efforts by Pierce and his LGBT psychology class resulted in a city-wide mobilisation. What started as a small class project evolved into an annual Pride Week celebration, where psychology students spearheaded events and activities that became safe spaces for the local LGBT+ community and allies. By its fourth year, Pierce and his LGBT+ psychology students, along with the university student council and student organisations, partnered with the local business sector, the local commission on human rights and department of health, and LGBT+ organisations. With the steady growth of this annual event, they tapped resources within and outside the university. As psychology students developed the tradition of organising the Pride Week celebration for the city, plans of action and budgeting were set to ensure week-long activities for the community could be sustained. For instance, Pierce and his students creatively tapped university funds, initiated fundraising activities (e.g. selling income-generating products such as rainbow-themed shirts, pins, stickers, flags), and established resource-sharing practices between the private and public sectors.

The experience in the Iloilo campus is similar: from teaching an LGBT Psychology module to leading a province-wide, psychologist-led mobilisation of the LGBT+ community. In 2015, when the LGBT Psychology module was first offered in the Iloilo campus, students went on social media to share a call for equality, inclusivity, social justice and a collective community. LGBT+ activists reached out and linked with us, having seen on social media that there was an LGBT+ module being taught at the university. Together we organised the first Pride March in Iloilo City in 2015, with about 200 people participating. Through continued collaboration with activists, this has now become an annual event, with more than 5,000 attendees in 2019, the largest Pride March in this part of the Philippines.

Furthermore, reflecting the sources of values such as vision, context, needs and action nestled within Community Psychology (Nelson & Prilleltensky, 2010), our alliance of psychologists and activists worked with key institutions and city officials, paving the way for the passage of two landmark anti-discrimination public policies, at the province level (2016) and at the city level (2018). These policies protect LGBT+ people in Iloilo from discrimination in employment, housing, social services, education and other settings. This policy also led to the establishment of an LGBT Affairs Office as part of the city government structure in 2019.

Social change, collective engagement and community-led political action are tethered tenets in the practice of Community Psychology (Kagan et al., 2020). In pursuit of social change, our engagement with LGBT+ activists towards policy development and formation has involved key tactics, such as crafting policy statements and sending amicus letters in support of proposed legislation. Bea and Eric have participated in parliamentary hearings for proposed national laws on anti-discrimination and on same-sex civil unions, in order to deliver the "official" perspective of the psychology profession. As a group we have also engaged with media by releasing public statements and using psychological science to challenge anti-LGBT+ stereotypes and biases through radio and television interviews. Across these domains, collaborating with the LGBT+ community to organise events and dialogues has been one of our effective tactics to gain momentum to enact social change. Guided by Community Psychology's principles of active collaboration, the curating of strategies at multiple levels, and recognition of the need for change (Moritsugu et al., 2014), our group has leveraged a critical mass of diverse and dedicated psychologists, academics, psychology teachers, students and mental health practitioners to collaborate directly with activists and the broader LGBT+ community.

Reflections as LGBT+ psychologists taking action

The three case studies presented above highlight the ways that we have worked, as LGBT+ psychologists, to advance LGBT+ rights and well-being in the Philippines. In this final section, we reflect on our work in this part of the world, drawing out broad principles that have underpinned and sustained our collective efforts.

Reaching out beyond academic spaces to build community collaboration

The first reflection point concerns the value, indeed the imperative, of collaborating with communities, including activists and organised groups. Here we take inspiration from the principle of "nothing about us without us" (Charlton, 1998). Originating from the work of disability rights movements in the 1990s, this principle refers to the idea that no policy about (or activity that purports to describe, analyse or create change in) the lives of a particular community should be decided without the participation and voice of members of that community.

We have applied this principle throughout our work in advancing LGBT+ rights and well-being. In developing and teaching the module on LGBT+ psychology, we have sought the voice and expertise of LGBT+ activists, in the form of guest resource persons, consultants for module content and delivery, and partners in knowledge exchange. We bring our students outside of the classroom and into spaces and places where they can engage LGBT+ communities, such as Pride events. In certain instances, this partnership has led to direct and sustained engagements with the community, as in the case of organising local Pride events and advocating for public policy alongside LGBT+ activists.

Diskarte: *creative problem-solving*

As LGBT+ psychologists in a context where psychology as a profession is relatively young, small and undervalued (Barron et al., 2020), we are conscious of working in a so-called resource-limited setting (Geiling et al., 2014). Indeed, there are considerable challenges in capacity, resources and knowledge in the Philippines, compared to other countries where LGBT+ psychology organising has had longer histories (Horne et al., 2019).

Throughout our work we apply the notion of *diskarte*, a Filipino concept referring to the process of creative problem-solving in the face of resource constraints and social inequalities (Morales, 2017). *Diskarte* involves elements of strategic improvisation and resourcefulness in order to navigate limited opportunities and uncertainties (Cajilig, 2017). We engaged in *diskarte*, for example, when faced with the lack of community events such as Pride celebrations for students to participate in. We guided them through the process of organising such an event, given the limited time and resources available to us. As another example, when faced with the dual problem of having no contextualised knowledge resources to support our teaching and not having a critical mass of trained academic researchers doing LGBT+ psychology research, we obtained funding and ran capacity building workshops on publishing LGBT+ studies, which led to the two special LGBT+ issues of the PJP, that later became the set of core readings for our classes.

Queering: playfulness and subversion

Another element that has enabled us to sustain our work is a sense of collective playfulness and subversion that can be referred to as *queering* (or in Filipino, *baklaan*). Here we use the notion of *queer* (as a verb) to mean an approach marked by "tactical frivolity [...] and playful building of a more emancipatory and caring world" (Shepard, 2010, p. 1). This playfulness can be used to subvert normative ways of thinking and doing, to uncover systems of power, to achieve group goals and possibly, "to mess up the desexualised spaces of the academy" and "to exude some rut" (Warner, 1993, p. xxvi). Observers of our LGBT+ psychologists' professional group's activities have remarked that ours are often full of laughter, theatricality, irony, wordplay, even flirtatious innuendo and erotic playfulness – often the very opposite of traditional notions of "professional". This is not to say that we do not take our work in psychology and LGBT+ rights seriously; if anything, we aim to take it so hyper-seriously that in doing so, we uncover and challenge normative ways of doing "proper psychology" – and have some fun along the way.

Doing LGBT+ Community Psychology and being LGBT+ community psychologists

One key factor in our work is that we position ourselves as members of the extended LGBT+ community, as lesbian or gay people or as heterosexual allies, alongside our professional identity as university-based psychologists. Professional identities such as "psychologist" or "academic" confer a certain degree of power, which we have at times taken advantage of in order to advance our social change agenda. In these instances, we have positioned ourselves as "psychologist" or "academic" or "representative of the PAP" in order to bring the authority of professional voice to the table, whilst at the same time, disrupting biased stereotypical notions of LGBT+ people. At the same time, we acknowledge that inhabiting these multiple identities (e.g. being gay *and* being a psychologist, being an academic *and* being a member of a sexual minority) does not necessarily confer a more "complete" perspective that can represent the views and lived experiences of the diverse spectrum of the LGBT+ community. This is precisely why we strive to work collaboratively, with each other and with activists as we build LGBT+ psychology in the Philippines.

Furthermore, we acknowledge that we have, in many respects, been engaged in the work of Community Psychology, without necessarily labelling ourselves as "community psychologists" or our work as "Community Psychology" explicitly (see also Harper & Wilson, 2017). As in many Asian countries, Community Psychology as a formal specialisation does not exist in the Philippines (Reich et al., 2017). However, our work resonates with many of the core principles, values and tactics that have been developed in Critical Community Psychology, including but not limited to: an explicit value base of equality, rights and well-being (particularly for LGBT+ people); an epistemology whereby knowledge is contextually built and given away for emancipatory ends; a vision of a "radically better society" (Fox, 2000); and tactics of working with a community that are simultaneously creative and responsive to resource constraints (in Filipino: *madiskarte*) as well as playful and subversive of conventional modes of doing and being (queering).

Conclusion

The aims of this chapter were to extend the analysis of gender as a systemic crisis to centre the less explored but related dimensions of *sexual orientation and gender identity/expression* (SOGIE) and to describe and reflect on our work and experiences as psychologists taking action for the rights and well-being of LGBT+ communities in the Philippines. We believe that by recognising and applying key principles, strategies and perspectives used by critical community psychologists, we can imagine – and create – social change that empowers lesbian, gay, bisexual, transgender and other gender and sexual minorities in the Philippines and beyond.

References

Abalos, J.B. (2017). Divorce and separation in the Philippines: Trends and correlates. *Demographic Research, 36*, 1515–48. https://doi.org/10.4054/DemRes.2017.36.50

Abinales, P.N., & Amoroso, D.J. (2017). *State and society in the Philippines* (2nd ed.). Rowman & Littlefield.

Anderson, J., & Holland, E. (2015). The legacy of medicalising "homosexuality": A discussion on the historical effects of non-heterosexual diagnostic classifications. *Sensoria: A Journal of Mind, Brain & Culture, 11*(1), 4–15. https://doi.org/10.7790/sa.v11i1.405

Atadero, O.E., Umbac, S.A., &Cruz, C.J.P. (2014). Kwentongbebot: Lived experiences of lesbians, bisexual and transgender women in the Philippines. In G. Poore & G. Cristobal, G. (Eds.), *Violence: Through the lens of lesbians, bisexual women and transgender people in Asia* (pp. 61–94). International Gay and Lesbian Human Rights Commission.

Barron, D., Khatib, N.A.M., & Lim, H.E.T.K. (2020). Psychology in the Philippines: An overview of the state of the discipline emphasising sociocultural, clinical, and health perspectives. In G.J. Rich, J.L.S. Jaafar, & D. Barron (Eds.), *Psychology in Southeast Asia: Sociocultural, clinical, and health perspectives* (pp. 14–32). Routledge. https://doi.org/10.4324/9780367823566

Bersola-Babao, T. (2013, March 11). Being gay. *Philippine Star.* www.philstar.com/entertainment/2013/03/11/918157/being–gay

Blondeel, K., de Vasconcelos, S., García-Moreno, C., Stephenson, R., Temmerman, M., & Toskin, I. (2018). Violence motivated by perception of sexual orientation and gender identity: A systematic review. *Bulletin of the World Health Organization, 96*(1), 29–41L. https://doi.org/10.2471/blt.17.197251

British Psychological Society. (2018). *Guidance for psychologists working with community organisations.* www.bps.org.uk/sites/www.bps.org.uk/files/Policy/Policy%20-%20Files/Guidance%20for%20 psychologists%20on%20working%20with%20community%20organisations%20%28Sep%202018%29. PDF

Butler, J. (1990). *Gender trouble: Feminism and the subversion of identity.* Routledge.

Cajilig, P.G. (2017). Designing life after the storm: Improvisations in post-disaster housing reconstruction as socio-moral practice. *AVANT, 8,* 79–88. http://doi.org/10.26913/80s02017.0111.0008

Calleja, K.S., Concepcion, N., de Jesus, J., Ramos, M., Fontanos, N., & Manglinong, Z. (2020). Struggling from the margins to the intersectionalities of power: The state of lesbian, gay, bisexual, transgender, intersex, queer (LGBTIQ) Filipinos from 2015 to 2020. In R.P. Ofreneo & J.F.I. Illo (Eds.), *Philippine NGO Beijing+25 report* (pp. 353–84). UP Center for Women's and Gender Studies.

Charlton, J.I. (1998). *Nothing about us without us.* University of California Press.

Commission on Elections. (2009, November). *Resolution in the matter of the petition for registration of Ang Ladlad LGBT Party for the party-list system of representation in the House of Representatives* (SPP no. 09-22). www.comelec.gov.ph/?r=Archives/RegularElections/2010NLE/Resolutions/spp09228

Cruz, C.J.P., & Mallari, R.B.C. (2007). Revisiting social acceptance of homosexuality among Filipino youth: Some theoretical and methodological implications. *Philippine Population Review, 6*(1), 45–70.

Dickey, L.M. (2020). History of gender identity and mental health. In E.D. Rothblum (Ed.), *The Oxford handbook of sexual and gender minority mental health* (pp. 25–34). Oxford University Press. https://doi. org/10.1093/oxfordhb/9780190067991.013.3

Docena, P.S. (2013). Developing and managing one's sexual identity: Coming out stories of Waray gay adolescents. *Philippine Journal of Psychology, 46*(2), 75–103.

Evangelista, Z.M., Dumaop, D.E., & Nelson, G. (2016). Journeying to a safe space: Sexual and religious identity integration of Filipino LGBT-affirmative church members. *Philippine Journal of Psychology, 49*(2), 101–33.

Florendo, M., Salinas-Ramos, T., & San Luis, M. (2013). Critical research in Philippine community psychology. *Annual Review of Critical Psychology, 10,* 784–800. https://thediscourseunit.files.wordpress. com/2016/05/philippines-ii-784-800.pdf

Flores, A. (2019). *Social acceptance of LGBT people in 174 countries: 1981 to 2017.* The Williams Institute. https://williamsinstitute.law.ucla.edu/wp-content/uploads/Global-Acceptance-Index-LGBT+-Oct-2019.pdf

Formby, E. (2019). *Exploring LGBT spaces and communities: Contrasting identities, belongings and wellbeing.* Routledge.

Fox, D. (2000). The critical psychology project: Transforming society and transforming psychology. In T. Sloan (Ed.), *Critical psychology: Voices for change* (pp. 21–33). Macmillan.

GALANG Philippines. (2013). *Social protection policies and urban poor LBTs in the Philippines.* Institute of Development Studies. https://opendocs.ids.ac.uk/opendocs/bitstream/handle/20.500.12413/ 2892/ER21Policy_Audit_Social_Protection_Policies_and_Urban_Poor_LBTs_in_the_Philippines. pdf?sequence=7

GALANG Philippines. (2015). *How Filipino LBTs cope with economic disadvantage.* Institute of Development Studies. www.ids.ac.uk/publications/how-filipino-lbts-cope-with-economic-disadvantage/

Garcia, J.N. (2013). Nativism or universalism: Situating LGBT discourse in the Philippines. *Kritika Kultura,* 48–68. https://doi.org/10.13185/kk2013.02003

Geiling, J., Burkle, F.M., Amundson, D., Dominguez-Cherit, G., Gomersall, C.D., Lim, M.L., Luyckx, V., Sarani, B., Uyeki, T.M., West, T.E., Christian, M.D., Devereaux, A.V., Dichter, J.R., & Kissoon, N. (2014). Resource-poor settings: Infrastructure and capacity building. *Chest, 146*(4), e156Se167S. https://doi.org/10.1378/chest.14-0744

GoSingco-Holmes, M. (1993). *A different love: Being gay in the Philippines.* Anvil.

Guevara, C.C.A. (2016). Life satisfaction among older Filipino sexual minorities and their experiences of support. *Philippine Journal of Psychology, 49*(2), 135–55.

Harper, G.W., & Schneider, M. (2003). Oppression and discrimination among lesbian, gay, bisexual, and transgendered people and communities: A challenge for community psychology. *American Journal of Community Psychology, 31*(3), 243–52. https://doi.org/10.1023/A:1023906620085

Harper, G.W., & Wilson, B.D.M. (2017). Situating sexual orientation and gender identity diversity in context and communities. In M.A. Bond, I. Serrano-García, C.B. Keys, &M. Shinn (Eds.), *APA handbook of community psychology: Theoretical foundations, core concepts, and emerging challenges* (pp. 387–402). American Psychological Association. https://doi.org/10.1037/14953-019

Horne, S.G., Maroney, M.R., Nel, J.A., Chaparro, R.A., & Manalastas, E.J. (2019). Emergence of a transnational LGBTI psychology: Commonalities and challenges in advocacy and activism. *American Psychologist*, 74(8), 967–86. https://doi.org/10.1037/amp0000561

Kagan, C., Burton, M., Duckett, P., Lawthom, R., & Siddiquee, A. (2020). *Critical community psychology: Critical action and social change* (2nd ed.). Routledge.

Kagan, C., & Lewis, S. (2015, May 19–22). *Community, work and family and the metamorphosis of social change* [Keynote address]. 6th Community, Work and Family Conference, Malmo, Sweden. http://eprints.mdx.ac.uk/17580/

Kloos, B. (2016). Cultivating community psychology for future generations: Symbiosis, synergy, and separation. *American Journal of Community Psychology*, 58(3–4), 303–8. https://doi.org/10.1002/ajcp.12105

Macapagal, R.A. (2013). Further validation of the Genderism and Transphobia Scale in the Philippines. *Philippine Journal of Psychology*, 46(2), 49–59.

Manalastas, E.J., Ojanen, T.T., Torre, B.A., Ratanashevorn, R., Choong, B., Kumaresan, V., & Veeramuthu, V. (2017). Homonegativity in Southeast Asia: A comparison of attitudes toward lesbians and gay men in Indonesia, Malaysia, the Philippines, Singapore, Thailand, and Vietnam. *Asia-Pacific Social Science Review*, 17(1), 25–33. http://apssr.com/wp-content/uploads/2018/03/2manalastas-053017-1.pdf

Manalastas, E.J., & Torre, B.A. (2016). LGBT psychology in the Philippines. *Psychology of Sexualities Review*, 7(1), 60–72.

McSherry, A., Manalastas, E.J., Gaillard, J.C., & Dalisay, S.N.M. (2015). From deviant to bakla, strong to stronger: Mainstreaming sexual and gender minorities into disaster risk reduction in the Philippines. *Forum for Development Studies*, 42(1), 27–40. https://doi.org/10.1080/08039410.2014.952330

Mendos, L.R., Botha, K., Lelis, R.C., de la Peña, E.L., Savelev, I., & Tan, D. (2020). *State-sponsored homophobia 2020: Global legislation overview update*. International Lesbian, Gay, Bisexual, Trans and Intersex Association. https://ilga.org/state-sponsored-homophobia-report

Miller, G.A. (1969). Psychology as a means of promoting human welfare. *American Psychologist*, 24, 1063–75. https://psycnet.apa.org/doi/10.1037/h0028988

Moore, M.R., & Stambolis-Ruhstorfer, M. (2013). LGBT sexuality and families at the start of the twenty-first century. *Annual Review of Sociology*, 39(1), 491–507. https://doi.org/10.1146/annurev-soc-071312-145643

Morales, M.R.H. (2017). Defining diskarte: Exploring cognitive processes, personality traits, and social constraints in creative problem-solving. *Philippine Journal of Psychology*, 50(2), 114–39.

Moritsugu, J., Vera, E., Wong, F., & Duffy, K. (2014). *Community psychology* (5th ed.). Routledge.

Muyargas, M.M., Manalastas, E.J., & Docena, P.S. (2016). The "I ♥ lesbian and gay rights" pin: An experiential learning exercise to understand anti-LGBT+ stigma. *Philippine Journal of Psychology*, 49(2), 173–88.

Nelson, G.B., & Prilleltensky, I. (2010). *Community psychology: In pursuit of liberation and well-being*. Palgrave Macmillan.

Ochoa, D.P., Sio, C.P., Quiñones, D.W., & Manalastas, E.J. (2016). A bond between man and woman: Religiosity, moral foundations, and same-sex marriage attitudes in the Philippines. *Philippine Journal of Psychology*, 49(2), 157–71.

Office of the United Nations High Commissioner for Human Rights (OHCHR). (2019). *Born free and equal: Sexual orientation, gender identity and se characteristics in international human rights law* (2nd ed.). www.ohchr.org/Documents/Publications/Born_Free_and_Equal_WEB.pdf

Ofreneo, M.A.P. (2013). Towards an LGBT-inclusive psychology: Reflecting on a social change agenda for Philippine psychology. *Philippine Journal of Psychology*, 46(2), 5–17.

Peplau, L.A., & Fingerhut, A.W. (2007). The close relationships of lesbians and gay men. *Annual Review of Psychology*, 58, 405–24. https://doi.org/10.1146/annurev.psych.58.110405.085701

Psychological Association of the Philippines. (2011). Statement of the Psychological Association of the Philippines on non-discrimination based on sexual orientation, gender identity and expression. *Philippine Journal of Psychology*, 44(2), 229–30.

Psychological Association of the Philippines. (2013, March 13). PH psychologists speak out on "Being Gay": "It's NOT a disease. It's NOT a disorder". *InterAksyon*. www.interaksyon.com/article/57043/statement-ph-psychologists-speak-out-on-beinggay-its-not-a-disease-its-not-a-disorder

Reich, S.M., Bishop, B., Carolissen, R., Dzidic, P., Portillo, N., Sasao, T., & Stark, W. (2017). Catalysts and connections: The (brief) history of community psychology throughout the world. In M.A. Bond, I. Serrano-García, C.B. Keys, &M. Shinn (Eds.), *APA handbook of community psychology: Theoretical foundations, core concepts, and emerging challenges* (pp. 21–66). American Psychological Association. https://doi.org/10.1037/14953-002

Rothblum, E.D. (2020). Introduction. In E.D. Rothblum (Ed.), *The Oxford handbook of sexual and gender minority mental health* (pp. 11–24). Oxford University Press. https://doi.org/10.1093/oxfordhb/9780190067991.013.1

Ruiz Austria, C.S. (2004). The church, the state and women's bodies in the context of religious fundamentalism in the Philippines. *Reproductive Health Matters*, *12*(24), 96–103. https://doi.org/10.1016/S0968-8080(04)24152-0

Salvador, D.S.A. (2016). An exploration of ethical and methodological challenges in trans-affirmative psychotherapy with Filipino transgender and gender non-conforming (TGNC) Clients. *Philippine Journal of Psychology*, *49*(2), 189–216.

Sanders, D. (2020). Sex and gender diversity in Southeast Asia. *Journal of Southeast Asian Human Rights*, *4*(2), 357–405. https://doi.org/10.19184/jseahr.v4i2.17281

Shepard, B. (2010). *Queer political performance and protest: Play, pleasure and social movement.* Routledge.

Silan, M.A.A., Rivera, M.A.F., & Chulipa, L.T. (2016). Trans on trains: Lived experiences of Filipina transgender women on the MRT. *Philippine Journal of Psychology*, *46*(2), 35–60.

UNDP, USAID. (2014). *Being LGBT in Asia: The Philippines country report.* United Nations Development Programme. www.undp.org/content/undp/en/home/librarypage/hiv-aids/being-lgbt-in-asia--the-philippine-country-report.html

Warner, M. (Ed.). (1993). *Fear of a queer planet: Queer politics and social theory.* University of Minnesota Press.

Wasco, S.M., & Bond, M.A. (2010). The treatment of gender in community psychology research. In J.C. Chrisler & D.R. McCreary (Eds.), *Handbook of gender research in psychology,* Vol. 2: *Gender research in social and applied psychology* (pp. 613–41). Springer Science + Business Media. https://doi.org/10.1007/978-1-4419-1467-5_26

Widmer, E.D., Treas, J., & Newcomb, R. (1998). Attitudes toward nonmarital sex in 24 countries. *Journal of Sex Research*, *35*(4), 349–58. https://doi.org/10.1080/00224499809551953

World Bank. (2020). *Philippines.* https://data.worldbank.org/country/philippines

Yarcia, L.E., de Vela, T.C., & Tan, M.L. (2019). Queer identity and gender-related rights in post-colonial Philippines. *Australian Journal of Asian Law*, *20*(1), 1–11. https://ssrn.com/abstract=3488543

8

PSYCHOSOCIAL ACCOMPANIMENT FROM A COMMUNITY APPROACH TO VICTIMS OF INTERNAL FORCED DISPLACEMENT IN COLOMBIA[1]

Claudia Tovar Guerra, Stella Sacipa Rodríguez and Laura Muñoz Restrepo

Abstract

This chapter is about the psychosocial accompaniment to victims of internal forced displacement in Colombia from a community perspective. The text has two main sections. In the first section, we present a characterisation of forced displacement in Colombia, offering an overview of its magnitude in figures and facts. Then, we draw attention to the new dynamics of uprooting in Colombia and its relationship with the reconfiguration of power on multiple scales, from the local to the global. In the second section, we go into the details of the psychosocial accompaniment perspective, addressing our working method with the communities from the first approach of familiarisation to the consolidation of psychological and recovery processes. Finally, we discuss the psychosocial consequences of forced displacement in terms of the emotional effects and the rupture of the social fabric. We suggest that due to the validity of the phenomenon it is needed to take preventive actions and a timely reaction facing the psychosocial risks.

Resumen

Este capítulo trata sobre el acompañamiento psicosocial a víctimas de desplazamiento forzado interno en Colombia desde una perspectiva comunitaria. El texto tiene dos apartados principales, el primero presenta una caracterización del desplazamiento forzado en Colombia, ofreciendo un panorama de su magnitud en cifras y hechos. también llama la atención sobre la nueva dinámica del desarraigo en Colombia y su relación con la reconfiguración del poder en múltiples escalas, desde lo local hasta lo global. En el segundo apartado, se adentra en los detalles de la perspectiva del acompañamiento psicosocial, abordando nuestro método de trabajo con las comunidades

DOI: 10.4324/9780429325663-11

desde el primer abordaje de familiarización hasta la consolidación de procesos psicológicos y de recuperación. Finalmente, discutimos las consecuencias psicosociales del desplazamiento forzado en términos de los efectos emocionales y la ruptura del tejido social. Sugerimos que por la vigencia del fenómeno es necesario tomar acciones y una reacción oportuna ante los riesgos psicosociales.

Forced displacement in Colombia

Of the nearly nine million victims left by the armed conflict in Colombia, it is estimated that more than 7,500,000 have been expelled from their territories and places of residence (Unit for Attention and Integral Reparation to Victims, UARIV, 2020). This figure places Colombia in the first place for internal forced displacement among all the countries in the world. Moreover, this figure alerts us to the violent conflict that exists in the country.

Technically, according to Colombian legislation,

> A displaced person is any that has been forced to migrate within the national territory, leaving their place of residence or usual economic activities, because their life, physical integrity, security, or personal freedom have been violated or are directly threatened, on the occasion of any of the following situations: internal armed conflict, internal disturbances, and tensions, generalised violence, massive violations of Human Rights, infractions of International Humanitarian Law or other circumstances arising from the previous situations that may alter or drastically alter public order.
>
> *(Law 387 1997, art. 1)*

Historical background

The long history of violent confrontations in Colombia has led to significant forced migration that can be traced back to the colony (Tovar, 2006). The civil wars of the late 19th and the early 20th century continued with the forced exodus of people. An important escalation of displacement happened in the so-called period of the Violence (1948–1964):

> In the period of the Violence of the mid-century, around 300,000 deaths were registered, and the number of internally displaced persons is estimated at two million, during profound restructuration processes of land ownership. A very high figure, which at the time corresponded to ten percent of the total population. But the history of this forced displacement has not even been written.
>
> *(Rojas and Romero, 2000, p. 6)*

Even so, the use of the term "internal forced displacement" and the first official records available in Colombia are very recent, having been in existence since 1985 (Episcopal Conference, recovered by CODHES in 1994) (CODHES and UNICEF Colombia, 1998) (RUT, the information system of the National Secretariat of Pastoral Social) and 1999 (Red de Solidaridad Social, now Acción Social). The current armed conflict is considered, by consensus, as the scene of the escalation of displacement in recent decades, which has drawn the attention of various social sectors that have given it not only visibility but also academic, media and legal existence as a social problem. Its most recognised causes are the struggle for land tenure, the control of political power and the generational transmission of hatred.

Over time, this scenario, with its actors, has led to a deep degradation that is widespread throughout the national territory. The irregular forces have impinged upon the political structure and the economic powers as never before anticipated. Furthermore, in the last two decades, the armed conflict has proven to be, more than an ideological dispute, a war of exile at the service of legal and illegal extractive economies. The proportion of displaced persons to the total number of victims in Colombia has increased to 84.8%.

Currently, the consequences of violence represent a serious ethical and humanitarian crisis, that is seen on the world stage as a highly complex conflict. Despite the recent peace process between the government and the *Fuerzas Armadas Revolucionarias de Colombia–Ejército del Pueblo* (FARC-EP; Revolutionary Armed Forces of Colombia–People's Army) in 2016, which resulted in a final peace agreement, we are witnessing a new escalation of violence. Although, it is recognised that the periods after peace agreements and the beginning of their implementation tend towards an escalation of violence, the scale of this has exceeded all forecasts. We need to seek how to understand the recent intensification of violence and forced displacement.

Forced displacement in the post-agreement period

The peace agreement promised, since its negotiation in Havana, Cuba (2012–2016), the reduction of the intensity of the armed conflict, which reached its lowest point between 2015 and 2016 (Jimenez, 2016). In that time, the FARC-EP changed its military strategy in preparation for the post-conflict. During that period, the guerrilla group chose to reduce confrontations with the public force and concentrated on rebuilding its social base in the territories (Fundación Paz y Reconciliación, 2014).

After the peace agreement, two possible scenarios depended on the political inclinations of the governments which followed. The first, which filled broad sectors of society with hope, consisted of the expansion of democracy with the social and political inclusion of ex-FARC combatants and the economic integration of the territories affected by the armed conflict and illicit crops. The second scenario, about which multiple national and international organisations warned, contemplated the escalation of violence against communities and social leaders in the dispute over the territories previously occupied and controlled by the FARC-EP.

To make the first scenario possible and to mitigate the second one, a strong institutional deployment of the state in the territories was necessary. However, the loss of the plebiscite held on October 2, 2016, and the electoral triumph of the opposition party in the 2018 presidential elections, meant a minimalist implementation of the peace agreement (Dejusticia, 2020).

A government that has not been interested in occupying the territories left by the FARC–EP has established the conditions that now exist following the peace agreement. Thus, there have been limitations to mechanisms for the protection of social leaders, failures in fulfilling the implementation of rural reform programmes and substitution of illicit crops, and a consequent deterioration of security and the resurgence of violence (Torres & Cruz, 2020).

Thus, the first semester of 2018 was considered the most violent semester of the last decade and confirmed the upward trend of violence against the civilian population in all its forms (CODHES, 2018). In the first two months of 2019, this trend continued, with nine events of massive, forced displacement that left 5,000 victims in the departments of Nariño, Norte de Santander, Antioquia and Córdoba (Pacifista, 2019). In total, by the end of 2019, forced displacements increased by 238%, rising from 266 cases in 2018 to 899 cases in 2019 (Fundación Paz y Reconciliación, 2019a); and murders against human rights defenders, increased by 50% in 2019 compared to 2018 (Colombia 2020, 2020).

The increase in forced displacements, homicides and massacres in the last four years responds to the reconfiguration of the armed actors that dispute the strategic territories and their illegal economies – drug trafficking and illegal mining – previously controlled by the FARC-EP. Thus, it continues to be confirmed that in Colombia there are displacements because there is war, but there are also war pretexts for displacement (Vega, 2012).

Leaving the territories, even temporarily, has meant that the displaced persons must remain in precarious conditions in the municipal capitals, generally in schools or improvised settlements provided through international cooperation. A return to the territories, once the confrontations have diminished, means facing the loss of crops, goods and living under the threat and domination of the armed actors, who also restrict the mobility of the populations. In 2019, the United Nations Office for the Coordination of Humanitarian Affairs registered 7,849 cases of confinement, which translates to an increase of 282% compared to the 2,055 registered in 2018 (Fundación Paz y Reconciliación, 2019b).

Researcher Ariel Ávila (Semana, 2020) has pointed out that there is a pattern of systematicity in the murder of leaders. Although the perpetrators have different origins and are generally hitmen, the profile of the victims is similar. He found that 70% of victims may be classified into the following categories of social and community work: presidents of community action boards; those who supervise the actions of councillors; those who inform against corruption; claimants of land and truth; environmental leaders; leaders of ethnic communities, indigenous peoples or Afro communities (Espinosa, 2020).

Although it is difficult to identify a unifying political project between the hitmen, their actions seek to deactivate local organisational processes that oppose or question the economic integration of the territories into a development model based on extractive economies and the concentration of land for agribusiness and livestock.

Forced displacement in the post-agreement time has been concentrated in the collective territories of indigenous and Afro-descendant communities. This is against their human rights and their collective rights over the territory. Long-term profound transformations can happen to the social organisation and ways of life that these groups have historically defended.

This shows that forced displacement is a current issue, and those accompaniment strategies for the people and communities that suffer from it are required more than ever. The community-based approach is considered by governmental (Victim Unit, Agency for Reintegration) and non-governmental institutions to be the most suitable and careful way of accompanying the processes of peacebuilding, reintegration and comprehensive reparation in these complex scenarios, given the political and collective nature of the violence associated with armed conflicts and inequities.

In this chapter, we want to present the experience of psychosocial accompaniment with a community perspective by bringing a paradigmatic case within our experience as a research group. Our work was strongly influenced by the teachings of *The Psychology of Liberation*, by Ignacio Martín Baró S. J., and the Latin American Community Psychology represented by, among other authors, Gabriel Restrepo and Maritza Montero. Undoubtedly, these perspectives were strengthened with values and methodologies from other disciplines such as sentipensante sociology by Orlando Fals Borda, popular education by Paulo Freire, and the popular political pedagogic proposal by the mathematician Germán Zabala.

Our guiding principles can be summarised as follows:

1. To generate processes of awareness and critical thinking in the communities, facilitating social, historical and cultural contextualised reflections.

2. To orientate the work not only towards the change in individuals and their relationships but also towards social change and the transformation of the conditions that generate violence and inequities.
3. To propose a relationship between the psychologist and the community that overcomes the traditional one-sidedness that leaves the psychologist as an active entity who possesses knowledge about reality and the community as a passive entity in the relationship.
4. To validate and prioritise the experiential knowledge of the people and their collective and ancestral knowledge.
5. To strengthen and enhance the community's agency to facilitate their processes of change and their social and political demands.
6. To respect and recognise the singularities of groups and individuals to avoid generalisations and homogenising interventions.
7. To work in coordination with other disciplines and with diverse social sectors.

Fieldwork methodology in psychosocial accompaniment

In 2001, our team of professors and students from the Peace Cultures Project, from the Faculty of Psychology of the Pontificia Universidad Javeriana, agreed to accept an invitation made by an ecology professor who worked with the Corporation for Education Development and the Peace (Cedepaz), an organisation of people who suffered forced displacement from their lands of origin and came to live in the outskirts of Bogotá. There, we had our first experience of psychosocial accompaniment to an organisation of victims of armed conflict with the focus of Community Psychology.

An ethical and political understanding of the armed conflict lived in Colombia guided our decision for a methodology committed to life. We had the conviction that building peace means working for social justice, promoting the dignity of people who suffer forced displacement, and starting from the perspective that accompanying means "being with, giving warmth of life, renewing trust, feeling the presence of the other, listening lovingly" (Sacipa, Tovar, & Galindo, 2005, p. 11). We found a community receptive to service but distrustful of its pain and suffering. Through conversation and accompaniment to its consolidation as an organisation, we showed them what we could offer as social psychologists (Sacipa, 2015), and as one of them would later say, little by little, "we were enchanted" with each other.

We opted for a multi-method methodology. We started with Participatory Action Research (PAR) (one of the bases of Community Psychology in Latin America), as a critical, liberating and dialogical process where the community is the subject of the process and a valid interlocutor of the professionals who share their knowledge. The field diary was the first tool we used, and with which we made the initial recognition of the area. We walked through the neighbourhood, chatted with the people with whom we were going to work, and we got to know the context in which they lived.

From the first visits, the team intended to weave ties with the community. When peasant families suffer forced displacement, they have been at the receiving end of multiple violence, which leads them to experience interactions with great mistrust. Aware of this, we sought to create bridges that would enable the building of a trusting psychosocial relationship aiming to touch the heart of the other with one's own (Sacipa & Tovar, 2002). Using the participant observation technique formulated by the PAR, we made a series of successive approaches. We regularly attended Cedepaz meetings and in a systematic psychosocial accompaniment process, we supported them in their organisational process.

In the second moment, we proposed to recover the history of their community organisation. Our conceptual framework started from the understanding that the psychosocial occurs in the interaction between the psychic and the social. It is the result of history and culture (Vygotski, 1973), and the person's "psychological" is built-in relationships, through social interaction. We share with Vygotski (1973) the centrality of the word "meaning", with Bruner (1991) the mediating role of meaning in symbolic activities, to build and make sense of the world and people themselves. We also share UNESCO's peace culture (1999) and its calling to create a movement aimed at initiating the transition from a war culture to a peace culture.

Once the community agreed, we used the oral history technique with open question interviews (Uribe, 1992, p. 34) to inquire through the language of the interviewees how they built their organisation. In their narrations, we found the meanings they constructed from living a common history. To give this history visibility, our psychology and design students integrated the narrations to make a book, the Cedepaz history book.

In the end, we gathered the entire community together in a workshop to return their history. We presented the book with the organisation's milestones and the meanings of their history using metaphors. Examples of these are: *the mirror*, to show the importance of each member of the organisation; *the sowing*, as the vital trajectory with its stages and difficulties; *the seed*, as the potential of the organisation to take care of life; and *the harvest*, as the moment of reward after all the efforts.

In the psychosocial workshop, we felt the strength of the solidarity bonds that helped the participants become active subjects in the building of their organisation. We also perceived the strength of their dignity, despite the monstrosity of the attacks during the war. In their verbal and bodily expressions, we confirmed the meanings that we had identified before in their narrations.

We found that, as a team, we had built the necessary trust with the community to address the third stage of the investigation, so in interviews through open questions, we summoned life stories of the forced displacement process. As Bruner (1991) did in his study, we designed the interviews to favour the production of meanings through the narratives. We generated the conditions that allowed displaced people, in a reflective movement, to give meaning to their experience and to resignify the displacement process to which they were subjected in armed conflict; therefore, the interviews were held in an ethical context where respect was the guiding value.

At the end of this stage, we held a workshop to return the personal stories. From a contextualised perspective, the workshop was designed to enable people to resignify the pain and repair their wounds from a perspective that builds non-violent cultures. We used three strategies. The first, through directed conversation, sought to break the silencing. The second involved the movement of the body. The third was the bodily release of emotions, wherein we worked through deep relaxation on the release of pain, on validation, and the release of anger, and fear management.

By collecting the memory of their experiences, in the narratives, with tears and smiles, each one of the participants recalled, named and resignified their experience of forced displacement. Sharing the life stories with their protagonists gave us the possibility of walking along other paths with them.

The results of the interviews also showed us the way to project new activities with the community. We combined an understanding of complexity in our research with community psychosocial support, drawing on dialogue between the team of teachers, interns and people from the community. We proposed that working with memories should be linked to practice, in spaces where people can share, give meaning and resignify the displacement experience, providing support to individuals and groups.

Our tools for community work

We used a number of tools in our work with communities, including active listening, activities organised by age and gender, and strengthening community organisation.

1. Active listening in informal spaces was an irreplaceable tool, both with women and men. In the context of urban political violence in which they lived, many psychosocial dynamics couldn't be expressed in public groups and were manifested quietly in the face-to-face encounter in private spaces with a companion (Sacipa & Tovar, 2004). With men in arranged meetings, whether at home, in the park or elsewhere, that would give them confidence. With women, in the visits to their home, the conversations took on a nuance of affective depth, were rich in details and allowed for redefining the meanings of the feelings of pain and disability.

   To promote advances in the accompaniment in these private spaces, without falling into the pathologisation of the experience, we based our work on theoretical approaches regarding conversational strategies that maintain the centrality of context and gave priority to the narrators' tools (Polkinghorne, 1988; Lieblich, 1998; Goncalves, 2002; Payne, 2000).

2. **Community meetings and activities were by designed gender and generation**. These were spaces designed to explore what it meant to be an uprooted peasant, expelled from Mother Earth. The peasant culture required us to speak its language, move in its rhythms and design the activities together (Sacipa & Tovar, 2004), thereby ensuring they were relevant and appropriate.

   a. **With women**: first, we sought the consolidation of bonds of trust between them and other members of the community, as well as the recognition of their personal and social potential to recover, develop a future with dignity, and of their capacity to support themselves emotionally (Sacipa & Tovar, 2004). We created group meetings where our work aimed to accompany them in the recovery from the wounds left by the displacement experience. These spaces were empowering and safe. The conversation became a significant tool to overcome the silencing and the paralysing fear, and to recover speech and constructive interaction (Pardo, 2003).

   b. **With young people**, we worked in role-playing games and openness to participation and expression of feelings through the body. According to Álvaro Restrepo (2003), those exercises allow a renewed understanding of the body as an essential element of the human condition and expression.

      Our interns, students of ecology and students of psychology carried out workshops with the young children of the members of Cedepaz where they integrated the body, the ecological look, the link with nature, respect, listening to each other and affectivity. They let their imagination fly, put it on stage while dramatizing and dancing, mapping the territory and seeking to go beyond fear.

      In the workshop design, we cared about the interplay of three elements: the construction of oneself (translated into the roles that they adopted); the construction of others (friendships, competition etc); and the contextual conditions that lead to constant change (choices and decisions). That interlinked game presented different dynamics to deconstruct and construct (Forero & Concha, 2003). In the psychosocial accompaniment of young people, we understood that the city had elements of additional violence. In addition to the control of the illegal armed group that had expelled them from their place of origin, they encountered in Bogotá, gangs and social cleansing groups who killed young people on the streets of the neighbourhood.

  c. **With the men**, in group meetings, we worked on memory through the recovery of their experiences of the peasant life. We accompanied them in rebuilding trust by listening to them in groups. We fine-tuned their communication channels, their ways of expression and validated their projects. We used meetings and games, such as shuffleboard, as tools to work on the recovery of their autonomy and placed emphasis on the value of unity among them.

3. **Strengthening community organisation**. We sought to empower Cedepaz members, as citizens, in the construction and autonomous management of themselves and their organisation. We gave priority to the initiatives and autonomy of the community in its recovery processes, renouncing the protagonist role of the psychologists in the project so that the voices of its members could guide their dynamics. At the same time, we worked on organisational autonomy through intentional activities guided by questions constructed to unleash ideas and proposals. In this way, we created conditions to facilitate the strengthening of community ties and the construction of relationships based on trust (Sacipa & Tovar, 2004).

Psychosocial consequences of forced displacement

Ignacio Martín Baró (1990) spoke of psychosocial trauma as a socially produced psychic wound in the war. In Colombia, millions of people forced into displacement have suffered this trauma, as well as disappearances, massacres, sexual assault, blackmail and extortion by armed groups. As a woman narrated it:

> *They killed my husband [...] I had to leave the children behind and that was very hard for me. Coming back after three months and finding these boys with very hard psychological trauma, has been very difficult for me [...] and for them to recover.*

Forced displacement causes the family ties to breakdown. *"We send the smallest child to a friend, we brought the other to the town"*, said another interviewee.

In line with Samayoa (1990), Martín Baró (1990), and Lira (1990), in our studies, we were able to corroborate that the psychosocial impact of sociopolitical violence in contexts of repression and war destroys opportunities to encounter others, breaks social ties and creates conditions for mistrust and dehumanisation. **The breakdown of social networks** is a violent mechanism used by armed groups to undermine the power of local movements, to gain control. A man interviewed stated: "*... today there is nothing because they killed many people of the organisation, [...] the president and other boys were killed [...] that's over*" (Sacipa and Montero, 2014).

The experience of the loss of territory is related to the meaning that displaced people give to their roots in Mother Earth. Men and women in their life stories repeatedly alluded to this rootedness:

> *"I like the countryside, and I think that the best thing that can happen to one ... is to have lived in the countryside." Others affirm: "there we always had all the food, cassava, plantain, beans, corn, sugarcane, coffee to collect." "That lagoon was very beautiful, it was clear and there were colourful fish." "Even the trees wave goodbye."*

The life memories in the countryside where they owned land, plants and animals are opposed to the reality they now live in the city, a space that is alien to them and where they face miserable conditions. The meanings that emerged in the life stories about the city show that it's lived as a place of danger: threats, robberies and sometimes death.

In several studies (Sacipa, 2003a; Sacipa, Vidales, Galindo, & Tovar, 2007), we have found that forced displacement generated serious consequences in people's lives. Some reported that as a result of this experience they presented revealing somatisations of affective burdens expressed in their bodies. A man once said:

> *"I did not feel like eating, [...] thinking one thing and then another, one does not want any-thing." Another man said, "when I was there, I felt very, very affected, [...] I couldn't sleep, I couldn't eat, I couldn't work." And one woman expressed "Oh, that was very difficult, I was going to die. Oh, I got skinny, really skinny and I didn't sleep or eat, that was running me out, I seemed like a little needle."*
>
> *(Sacipa, 2003b, p. 5)*

People have been exposed to the intense experience of pain due to the violence they have suffered in their bodies, or that's been lived by their loved ones, either due to their murder before, during or after displacement, or due to the separation of the youngest members of the family forced to join the armed groups. These losses were signified as painful events, as a woman narrated, *"in this situation of violence because I suffered a lot [...] they took away my husband and children"*.

Sadness ran through several stories: *"for me it was very sad to have three daughters to feed and not have anything to give them"*, a woman told us. Another woman related:

> *I arrived here with great sadness, I said what should I do? My husband without papers and here everywhere asked for papers, but when you are running, who is going to be thinking about shoes, papers, or anything. You hug your children and see how it comes out.*

The narrators spoke of the **fear** associated with dangerous situations due to sociopolitical vio-lence. This is expressed as a state of alert for the presence of actors in the conflict, *"that way of living of one is tenacious, it is distress every day, it is horrible"*. Regarding the fear that persists when they arrive in the city, a man said: *"They took us to the park and you looked everywhere to see if there were people like that, the park made me afraid because someone could have looked at me and hurt me."* Also, a woman affirmed, *"At the beginning in public transport, if a young man stared at me a lot, I preferred to lose the ticket, [I thought] 'run from here, that's must be the paramilitaries that sent me the plague, so run.'"*

Fear immobilises and hinders action: *"I did nothing because I was closed, I did not look fur-ther, I could have taken courses, but out of fear I did nothing."* Another participant talked about the **silence** as a result of the daily experience of fear: *"I felt bad, for me it was very hard ... some colleagues commented on their case and cried, I was afraid to tell."* The silencing also comes from the **weakening of trust**, due to the armed forces, as stated by one interviewee:

> *One does not trust anyone, if someone approached me a lot, I thought, could it be that there are paramilitaries here? As in the mayor's office of my town, there are, as in the governorate of my department there are, why wouldn't they be in another institution? I thought, should I speak or not, should I tell my problem or not?*

Upon emerging from the psychosocial activities, feelings gradually became strong elements in the recovery process of the people we accompanied (Sacipa, Vidales, Galindo, & Tovar, 2007).

This is expressed by the interviewee who spoke of not trusting anyone: "In the workshops, in the dialogues, one begins to see that there are still good people who can help one overcome this problem, listen to it and give one advice in time", and another reaffirmed, "there is already trust." Even the pain that emerges opens the possibility of alleviating suffering:

> *The psychosocial part was a space to cry, to mourn that situation, the opportunity to remember that difficult moment allowed us to gain strength to get ahead and say: "I can't get stuck in this". The first workshop we had was hard, painful, but at night I felt drained. One day I cried a lot, but later, although the memories would return and sometimes moments of tears would return, that pain was a more bearable pain, I said: "I'm not alone."*

One interviewee related how he freed himself from fear:

> *In the end, I gained confidence and said: "I have to move forward" and so with this help that they give me, all problems are taken forward, commenting on them in front of people; Nowadays I comment on anything and it doesn't scare me, and you get used to the fact that you have to be what you are now, that if you go back to the past, then you will never get out of that situation [...] those activities made me lose fear, feel safe; I said to myself: "what I aim I can do through that person who is guiding me."*

However, it is important to highlight that many of them continued to feel fear, as enunciated by Heller (1980), a form of anxiety linked to public spaces. Others experienced chronic fear, which Lira (2004) referred to. This is an understandable situation since in Colombia the conflict takes wicked forms in our cities.

Solidarity was a value that emerged in personal stories, giving a privileged place to affection and the importance of a closer knowledge between members of a community. The creation of **community organisations** is a solidarity event that arises from the need for better living conditions, bearing in mind the importance of working collectively.

The people in a situation of displacement who were interviewed opted for **non-violence** as a lifestyle. They created tools to build a cultural condition of coexistence, involving all areas of social action. They focused on conflict resolution, justice strengthening and key transformation, in the pursuit of the defence of life and human dignity (Sacipa, 2003a). In the narratives traversed by the pain of violence, tinged by physical and symbolic deaths, people in a situation of displacement expressed **love for life**, stronger than any threat, than any weapon, than any displacement.

This constitutes hope, as Martín-Baró declared:

> A mentally healthy person is a person capable of working and loving, and love, which is ultimately the union and mutual surrender, is blocked by personal and social lies, by the violence that corrodes the personal closeness between members that is experienced as the possibility of opening space for trust, which makes it possible to generate and maintain activities together.
>
> *(1990, p. 31)*

War followed them to the outskirts of Bogotá

Unfortunately, as a result of the territorial expansion of the conflict, paramilitaries arrived in the area. After the killings of young people, several families of Cedepaz moved again and experienced their third or fourth displacement. The recovery of territories by paramilitary control tells us about a strategy that uses fear, hatred, deception, pain and humiliation, where, as affirmed by the Chilean psychologist Elizabeth Lira (1990), the objective is to control the minds of the population, transforming the danger and vital threat into a permanent situation.

We confirm again, what we have repeatedly said (Sacipa & Tovar, 2002; Sacipa, 2003, 2005), that if we don't want to fall into the realm of naivete and psychological reduction, it is essential to recognise that these processes also require non-psychological conditions. They require economic conditions that allow displaced peasant people to live in dignity through work. Furthermore, they require sociopolitical conditions that guarantee the lives of these citizens, today threatened by armed groups, as well as their participation in the construction of the city and the country. In terms of Galtung (1998), it is necessary to defeat structural violence.

Despite the latest displacement of the leaders and their families and the adverse conditions in the territory, several women who remained in the area took over the leadership of Cedepaz and continued the work in the community, showing great strength in the decision to build a new story for themselves, their families and their community.

Finally at the end of the community work, we did another investigation to assess the accompaniment process. We studied its scope and what our work meant for the people who suffered forced displacement. We did this with an ethical perspective that led us to build with the community, in a process that, far from intervening to make changes, tried to accompany them to find a new collective sense of their experience (Sacipa & Tovar, 2004). Although we have already discussed some of its results here, they also can be found in Sacipa et al. (2007), and Sacipa (2015).

Our research demonstrated that community-based psychosocial work – accompaniment – in places of internal forced displacement can be carried out as a preventive strategy, and for personal and collective strengthening, in cases of threat or risk. The legacy gathered in the experiences of working with people, families and organisations that suffered displacement, has allowed us to establish a dialogue with the territorial initiatives of peaceful resistance about a series of psychosocial strategies for community environments, which constitutes our current work (Sacipa, 2015; Tovar, 2019; Tovar et al., 2019).

Note

1 This chapter is a product of the reflections derived from the work of psychosocial accompaniment and academic research of the authors as professors of the group Lazos Sociales y Culturas de Paz and an intern student of psychology of the Pontificia Universidad Javeriana of Bogotá, Colombia.

References

Bruner, J. (1991). *Actos de significado*. Madrid: Alianza.

CODHES. (2018, July). CODHES informa. *Boletín Informativo*, 94. [boletín n° 94] CODHES.

CODHES, & UNICEF Colombia. (1998). *Esta guerra no es nuestra*. Niños y desplazamiento forzado en Colombia. www.unicef.org/colombia/pdf/esta-guerra.pdf

Colombia 2020. (2020, February 26). En 2019 hubo 36 masacres en Colombia, la cifra más alta desde 2014: ONU. *El Espectador*. www.elespectador.com/colombia2020/pais/en-2019-hubo-36-masacres-en-colombia-la-cifra-mas-alta-desde-2014-onu-articulo-906492/

Congreso de la Republica de Colombia. (1997, July 8). Ley 387. Por la cual se adoptan medidas para la prevención del desplazamiento forzado; la atención, protección, consolidación y esta estabilización socioeconómica de los desplazados internos por la violencia en la República de Colombia.

Dejusticia. (2020, November 4). Cuatro años del acuerdo de Paz. www.dejusticia.org/cuatro-anos-del-acuerdo-de-paz/

Espinosa, Z. (2020, September 7). Colombia y su apartheid geografico: genocidio de líderes sociales. Pressenza. www.pressenza.com/es/2020/09/colombia-y-su-apartheid-geografico/

Forero, C., & Concha, M. (2003). *Cambios en los escenarios cotidianos de un joven, durante el proceso de acompañamiento psicosocial.* Facultad de Psicología, Pontificia Universidad Javeriana. Informe Final Práctica Culturas de paz.

Fundación Paz y Reconciliación. (2014). Lo que hemos ganado, han disminuido los combates, las muertes, los heridos, los muertos y los desplazamientos. https://www.pares.com.co/wp-content/uploads/2015/04/Informe%20Lo%20Que%20Hemos%20Ganado.pdf

Fundación Paz y Reconciliación. (2019a, March 7). Fumigar a los campesinos no ha funcionado. https://pares.com.co/2019/03/07/cultivos-ilicitos-fumigar-campesinos-no-ha-funcionado/

Fundación Paz y Reconciliación. (2019b, August 10). Carteles mexicanos en el Choco, más leña para el fuego. https://pares.com.co/2019/08/10/carteles-mexicanos-en-el-choco-mas-lena-para-el-fuego/

Galtung, J. (1996). Cultural peace: Some characteristics. What is a culture of peace and what are the obstacles? In UNESCO (Comp.). *From a culture of violence to a culture of peace.* https://unesdoc.unesco.org/ark:/48223/pf0000105136

Galtung, J. (1998). *Tras la violencia, 3R: reconstrucción, reconciliación, resolución. Afrontando los efectos visibles e invisibles de la guerra y la violencia.* Gernika Gogoratuz.

Gonçalves, F. (2002). *Psicoterapia cognitiva narrativa.* Desclèe.

Heller, A. (1980). *Teoría de los Sentimientos* (1ª ed.). Fontamara.

Jimenez, S. (2016, August 29). ¿Ha servido el proceso de paz para reducir la violencia en Colombia? CNN Latin America. https://cnnespanol.cnn.com/2016/08/29/ha-servido-el-proceso-de-paz-para-reducir-la-violencia-en-colombia/

Lieblinch, A., Tuva-Mashiache, R., & Zilbert T. (1998). *Narrative research.* SAGE.

Lira, E. (1990). *Guerra psicológica: intervención política de la subjetividad colectiva.* In: I. Martín Baró (Comp.). *Psicología social de la guerra* (pp. 137–58). UCA Editores.

Lira, E. (2004). Consecuencias psicosociales de la represión política en América Latina. In L. De la Corte, A. Blanco, & J. Sabucedo (Comp.). *Psicología y Derechos Humanos* (pp. 221–47). Icaria.

Martín Baró, I. (Comp.) (1990). *Psicología social de la Guerra* (pp. 137–58). UCA Editores.

PACIFISTA!. (2019, April 5). Tortura, homicidios y desplazamientos, todos aumentaron en el 2019. https://pacifista.tv/notas/tortura-homicidios-y-desplazamientos-todos-aumento-en-2019-onu/

Pardo, V. (2003). *Cambios de una mujer de Cedepaz en la narración de si misma, a partir del acompañamiento psicosocial.* Facultad de Psicología. Pontificia Universidad Javeriana. Informe final de la práctica Construcción de culturas de paz.

Payne, M. (2000). *Terapia Narrativa.* Paidos.

Polkinghorne, D. (1988). *Narrative knowing and the human sciences.* State University of New York Press.

Restrepo, A. (2001). El colegio del cuerpo: danzar la vida. In *Educar en medio del conflicto: Experiencias y testimonios. Retos de esperanza* (pp. 47–54). World Bank – Gobernación de Antioquia.

Rojas, J., & Romero, M. (2000). *Esta guerra no es nuestra. Niños y desplazamiento forzado en Colombia.* Codhes-UNICEF.

Sacipa, S. (2003a). Lectura de los Significados en Historias del Desplazamiento y de una Organización Comunitaria por la Paz. *Universitas Psychologica.* Bogotá (Colombia), *2*(1, enero-junio), 49–56.

Sacipa, S. (2003b). *Hacer paz en medio de la guerra.* Significados culturales. Ponencia 24 Congreso de la Sociedad Internacional de Psicología Política.

Sacipa, S. (Comp.) (2015). *Acompañamiento Psicosocial a Personas Víctimas de Desplazamiento forzado, Acercamientos metodológicos.* California Edit.

Sacipa, S., & Tovar, C. (2002). *Una propuesta para pensar la paz en la vida comunitaria.* Presentation at III Congreso Iberoamericano de Psicología, Bogotá (Colombia), held between July 21st and 27th, 2002.

Sacipa, S., & Tovar, C. (2004). Acompañamiento psicosocial a una comunidad en situación de desplazamiento. In A. Ospina (Ed.). *Enfoques y metodologías de atención psicosocial en el contexto del conflicto socio político colombiano* (pp. 139–50). Unión Europea, Terre des hommes.

Sacipa, S., Tovar, C. & Galindo, L. (2005). *Guía de Orientaciones para el acompañamiento psicosocial a población en situación de acompañamiento.* CHF internacional Colombia.

Sacipa, S., Vidales, R., Galindo, L., & Tovar C. (2007). Sentimientos asociados a la vivencia del desplazamiento (Colombia). In *C@hiers de Psychologie politique*, no. 11. http://lodel.irevues.inist.fr/cahierspsychologiepolitique/index.php?id=704

Sacipa-Rodriguez, S., & Montero, M. (Eds.). (2014). *Psychosocial approaches to peacebuilding in Colombia* (Peace Psychology Book Series). Springer International Publishing. https://doi.org/10.1007/978-3-319-04549-8

Samayoa, J. (1990). Guerra y deshumanización: una perspectiva psicosocial. In I. Martín Baró (Comp.). *Psicología social de la guerra* (pp. 41–65). UCA Editores.

Semana. (2020, August 28). A los líderes los matan por la impunidad en las regiones: Ariel Ávila. www.semana.com/nacion/articulo/entrevista-con-ariel-avila-sobre-asesinatos-de-lideres-sociales/697951/

Torres, N., & Cruz, F. (2020, November 23). Los PDET y el PNIS la guerra, la coca y la paz transformadora. Dejusticia. www.dejusticia.org/column/los-pdet-y-el-pnis-la-guerra-la-coca-y-la-paz-transformadora/

Tova, C., Morales, R., Campagnoli, M., Giovannetti N., Gómez, L., & Grupo Juvenil Prodesarrollo de Micoahumado. (2019). *Plan de formación para el liderazgo*. Micoahumado, Sur De Bolívar.

Tovar, C. (2019). Subjetividad política para la vida y liderazgo juvenil: una iniciativa de paz desde el territorio. In A. Gómez & A. Bravo (Eds.), *Psicología política y procesos para la paz en Colombia* (pp. 201–44). Editorial Universidad ICESI y Ascofapsi.

Tovar, H. (2006, March). Emigración y éxodo en la historia de Colombia. *Les Cahiers Amérique Latine, Histoire et Mémoire.* 7. http://alhim.revues.org/index522.html.

UNESCO. (1999). *Movimiento mundial para la cultura de paz y no violencia*. Ediciones UNESCO.

Unidad para la Atención y la Reparación Integral a las Víctimas. (2020). Cifras unidad de víctimas. www.unidadvictimas.gov.co/. 1 de 1 de 2020. https://cifras.unidadvictimas.gov.co/Home/General.

Uribe, M.T. (1992). *Los Materiales de la Memoria, en La Investigación Cualitativa*. ICFES-INER.

Vega, R. (2012). Colombia, un ejemplo contemporáneo de acumulación por desposesión. *Theomai, 26*. Segundo semestre 2012.

Vygotski, L. (1973). *Pensamiento y Palabra*. Pleyade.

9

COMMUNITY TRUST AND COMMUNITY PSYCHOLOGY INTERVENTIONS

Caterina Arcidiacono, Immacolata Di Napoli,
Ciro Esposito and Fortuna Procentese

Abstract

The present chapter examines community trust, considered as the positive expectations of community members towards their local community, with local community being defined as the place where people live and interact. Specifically, this contribution examines the crisis in participation and how community trust is the basic resource for community development and social empowerment of specific places; how it contrasts the crises of participation and social togetherness. This aim was pursued through the description of an action research project strengthening the building of community trust through multifaceted interaction among people, their place of belonging and their social attitudes.

Resumen

El presente capitulo examinó la confianza de la comunidad. Por confianza entendemos las expectativas positivas de los miembros de la comunidad en la propia comunidad local, definiéndose la comunidad local como el lugar donde las personas viven e interactúan. Específicamente, esta contribución ha examinado la crisis de la participación y también cómo la confianza comunitaria es el recurso básico para el desarrollo comunitario y el empoderamiento social de lugares específicos; la confianza de la comunidad contrasta la crisis de participación y de convivencia social. Estos objetivos se persiguieron mediante un proyecto que profundiza la construcción de la confianza de la comunidad a través de interacciones multifacéticas entre las personas, su lugar de pertenencia y sus actitudes sociales.

Introduction

Literature recognises trust as a central theme for all scholars who deal with individuals in their life contexts. In fact, trust assumes great importance for those who deal with politics, economics, social bonds and in broader terms for individual and collective well-being. Trust is recognised as an important dimension in community life and, in fact, it aligns well with both subjective well-being (Growiec & Growiec, 2016; Fu, 2018) and social justice (Colquitt & Rodell, 2011).

DOI: 10.4324/9780429325663-12

In addition, recent studies involving European countries have specifically highlighted the role of trust in increasing not only the subjective well-being but also the happiness of communities (Glatz & Eder, 2019). In the Edelman Trust Barometer Global Report (2019), trust is considered to be a forward-looking metric and an indicator of support of the citizens to the present and future initiatives that institutional bodies and associations promote.

Furthermore, Liu et al. (2018) proposed a Global Trust inventory as an indicator of trust in others that interconnected forms of trust into a global system of meaning (Sibley & Liu, 2013), represented by governmental institutions, governing bodies, security, financial institutions and corporate knowledge producers, but also by the community and close relations. The inventory culminated in four profiles of trust: Low institutional Trust, Low Trust, Moderate Trust and High Trust.

The survey showed that in the democratic Western and Catholic/European countries, Moderate Trust and High Trust profiles are more prevalent. Furthermore, additional cross-national studies have found a strong decline in confidence in political institutions in Southern Europe (Algan et al., 2017) where the effects of the social and economic crisis and unemployment are highest (Eurofound, 2018). Mingo and Faggiano (2020) also highlighted that the most influential elements on trust in political institutions, both national and international, are some subjective aspects and in particular a variable connected to the perception of the surrounding reality, namely, satisfaction with the conditions of one's own country (economic, governance, democracy, education, health).

Surveys carried out in Europe and all over the world were conducted to detect the level of trust with respect to significant others, political institutions and legal systems as well as security systems (e.g. the police). These studies especially highlighted that the low trust in institutions is a critical aspect which is reflected in the absence of participation and involvement in the political life of the country (Ortiz-Ospina & Roser, 2016; Eurostat, 2013).

Upon a closer examination of the scientific literature, it is evident that trust has been more carefully investigated and its various aspects have been separately theorised. Below, we share some definitions of trust, and in this chapter, we are particularly concerned with community trust. *Social trust* means a positive expectation regarding a cooperative exchange of behaviour with others (Putnam, 1993; Foddy & Dawes, 2008). This develops the participants' commitment to the exchange (Morgan & Hunt,1994) along with a sense of interpersonal goodwill. Social trust has two distinct components (Uslaner, 2002): particularised social trust – towards a specific person or social group (Bjørnskov, 2006) – and generalised social trust – directed towards others not directly known (Nannestad, 2008; Hamamura et al., 2017).

Conversely, *institutional trust* merely expresses the people's judgement with respect to whether the performance of the institutions such as the government meets their expectations (Kong et al., 2014), and *political trust*, which is directed towards the political legitimacy of governments, which are assumed to develop laws that are fair and do "the right thing" (Schneider, 2017; Andrè, 2014). Liu et al. (2018) suggested that trust in government may be culture specific, as the meaning of government varies according to the social system it leads.

Furthermore, *community trust* was introduced as a particularised trust towards neighbourhood (Wallman, Lundåsen & Wollebæk, 2013). Jachimowicz et al. (2017) specifically defined the concept of community trust, but they refer to the individual's interactions with his or her immediate surroundings and not with the general environment as a whole, as is the case for generalised trust. Community trust, in this sense, is based upon both personal experiences as well as elements of collective memory shared in a lived territorial space (Wollebæk et al., 2012). Moreover, in this sense, the level of trust towards people in one's own community is considered to be decisive for the general perception of trust (Wallman Lundåsen & Wollebæk, 2013).

Building on the definition of community trust described above, we propose an alternative form of community trust, specifically related to the place and its relational symbolic and cultural organisation. It concerns the positive expectations towards the opportunities offered as well as those envisaged, attributed and perceived in the territorial context of belonging for the realisation of personal and collective life projects. To address this new definition of community trust, we propose a new conceptualisation.

Community trust: fitting places to people's needs

In the early 1990s, our team detected among Neapolitan youth rage and refusal to invest energy in projects for social change (Arcidiacono, 1999). A widespread sense of impotence, powerlessness and feelings of helplessness were dominant among these youths. Their collaboration to invest energies in projects of social change was minimal.

In our research this has emerged as a very significant issue in the Southern Italian context. The whole team have carried out research in different contexts of Southern Italy (i.e. Arcidiacono et al., 2007; Arcidiacono et al., 2011), facing also different issues: migrants' inclusion (Arcidiacono et al., 2017; Mannarini & Procentese, 2018; Procentese et al., 2021), women's participatory actions (Di Napoli et al., 2019c), local cohesion and shared goals (Arcidiacono, 2004; 2017), youth engagement and future planning (Natale et al., 2016; Procentese et al., 2019a, 2019b; Carbone et al., 2021).

Our writing team for this chapter is made up of two senior researchers, one young researcher and a PhD student, all working at the Federico II Naples University that is active in training, research and social projecting characterised by close collaboration with NGO and non-profit organisations (www.communitypsychology.eu; Arcidiacono & Esposito, 2017; Esposito et al., 2020). We are intensely involved in urban projects for social renewal, introducing people's and associations' voices into the public governance of the town district. Our competence in maintaining networks and pursuing social interaction as well as developing shared and community social projects is an added value for all the social interactions we are dealing with (Arcidiacono et al., 2016). Our background in Community Psychology (CP) gave us the methodological tools for social intervention at individual, relational and organisational levels. Arcidiacono and Procentese were leading projects related to their experience of action and research with youth of the Naples area (Arcidiacono, 1999; Arcidiacono & Procentese, 2005), Di Napoli enriched the team with her research background on community trust issues and lastly, Esposito, based on his social research on inequality and well-being, was able to interact at a local level in the Sanità district. As members within the whole team were part of social action networks, we brought our knowledge to understand, support and empower ongoing best practices. For this chapter, Arcidiacono and Procentese introduced general aims of their CP engagement, Esposito described the action research experienced in the Sanità district and Di Napoli especially highlighted the importance of community trust in local change, describing its role in organisational social networking and in the interaction with local people.

In our field activity we detect the importance of the value of community trust as social glue and its action in social life acting as "*a solution to the problems caused by social uncertainty*" (Yamagishi & Yamagishi, 1994, p. 131, emphasis in original). Indeed, CP is an approach that collects a cultural and social vision, together with organisational issues as well as the consideration of individual needs, aspirations and motivations. Last but not least, its intervention is from an interactive and bottom-up perspective. Therefore, citizen participation and expression are at the same time a value and an aim.

We first started to explore networks and territorial communities through some leading concepts of CP such as sense of community, place attachment and place identity (Arcidiacono et al., 2007; Arcidiacono, 2001). From this viewpoint, we understood the psychological interactions that people establish with their territorial communities of residence. In particular, we further looked at sense of community (SoC), defined by McMillan and Chavis (1986) as: "*the feeling that members have of belonging to a place, mattering to one another and to the group, together with the hopeful belief that one's own needs will be met through their commitment to being together*" (p. 9, emphasis in original).

Until 2010, we considered SoC for its centrality in the studies on community engagement (Arcidiacono & Di Napoli, 2010), but we also agreed that the association between the sense of community and citizen participation was still unclear (Talò et al., 2014). Indeed, research has highlighted the role of strong feelings of belonging, memory, beliefs, norms, emotions and shared values (Oyserman, 2015); these can all be seen as social glue, but at the same time in some places and circumstances, there was evidence that the trustworthiness of common goals and projects was still lacking, and moreover people's unwillingness to share their own goals was clear.

This led us to detect evidence of a sort of people's detachment from the collective sphere, specifically related to the contextual features and not to merely individual values. Moreover, the lack of trust in the context of life and the perception of poor social and territorial support induces individuals to fall back on their own individual resources for their personal planning (Wallace & Kovatcheva, 1998) and also to reduce their individual future perspectives. The literature then highlighted the missing fit of people's needs and aspirations with contextual opportunities. This remarkable, but somehow invisible dimension, brings about disengagement towards community participation and, consequently, feelings of isolation and lack of interest as well as distrust towards the place of belonging (Di Blasi et al., 2016; Di Napoli et al., 2019a; Di Napoli et al., 2019b). Isolation from social life and the pursuit of mainly personal and familial interests is evident and, according to Kintrea et al. (2015), personal aspirations towards the future and attitudes towards personal development and one's own work are detached from the place of belonging and invested in family ties instead.

Starting from these premises, we introduced a global indicator of community trust to promote personal and collective planning in one's own territorial community. This indicator is based on:

a) trust based on performance of local institutions, associations and of other inhabitants, as well as in their own abilities; and
b) trust as a positive expectation of resources in the future community (Di Napoli & Arcidiacono, 2013; Di Napoli et al., 2019a).

In accordance with Yamagishi and Yamagishi (1994), we first highlighted that trust differs from any form of assurance, because it always involves an assumption of risk that what is expected may not be realised or obtained.

More specifically, community trust as a composite indicator reflects in two domains: Community Action Orientation (CAO) and Community Future Orientation (CFO).

CAO expresses citizens' trust towards the resources in his/her community of residence in the present; this domain is reflected in the following dimensions:

a) Trust in the competence and efficacy of the territorial community is related to citizens' trust towards the competence and efficacy of all those that can promote community well-being such as public institutions and other citizens as well as themselves. This dimension considers the conditions that can improve community trust: the authentic interest of public institutions in offering services to support the realisation of citizens' life plans and their engagement in community life; the initiatives of other citizens to promote community well-being and one's own engagement in favour of this collective purpose;

b) *Trust in personal and collective potential* expresses both one's willingness to participate in the improvement of one's own territorial community together with other citizens and recognising oneself as capable of actively contributing to the construction and planning of interventions aimed at one's own community; and

c) *Trust in territorial community as a selected place for personal pleasure* refers to trust towards one's own territorial community as a place in which to realise one's own social and creative life. The latter is, especially among the young generation, a new social need that influences their behaviours. In fact, according to our research (Carbone et al., 2021) trust in entertainment and relational opportunities plays an important role in defining one's own local context as a place of pleasure in which aspire to live, to spend one's free time and to talk about the main topics for personal concern with other citizens.

On the other hand, the domain of CFO introduces a future-based perspective; it stimulates a person to compare his/her present state of affairs with a probably completely different expectation that lies in the future. Two dimensions are included:

a) *Trust in one's own social realisation and quality of* life, which concerns the citizen's expectations related to the resources (safety, housing, school and work opportunities) that the territorial community can guarantee in the future. In particular, the resources considered are related to citizens' rights such as safety, taking part in decision-making and one's own professional realisation; and

b) *Trust in social opportunities and relationships in one's own community*, which concerns the possibility of accessing the resources of territorial community near and far from one's own territorial one. In a way, it includes the future possibility of personal mobility.

Community trust at stake

CP is strongly rooted in an ecological model; therefore, it is a discipline capable of understanding the interactions among individuals, their relational contexts and more generally the cultural and organisational feature of whole societies and their troubles (Kagan & Burton, 2015; Prilleltensky et al., 2001; Kagan & Lewis, 2015; Esposito et al., 2015). Each single individual is located at the boundaries between such different dimensions, and therefore oneness is complex and multifaceted (Amerio, 2013). However, only by tracing these different material and immaterial paths we will be able to intervene for individual and social well-being in neglected areas, highlighting values, methods and strategies.

Context

Italy, in line with other European countries, is recording a decline in trust in institutions compared to 2019 (Eurispes Report, 2020). In fact, only 26.3% of Italians declare themselves confident compared to 32.5% of the previous year. The Gallup poll (2018) placed Italy among the most pessimistic countries.

Furthermore, recent national studies (Bigoni et al., 2019) have revealed that citizens living in Southern Italy have more pessimistic beliefs with respect to the cooperation of other citizens than those living in the north. Together with the lack of trust in others' cooperation, in the southern area of Italy there is also higher hostility towards social risk, also due to a perception of southerners of being cheated. Bigoni et al. (2019) argue that the critical feature of Southern Italy is distrust in possible cooperation with others, which influences engagement on a collective level. This distrust underpins Banfield and Fasano's (1958) claim that individual pro-social preferences push Italians residing in Southern Italy to prefer the family system over the collective context. According to these authors, an interesting implication of these studies is the need to create greater trust in others and to enhance the expectations of collaboration, and to increase the accessibility of resources in the areas of Southern Italy.

In order to honour this understanding of social interaction and human planning, and to further deepen this topic, we present a short vignette of a local experience of youth and citizen engagement in the south of Italy. This vignette allows us to summarise some useful principles for social participatory actions that we share with readers of different countries and various backgrounds. The following case study highlights the practical implications of community trust through shared social experiences. It is focused on the role of local associations in encouraging citizen engagement and bridging citizens and interactions with public bodies.

The Sanità miracle: community trust as social glue

In some Italian contexts characterised by degradation, poverty and delinquency, there is often a lack of social cohesion and citizens do not trust local and national institutions (Sgueglia, 2012). This lack of cohesion orients people towards the family private system, leading citizens to distrust the opportunities of the community as well as feel not protected by the institutional system. This leads to citizens considering institutions as unfriendly or even as enemies. Indeed, trust is an expectation that implies opening up to the other, letting the other enter into something of one's own and is limited by the absence of positive knowledge of the other. Trusting the institutions for the citizens of some neighbourhoods would mean, in other words, letting a stranger or even an "enemy" into one's home. How, then, can the trust of individuals in social institutions and, ultimately, in the community as a whole be enhanced?

To answer this question, we conducted a research intervention in a particular context of Southern Italy, a district of the city of Naples, named Rione Sanità, where, in recent years, social engagement has led to the so-called Sanità miracle (Loffredo, 2013).

The Rione Sanità is a very large area of the Stella district, one of the main districts of the III Municipality of the city of Naples located within a valley, excluded from the connections that cross the city (ring road, subway etc). The heart of Sanità (as the district is commonly named) develops below the Maddalena Cerasuolo bridge, built in the nineteenth century at the behest of Gioacchino Murat. This bridge acts as a link between the historical centre of the city and the Capodimonte area, crossing the neighbourhood, in the sense of going beyond it by eliminating it.

This geographic location of the neighbourhood has favoured the vision of its own health, both of those who live there and of those outside it, as a closed neighbourhood separated from the rest of the city.

Its territorial closure is not only geographical, but also cultural. Remains of the urban conviviality of an archaic society remain in a place rich in cuisine (pizza, tripe, "snowflake") and vestiges of ancient monuments and rites. The immense historical-cultural value of the area, such as the Fontanelle cemetery and the catacombs of San Gennaro, promote a constant flow of visitors and tourists. However, high unemployment, low socio-economic conditions and a massive presence of organised crime characterise the neighbourhood. The immense artistic and cultural material and immaterial beauty of Sanità is thus characterised by strong social degradation mixed with the fruitful seeds of social change activated by associations for local development. Specifically, the San Gennaro Foundation is a sort of umbrella association that acts as a local multiplier of the specific actions of connected associations. In fact, the Foundation has gathered different associations working in different social domains into a whole political and cultural unit aimed at the reuse of the facilities and the monuments of the area for tourism, supporting children and youth in school attendance, vocational development, and introducing them to music and theatre (Arcidiacono & Esposito, 2017).

> *Everything starts from the problem of institutions. The lack of institutions is the basis of the deterioration of the neighbourhood. People here feel abandoned, because they have trusted the institutions but they have only obtained empty promises. Promises that deceive families and that make them lose hope.*
>
> *(G. male, 55 years old, resident of the Sanità)*

In this critical context, characterised by an institutional vacuum, many of the inhabitants of the neighbourhood perceive the municipal and state institutions as distant and disinterested.

> *We aim to combat educational poverty and give the opportunity to disadvantaged children, who do not have the opportunity to participate in activities such as sports, music [...] we try to give them the opportunity to be welcomed in safe places, run by people they can trust ... the aim is to support their growth, not in a welfare manner, but in order to start a process that gives new opportunities.*
>
> *(A., male, 27 years old, volunteer worker)*

At the same time the massive presence of organised crime in the district promotes feelings of neglect and fear in the inhabitants of the neighbourhood, and people feel abandoned by state institutions.

Discomfort has led some inhabitants to take action for the creation of an alternative welfare system, formed by a dense network of volunteer associations. These provide daily support to families in economic need, training for young people in difficulty, and also manage to protect and enhance the artistic and cultural heritage of the district, increasing the traffic of external visitors, by organising public recreational, cultural and social events.

From a careful observation of these dynamics within the community, also carried out through focused interviews conducted with inhabitants and members of associations, it has emerged that the mechanism that leads citizens, especially mothers, to trust the operators of the associations, starts from the feeling that something or someone in the local context is addressing their needs. First, there is the need to entrust their children to someone during work hours, but also the need to have offers to enable their children to see the prospect of valid alternatives; recognition by someone who helps them understand that they are not destined to spend their lives in a disadvantaged context and therefore, that the possibility of improvement is not only to become a criminal.

> *Knowing that there are these associations that improve the lives of local children, makes us parents feel more serene [...] it makes us feel that something is changing in the neighbourhood and at this rate it will get better and better.*
>
> *(G. female, 39 years old, parent)*

Trust in these associations is made possible by the fact that the volunteers live and operate within the context; they are seen as part of the community and not perceived as external, in contrast to what happens for state institutions.

Understanding the dynamics of this relationship of trust, our intervention focused on making the operators of the volunteer associations aware of their role of mediation between individual citizens and organisations. In this way it was possible to obtain a "shift" of trust from individuals to associations, and then from associations to local institutions. This last transition was created by increasing collaboration with local and national institutions, developing their awareness of local needs and finally inducing their prompt intervention.

In this way, the associations were no longer seen by citizens as alternative institutions to official ones, but as the "guarantors" of the good will and actions of official institutions.

This mediation carried out by the associations ultimately allows the inhabitants of the neighbourhood to trust the institutional representatives and no longer perceive them as enemies or an obstacle to be circumvented, but rather as an entity to involve in projects and initiatives for local well-being.

The intervention of our research team consisted in supporting and amplifying the work of associations so that the trust conferred to them by citizens could be further extended to local and state institutions.

The research-intervention method we used is part of the set of practices called Community-based Participatory Research (CBPR) (Israel et al., 2012), which are based on the involvement of researchers and community members in a collaborative process, with a reciprocal exchange that allows the development of the skills of all the partners involved. CBPR practices, provided that the recipients of the intervention are active operators in the development of a community, are able to promote the empowerment of individual members of the entire community (Minkler & Wallerstein, 2003).

In the context of the Rione Sanità, this process of empowerment implemented through the active involvement of the paid and voluntary workers within associations, implied that they took responsibility for the trust bestowed on them by the citizens and that the citizens, in turn, would participate in community development. In this way, trust ceased to be characterised as a mere request for reassurance and therefore substantially of delegation, and was instead transformed into an active attitude of assuming the common risk by the citizens, by the operators, by the state institutions and by the researchers alike.

The intervention implemented has in this way increased the opportunity to create projects at a local level through reciprocal relationships between inhabitants, social operators (i.e. the workers and volunteers) and representatives of state institutions; the whole process was characterised by trust in the development opportunities for the territory, of its entrepreneurial and cultural activities and of the whole community.

The achievement of this climate of community trust has in fact improved the quality of life of the inhabitants of the neighbourhood. Over time, the network of associations, together with commercial activities and due to some state interventions, has managed to give new life to the neighbourhood, organising events that have brought visitors and tourists to the area, proposing cultural initiatives that have favoured the economic development of small commercial activities, and giving the young people of the neighbourhood the opportunity to study, to enter the job market and to live in an environment with greater well-being and community trust.

The specific intervention of our teams consisted in interviewing members of the associations and users of association services as well as the general citizens of the area. They were interviewed in order to understand what was the meaning of Fondazione San Gennaro for them. We detected that the main role played by this foundation in the area was its commitment to networking among people, people and associations, citizens, associations and the town municipality (Di Napoli et al., 2019b). Therefore, all the associations had a twofold role: they promoted shared trust and created community hope.

Discussion

This intervention outlines the positive action of community trust in a specific territorial context, showing the invisible strength that it gives to local action and highlighting how effective actions in a specific district created a new trust in future change.

We learnt from this how important it is to build trustworthiness into the potentiality of a place to improve its liveability and to create new job opportunities.

Public trust, namely in our cases, community trust, is the invisible glue that allowed community action interventions. Therefore, participatory local action is a way to give voice to people's needs and demands.

Martin-Baró (1994) pointed out the need to build a bottom-up psychology *"in which central place would be given to the needs, aims and experiences of the oppressed"* (p. 8).

His thought let us understand that the lack of community and public trust is a defensive form of resilience purposely used by excluded people for their own survival. Taking into account the lack of community trust entails considering the existential fatalism that in an oppressed community is strictly connected *"with the structural forces that oppress them, deprive them of control over their own existence, and force them to learn submission and expect nothing from life"* (Martin-Baró, 1994, p. 27, emphasis in original).

Indeed, the awareness of the lack of trust is the first step in creating contextual shared goals, developing reciprocal trust and pursuing community goals. We are convinced that any conscientisation action is the turning point for starting every shared contextual action.

CP through shared actions plays a role in creating fruitful interactions that transform desires into facts. Gathering the existing associations into a shared project of renewal of an area should be a CP priority. The endeavours of different stakeholders (associations, shop dealers, public institutions and citizens) should be supported in their finding shared solutions for the improvement of the context: that is, access to a closed green area, rules for a street market, projects of shared use of public spaces. Therefore, energy is usefully spent in pursuing meetings of associations and with public authorities concerning possible community renewal.

Conclusion and implications for the future of Community Psychology

Pessimism about the future and feelings of being immersed in an anomic context together with a sense of inability to control one's life, a low sense of agency and fatalism of areas that are characterised as the poorest and most powerless throughout Europe (Salvatore et al., 2018) are ongoing challenges for community psychologists.

Intervening in such contexts, from an ecological perspective, on the one hand, aims to increase citizens' recognition of all the opportunities offered by the different systems within their own life context; and on the other, to implement the possibility of realising citizens' individual and collective projects. An intervention aimed at building community trust, as already reported above, implies activating the participation of citizens, institutions and bodies present in the community to take on board the risks associated with not knowing the outcomes of such participation, and in identifying, supporting and strengthening current or expected resources and opportunities. It involves both community action and community future orientations.

Salvatore (2018), in a wide investigation at European level, found out that social cohesion is a significant dimension related to low social engagement, and therefore community trust becomes the social glue that activates the exchange, recognition and enhancement of those opportunities present in a community to support individual and collective projects.

In this way, community trust becomes an activator of awareness-raising processes, ways of overcoming resignation and of enhancing expectation of opportunities.

The preliminary objective of a CP intervention focused on activating trust in the community is to promote the recognition of opportunities; to activate participation and cooperation among inhabitants, associations and local institutions; and to detect the expectation of living opportunities for that public unused space, according to their personal and collective needs and expectations. Here, the intervention moves away from the wishful narrative of strategic visioning to the concrete reality of implementation, building the opportunities for the inhabitants to cooperate in defining the regeneration of the whole community. It is fundamental when working in the poorest and most powerless contexts to create a dialogue with the institutions. A necessary priority for implementing trust in institutions is especially promoting the passage from seeking reassurance, through the ability for delegation to the assumption of risk and responsibility for promoting collective change.

The role of CP is to help people in their awareness of feelings and 'mattering' of places and of their own desires. It is a significant experience for residents to have the opportunity to be the actor in local transformations.

According to the Quadruple Helix Innovation model (Campbell, Carayannis, & Rehman, 2015), which outlines interaction among universities, business, citizens and government on common projects, the CP emphasis will be on a shared project unifying different social actors in a joint endeavour.

Here, the CP competence is in creating interaction among different bodies as the backbone that structures the whole project, with community trust as the petrol that animates the whole process.

From an ecological point of view, a future perspective will be to emphasise the contextual dimension with respect to its implications for the individual sphere, and future research will investigate how the expectation of opportunities in one's community of residence affects the general state of well-being in addition to the individual level of hope. In particular, with respect to hope, this line of research of the interconnection between contextual and individual dimensions will be even more interesting.

In fact, strong criticism directed at studies on hope highlights that this construct is examined exclusively from an individualistic view, which does not adequately contemplate the dimensions of the context in which individuals live (Aspinwall & Leaf, 2002), and ignores the impact of supportive experiences of social networks (Jason et al., 2016). This view is echoed by these authors: *"Community psychology provides a unique framework from which to examine contextual influences on feelings of hope"* (Jason et al., 2016, p. 335, emphasis in original).

As Scioli (2020) suggested, hope is a complex feeling that includes attachment, survival and spiritual elements; it is essential for understanding fears and aspirations as well as the vulnerabilities and strengths of individuals, and in particular of specific populations; it is the pillar for every action based on community trust.

Lastly, we recall Antonio Genovesi (1765–1767), the famous Neapolitan Enlightenment author, who already in the eighteenth century pointed out the need to contrast the condemnation of the impotence of the nature of things with the affirmation of the need to overcome the inertia *nonsipuotismo*, the philosophy of "cannot be done".

Genovesi himself introduced the concept of public happiness, to be achieved by freeing mankind from its state of "obscurity". The first chair of economics at Naples University is named after him and his thought can be considered a prestigious legacy for scholars and activists aimed at pursuing public virtues. Public trust, social cohesion and conviviality are values that create public happiness. Our CP action research team, in this vein is presenting this trustfulness participatory action that pursues shared community goals acting as levers for social change.

References

Algan, Y., Guriev, S., Papaioannou, E., & Passari, E. (2017). The European trust crisis and the rise of populism. *Brookings Papers on Economic Activity*, *48*(2), 309–400. www.jstor.org/stable/90019460

Amerio, P. (2013). *L'altro necessario*. Il Mulino Editore.

André, S. (2014). Does trust mean the same for migrants and natives? Testing measurement models of political trust with multi-group confirmatory factor analysis. *Social Indicators Research, 115*(3), 963–982. https://doi.org/10.1007/s11205-013-0246-6

Arcidiacono, C. (1999). *Napoli: Diagnosi di una città*. Magma Edizioni.

Arcidiacono, C. (2001). Sense of community: Avoidant attachment and belonging. further comment on a psychological profile of Naples, a metropolis in the south of Italy. *Gemeinde Psychologie, Rundbrief, 2*(7), 35–45.

Arcidiacono, C. (2017). *Psicologia di comunità per le città. Rigenerazione urbana a Porta Capuana*. Liguori Editore.

Arcidiacono, C., & Di Napoli, I. (2010). Crisi dei giovani e sfiducia nei contesti locali di appartenenza. Un approccio di psicologia ecologica. In E. Shafroth, C. Schwarzer, & D. Conte (Eds.), *Krise als Chance aus historischer und aktueller Perspektive* (pp. 235–50). Athena Verlag.

Arcidiacono, C., Di Napoli, I., & Sarnacchiaro, P. (2007). Puddifoot community identity and juvenile community action orientation. In A. Bokszczanin (Ed.), *Social change in solidarity: Community psychology perspectives and approaches* (pp. 93–108). Opole University Press.

Arcidiacono, C., & Esposito, C. (2017). Benvenuti alla Sanità. In U.M. Olivieri (Ed.), *Lavoro, volontariato Dono* (pp. 263–83). Milella Editore.

Arcidiacono, C., Grimaldi, D., Di Martino, S., & Procentese, F. (2016) Participatory visual methods in the "Psychology loves Porta Capuana" project. *Action Research, 14*(4), 376–92. https://doi.org/10.1177/1476750315626502

Arcidiacono, C., Natale, A., Carbone, A., & Procentese, F. (2017). Participatory action research from an intercultural and critical perspective. *Journal of Prevention and Intervention in the Community, 45*, 44–56. https://doi.org/10.1080/10852352.2016.1197740

Arcidiacono, C., & Procentese, F. (2005). Distinctiveness and sense of community in the historical center of Naples: A piece of participatory action research. *Journal of Community Psychology, 33*(6), 631–8. https://doi.org/10.1002/jcop.20074

Arcidiacono, C., Procentese, F., & Di Napoli, I. (2007). Youth, community belonging, planning and power. *Journal of Community and Applied Social Psychology, 17*, 280–95. https://doi.org/10.1002/casp.935

Arcidiacono, C., Procentese, F., & Paolillo, M.G. (2011). Identity, traditions and lack of environmental behaviour. *Journal of Environmental Science and Engineering, 5*(3), 365–380.

Aspinwall, L.G., & Leaf, S.L. (2002). In search of the unique aspects of hope: Pinning our hopes on positive emotions, future-oriented thinking, hard times, and other people. *Psychological Inquiry, 13*(4), 276–88.

Banfield, E.C., & Fasano, L. (1958). *The moral basis of a backward society*. The Free Press.

Barometer, E.T. (2019). Edelman trust barometer global report. Edelman. www.edelman.com/sites/g/files/aatuss191/files/2019-02/2019_Edelman_Trust_Barometer_Global_Report_2.pdf

Bigoni, M., Bortolotti, S., Casari, M., & Gambetta, D. (2019). At the root of the North–South cooperation gap in Italy: Preferences or beliefs? *The Economic Journal, 129*(619), 1139–52. https://doi.org/10.1111/ecoj.12608

Bjørnskov, C. (2006). The multiple facets of social capital. *European Journal of Political Economy, 22*(1), 22–40. https://doi.org/10.1016/j.ejpoleco.2005.05.006

Campbell, D.F., Carayannis, E.G., & Rehman, S.S. (2015). Quadruple helix structures of quality of democracy in innovation systems: the USA, OECD countries, and EU member countries in global comparison. *Journal of the Knowledge Economy, 6*(3), 467–93. https://doi.org/10.1007/s13132-015-0246-7

Carbone, A., Di Napoli, I., Procentese, F., & Arcidiacono, C. (2021). Close family bonds and community distrust. The complex emotional experience of a young generation from Southern Italy. *Journal of Youth Studies*, https://doi.org/10.1080/13676261.2021.1939283

Colquitt, J.A., & Rodell, J.B. (2011). Justice, trust, and trustworthiness: A longitudinal analysis integrating three theoretical perspectives. *Academy of Management Journal, 54*(6), 1183–206. https://doi.org/10.5465/amj.2007.0572

Di Blasi, M., Tosto, C., Marfia, A., Cavani, P., & Giordano, C. (2016). Transition to adulthood and recession: A qualitative study. *Journal of Youth Studies, 19*(8), 1043–60. https://doi.org/10.1080/13676261.2015.1136055

Di Napoli, I., & Arcidiacono, C. (2013). The use of self-anchoring scales in social research: The Cantril scale for the evaluation of community action orientation. In C. Davino and L. Fabbris (Eds.), *Survey data collection and integration* (pp. 73–85). Springer.

Di Napoli, I., Dolce, P., & Arcidiacono, C. (2019a). Community trust: A social indicator related to community Engagement. *Social Indicators Research, 145*(2), 551–79. https://doi.org/10.1007/s11205-019-02114-y

Di Napoli, I., Esposito, C., Candice, L., & Arcidiacono, C. (2019b). Trust, hope, and identity in disadvantaged urban areas. The role of civic engagement in the Sanità District (Naples). *Journal of Community Psychology in Global Perspective, 5*(2), 46–62. https://doi.org/10.1285/i24212113v5i2p46

Di Napoli, I., Procentese, F., & Arcidiacono, C. (2019c). Women's associations and the well-being of their members: From mutual support to full citizenship. *Journal of Prevention & Intervention in the Community, 48*(2), 189–205. https://doi.org/10.1080/10852352.2019.1624357

Esposito, F., Ornelas, J., & Arcidiacono, C. (2015). Migration-related detention centers: the challenges of an ecological perspective with a focus on justice. *BMC International Health and Human Rights, 15*(1), 13, 1–15. https://doi.org/10.1186/s12914-015-0052-0

Esposito, F., Ornelas, J., Scirocchi, S., Tomai, M., Di Napoli, I., & Arcidiacono, C. (2020). "Yes, but somebody has to help them, somehow": Looking at the Italian detention field through the eyes of professional nonstate Actors. *International Migration Review, 55*(1) 166–194. https://doi.org/10.1177/0197918320921134

EURISPES. (2020). 32° Rapporto Italia. Percorsi di ricerca nella società italiana, Bologna, Minerva, 2020. *Geostorie. Bollettino e Notiziario del Centro Italiano per gli Studi Storico-Geografici, 28*(2), 127–127.

Eurofound. (2018). *Living and working in Europe 201–-2018.* Eurofound.

Eurostat. (2013). Quality of life in Europe – facts and views – governance. https://ec.europa.eu/eurostat/statistics-explained/index.php?title=Quality_of_life_in_Europe_-_facts_and_views_-_governance

Foddy, M., & Dawes, R. (2008). Group-based trust in social dilemmas. In A. Biel, D. Eek, T. Gärling and M. Gustafsson (Eds.), *New issues and paradigms in research on social dilemmas* (pp. 57–71). Springer. https://doi.org/10.1007/978-0-387-72596-3_5

Fu, X. (2018). The contextual effects of political trust on happiness: Evidence from China. *Social Indicators Research, 139*(2), 491–516. https://doi.org/10.1007/s11205-017-1721-2

Gallup International Association. (2018). Hope & optimism on global peace. https://www.gallup-international.com/surveys/hope-optimism-global-peace/

Genovesi, A. (1765-67/2005). *Delle Lezioni di Commercio o sia di Economia Civile.* Istituto Italiano per gli Studi Filosofici.

Glatz, C., & Eder, A. (2019). Patterns of trust and subjective well-being across Europe: New insights from repeated cross-sectional analyses based on the European Social Survey 2002–2016. *Social Indicators Research, 148*, 417–439. https://doi.org/10.1007/s11205-019-02212-x

Growiec, K., & Growiec, J. (2016). Bridging social capital and individual earnings: Evidence for an inverted U. *Social Indicators Research, 127*(2), 601–31. https://doi.org/10.1007/s11205-015-0980-z

Hamamura, T., Li, L.M.W., & Chan, D. (2017). The association between generalized trust and physical and psychological health across societies. *Social Indicators Research, 134*(1), 277–86. https://doi.org/10.1007/s11205-016-1428-9

Israel, B.A., Eng, E., Schulz, A.J., & Parker, E.A. (Eds.). (2012). *Methods for community-based participatory research for health.* John Wiley & Sons.

Jachimowicz, J.M., Chafik, S., Munrat, S., Prabhu, J.C., & Weber, E.U. (2017). Community trust reduces myopic decisions of low-income individuals. *Proceedings of the National Academy of Sciences, 114*(21), 5401–06. https://doi.org/10.1073/pnas.1617395114

Jason, L.A., Stevens, E., & Light, J.M. (2016). The relationship of sense of community and trust to hope. *Journal of Community Psychology, 44*(3), 334–41. https://doi.org/10.1002/jcop.21771

Kagan, C., & Burton, M. (2015). Towards and beyond liberation psychology. In T. Afuape & G. Hugues (Eds.), *Liberation practices towards emotional wellbeing through dialogue* (pp. 211–221). Routledge.

Kagan, C., & Lewis, S. (2015). *Community, Work and Family* and the metamorphosis of social change. Invited keynote paper presented to the *Community Work Family Conference*, Malmo, 2015. http://eprints.mdx.ac.uk/17580/1/malmo_Cwf_paper.pdf

Kintrea, K., St Clair, R., & Houston, M. (2015). Shaped by place? Young people's aspirations in disadvantaged neighbourhoods. *Journal of Youth Studies, 18*(5), 666–84. https://doi.org/10.1080/13676261.2014.992315

Kong, D.T., Dirks, K.T., & Ferrin, D.L. (2014). Interpersonal trust within negotiations: Meta-analytic evidence, critical contingencies, and directions for future research. *Academy of Management Journal, 57*(5), 1235–55. https://doi.org/10.5465/amj.2012.0461

Liu, J.H., Milojev, P., Gil de Zúñiga, H., & Zhang, R.J. (2018). The global trust inventory as a "proxy measure" for social capital: measurement and impact in 11 democratic societies. *Journal of Cross-Cultural Psychology, 49*(5), 789–810. https://doi.org/10.1177%2F0022022118766619

Loffredo, A. (2013). *Noi del rione sanità*. Mondadori.

Mannarini, T., & Procentese, F. (2018). Identity and immigrant stereotypes: A study based on the ego-ecological approach. *Identity, 18*(2), 77–93. https://doi.org/10.1080/15283488.2018.1447480

Martin-Baró, I. (1994). *Writing for a liberation psychology* (A. Aron & S. Corne, Eds.). Harvard University Press.

McMillan, D.W., & Chavis, D.M. (1986). Sense of community: A definition and theory. *Journal of Community Psychology, 14*(1), 6–23. https://doi.org/10.1002/1520-6629(198601)14:1%3C6::AID-JCOP2290140103%3E3.0.CO;2-I

Mingo, I. & Faggiano, M.P. (2020). Trust in institutions between objective and subjective determinants: A multilevel analysis in European countries. *Social Indicators Research, 151*, (3), 815–39,https://doi.org/10.1007/s11205-020-02400-0

Minkler, M., & Wallerstein, N. (2003). Part one: introduction to community-based participatory research. In M. Minkler and N. Wallerstein (Eds.). *Community-based participatory research for health* (pp. 5–24). Jossey-Bass.

Morgan, R. M., & Hunt, S. D. (1994). The commitment-trust theory of relationship marketing. *Journal of Marketing, 58*(3), 20–38. https://doi.org/10.1177%2F002224299405800302

Nannestad, P. (2008). What have we learned about generalized trust, if anything? *Annual Review of Political Science, 11*, 413–36. https://doi.org/10.1146/annurev.polisci.11.060606.135412

Natale, A., Di Martino, S., Procentese, F., & Arcidiacono, C. (2016). De-growth and critical community psychology: Contributions towards individual and social well-being. *Futures, 78*, 47–56. https://doi.org/10.1016/j.futures.2016.03.020

Ortiz-Ospina, E., & Roser, M. (2016). World population growth. *OurWorldInData.org*. https://ourworldindata.org/world-population-growth

Oyserman, D. (2015). Values, Psychology of. In J. D. Wright (Ed.), *International Encyclopedia of the Social & Behavioral Sciences* (2nd ed.; Vol. 25, pp. 36–40). (Elsevier).

Prilleltensky, I., Nelson, G., & Peirson, L. (2001). The role of power and control in children's lives: An ecological analysis of pathways toward wellness, resilience and problems. *Journal of Community & Applied Social Psychology, 11*(2), 143–58. https://doi.org/10.1002/casp.616

Procentese, F., Candice, L., Arcidiacono, C., Esposito, C., & Di Napoli, I. (2021). Place identity, hope and expectations of decent work in Italian youths moving to London. *Journal of Prevention and Intervention in the Community*. https://doi.org/ 10.1080/10852352.2021.1935196

Procentese, F., & Gatti, F. (2019a). Senso di Convivenza Responsabile: Quale Ruolo nella Relazione tra Partecipazione e Benessere Sociale? *Psicologia Sociale, 14*(3), 405–26. https://doi.org/10.1482/94942

Procentese, F., Gatti, F., & Falanga, A. (2019b). Sense of responsible togetherness, sense of community and participation: Looking at the relationships in a university campus. *Human Affairs, 29*(2), 247–63. https://doi.org/10.1515/humaff-2019-0020

Putnam, R. (1993). The prosperous community: Social capital and public life. *The American Prospect, 13*(4, Spring). www.prospect.org/print/vol/13

Salvatore, S., Fini, V., Mannarini, T., Veltri, G. A., Avdi, E., Battaglia, F., & Kadianaki, I. (2018). Symbolic universes between present and future of Europe. First results of the map of European societies' cultural milieu. *PloS One, 13*(1), e0189885. https://doi.org/10.1371/journal.pone.0189885

Schneider, I. (2017). Can we trust measures of political trust? Assessing measurement equivalence in diverse regime types. *Social Indicators Research, 133*(3), 963–84. https://doi.org/10.1007/s11205-016-1400-8

Scioli, A. (2020). The psychology of hope: A diagnostic and prescriptive account. In S.C. van den Heuvel (Ed.), *Historical and multidisciplinary perspectives on hope* (pp. 137–63). Springer. https://doi.org/10.1007/978-3-030-46489-9_8

Sgueglia, L. (2012). Una comunità rionale di Napoli: donne e uomini tra subalternità e soggettività. *La camera blu. Rivista di studi di genere, 6*, 25–45. https://doi.org/10.6092/1827-9198/1237

Sibley, C.G., & Liu, J.H. (2013). Relocating attitudes as components of representational profiles: Mapping the epidemiology of bicultural policy attitudes using Latent Class Analysis. *European Journal of Social Psychology, 43*, 160–74. https://doi.org/10.1002/ejsp.1931

Talò, C., Mannarini, T., & Rochira, A. (2014). Sense of community and community participation: A meta-analytic review. *Social Indicators Research, 117*(1), 1–28. http://dx.doi.org/10.1007%2Fs11205-013-0347-2

Uslaner, E.M. (2002). *The moral foundations of trust.* Cambridge University Press.

Wallace, C.D., & Kovacheva, S. (1998). *Youth and society: The construction and deconstruction of youth in West and East Europe.* Palgrave Macmillan.

Wallman Lundåsen, S., & Wollebæk, D. (2013). Diversity and community trust in Swedish local communities. *Journal of Elections, Public Opinion & Parties, 23*(3), 299–321.

Wollebæk, D., Wallman Lundåsen, S., & Trägårdh, L. (2012). Three forms of interpersonal trust: Evidence from Swedish municipalities. *Scandinavian Political Studies, 35*(4), 319–46. https://doi.org/10.1111/j.1467-9477.2012.00291.x

Yamagishi, T., & Yamagishi, M. (1994). Trust and commitment in the United States and Japan. *Motivation and Emotion, 18*(2), 129–66. https://doi.org/10.1007/BF02249397

10

THE OTHERS

Discovering and connecting community life

Moisés Carmona Monferrer and Rubén David Fernández Carrasco

Abstract

Why do the same people always participate? Is there no community life beyond the partners we usually work with? These are some of the questions we hear constantly in community actions in which we participate, as professionals or as citizens, as promoters or as participants. In this chapter we present a methodological proposal which proposes five stages for knowing about and connecting to that community life that escapes the formality of community action processes promoted by public administrations or formal associations. Our discussion is the result of two years of work in two action-research processes carried out in the neighbourhoods of Trinitat Nova and Verneda Alta in the city of Barcelona.

Resumen

¿Por qué siempre participa la misma gente? ¿No existe vida comunitaria más allá de las asociantes con las que trabajamos habitualmente? Estas son algunas de las preguntas que escuchamos constantemente en acciones comunitarias en las que participamos, como profesionales o como ciudadanos, como promotores o como participantes. En este capítulo presentamos una propuesta metodológica que propone 5 fases para conocer y conectar con la vida comunitaria que se escapa de la formalidad de los procesos de acción comunitaria promovidos por las administraciones públicas o asociaciones de carácter más formal. Es el resultado de dos años de trabajo en dos procesos de investigación-acción llevado a cabo en los barrios de Trinitat Nova y la Verneda Alta en la ciudad de Barcelona.

Introduction

The purpose of this chapter is to offer a methodological resource for people, organisations and institutions interested in deepening strategies to stimulate and promote community actions with those social actors who usually do not participate in more formal community processes and actions. We refer to people and groups that are involved in activities that contribute to the creation of a neighbourhood or community. In particular we refer to people who give meaning to community life; who contribute to the creation of a collective identity and relationships of trust

DOI: 10.4324/9780429325663-13

with their neighbours; who support neighbours or allow themselves to be helped by them; and who make us feel that we do not live alone in the city. Ultimately, we are talking about people who connect, relate and weave cooperation with other people and groups. These people and groups are often unknown or not very visible in the framework of the more "formal" community action that is promoted via the social policies of public administrations or from the usual associative web of relationships that participates (Whitham, 2012).

In short, we offer a methodological approach for people who have an interest in creatively moving beyond those usual participants who define themselves as community leaders, to incorporate new actors, thereby expanding the histories to be told, and generating new energy and impetus for the initiation of community actions (Foster-Fishman et al., 2013).

This chapter is also the result of the collaboration between the Social Interaction and Social Change Research Group (GRICS) of the University of Barcelona and the Community Action Services of Barcelona City Council. It takes place within the public policy framework, "Towards a public policy of community action. Conceptual, strategic and operational framework" (Adjuntament de Barcelona, 2017). This underpins Barcelona's community action strategy, with the aim of providing a greater social base for community projects in the City since 2015. It represents a break with the traditional drive for community actions, which were based on the participation of service providers and the historic and formally recognised organisations present in neighbourhoods. This rupture represents four challenges: for professionals who must learn how to connect with these "new" groups; for traditional associations that can see these actors as new energy or as a threat to their leadership; for the city council that has to assume and manage the rich diversity that emerges in each neighbourhood of the city; and finally for those "new" participants, who have to learn to interact and collaborate with other actors in the community.

The chapter draws on the implementation of two cycles of action research in which we were involved between 2016 and 2018 in the neighbourhoods of La Verneda Alta and Trinitat Nova, both in the city of Barcelona.

People and groups that contribute to social and community life beyond formal groups and mechanisms for participation

In energising and promoting community action, it is quite common to ask the following question: how can those people who do not usually participate in organisations or other formal participation channels be reached? This is a highly relevant issue for a participative Community Psychology, since it is known that the majority of the population does not participate in these formal channels. It is not so easy to answer the question.

Intuitively we know that interacting with other people to do things that interest them jointly in a neighbourhood, happens largely outside formal associative life, and outside the participation exercises carried out through the formal channels proposed by the local administration.

When we speak of community, we speak of groups that contribute to generating a group identity, "we" rather than "I" (Jetten et al., 2020); groups that meet the needs of its members and that are based on relationships of exchange, reciprocity, friendship or family ties, and shared interests. They include, for example, playing sports, sharing children's playgrounds, making music, going for a walk, walking the dog and so on. We argue that it is these non-formal groups that are key drivers of community and of community engagement (Whitham, 2019; Wang et al., 2020).

Building community is a process that is largely based on the social action of people and groups, mostly non-formal, that help shape and signify social and community life in a given context (Carmona & Rebollo, 2009). From our perspective, it is not possible to speak of community in the absence of interconnected people and groups, shared projects and motivation. For us, *community action*, then, is best understood as an intentional action for energising cooperative social relations between the members of a certain area or space of coexistence in the city (from neighbourhoods to individual building communities, educational and health centres or projects, sports etc) to improve the daily well-being of people (Carmona & Rebollo, 2009, p. 14).

Paradoxically, most of the public policy strategies that promote community actions are based on organisations and formal participation channels. Whilst this may seem like an agile response and efficient use of resources in the face of the momentum for community actions, it is at the same time a limitation that renders invisible enormous knowledge and potential regarding the social life of a particular community in its own context (Morales & Rebollo, 2014).

Two dimensions underpin community action: the substantive (or what is to be transformed), and the relational (the way to do it) (Carmona, 2011). In neighbourhood work, attention to both these dimensions is needed in order to mobilise people for change. The nexus of community action in a neighbourhood will be made up of small, informal groups, who constitute the building blocks of the community, both in terms of what they want to do and how. These non-formal groups, then, those we want to reach with this methodology, have two characteristics:

- they make it possible to satisfy one or more of the needs felt by their members, such as, for example, accompanying each other (for example, to take bicycle rides along river); being able to do activities (for example, play a soccer game or a trip to the zoo with other families from the school); or learn skills (for example, to play a guitar or any other musical instrument);
- they provide a collective group identity, a "we", which acts as a mediator between the "I" and the community (or neighbourhood) where people live.

In the context of this project, we understand *the community* as a physical space or a geographical environment, which can present different mechanisms and processes, more or less formalised, of interaction and social support, providing opportunities for mutual bonding and daily reciprocity. Within any specific community context, the various actors may have different degrees of motivation to work on shared objectives with other actors in the same context. Where they do, we have the potential for collective community actions: actions based on the interest of and relevance to those involved.

Because these small groups are likely to be concerned with their own interests, they tend not to look out towards the rest of the community. The groups themselves present very diverse and autonomous forms of organisation and operation and constitute what Llena and Ucar (2006) describe as Type 1 community actions – the community actions of everyday life. (This is in contrast to Type 2 actions, which are those involving the formal institutions and agencies). The different forms and constellations of community groups in a neighbourhood suggest two different kinds of social capital – social group capital and social community capital (Durston, 2002; Garrido, 2015).

Social group capital refers to the existence or not of groups (formal and non-formal) within a physical space such as a neighbourhood, that can support or solve specific needs of members of this community. Thus, social group capital is the store of capital to meet the everyday needs of people sharing the space and determines what it is like to live as part of it.

Social community capital, on the other hand, refers to the existence or not of groups (formal and non-formal) interconnected within the community (or neighbourhood), and to the capacity that individuals, groups, entities, associations and services have to be able to find shared objectives, beyond those of the individual group, in order to be able to work together. Thus, we could say that a neighbourhood has a strong *social community capital* when it encounters a rich network of individuals and groups with the experiences, traditions and ability to work together to achieve joint objectives. Social community capital could be understood as the relational dimension of community action, when social ties are based on interdependence, whereas social group capital arises from ties based on affection and affiliation (Kagan et al., 2020).

Examples of *social group capital* include:

- Adolescents and young people who go repeatedly to the sports courts and organise matches and competitions that generate bonds of friendship and rivalry.
- Older people who go out to walk together periodically.
- Groups of mothers and (some) fathers who meet at the same time in the park with their sons and daughters, and keep each other company while they take care of them.
- People who exchange knowledge, for example, learning to play musical instruments.

Examples of *social community capital include*:

- People, groups and entities that work together to organise the Sports Week in the neighbourhood.
- A platform that brings together entities, groups and people who work to support a food bank in a neighbourhood.
- People, groups, entities and public services that work within the framework of a community plan.

A neighbourhood or territory will become a community if it promotes and energises its social group capital. However, a neighbourhood or territory will become an empowered community if it promotes social community capital (Kim, 2018).Social group capital can become social community capital if alliances and relationships between interest groups are forged.

In the Barcelona context, formal community action has been more oriented towards promoting social community capital, and has neglected the potential of directing its energy to promote social group capital, thereby excluding many people from community action. This proposal aims to help turn this situation around.

The role of non-formal social and community life in energising and promoting community action

As a critical reflection on our own practices working in urban settings in Barcelona, we recognise that on some occasions we have mapped these people and non-formal groups but we have not been able to (or known how to) dedicate the time or energy necessary to incorporate them into community actions. On other occasions, we have had a tendency to accept that the formal organisations within an area are representative of the population as a whole, or to believe that the traditional (often self-selected) social actors are sufficiently representative of the diversity of an area, without adequately assessing the evolution of populations or their growing diversity (Pindado, 2008). On other occasions we have tended to streamline community actions by mobilising the most visible, accessible and participatory social actors, taking what is, in effect, the easiest way to work in the neighbourhood (which is understandable given constraints on time and resources).

We now propose that non-formal social and community life must be taken into account for the catalysing and promoting of community action. Non-formal people and groups are citizens and must be recognised as a potentially active part of communities. Indeed, non-formal groups are the building blocks of communities: without these groups there are no communities, and the most cohesive and resilient communities are those that welcome and interconnect with a larger diversity of actors and groups.

Guaranteeing community work with individual citizens and informal groups does not exclude work with more formal associations and entities: both are needed to enable us to better understand the community context where community actions are to be promoted.

In short, in our work we are going to look for those people and non-formal groups who, in the main, do not participate in formal associations. If we are successful, then we will be able to incorporate a wider variety of actors into community action. We will be able to promote a range of different visions about the history; social and community life; organisation; problems; and opportunities within the neighbourhood in which we are working. In short, we will be able to be more inclusive and be in a better position to animate and support the engagement of more, diverse people.

We will now go on to suggest a methodology for getting to know the complex web of interests and actors in neighbourhoods.

A methodological framework for including non-formal groups

Getting to know non-formal social and community life provides opportunities for community actions (Kagan et al., 2020). But it can be more important whenever the promoters of community action are working in one of the following situations.

- Areas where there are no active formal associations or organisations.
- Areas where formal associations and organisations are scarce and apparently weak or not representative of the diversity of the population as a whole.
- Areas where there are few and unconnected groups involved in community life, where there is potential to promote a strategy to strengthen the set of groups that are present, in order to contribute to a more inclusive and diverse community network or system.

To learn about non-formal social and community life, we propose a set of methodological principles for flexible application:

a) Be intentional and proactive, that is, to be clear about our intentions and have positive strategies for seeking out and engaging these different groups. We cannot wait for non-formal groups to come to us and we need to include time and energy in our daily diary get to know people and the patterns of daily life.
b) Modify our usual ways of working, that is, different ways of working need to be found to achieve these new goals. These will include detailed observation, informal conversations and careful listening to diverse people, particularly those with wide sets of local relationships or community knowledge, such as traders, bar tenders, estate agents, the halal butcher, delivery people. It also includes informal conversations with strangers in different community spaces.
c) Have presence and patience, guaranteeing the time, flexibility and necessary resources required to energise people and non-formal groups in community settings or, to use a culinary metaphor, "the good dish calls for a slow fire". This will require spending time in a place.

d) Getting to know a community cannot be rushed. Paradoxically, by being patient and taking the time to see, understand and follow the rhythms of life in the community, we can get to where we want to, earlier. In taking time to discover and learn to be more patient; to learn to look and understand more fully; to get to know the people and the groups in the neighbourhood, we are absorbing a new reality. This reality is one of diverse and unheard perspectives, and it is only with time that we can make this our own.

e) Welcome constant learning or look at and listen to others to learn and incorporate their knowledge. This requires a full and conscious learning attitude towards the diversity and complexity of the environment in which community action will take place, leaving aside our expectations and prejudices regarding the potential for participation. This means we must be open to learning from the actors and organisations with whom we interact in different social settings.

f) Respect the intimacy and privacy of non-formal groups – consider the possibility that they don't want us around and their motivations for change differ from ours. Whilst our interests might be to articulate and connect various groups, they themselves might wish to remain as they are. Connections cannot be forced and the reasons to connect must be relevant to the group. We must take time to get to know and respect the rhythms of individuals and non-formal groups: perhaps going for a walk together is enough, for now.

Understanding the complex web of connections within a neighbourhood is the first step to moving from social groups to social communities.

Transformation of social group capital to social community capital

In this section we will discuss our work in the two neighbourhoods of Barcelona and illustrate the stages of getting to know the community and in particular the non-formal groups within the neighbourhood. In order to move from a neighbourhood with disconnected small groups to one that is well connected and has the potential for community development, beyond that produced in formal participation, we suggest a cyclical and iterative five-stage approach. This includes establishing the starting point, familiarisation, walking and looking around, holding conversations with non-formal groups and feedback in context. Each stage itself has four phases. Table 10.1 summarises the stages and phases of the approach. It is important to note that this is not necessarily a linear process: each stage or each Place identity, hope and expectations.

(1) Establishing the starting point

Questions/objectives to be addressed

The first step in the process is the most strategic. It consists of establishing our starting point. The questions or objectives that we need to work on are:

- Why and for what do we want to know community life beyond formal participation? or What is the agenda of those involved in the process?
- What resources will be allocated to this project (leadership, time, professional resources, materials)?
- And, assuming that it is an action linked to a previously existing community action, how does this initiative fit into the community action already taken?

Table 10.1 Stages and phases of non-formal neighbourhood work

Stage	Phase
1. Establishing the Starting Point	a) Questions/objectives to work on in this phase. b) Main actions to take. c) Ideal timescale. d) Lessons from our previous experience in Verneda Alta and Trinitat Nova.
2. Familiarisation	a) Questions/objectives to work on in this phase. b) Main actions to take. c) Ideal timescale. d) Lessons from our previous experience in Verneda Alta and Trinitat Nova.
3. Walking and Looking Around	a) Questions/objectives to work on in this phase. b) Main actions to take. c) Ideal timescale. d) Lessons from our previous experience in Verneda Alta and Trinitat Nova.
4. Conversations with Non-formal Groups	a) Questions/objectives to work on in this phase. b) Main actions to take. c) Ideal timescale. d) Lessons from our previous experience in Verneda Alta and Trinitat Nova.
5. Feedback in Context	a) Questions/objectives to work on in this phase. b) Main actions to take. c) Ideal timescale. d) Lessons from our previous experience in Verneda Alta and Trinitat Nova.

Main actions to be taken

- Address initial questions: The above questions must be addressed and shared with potential project partners, for example, by organising meetings with professionals from the neighbourhood's public services or with neighbourhood networks with whom we collaborate regularly. These meetings are an opportunity to publicise the project (and its area of interest) and to recognise and incorporate the knowledge of the community actors with whom we usually work.
- Establish a shared proposal: Once these starting questions have been worked out, from the leadership of the process, a shared proposal must be established where the objectives agreed between the promoters and the main allies in the context are detailed. That is, we have to have a contextualised proposal that indicates the time, the boundary of the geographic area, the necessary and available resources and the steps to reach the end of the road.

Ideal timescale

Between 15 days and a month and a half. It depends on the number of meetings that we have to have with community actors.

Lessons learnt from previous work

The first thing to consider in this phase is the energy required by the team of people needed to carry out the project. As far as possible, it is better that it be a team and not a single person who carries out the entire project. Many of the tasks are better carried out in pairs, for example.

The second, is that resources are needed to carry out the project: this work takes time and effort, which cannot be added to the daily work we do. In this way, either internal resources must be freed up to carry it out or external resources are added. In either case, we understand that the ideal team is one that incorporates the following skills and provisions:

- Knowledge of community-based and participatory intervention and analysis strategies and techniques, and the ability to guarantee a balance between rigour, adaptability and innovation before their implementation.
- Social and communication skills, in particular the willingness and confidence to strike up conversations with a range of different people in the neighbourhood
- Ability to synthesise the information generated.
- Ability to work in a team.
- Negotiation skills between various community actors.
- Provision of the time necessary to assume the tasks required throughout the process.

This intervention, like all those linked to community action, implies interacting with many people and groups, and building relational capital, which will be the basis for subsequent community actions. Ideally, this capital remains among the team who will later facilitate community action in the context. Two strategies can help achieve this. The same team that generates the links with informal groups should later be the ones to carry out the community actions. Alternatively, teams could be mixed teams of external professionals and actors from the territory, guaranteeing spaces for transfer of skills and facilitating the transfer of relational capital from one to the other.

(2) Familiarisation

Questions/objectives to be addressed

The second phase of the process has as its main objective that the team begins to absorb the nature of the place and its social and community life, making the unknown known. We understand familiarisation as an essential ingredient of community action and as a preliminary step in the exhaustive investigation of groups and people who make up the community non-formally, that is, who make neighbourhood life (Montero, 2006).

Main actions to be taken

Obtain maps of the territory or the physical space under investigation. These maps have to allow us to write down what we take in, in the first walks we make through the neighbourhood: distances, hot points of community activity and so on. The larger the map, the easier it will be to add detail to the spaces and share it with the whole team.

Define a system for recording the impressions that will be generated from this first familiarisation with the territory under exploration. For example, in the case of the project work, it was decided to identify the zones and distances within and between the maps of the neighbourhoods.

Furthermore, some initial photographs were also taken with mobile phones, and these were shared amongst the work team.

First contacts with the area: The team can make two or three free walks to familiarise themselves from the maps available and to know the topography, the real walking distances, public spaces, parks, main facilities and services, shops, bars, transportation and so on.

Establish reference zones for observation: From the first walks, the team can generate initial ideas about the main areas of the neighbourhood or territory where social and community life takes place. These walks enable us to develop criteria to identify different relevant divisions, for example, areas that can be observed in two hours of walks or areas that concentrate a higher density of social activity and interactions.

Walking with someone: After the free walks, it can be interesting to walk once or twice accompanied by key informants, to do community walks (Kagan et al., 2020). We understand that, as key informants, the people who live or work in the delimited area are experts in their social and community life. Then, familiarisation begins to incorporate a narrative dimension based on the stories about the territory shared by key informants: stories, community experiences, experiences about changes over time and discovery of the actors who play a leading role in social and community life. Different informants, by virtue of their different tacit knowledge, will produce different information.

Contrast the impressions and information generated in this phase of the process with more formal sources of information, such as services providers' reports and socio-economic data, to finish expanding our understanding.

We will finish this first approximation of understanding the place when we have an initial idea of: the diversity of views of what the area or neighbourhood to be explored means; as well as a first set of ideas about how we can divide the area, meaningfully, in order to organise the deployment of subsequent observations. We will also have identified areas where there is a social and community life that must be observed and learned more deeply.

Ideal timescale

This phase of familiarisation is worth time and effort. If this stage is over too quickly or we rush it in order to start "doing things", we may jeopardise relationships and have an inadequate understanding of the neighbourhood. We estimate between three and six weeks to complete this stage, depending on the size of the area to be explored and the number of team members participating in the project.

Lessons learnt from previous work

The activities require slow and organic rhythms. It is worth spending time on this first familiarisation: it is not only about spending hours to become familiar with the environment (walking, looking, listening, feeling, discovering, being surprised), but also allowing enough time to pass so that we assimilate what we are seeing and feeling. We are at a time when what we do is an insertion into an ecosystem that affects and cuts across us. It is not about going every day, morning, afternoon and night (because there comes a point where we do not see anything new) but about interspersing mornings, afternoons and nights on different days.

The attitude of familiarisation with community settings should be inherent in any effort to promote community action. We say this because frequently it is not. We often start our community actions by "convening" community actors, expecting them to participate in the spaces we propose to them. Seldom, before convening, do we allow ourselves an exercise of direct familiarisation with the real context where we want to promote our community actions. We have learnt, through the development of these projects, that familiarisation is a good place to start for a community action.

The division (or not) of the area to be explored by zones has to be flexible. We have learned that in order to be comprehensive and systematic in our observations, it is sometimes necessary to segment or divide the territory into more encompassing areas. Perhaps it is necessary to enable smaller areas to make the investigation task more operational. The criteria for creating these zones are marked by two variables: the extension of the zone and the degree of observable social and community activity.

Ideally, the initial walks are done in pairs or as a team. The first familiarisations with the territories can be enriched if the team dimension is considered; walking in pairs, at least, allows us to contrast what we observe and, later, put to the test the instruments that we have been creating to collect the information related to the project. This is an exercise that represents an opportunity to improve and adjust the project and its instruments to the reality we are trying to understand.

(3) Walking and looking around

Questions/objectives to be addressed

The third phase of the process aims at intense and extensive observation of the social and community life of the environment to be explored. These observations can be carried out through non-participatory observations (Guasch, 1997),at a certain distance, without coming into contact with people, a technique similar to the psychogeographical "dérive" (Debord, 1958) – more colloquially known as strolling or wandering.

The objective of this stage is to establish a systematic map of the community environment in which the non-formal groups with whom we will talk in the next stage of the project are detected.

Main actions to be taken

Firstly, the systems used to record the information generated must be defined. An example could be to combine three ways of recording the information:

- Two online forms, of the Google Form type, to be able to record the information and reflections resulting from the walks (non-participant observations): the first form records the information related to the non-formal groups under observation; and the second collates the global reflections about the walk or the observations, collected at the end of each session.
- A programme or application that allows to record the movements carried out in the community environment. We can use, for example, an application used by runners.
- Taking photographs of the non-formal groups detected or of the spaces with more social and community life. The photographs can be taken with any mobile phone and linked to the programme or applications used to record the walks.

Secondly, a schedule of observations must be created. For example, this could include a table with the hours, zones and people of the team to guarantee systematic observation of the community environment. Mornings, afternoons and nights on weekdays and also on weekends must be covered.

Thirdly, data from interviews with key informants in the community must be organised to complement the field trips. For example, the people interviewed may be waiters and waitresses in bars, shop assistants in pharmacies or markets, postmen and postwomen, or drivers of the neighbourhood bus. In short, these are people who have access to information about non-formal groups in the community, either because they can talk to many people throughout the day or because they move and see them every day.

Lastly, ensure that the systematisation and visualisation of non-formal groups is presented clearly and comprehensively. To finish this stage, we would have to systematise a list of spaces, times and groups observed, and collate and analyse the data collected in understandable way that is meaningful for the project.

Ideal timing

We calculate between four and eight weeks for walking and looking around, depending on the size of the neighbourhood, the energy of the team and what we find. As far as possible, it would be good to be able to collect field data in winter and summer, since community life in neighbourhoods can be quite different in these two seasons and, by extension, so would the findings of our research.

Whenever possible, it is better to carry out the walks in a staggered manner (spaced in time) and to be able to share the impressions that are generated with the team, since this will allow us to adjust the protocol of observations, of areas to observe, of schedules and so on.

This phase is the one that requires the most time and energy of the entire project and it is important that we be exhaustive in the systematic observation of the entire neighbourhood.

Lessons learnt from previous work

Walking does not mean going out desperately to meet people in the community environment. Low-key strolling is not compatible with quickly searching for targets to observe. Essentially, it means letting go organically, collecting ourselves and being calm and focused on what we do. In this way we are able to observe who and what we see, and what we hear and feel. Strolling could mean sitting on a bench to soak up the life that surrounds us, for example. This slow and informal way of working has to be learnt, because we are more used to moving quickly through city spaces and making instant judgements about what we experience. Walking also requires a space for reflection afterwards. It is necessary to provide spaces for reflection with the team, during and after the walks. Reflection makes it possible to adjust the walking strategy ad hoc, since it adapts to the knowledge that is being generated.

Walking implies a certain flexibility. Despite establishing routes for the walks, we have to adopt a criterion of flexibility in the face of situations that may be of interest, such as observing the groups that pass from one neighbourhood to another or that arrive at a public space at the moment the observation finishes, for example.

Before going for a walk, make sure that everything is ready. Before the walk, check that all recording systems are ready: including batteries and memory cards. It is necessary to be properly equipped, with appropriate clothing to take account of the climactic conditions of the season and the place. In this way, walks are enjoyable and not a trial.

(4) Conversations with non-formal groups

Questions/objectives to be addressed

The fourth phase that we propose has the fundamental objective of establishing conversations (Christens, 2010) with the non-formal groups identified in the previous stage. It embraces participatory observation (Guasch, 1997), because the team will access the daily situation of the groups and will seek to start and maintain conversations to learn about activities undertaken and their contribution. A door-to-door strategy could be implemented, involving previously identified groups and (also) with other community actors that may be of interest to us. In our work in the two neighbourhoods, we have used this stage to establish and follow a more expansive and comprehensive strategy, aimed at conversing with neighbours in general.

Main actions to be taken

Once more, it is necessary to define the systems that will generate and record the content of the conversations. Two systems have been found to be useful: a protocol of questions to ask during conversations, and a method of recording conversations with informed consent.

In order to talk with them, we must find non-formal groups. The non-formal groups previously identified in the community setting must be systematically searched for and talked to. We have to say that in the two projects on which we based this experience, if it is impossible to contact all the groups previously detected, this does not mean that we are not doing well. The challenge is to get a good spread of groups and informants, not to talk to absolutely everyone in a neighbourhood.

The actions of conversing with the non-formal groups detected can be complemented with non-formal conversations with residents of the community environment (who may or may not be a member of a group). With the desire to expand the stories about social and community life, we can take advantage of this stage of the process to establish conversations with people who pass through the community environment. We will illustrate ways in which this can be done by presenting two of the strategies we use, in order to include people in our neighbourhood work.

The first strategy was to deploy our students of Community Psychology at the University of Barcelona. They were dispersed throughout the neighbourhood and they established and recorded conversations with people who were in the street. These conversations extended over the following two weeks with groups of between eight and ten students who had more conversations with neighbours in the mornings and afternoons. In total, 423 conversations were recorded.

The second strategy was to undertake street-based sofa conversations. Two sofas were placed in the morning, afternoon and evening for three weeks in various locations of the neighbourhood. The neighbourhoods were identified from earlier stages of getting to know the community. A team of three people for each sofa invited neighbours to sit down and talk about the neighbourhood and its social and community life. In total, 653 conversations were recorded.

Once all the information has been generated, at this stage of the project it will have to be systematised for analysis and subsequent feedback (Kagan et al., 2020). For example, in the case of recorded conversations with non-formal groups, you can choose to transcribe the audio files (created either within the team or done professionally outside the team) and perform the analysis with qualitative data analysis techniques, such as thematic analysis (Braun & Clarke, 2006).

This analysis makes it possible to generate maps with the main issues identified in the information obtained and to make everything that we have found in the project more understandable.

In the case of unrecorded conversations, expect the people who have them to fill out a questionnaire right after they have occurred. In this questionnaire they will write down the main ideas collected; these data can also be analysed by applying the thematic analysis technique or the analysis that is considered appropriate. Kagan et al. (2020, p. 200) describe the process of systematisation as follows: "The idea is that the recording, recuperation and sharing of people's different interpretations of common experiences leads to new insights [...] and new ways of understanding and theorising about the world – all based on concrete action sand experiences".

Ideal timescale

This stage of conversations can last between one and two months, depending on whether we restrict our conversations to previously detected groups (and then the number of groups) or whether we take the opportunity to organise conversations with the general public as well.

Lessons learnt from previous work

Sometimes the people we meet don't want to talk. Starting a conversation with a person or people we do not know is not easy. We need to introduce ourselves, make it clear what the objectives of the conversation are and why we want to talk. In general we have found that we will be well received, but we must bear in mind that there are people who do not want to talk to us; in this case, we must respect their disposition and appreciate their frankness.

Talking does not mean taking a survey. Although there is a protocol of questions that can inspire us for conversations, the attitude to have in these conversations is one of openness and flexibility. It is necessary to contribute to generating a relaxed atmosphere and active listening that allows a respectful and generative interaction between the team and the people with whom they talk.

The act of conversation can be trained. It is recommended that the team role-play the conversations before carrying out the first ones. Likewise, it is advisable to create a space for reflection and learning within the team about the conversations held, with the aim of gradually improving and generating knowledge.

Talking with citizens can be an opportunity to incorporate other actors into projects. In the work that we have carried out in Trinidad Nova and Verneda Alta, we have incorporated around 90 students of the degree of psychology to talk with neighbours. What about incorporating students from the neighbourhood school? Or members of the community network with whom we usually interact? Or professionals of the service providers of the neighbourhood?

(5) Feedback in context
Questions/objectives to be addressed

The objective of this phase is to be able to organise the return of the information generated, make the analysis and extract the main conclusions that have been reached within the framework of the project. It is about "closing to open", that is, closing the work that we have done to open up the possibilities to work with this community life that we have "discovered" and potentially enrich the community actions that we are carrying out. From this perspective, such sharing must allow for:

- Recognising the contribution of all the people who have offered their ideas, opinions and experiences. For example, inviting them to be part of this space and to be the protagonists.
- Ensuring that the different information generated by the project is shared in an understandable and assimilable way. For example, using different ways of communicating research results in a variety of different ways.
- Facilitating the people attending the feedback sessions to articulate their reactions. It is necessary to think of dynamics to interconnect the people who attend the feedback. That involves including ways in which they can meet and find common ground with each other, formally (in participatory small group dynamics, for example) or non-formally (having a juice or a coffee).
- Being a link or transfer point between the end of the search for non-formal community groups and the future derived community action.

Main actions to be taken

There are four key actions in this stage.

- Prepare the results of the information analysis and the conclusions in accessible and understandable formats for the general public. Use different formats for different audiences.
- Convene the people who have stated that they want to know the results of the projects. For this reason, it is important that beforehand some type of agile communication channel has been set up, for example, email or mobile phone.
- Design and organise the event in a space in the community environment ideal for a dynamic and creative feedback session. Remember that, as we said at the beginning, if we want different things to happen, we have to do different things.
- Take advantage of the feedback session to collect new contributions from participants who contribute to further strengthening the social and community life of the community environment.

Ideal timescale

Between 15 days and a month, depending on whether we have one or more feedback sessions and the ability to prepare the information generated in the previous stage of the conversations.

Lessons learnt from previous work

Close and comfortable feedback spaces must be guaranteed. In the previous stage we created a comfortable space to talk, and we try to maintain this same spirit in this final stage. We promote recognition and active listening, a warm and welcoming climate and, above all, an organic rhythm, a parenthesis in the hurry of every day.

We need to get closer to where the non-formal groups are. Since we are talking about groups that have particular, "other" forms and places of participation, if we want to make it easier for them to be protagonists of the feedback, and take community building forward, we have to bring it closer to their contexts. Rather than holding the session in the civic centre or the local residents' association, for example, we could approach the park, the sports courts or the other identified spaces where community life converges.

Final thoughts

We have outlined a method of working to identify and include non-formal groups and residents in understanding a community, with a view to engaging a wider number of people in community actions, beyond formal associations. This is not the end point; rather, it lays the foundation for exploring the potential of moving from a collection of social groups to a social community – one that is connected and resilient, able to participate in further actions for change. We do not want to end this chapter without sharing the fulfilment that discovering that there is community life beyond formal participation in our neighbourhoods has brought us. This is a communitarian life, normally forgotten and marginalised by the public imposition of a particular type of communitarian action. We still have strong "bricks" which constitute and can be used to build community in our districts. These form life that is organised in a small-scale, diverse and creative way, oriented to the satisfaction of basic and daily needs, and that contributes to bringing public space to life. These elements build an "us" to lean on, beyond a collection of "me's" in our neighbourhoods and cities. We think we still have a lot of learning to do, which will require commitments of time, energy and resources. Finding and growing these building blocks is our best future for community life in the kinds of neighbourhoods we want to live in.

References

Adjuntament de Barcelona (2017). *Hacia una política pública de acción comunitaria: marco conceptual, estratégico y operativo*. Direcció de Serveis d'Acció Comunitària de Drets de Ciutadania, Participaciói Transparència.

Braun, V., & Clarke, V. (2006). Using thematic analysis in psychology. *Qualitative Research in Psychology, 3*, 77–101.

Carmona, M. (2011). *Construyendo acción comunitaria: significados y estrategias para su promoción a partir de las experiencias de Barcelona*. [Tesis doctoral]. Universidad de Barcelona.

Carmona, M., & Rebollo, O. (2009). *Guía operativa de la acción comunitaria*. Ajuntament de Barcelona.

Christens, B.D. (2010). Public relationship building in grassroots community organising: Relational intervention for individual and systems change. *Journal of Community Psychology, 38*(7), 886–900. https://doi.org/10.1002/jcop.20403

Debord, G. (1956). Theory of the dérive. In K. Knabb(Ed.), *Situationist international anthology* (pp. 50–4). Bureau of Public Secrets.

Durston, J. (2002). *El capital social campesino en la gestión del desarrollo rural. Díadas, equipos, puentes y escaleras*. CEPAL.

Foster-Fishman, P.G., Collins, C., & Pierce, S.J. (2013). An investigation of the dynamic processes promoting citizen participation. *American Journal of Community Psychology, 51*(3–4), 492–509. https://doi.org/10.1007/s10464-012-9566-y

Garrido, M. (2015). *Capital social comunitario: fuentes y dinamismos en redes inter-organizacionales de barrios urbanos desfavorecidos: el caso de Tres Barrios-Amate*. [Tesis doctoral]. Universidad Pablo de Olavide.

Guasch, O. (1997), *Observación participante. Cuaderno smetodológicos*. CIS.

Jetten, J., Reicher, S.D., Haslam, S.A., & Cruwys, T. (2020). *Together apart: The psychology of COVID-19*. SAGE. https://socialsciencespace.com/2020/05/addressing-the-psychology-of-together-apart-free-book-download/

Kagan, K., Burton, M., Duckett, P., Lawthom, R., & Siddiquee, A. (2020). *Critical community psychology: Critical action and social change* (2nd ed.). Routledge.

Kim, H.Y. (2018). Effects of social capital on collective action for community development. *Social Behavior and Personality, 46*(6), 1011–28. https://doi.org/10.2224/sbp.7082

Llena, A., & Úcar, X. (2006). Acción comunitaria: miradas y diá logos interdisciplinares. In X. Úcar & A. Llena (Eds.), *Miradas y diálogos entorno a la acción comunitaria* (pp. 11–57). Graò.

Montero, M. (2006). *Hacer para transformar: el método oen la psicología comunitaria*. Paidós.

Morales, E., & Rebollo, O. (2014). Potencialidades y límites de la acción comunitaria como estrategia empodera dora en el contexto actual de crisis. *Revista de Treball Social, 203*, 9–22.

Pindado, F. (2008). *La participación ciudadana es la vida de las ciudades*. Ediciones del Serbal.

Wang, Z., Zhang, F., & Wu, F. (2020). The contribution of inter group neighbouring to community participation: Evidence from Shanghai. *Urban Studies*, *57*(6), 1224–42. https://doi.org/10.1177/0042098019830899

Whitham, M.M. (2012). Community connections: Social capital and community success. *Sociological Forum*, *27*(2), 441–57. https://doi.org/10.1111/j.1573-7861.2012.01325.x

Whitham, M.M. (2019). Community entitativity and civic engagement. *City and Community*, *18*(3), 896–914. https://doi.org/10.1111/cico.12385

11

A CALL FOR A DIGITAL COMMUNITY PSYCHOLOGY

Jenna Condie and Michael Richards

Abstract

Community Psychology has seemingly been left behind on the digital front. For one reason or another, the connections between Community Psychology, digital technologies and social media remain unplugged. We are calling for a new "Digital Community Psychology". In this chapter, we apply a digital autoethnographic method to generate knowledge about Community Psychology, social media and digital technologies. We reflect on what "Digital Community Psychology" might entail in email "call and response" exchanges. We use our emails to one another as data to explore and outline the disconnect between Community Psychology, digital technologies and social media. Second, we examine Community Psychology's existence against "mainstream psychology" to make the case for critical forms of psychology to interrogate and render accountable the powerful advances in the digitalisation and datafication of society, institutions and social practices. To push community psychological work around human–technology relations further, we draw upon ideas and concepts from transdisciplinary fields of knowledge, mainly from the scholarly work that is being badged together as feminist new materialism and posthumanism. Then we theorise social media communities: what are they becoming and what new subjectivities reflect our networked lives? Lastly, we include a case study that highlights how making social media for social activism falls within the remit of practicing Digital Community Psychology.

Resumen

En este capítulo, aplicamos un método autoetnográfico digital para generar conocimiento sobre la psicología comunitaria, medio social y tecnologías digitales. En primer lugar, reflexionamos sobre lo que una nueva "psicología de la comunidad digital" podría implicar por intercambios de "llamadas y respuestas" por correo electrónico. Usamos los correos electrónicos entre nosotros como datos para explorar y delinear la desconexión entre la psicología comunitaria, las tecnologías digitales y las redes sociales. En segundo lugar, utilizamos la existencia de la psicología comunitaria contra la "psicología convencional" para reclamar las formas críticas de la psicología para interrogar y rendir cuentas de los poderosos avances en la digitalización y datificación de la sociedad, las instituciones y las prácticas sociales. Para impulsar aún más el

DOI: 10.4324/9780429325663-14

trabajo psicológico comunitario en torno a las relaciones entre humanos y tecnología, utilizamos nuevos conceptos, ideas y la explosión de la producción de nuevos conocimientos desde nuevos campos transdisciplinarios del conocimiento, principalmente del trabajo académico que se está identificando como nuevo materialismo feminista y posthumanismo. Luego teorizamos las comunidades de medios sociales: ¿en qué se están convirtiendo y qué nuevas subjetividades reflejan nuestras vidas en las redes? Por último, incluimos un estudio de caso que destaca cómo hacer medios sociales para el activismo social entra dentro del ámbito de la práctica de la Psicología Comunitaria Digital.

Introduction

The possibilities and implications of our digitalising society require disciplinary and practice-based attention within Community Psychology. We argue that, to date, Community Psychology has seemingly been left behind on the digital front, particularly when compared to other disciplines and some of the new and emerging fields of knowledge. In this chapter, we apply "writing as inquiry" (Richardson & St Pierre, 2005) as a digital autoethnographic method to generate new knowledge about Community Psychology, social media, digital technologies and social justice/activism. This is a methodological approach that Jenna, an author of this chapter, has applied with colleagues elsewhere to examine their involvement in public housing activism (Chatterjee et al., 2019). "Writing as inquiry" works in a post-qualitative mode (St Pierre, 2018) where living with critical theories and working against "mainstream psychology" are the positions from which we have come to know Community Psychology and what it is (and invariably what and who we are) in the processes of becoming. Our email exchanges of "just writing" (Linnell & Horsfall, 2016) to one another provide us with qualitative data, which we use to map out the opportunities and challenges of digital technologies and social media for Community Psychology and relatedly, social justice.

This chapter exists to ensure a technological and digital dimension was included in this handbook. Initially Jenna planned to contribute a chapter about making social media in housing activism. However, this plan changed through a dialogue between Jenna (as contributor) and Michael (as co-editor) about the possibilities and implications of a Digital Community Psychology. What does that look like? How will it come about? Why does that matter? And who are "we" to conjure it up?

Jenna:

I must locate myself when I offer this analysis and why I am compelled to configure the possibilities and implications of social media and digital technologies for Community Psychology with you. My first discipline was what we refer to as "mainstream psychology". I moved into the more critical forms of "mainstream psychology" and towards qualitative methodologies during my PhD research. I do not identify as a community psychologist or any kind of psychologist anymore to be honest. However, I do feel as though I might always be on the very edges of the discipline as I venture in and out of the discipline in "nomadic" (Braidotti, 2019a) mode when it is conceptually necessary to do so. In my scholarship, I hope to make my location in the margins of Psychology both productive and activist, and so here I am speaking up about making social media within community psychological work.

Michael:

Similarly, I have not worked in a Psychology department since 2014 and I knew at the time that I would start to move away from Psychology, and I see myself on the fringes too. When I put my PhD together, it was interdisciplinary and a big part of it was around [Rosi] Braidotti and the posthuman, and I love that stuff and I am trying to write more about how psychology can learn more from posthuman thinking through the lens of people with disabilities. So, maybe as we introduce the chapter and locate ourselves, we can put those thoughts together to show that we are on that edge, dipping in and out. I have suggested that's what community psychologists need to do anyway going forward rather than being entrenched into a "division" or "section" like at the British Psychological Society, UK. It's interesting isn't that we worked in quite a mainstream, straight down the line Psychology department at Salford, UK, and then 6–7 years later, unbeknown to us, we have journeyed to the edges of Psychology and beyond.

Throughout the chapter, we include direct quotes from our emails to show the trajectory of our arguments and where our points are going. From this point on, we do not always denote who is speaking as we felt that it does not matter so much as we have co-produced this piece. Also, by threading our email data into our "chapter voice", we seek to offer a "multi-voicedness" and "polyphony" of voices (Bakhtin, 1984) so that we can speak from subject positions that may otherwise be less available, perhaps even unavailable. We did not aim to write a finalising monologue on Community Psychology, what the discipline is and what it is becoming with technologies. We want to be a part of, and encourage an "unfinalising approach to social science scholarship" (Cooper & Condie, 2016, p. 39) and have used "writing as inquiry" as a creative, reflexive method to do so.

I started writing my reply into a first draft of our chapter, but I find writing for email provides greater freedom to say what I need to say in comparison to writing straight up in "chapter voice". So everything is here instead.

"Writing as inquiry" sounds good to me, and forgive me if I keep tinkering with it in such a way that formalises it like a normal chapter, but that might link with the response above to your "position" about being in and out of Psychology, because I am the same, and I always seem to be straddling between the formalities and structured ways that I have been taught to write in Psychology, and yet, wanting to be creative and different, like much of the research I have actually done.

While we may be attempting a more creative approach to academic writing, there is always the pull back to the trained ways of being academic. Even writing emails to one another is very academic! Our work here is always tied – tied to tradition while we attempt to pull away, and tied to what we are calling here "mainstream psychology" while we attempt to critically re-orientate ourselves as well as Community Psychology as a sub-discipline.

In what follows, we firstly explore and outline the disconnect between Community Psychology, digital technologies and social media. Second, we use Community's Psychology's existence against "mainstream psychology" to make the case for critical forms of psychology to interrogate and render accountable the powerful advances in the digitalisation and datafication of society, institutions and social practices. To push community psychological work around human–technology relations further, we draw upon new ideas and concepts from scholarly work that is being badged together as feminist new materialism and posthumanism. Then we theorise social media communities: what are they becoming and what new subjectivities reflect our networked lives? Lastly, we conclude with the materialities of making social media for social activism and justice within the remit of researching within and practicing Community Psychology.

The disconnect between Community Psychology, digital technologies and social media

For one reason or another, the connections between Community Psychology, digital technologies and social media have yet to be made even though our lives have always been technologically enmeshed and now digital technologies "saturate" everything (Ruppert, Law, & Savage, 2013). Whilst papers have been published that promote the use of social media and media networks under the umbrella of Community Psychology (for example, Siddiquee & Kagan, 2006; Sichel et al., 2020), and promote the benefits of online communities (De Meulenaere, Baccarne, Courtois, & Ponnet, 2020), the literature is scarce in linking Community Psychology and digital technologies together. This scarcity is alarming, given the explosion of online networks, the mobilising role of social media in social movements (Brown, Ray, Summers & Fraistat, 2017), and the imbalances of power and social inequalities that are materialised through digital means (Noble, 2018; Schradie, 2018). Community Psychology must have something to say.

The digitalisation and datafication of society, its institutions and its social life should be somewhere near centre stage within contemporary "Community Psychology". Long-standing social inequalities manifest anew as new digital systems, practices and technological infrastructures marginalise, oppress, exclude and punish some people to the benefit of others (Eubanks, 2017; Noble, 2018). Social media are perhaps well described as a double-edged sword. Our new digital platforms where much of our sociality is now entwined, have positives and negatives, advantages and disadvantages, and gains and losses. Indeed, social media are proving to be complex and contradictory spaces (Locke, Lawthom, & Lyons, 2018). Social media has certainly opened up new opportunities for civic engagement, community participation, dialogue and action. But who gets to participate, and on what grounds do they stand upon in order to instigate change? While our increasingly digitalised sociality forms part of "society's institutional fabric" (van Dijck, 2013, p. 6), not everyone is part of the tapestry currently being made. Some people, groups and communities might be likened to loose threads in the digital tapestry, or are falling through the holes in that they are not woven into the fabric at all. For example, whilst it should not be assumed that people with intellectual disabilities cannot engage with social media, as many do, there are many challenges such as not being able to read or write, or not being able to afford the Internet and use social media on a regular basis, ensuring that only certain groups are "allowed" to engage.

Like you, I am also surprised that there are not yet the key "go to" pieces of writing that we wish there were by community psychologists, which connect Community Psychology, social media and digital technologies. A Google Scholar search brings up a handful of articles about applying digital technologies for community psychological work and using social media for research dissemination, but nothing substantial nor particularly critical nor with any notable calls to action. That said, I am also unsurprised as many disciplines have been slow to social media and are struggling to grapple with the impacts of digital technologies for their respective fields. Slowness is not necessarily bad and a hesitance to jump on the social media bandwagon may well be justified. Social media and our new technologies are not turning out to be the utopian democratic equalising technologies they were purported to be in the early days of the web. Far from it.

In her book *Pressed for Time*, Judy Wajcman (2015) argues that things are not moving so quickly if you get some perspective on the historicity of technological change within society. The slower-moving disciplines can therefore put technological change into perspective. For example, the workings of communities are in many ways a continuity of what has come before the digitalisation of social networks and relations. Working at a slower pace also stands at odds with the contemporary university machine, and our current state of advanced cognitive capitalism (Braidotti, 2019b). Going more slowly, therefore, fits with the description of Community Psychology as resisting neoliberalism and the status quo (i.e. the accelerated pace of our times). Marginalisation and oppression are centuries in the making; so too is social media if you take a more historical perspective.

It is important not to get carried away and lost to the hurried pace that characterises technologically induced change and "innovation". Actually, the technology industry now turns towards longer-standing disciplines for answers to the social problems it has embedded in code and amplified through digital platforms, and to address the economic, political, cultural, ethical and unjust implications of their creations. Flipping things on its head, Community Psychology could make an important contribution to the technology industry, and not vice versa. A question for community psychologists is what can you/must you bring to social media and digital technologies to ensure they work for marginalised communities and against structural inequalities?

Community Psychology is relevant to social media and digital technologies – without the social relations between people and the groups that people make up, much of the web is completely defunct. Facebook, Twitter, Instagram, TikTok, WhatsApp, WeChat and so on are completely inseparable from communities.

> *Without communities, there is no platform. A community psychology of social media needs theorising. Perhaps I can be as bold as to say we are making a start here?*

Perhaps our concern is less with why Community Psychology has not boldly ventured into the digital realm and more with what could be gained if and when it does. We draw from new highly productive and generative interdisciplinary fields of inquiry that are examining the digital more prominently such as the Critical Posthumanities (Braidotti 2019a), Critical Data Studies (Dalton & Thatcher, 2014), and Critical Disability Studies (Goodley, Lawthom & Runswick, 2014; Goodley et al., 2019) for scholarly ideas and practical support.

Countering "mainstream psychology's" technological power and persuasive design

Community Psychology challenges the pathologising, individualising and neoliberalising ways of "mainstream psychology" with a framework that seeks to collaborate with those who are most marginalised by society. Community Psychology is ethically focused, participatory driven and committed to social justice and forging long-standing alliances across communities and disciplines. Unlike the medicalised underpinnings of "mainstream psychology", reflexive practices underpin community psychological work. Thus creative and visual methods are often employed, and the controlled, clinical, scientised experiments that take place in laboratories and other controlled conditions are resisted and rejected. Community Psychology is about how people think, experience, feel and act in their struggles to create better communities, lives and livelihoods for themselves and others (Burton, Boyle, Harris, & Kagan, 2007). However, as we have pointed out, the values that underpin much of Community Psychology do not directly connect with digital technologies in a way that one would expect. And, perhaps a key reason for Community Psychology to take on social media and digital technologies is that "mainstream psychology" is doing so and therefore particularly appeals to the technology industries.

> *For me, one of the most notorious and notable examples in recent years is the Facebook Cambridge Analytica data privacy scandal where the data analytics company harvested data from around 87 million Facebook users' profiles without their consent (Cadwalladr, 2018). The data was used to create tailored political advertising based on personality-based predictions so as to influence voting during the 2016 US presidential elections. The personality work came from a University of Cambridge graduate working for the data company. The misuse of power and issues of ethics, privacy, and data rights abound. But people don't really care too much about data privacy and breaches from Facebook even after such a scandal (e.g. Hinds, Williams, & Joinson, 2020). Apathy? Helplessness? Or is it that the platforms provide so much pleasure that their problems are ignored?*

"Mainstream psychology" can be a very problematic field when applied to technology, and its tools can be used to influence, persuade, manipulate and harm. Indeed, research on the culture of the Silicon Valley technology industries where many of our platforms, apps and digital products originate, shows that there is a keen interest in, and use of, the psychology of addiction, motivation and persuasion (Cook, 2020). New digital products are being designed and built in ways that tap into our "psychological make-up" (Brennan, 2020) to get us to do things such as download apps, upload data, play games, buy products, check in, check out, stream content, post content, share content, take photos, like photos, comment on photos, make videos, use filters, swipe left and right, talk to friends, talk to strangers, and so on. Known as "persuasive design", such application of psychological knowledge is highly contentious and ethically contestable (Brennan, 2020).

> *The apps and platforms, phones and devices are all needy for our attention. Look at me, look at this, so-and-so waved at you, so-and-so messaged you, so-and-so checked in, look at me. LOOK! Feel this way. Want this, want that. Look at what they have? Look at their life? Look at yours? Loook!*

Our digital actions are generating increasingly more data about ourselves that is worth something and has value. Jenna has previously considered the implications of profit-driven platforms structuring human–technology interactions in the context of digital dating practices where companies are capitalising on our most intimate relationships of all (Condie, Lean, & James, 2018). By gamifying and simplifying intimate dating practices, the apps are not working ethically in many ways, especially when we centre race, gender, class, sexuality, age and ability in analysing new dating technologies. The dating app industry has been encouraging a commodification of people through its designed marketplace of people, which is resulting in toxic interactions and unsafe encounters for many of those involved. If apps are reworking even our intimate relations, is there anything left untouched?

> *Then there is the creation of new apps as solutions to treat mental health and make profit from "life itself" (Rose, 2007). Got low self-esteem? Try this app. Can't sleep? Track your sleep/ wake cycle here! Want your welfare check? Insert your data here.*

Take another intimate realm, that of mental health. Telehealth technologies and mental health apps are growing, especially under present pandemic conditions (Cosgrove, Karter, Morrill, &

McGinley, 2020). De Vos (2021) notes that the "digitalisation of counselling and psychotherapy played right into the hands of official policies" (pp. 12–13) to push mental health services into the digital realm permanently. Such digital interventions in mental health matters require caution and interrogation given the ethical challenges they pose and the agentic constraints they can put on the people who use them. If an app evidences a person's mental health distress, what are the implications and consequences? Who is told (or not told)? Who becomes responsibilised by the technologies capacity to report and inform? What data is being collected and how might it be used against somebody? More pressing still is how a person's psychological/mental health data might be used to predict and shape their thoughts, behaviours and desires (Cosgrove, Karter, Morrill, & McGinley, 2020). Money talks and "mainstream psychology" rarely ventures into untangling the technology from its revenue streams to consider how it might look if designed without profit in mind.

Methodologically, "mainstream psychology's" preference for experimental and quantitative methods aligns with the huge volumes of digital data being generated by our technological activities. The datafication of society fits well with the quest to quantify and know all that there is to know about the individual. How this data might be used by societal institutions, government services and private corporations, as well as the person's rights to personal data ownership, are some of the biggest questions of our time. The implications of "big data" in Psychology require critique.

> *In contrast to my earlier Google Scholar search for "Community Psychology and social media", a Google Scholar search for "big data Psychology" returns some clear and obvious "go to" publications on this topic.*

The issues are plentiful – psychological knowledge being used to create powerful (*monstrous*) social media and digital technologies, psychological research pathologising and essentialising digital behaviours, and psychological methodologies and analytical approaches aligning with the digitalised profit making of every single aspect of people's everyday lives. What is being stirred up within digital technologies and social media right now is far from "good compost" (Haraway, 2016). The situation is quite dire as we write it out here. Do community psychologists have the capacity to step into this mess?

Yes!

Community psychologists are well positioned to tackle this mess because with the ethically driven, emancipatory and inclusive approach that Community Psychology proposes, we can begin to tackle the scientific, experimental and psychologised dimensions of the digital that "mainstream psychology" is manifesting within itself, the technology industries and beyond. This is crucial because as we have seen in the recent pandemic, COVID-19 was psychologised and linked strongly to digitalisation. For example, De Vos (2021) pointed out that this pandemic forced people to engage more with people in digital spaces, socially, for work, to learn at a school and so on. The mixing of the digital and the psychologising proposition that this is "good for us" has impacted on people's mental health, isolating and marginalising people maybe more than ever before (De Vos, 2021). An ethically driven, inclusive and emancipatory Digital Community Psychology might just be the way to tackle some of those disturbing consequences of "psychodigitalisation".

> *I like the term "psychodigitalisation", it seems apt for us.*

New ideas and practices from feminist new materialism and posthumanism

I use Rosi Braidotti's work on the posthuman a lot as it is so productive for thinking and doing scholarship differently. It gives me more confidence to be a scholar-activist. It gives me more confidence to challenge the status quo. A materialist perspective enables me to say/do more than a social constructionist stance ever did.

Community Psychology can utilise ideas and concepts about humans and technologies from feminist new materialism and posthumanism (Barad, 2003, 2007; Bennett, 2010; Braidotti, 2013, 2019; Coole & Frost, 2020; Fox & Alldred, 2015; Haraway, 2016). It is challenging to trace the impacts of posthumanism and feminist new materialism within Community Psychology given the interdisciplinary aspects of the field and its practitioners. Community Psychology probably already does make use of feminist new materialist and post-humanist ideas as they are part of the broader "material turn" (Mukerji, 2015), especially as Community Psychology already decentres the human somewhat by accounting for how our conditions and social structures impact the political, economic, environmental and colonial contexts within which we live, shape people and communities (see Sonn & Baker, 2015). It is only one step away from considering humans in assemblages with other human and non-human actors (technologies, institutions, structures, animals, places).

Although am I right in saying that our technological and digital conditions are not typically brought into the fold as yet? I turned towards Feminist New Materialism and Posthumanism to think differently about digital life when my home disciplines were not offering the necessary complexity and new subjectivities required to understand the relationship between humans and technologies.

Post-humanist and new materialist philosophies offer ways to think differently about the human and replace dominant binary constructs – the human/non-human, body/machine, online/offline, self/other, people/places, digital/material – that reinforce boundaries between what should be considered intra-acting phenomena (Barad, 2003). In other words, there is clear split or boundary between one person and the next. Who we are is because of the other – human, machine, otherwise. Jenna has drawn upon feminist new materialism the most to better understand her participation in the "rush of research" on dating apps (Condie, Lean, & James, 2018), arguing that anthropocentrism abounds in research on digital dating practices where agency is often located firmly within the person (also called the "user") and therefore technology's capacity to act and produce phenomena is dangerously downplayed. Motivations and gratifications, personality traits, antisocial behaviours and gender differences in dating practices are "mainstream psychology's" foci. These studies demarcate the human from the non-human, the subject from the object, the man from the woman and so on. This is reductive, essentialist, finalised and contributes to othering. Technology and its ability to act with people in the productions and performativities of bodies, things and power, should be in focus.

I do love this posthuman perspective, thinking about technology, identities and how we think about what a "human" is. I have written similar stuff in relation to disabilities, so going beyond the binary of disabled vs. non-disabled. This is powerful and maybe Psychology and Community Psychology needs to embrace the ideas behind these newer perspectives more. Here's a link a to a very blunt paper I published about myself and it links in with posthumanism later on, only a short paper (Richards, 2016), but I am clear enough when I say that "it is becoming more difficult to define what people are or are not as we move further into the twenty-first century." (Richards, 2016, p. 1304)

One of the things that strikes me from your paper is the power of labelling and how technology can be co-opted for that labelling process and used by institutions to digitally flag, mark, categorise and label people. In this way, technology and our digital systems are harming and killing people.

The posthuman is not only about new concepts and ways of thinking about humans, communities, places, spaces, inequalities and justice, but also new ways of doing research and new ethical praxis. Karen Barad (2007) intertwines questions of ethics, knowing (epistemology), and being (ontology) with the new materialist concept of "ethico-onto-epistemology" to situate research as a complex "intra-action" with no clear boundaries between theory, method and ethics. When does research start and end when you have a phone in your hand and you are already becoming-with a community of people in a digital space? The term "intra-action" is proposed to go beyond "interaction" to understand that binaries and entities (e.g. human/non-human, online/offline, digital/material, male/female) were always one and becoming together. A new materialist approach sees digital technologies performing with people "and these performances take place somewhere" (Condie, Lean, & James, 2018). New materialism takes on the struggles and strengths of feminist, postcolonial, anti-racist and queer theories in resisting binaries and finalising categorisation, and examining the boundary-making practices of research and knowledge production (Haraway, 2016). Community psychologists in the main will also claim to take a similar stance. For instance, Community Psychology is well placed to make use of, research and agitate for change with social media given its arts-based practices and creative, ethical ways of working with communities, and with its strong links to participatory action research approaches too.

With digital platforms rearranging our work and lives, we need to rethink the way we do our research, and "reassemble" our "social science apparatus" (Ruppert, Law, & Savage, 2013). Community Psychology is well placed to engage with this through its creative and inter/intra-disciplinary connections. The rules of research demand to be rewritten when the field is your laptop or smartphone and you are already becoming a researcher through your networked, located, digitalised existence. Creativity is therefore key when embracing the complexities of mobile technologised lives, to make the technology accessible and engaging for all, including for people from oppressed groups such as those with disabilities, and to do this, community psychologists must work across disciplines and continue to create space for other ways of knowing about the world and doing our human-technology-society research.

Understanding social media communities: what are "we" becoming?

I think I need to write something on the current state of social media communities and how communities are starting, forming, reinforcing, changing, instigating, agitating, and ending. What are communities now? Who is "we"?

We are conscious that almost by default, encouraging Community Psychology to engage with digital technologies might instigate somewhat individualising processes. For example, Reich (2010) recognised that people switch social networks frequently rather than remain in a community, which has been theorised as "networked individualism" (see Wellman et al., 2003). This might lead to less face-to-face contact, weaker relationships, less community spirit and togetherness amongst people and communities. Indeed, when the Internet and digital technologies emerged, there was a moral panic that communities would be lost altogether because amongst other things, the individualised nature of digital technology might cause communities to split and be divided (Hampton & Wellman, 2018). Whilst there was a moral panic feel to these claims, it can be argued that digital technologies do strip away the complexities of communities or social networks by enabling one-to-one interactions so that there is less accountability to a group or wider social relations for a person's behaviour. Such individualising and separating designs enable problematic encounters that capitalise on the power inequalities and differing vulnerabilities between people in their digitally mediated interactions (James, Condie, & Lean, 2019).

> *Dating apps provide the example here again where swiping generates "matches" with people who you cannot situate within your networks because the information has been taken away or is not allowed due to data privacy policies. Any mutual friends or connections? You have to get more information and go looking on other social media platforms for more details to verify a person. Those who are less safe in new encounters have to do more digital labour to figure out if they are good and safe to meet.*

With those thoughts in mind, we started to consider perspectives from feminist new materialism and posthumanism. These perspectives confront the humanist notions of the individual and the human by stretching the dominant ways of understanding subjectivity in new directions (Connolly, 2013), by decentring the human and recognising the agency of the material world. As previously stated, community psychologists, especially the more critical kind, are already there in some ways. Our digital systems add another component to the assemblage of communities and are structuring and shaping how social groups form, change and grow. However, the echoes of "mainstream psychology" and the tie to the human as a distinct and superior entity remain (Brinkmann, 2017). Yet, as Michael has argued elsewhere (Richards, 2016), this is problematic, particularly when thinking about "disabilities". For example, instead of being caught up in a "battle of the binaries", of deciding whether someone is disabled or not, or autistic or not, we instead should consider disabilities and humanities as a productive relationship that challenges norms, labels and sameness. This may help ensure that we see disabilities not through a medicalised gaze but through theoretical, practical and political lenses, which might break down the barriers that those traditional binaries enforce (see Goodley, Lawthom, & Runswick-Cole, 2014; Goodley & Runswick-Cole, 2016; Goodley, Runswick-Cole, & Liddiard, 2016).

> *I really like the notion of "a battle of binaries" in terms of individual identities equally applies to communities. Also this point "it is becoming more difficult to define what people are or are not as we move further into the twenty-first century" (Richards, 2016 p. 1304). New technologies and social media are making it more difficult to define communities and are also influencing what communities in the process of becoming. They are making new formations and configurations possible that comprise not just of humans but also non-human agents like code, algorithms, signals and bleeps.*

> *We have a situation where boundaries are confused and less easily held up and so at the same time, dogmatic processes are trying to pin people down – it's a constant struggle. Communities and the discourses that take place within digital spaces evidence this "battle of binaries". To give an example, I've seen it recently in pregnancy/labour/birth/parenting social media spaces where group members exert their cisgendered power to exclude trans and non-binary parents and maintain cisgendered women's divine, spiritual power as mama/woman/birthing goddess.*

Communities "implode" (Chatterjee et al., 2019) but out of that, new communities or collectives can shoot out and form something new, unique, and way more necessary for our urgent times. But something needs to keep the new things going and that something is people. Vibrant digital spaces do not run themselves. Individual people matter in digital-material communities.

Any research that is working with people cannot ignore how those people live and breathe in digital-material form. You might be doing research in a particular neighbourhood – how does that neighbourhood map in a digital-material way, how do the people living there make place through digital-material intra-actions? How are social relations in place captured in digital form? The digital is already there in research; it is ever present and has something to say, something to do for and within communities. It cannot be ignored.

So, in researching and working with "online communities", those communities, while appearing to be digital, are also grounded, located and placed. Feminist new materialism and posthumanism encourages us to consider the materiality of the digital – the virtual is real, the digital is material, the binary distinction between online/offline and human/technology is produced just as the binary distinction between individual/community, agency/structure is, and so on. The digital-material "communities" of the present take place somewhere; they are real. When thinking of "online communities" in a materialised framework, the matters of social media matter more.

Making social media within social activism

We have argued that community psychologists have, in general, been slow to pick up on the importance of digital technologies both in terms of the possibilities of bringing people together in communities but also the further deepening of social inequalities, marginalisation and oppression. Community Psychology has much to offer communities as they traverse digital and physical spaces (Stein et al., 2019). After all, a primary focus of Community Psychology, whatever the approach or region or country, is social justice, with explicit values and principles and action strategies that seek to promote social justice and the voices, knowledges and interests of the most marginalised within society (Kagan et al., 2020).

A central tenet of all forms of Community Psychology is social justice (Kagan et al., 2011; Kagan et al., 2020) in recognition of the inequalities many groups and people face at ALL levels, by oppressive and exclusionary aspects of communities and societies. The general concern for community psychologists has been that "mainstream psychology" has not contributed enough to social justice where the dominant, clinical, individualising and psychologising ideologies that underpin medical models mean that psychologists and psychology researchers are not so concerned with the day-to-day issues faced by oppressed people. However, as Kagan and Burton (2015) have pointed out, whilst Community Psychology concerns transformational change, with a view to changing the conditions that people face, it is easier to dream of that happening and much harder to implement change to tackle social justice issues. After all, community psychological work is often localised and small scale, ensuring that community psychologists are detached from wider social movements, meaning change remains ameliorative rather than transformational. And methods that are used by community psychologists, whilst varied (Richards et al., 2018), do not really connect at a societal level like the big social justice issues that have emerged vividly during the COVID-19 pandemic. With this in mind, it would be useful for community psychologists to engage with a more societal-level tool such as social media and other digital technologies, as a way to engage with local, regional, national and global networks and communities all at once while working towards social justice.

As noted, Community Psychology and social justice come hand-in-hand, and social media can have an impact on civic participation, as we have seen during the COVID-19 pandemic and protest movements such as the Black Lives Matter campaign and School Strikes for Climate, for example. People have come together with shared values and sought to take action on racial and climate justice. Online technologies can be used as a tool for change and bring people together in ways that were not always possible before digitalisation. However, whilst there are many possibilities with the use of social media for community action, there are also some obvious barriers and issues. For example, many people do not have the technology, the money or the resources required to succeed on corporate commercialised digital platforms. Indeed, there is often much at stake when a community action group creates itself a digital presence and starts to operate across mainstream social media.

In her scholar-activist practices, Jenna witnessed and felt the complexities of making social media within housing activism, and participated in the behind-the-scenes making of social media content, strategies and groups, as well as the digital-material communities they generate, administrate, moderate, manage and galvanise for collective action. This case study outlines some of the intricate issues and possibilities that can emerge in making social media for social activism.

> *I've been wanting to write about making social media in housing activism for years now but time flies and academic thoughts get left behind, forgotten and misremembered as social media and life in general moves at an accelerating pace. My two worlds of housing studies and using social media for community engagement first collided a decade ago now when I did some consultancy work for a social housing organisation in the UK. The organisation's Director was keen to use social media for tenant engagement but wanted to move forward professionally, establishing both protocols and good practices. In 2011, I was also hopeful that social media would be really good for social housing communities. I was championing social media use for community building across all aspects of my work – teaching, learning, research and engagement/consultancy.*
>
> *The social housing organisation were keen for their Facebook Page to be used by tenants to report faults and request maintenance and repairs. I ran a workshop with staff to unpick their perceptions of social media. We produced a Facebook Guide for residents (not staff, funnily enough). As I'm writing this, I still have the Facebook Guide in my files. It returns on a quick computer search for the organisation. It is a step-by-step guide to signing up to Facebook, it was very, very basic. Other sections of the Facebook Guide include how to find the organisations Page and how to manage personal privacy settings. I remember when the Page got to 100 likes and the housing staff were over the moon. A decade later, the Page is still in use and they have over 1000 followers. What you create on social media platforms tends to stick around…unless of course someone deletes it (more on this later).*
>
> *A couple of years later I moved to Australia and commenced a study on the use of social media by social housing organisations with a "new staff" research grant from my University. I collected a lot of data from housing representatives in New South Wales. I still have this data and would like to do something with it but I worry it is out of date – a reoccurring issue with researching social media that I haven't quite figured out yet. In generating these datasets, I realised I didn't understand social housing well enough from a sociological/economic perspective to critically analyse how social media platforms were being used by housing providers. Long story short, the tenants of social housing were not at the centre of social media engagement. The commercial interests of new community housing providers often took precedent and social media use was more about branding and attracting philanthropic support and corporate partnerships, which are all symptomatic of the neoliberal housing system.*

It was then when I realised that the UK was a couple of steps ahead with "social housing" and in Australia, the sector was still "public housing" and "community housing" with the push to transfer public housing stock to community housing providers well underway. It was here where I also realised that the ways in which the social housing organisation I was working with in the UK were using (or intending to use) social media for tenant engagement were not resonating loudly elsewhere. Tenant voices were not there and moreover, they were being silenced by the corporate social media machine in play. This is why community psychologists need to be really careful when thinking of social media as a tool of empowerment and for hearing voices. The corporate machine is embedded within social media. Voices often get buried under an avalanche of content.

I did talk about my research on social media use for tenant engagement in various places. Such talking/networking led to a meeting with Clare Lewis in early 2016. Clare had started up a social action project called #WeLiveHere2017 in response to the New South Wales (NSW) government's announcement that the large inner city public housing estate in Waterloo, Sydney, would be demolished and redeveloped to make way for a new "socially mixed" estate of predominantly private (70%) and social housing (30%). We have written on #WeLiveHere2017 project (Condie & Lewis, 2017; Chatterjee et al., 2020) and it was probably the most successful action project of the groups I was involved in as the resulting documentary and public art work where the estates towers were illuminated in colourful lights to show "the lights are on, somebody's home" attracted a lot of media attention and could even have gone someway to slowing down the redevelopment? The estate is still standing at least but residents have experienced 6 years of uncertainty now. Our government's approach to people's homes and neighbourhoods is cruel.

I joined the #WeLiveHere2017 team as a social researcher, but Clare also introduced me to other groups in the area. One group was organised and led by tenants and I was one of the first outsiders through the door to attend one of their meetings. I felt really at home as I grew up on a council estate in the North of England, and also really inspired by a diverse group of tenants that were talking about taking the government on. Really powerful rhetoric, really radical goals – at first. This group is where I learned a lot of lessons around "community building" and making social media in activism.

A lot of the time when people look at the social media content generated by a group, movement or organisation, they just see what is on the page, they don't see the amount of work and the complexities involved in making that social media. How a post comes to fruition and gets posted and remains on the Page or account of a group involves a complex web of interpersonal relationships and power sharing. What gets posted often represents the collective voice of a group, a singular voice for a group of diverse people. Doing this digital work is rife with issues and these issues can derail activism. It is very difficult territory to navigate.

In this group, making social media for activism was even more difficult as many of the group members were older, using older "non-smart" mobile devices (some without Internet access), were not on social media, and had overly cautious reactions to it. We had to get back to basics in a workshop that was initially about setting up a social media team and generating digital campaigns. But as it happened, we were helping people sign up to Facebook, work out their forgotten passwords, access their emails, and pinch a smartphone screen. At the close of one of the workshops, we had abandoned the challenge of social media and had committed instead to creating a paper-based flyer to post through people's doors. That was deemed more relevant. It was!

So the social media duties and in turn the voice of the group often fell to me and other outsiders, private renters living up the road not public housing tenants directly affected by the proposed housing redevelopment. This was tricky, but some tenants did speak up. Sometimes what got shared on the page disappeared – it had been deleted if what was posted was seen as *too outspoken, something that might get the group into trouble. Often, not much action was happening through social media. But this experience exemplifies to me how organised and diverse groups, communities and networks of people need to be in order to navigate the complexities of social media for social activism and justice. And an important point is that while some posts may have been deleted and some people have come and gone, Facebook Pages and Groups, Instagram and Twitter accounts remain. To me, this represents some continuity, some permanency within an increasingly transient and temporary world. For the record, these groups existed and resisted the government's unjust housing developments and policies.*

Another related action group I helped establish was one comprised only of women (and their allies) who successfully campaigned with social media to save the local Library. However this group was largely made up of middle-class white women with professional networks and media experience. This group had more power to see action happen fast. The group above led by public housing tenants did not have quite the same visibility, voice and power. It is perhaps harder to take up the identity of activist so visibly and permanently on social media when your home is threatened by the government's planning department. Public housing has been successfully stigmatised and its tenants marginalised – going mainstream on social media to support the calls for more public housing is by no means an easy feat either. As more and more people face housing inequality and realise that the current housing model does not and will not serve them, we may see more connective and powerful social media activism for housing justice.

The experience Jenna has faced in relation to housing activism and social media, is that social media matters in social activism and social justice. We are only just beginning to document and work out what is going on and how to use digital technologies and social media for communal gains but at the same time resist vested corporate and government stakes, interests and manipulations. Community psychologists could be operating in ethical ways to support groups, communities and social networks to organise, mobilise and galvanise support through social media platforms. This case study shows the complexities of communities and how communities are becoming action groups and social movements with digital technologies and social media. Community psychologists should not be so far away. The interpersonal dynamics of groups and the power differentials that characterise society, always come into play.

Conclusion

This chapter calls for a "Digital Community Psychology" which recognises that despite Community Psychology seemingly being slow off the mark, there are many opportunities for community psychologists to work with social media and digital technologies more. In fact, it is needed for Community Psychology's commitment to social justice. Through the chapter we applied a digital autoethnographic method to generate knowledge and explore how Community Psychology and its central value of social justice connects with social media and digital technologies. This enabled us to say what we needed to say and take more risks in what we are saying, allowing us to generate viewpoints on where Community Psychology is and where it can go in a digitalising society.

We outlined the disconnect between Community Psychology, digital technologies, and social media and considered why Community Psychology has not been as technologically forthcoming as would be expected due to digitalisation. We concluded that Community Psychology is well placed to challenge the already well-established use of "mainstream psychology" within social media and digital technologies that continue to pathologise, problematise and psychologise and maintain the continued marginalisation of the most excluded in society, meaning that new technologies are being used to further disempower and silence voices. Community psychologists are already set up and ethically equipped to counter the manifestations of "mainstream psychology" within new technological systems and practices, and must embrace their responsibility to address the domination of "mainstream psychology".

We also suggested that social media is changing communities and how we participate in and belong to groups, which means what we know to be human is not the same as it was. We drew on ideas and concepts that have influenced the new knowledges that have emerged from different interdisciplinary fields. We concluded that the materialities of making social media for social activism and justice is an essential part of the remit for Digital Community Psychology to flourish into the future.

> *It will be weird when I don't write to you every day about a Digital Community Psychology. We should probably keep it going!*

References

Bakhtin, M. (1984). *Problems of Dostoevsky's poetics* (C. Emerson, Trans.). University of Minnesota Press.

Barad, K. (2003). Posthumanist performativity. Toward an understanding of how matter comes to matter. *Signs, 28*(3), 801–31.

Barad, K. (2007). *Meeting the universe halfway: Quantum physics and the entanglement of matter and meaning.* Duke University Press.

Bennett, J. (2010). *Vibrant matter: A political ecology of things.* Duke University Press.

Braidotti, R. (2013). *The posthuman.* John Wiley & Sons.

Braidotti, R. (2019a). A theoretical framework for the critical posthumanities. *Theory, Culture & Society, 36*(6), 31–61.

Braidotti, R. (2019b). *Posthuman knowledge.* Polity Press.

Brennan, J. (2020). Trust as a test for unethical persuasive design. *Philosophy & Technology,* 1–17.

Brinkmann, S. (2017). Humanism after posthumanism: Or qualitative psychology after the "posts". *Qualitative Research in Psychology, 14*(2), 109–30.

Brown, M., Ray, R., Summers, E., & Fraistat, N. (2017). #SayHerName: A case study of intersectional social media activism. *Ethnic and Racial Studies, 40*(11), 1831–46.

Burton, M., Boyle, S., Harris, C., & Kagan, C. (2007). Community psychology in Britain. In S. Reich, M. Riemer, I. Prilleltensky, &M. Montero (Eds.), *International community psychology: History and theories* (pp. 219–37). Kluwer Academic Press.

Cadwalladr, C. (2018, April6). Facebook suspends data firm hired by vote leave over alleged Cambridge Analytica ties. *The Guardian.* www.theguardian.com/us-news/2018/apr/06/facebook-suspends-aggregate-iq-cambridge-analytica-vote-leave-brexit

Chatterjee, P., Condie, J., Sisson, A., & Wynne, L. (2019). Imploding activism: Challenges and possibilities of housing scholar-activism. *Radical Housing Journal, 1,* 189–204.

Chatterjee, P., Sisson, A., Condie, J., Wynne, L., Lewis, C., & Skipper, C. (2020). Documentary and resistance: There goes our neighbourhood, #WeLiveHere2017 and the Waterloo estate redevelopment. *International Journal of Housing Policy,* 1–18.

Condie, J., Lean, G., & James, D. (2018). Tinder matters: Swiping right to unlock research fields. In C. Costa & J. Condie (Eds.), *Doing research in and on the digital: Research methods across fields of inquiry* (pp. 102–15). Routledge.

Condie, J.M., & Lewis, C. (2017). The lights are on, somebody's home. *Around the House: The Newsletter of Shelter NSW, 108,* 18–20.

Connolly, W. (2013). The "new materialism" and the fragility of things. *Millennium: Journal of International Studies.* https://doi.org/10.1177/0305829813486849

Cook, K. (2020). *The psychology of Silicon Valley: Ethical threats and emotional unintelligence in the tech industry.* Springer Nature.

Coole, D., & Frost, S. (Eds.). (2020). *New materialisms: Ontology, agency, and politics.* Duke University Press.

Cooper, A.M., & Condie, J. (2016). Bakhtin, digital scholarship and new publishing practices as carnival. *Journal of Applied Social Theory*, *1*(1), 26–43.

Cosgrove, L., Karter, J. M., Morrill, Z., & McGinley, M. (2020). Psychology and surveillance capitalism: The risk of pushing mental health apps during the COVID-19 pandemic. *Journal of Humanistic Psychology*, *60*(5), 611–25.

Dalton, C., & Thatcher, J. (2014, May 12). What does a critical data studies look like, and why do we care? Seven points for acritical approach to "big data". *Society + Space*. www.societyandspace.org/articles/what-does-a-critical-data-studies-look-like-and-why-do-we-care

De Meulenaere, J., Baccarne, B., Courtois, C., & Ponnet, K. (2020). Disentangling social support mobilisation via online neighbourhood networks. *Journal of Community Psychology*, *49*(2), 481–98.

De Vos, J. (2021). A critique of digital mental health via assessing the psychodigitalisation of the COVID-19 crisis. *Psychotherapy and Politics International*, *19*(1). https://doi.org/10.1002/ppi.1582

Eubanks, V. (2018). *Automating inequality: How high-tech tools profile, police, and punish the poor*. St. Martin's Press.

Fox, N.J., & Alldred, P. (2015). New materialist social inquiry: Designs, methods and the research-assemblage. *International Journal of Social Research Methodology*, *18*(4), 399–414.

Goodley, D., Lawthom, R., & Runswick, C.K. (2014). Posthuman disability studies. *Subjectivity*, 7, 342–61.

Goodley, D., Lawthom, R., Liddiard, K., & Runswick-Cole, K. (2019). Provocations for critical disability studies. *Disability & Society*, *34*(6), 972–97.

Goodley, D., & Runswick-Cole. K. (2016). Becoming dishuman: Thinking about the human through dis/ability. *Discourse: Studies in the Cultural Politics of Education*, *37*(1), 1–15.

Goodley, D., Runswick-Cole, K., & Liddiard, K. (2016). The dishuman child. *Discourse: Studies in the Cultural Politics of Education*, *37*(5), 770–84.

Hampton, K.N., & Wellman, B. (2018). Lost and saved … Again: The moral panic about the loss of community takes hold of social media. *Contemporary Sociology: A Journal of Reviews*, *47*(6), 643–51.

Haraway, D.J. (2016). *Staying with the trouble. Making kin in the Chthulucene*. Duke University Press.

Hinds, J., Williams, E.J., & Joinson, A.N. (2020). "It wouldn't happen to me": Privacy concerns and perspectives following the Cambridge Analytica scandal. *International Journal of Human-Computer Studies*, *143*, 102498.

James, D., Condie, J., & Lean, G. (2019). Travel, Tinder and gender in digitally mediated tourism encounters. In C.J. Nash & A. Gorman-Murray (Eds.), *The Geographies of Digital Sexuality* (pp. 49–68). Palgrave Macmillan.

Kagan, C., & Burton, M. (2015). Theory and practice for a critical community psychology in the UK. *Psicología, Conocimiento y Sociedad (Psychology, Knowledge and Society)*, *5*(2), 182–205. https://www.researchgate.net/publication/286025156_Theory_and_practice_for_a_critical_community_psychology_in_the_UK

Kagan, C., Burton, M., Lawthom, R., Duckett, P., & Siddiquee, A. (2020). *Critical community psychology: Critical action and social change*. Routledge.

Kagan, C., Duggan, K., Richards, M., & Siddiquee, A. (2011). Community psychology. In P. Martin, F. Cheung, M. Kyrios, L. Littlefield, M. Knowles, B. Overmier, & J.M. Prieto. (Eds.), *The IAAP handbook of applied psychology* (pp. 471–500). Blackwell.

Linnell, S., & Horsfall, D. (2016). Disturbing professional practice discourse: re: writing practices. In J. Higgs & F. Trede (Eds.), *Professional practice discourse marginalia* (pp. 83–90). Brill Sense.

Locke, A., Lawthom, R., & Lyons, A. (2018). Social media platforms as complex and contradictory spaces for feminisms: Visibility, opportunity, power, resistance and activism. *Feminism and Psychology*, *28*(1), 3–10.

Mukerji, C. (2015). The material turn. In R.A. Scott, S.M. Kosslyn, & M.C. Buchmann (Eds.), *Emerging trends in the social and behavioral sciences: An interdisciplinary, searchable, and linkable resource* (pp. 1–13). Wiley.

Noble, S.U. (2018). *Algorithms of oppression: How search engines reinforce racism*. NYU Press.

Reich, S. (2010). Adolescents' sense of community on MySpace and Facebook: A mixed-methods approach. *Journal of Community Psychology*, *38*(6), 688–705.

Richards, M. (2016). "You've got autism because you like order and you do not look into my eyes": Some reflections on understanding the label of "autism spectrum disorder" from a dishuman perspective. *Disability & Society*, *31*(9), 1301–5.

Richards, M., Lawthom, R., & Runswick-Cole, K. (2018). Community-based arts research for people with learning disabilities: Challenging misconceptions about learning disabilities. *Disability and Society*, *34*(2), 204–27.

Richardson, L., & St. Pierre, E.A. (2005). Writing: A method of inquiry. In Norman K. Denzin and Yvonna S. Lincoln (Eds.), *The SAGE handbook of qualitative research* (1st ed.) (pp. 959–78). SAGE.

Rose, N. (2007). *The politics of life itself: Biomedicine, power and subjectivity in the twenty-first century*. Princeton University Press.

Ruppert, E., Law, J., & Savage, M. (2013). Reassembling social science methods: The challenge of digital devices. *Theory, Culture & Society*, *30*(4), 22–46.

St. Pierre, E.A. (2018). Writing post qualitative inquiry. *Qualitative Inquiry*, *24*(9), 603–8.

Schradie, J. (2018). The digital activism gap: How class and costs shape online collective action. *Social Problems*, *65*(1), 51–74.

Sichel, C.E., Javdani, S., Shaw, S., & Liggett, R. (2020). A role for social media? A community based response to guns, gangs and violence online. *Journal of Community Psychology*, *49*(3), 822–837.

Sonn, C., & Baker, A. (2016). Creating inclusive knowledges: Exploring the transformative potential of arts and cultural practice. *International Journal of Inclusive Education*, *20*(3), 215–28.

Stein, C.H., Hartl-Majcher, J., Froemming, M.W., Greenberg, S.C., Benoit, M.F., Gonzales, S.M., Petrowski, C.E., Mattei, G.M., & Dulek, E.B. (2019). Community psychology, digital technology and loss: Remembrance activities of young adults who have experienced the death of a close friend. *Journal of Community and Applied Social Psychology*, *29*(4), 257–72.

van Dijck, J. (2013). The culture of connectivity: A critical history of social media. Oxford University Press.

Wajcman, J. (2015). *Pressed for time: The acceleration of life in digital capitalism*. University of Chicago Press.

Wellman, B., Quan-Haase, A., Boase, J., Chen, W., Hampton, K., & de Diaz, I. (2003). The social affordances of the Internet for networked individualism. *Journal of Computer Mediated Communication*, *8*(7). https://doi.org/10.1111/j.1083-6101.2003.tb00216.x

12

THE INTERFACE OF COMMUNITY AND WELL-BEING IN CHILDHOOD

A critical perspective[1]

Jaime Alfaro and M. Isidora Bilbao-Nieva

Abstract

This chapter seeks to contribute to the theoretical development of a community perspective of well-being in childhood. Furthermore, it focuses on the relevance of relational frameworks from which well-being in childhood is defined as a subjective experience mostly of a social nature.

Theoretical notions that contribute to the development of a community and relational perspective of well-being in childhood are reviewed and presented. Two social theories are introduced – The New Sociology of Childhood and the Intersectional Approach – highlighting the central ideas that contribute to a critical perspective of well-being in childhood.

A community-based and critical perspective is suggested that problematises the homogenisation of well-being, as well as grounding it as a socially constructed subjective experience, including the relevance of voice and agency of children. It also differentiates challenges and demands that this kind of perspective has with regard to the methods and tools of the study.

Resumen

Este capítulo busca aportar al desarrollo de una perspectiva comunitaria del bienestar en la infancia, poniendo foco en la relevancia de los entramados relacionales desde donde éste se define como un emergente subjetivo, básicamente de carácter social.

Se revisan y exponen nociones teóricas que contribuyen al desarrollo de una perspectiva comunitaria y relacional del bienestar en la infancia. Se introducen dos teorías sociales –La Nueva Sociología de la Infancia y el Enfoque Interseccional – destacando las ideas centrales que aportan a una perspectiva crítica del bienestar en la infancia.

Se propone una perspectiva con base comunitaria y crítica que problematiza la homogeneización del bienestar, así como fundamenta una concepción de él como emergente subjetivo socialmente construido, incluyendo la relevancia de la agencia y las voces de los niños, niñas y adolescentes, y finalmente distingue desafíos y exigencias que una perspectiva de este tipo tiene a nivel de los métodos y herramientas de estudio.

DOI: 10.4324/9780429325663-15

Introduction

The study of children's well-being has gained academic and political importance. Well-being has been recognised as a key psychological strength, linked to a wide range of indicators of emotional health and social functioning, and of great relevance for the promotion of childhood development (Proctor et al., 2009). Well-being is a fundamental contribution to the development of public policies, especially within the framework of mandates of international organizations such as the Organisation for Economic Co-operationand Development (OECD, 2013) and the World Health Organization (OMS, 2013), both of which propose well-being as the goal of their respective missions.

An impetus of great relevance for the study and promotion of well-being was given by the adoption of the Convention on the Rights of the Child (CRC), which recognises children as active participants in decisions that affect their lives (Earls, 2011; Gómez & Alzate, 2014). Therefore, the study of well-being has become a priority, as a way of visualising and legitimising the voice of children through the study of their opinions, attitudes and perceptions of issues that affect them (Newton & Ponting, 2013).

The recommendations of the CRC have encouraged debates that challenge and expand childhood research. They have contributed to the analysis of the notions of childhood as a socially and culturally situated category (Gómez & Alzate, 2014; Gaitán, 2010) which assigns to children the status of citizens who are holders of rights and endowed with agency (Fegter et al., 2010; Dockett & Perry, 2011). These new forms of analysis highlight the relevance of studying the voices and everyday practices of children, as well as the effects of their position on structures of power distribution and participation within society (Gaitán, 2010).

These new approaches also challenge the way the study of well-being in childhood has been done thus far, allowing the emergence of community-based analysis and perspectives. In other words, it focuses analysis on contextual, social and systemic levels, rather than the individual level. Within this approach, well-being is a socially constructed, subjective experience, rather than a universal or uniform one, in which relational dynamics are at the centre of the study, inherently linked to social context. This framework provides the basis for a critical analysis of this field of study. It explicitly enables paying attention to and making visible the risks that traditional notions of well-being have regarding their effect on representation and recognition of certain social groups, particularly those that are not part of dominant groups: men, white people, cisgender and Westerners.

This chapter describes approaches to the study of children's well-being. These approaches concur with a relational perspective that understands well-being as subjective and inherently linked to the dynamics of social exchange, rooted in a particular time and place. Well-being is understood here as located territorially and materially, and it is both a product and a producer of social practices that include political, economic and cultural dimensions.

Secondly, the chapter presents a deeper examination of the analytical implications of this relational perspective of well-being in childhood. To do this, distinctions and concepts from the New Sociology of Childhood and Intersectionality are reviewed. The aim of this section is to develop a critical approach to the homogenisation of well-being and to provide theoretical foundations for its comprehension as a socially constructed, subjective experience. In addition, it highlights the relevance of children's agency, and voices, for the study of well-being. Challenges and demands that emerge from this perspective are identified from theoretical and methodological points of view.

The authors have worked together on different research projects about social dimensions of children and adolescent well-being. This chapter emerges from the reflections of doing this work pursuing a Community Psychology view of well-being.

Theoretical approaches to well-being from relational perspectives

In recent years, different authors have delved into ways in which individuals relate and interact with contextual structures and dynamics, locating a fundamental basis upon which experiences of well-being of children is rooted (Ben Arieh et al., 2014; Casas et al., 2007). Initially, these new approaches were based on empirical studies that provided important evidence of the positive correlation between well-being and higher levels of life satisfaction, the quality of exchanges with friends and family, and the degree to which they contribute to better self-esteem and to strategies for better facing life in general (Casas et al., 2007).

Among these studies, those referring to broader levels of interactions have also been considered, such as those including school and relationships and dynamics that occur within it. These have focused on teaching and learning processes, and the relationships of coexistence between all of the participants from within these contexts (Casas et al., 2014). In the same group of studies focused on broader levels of exchange, Sarriera and Bedin (2015) have proposed a socio-community model of well-being that includes variables associated with the feeling of belonging to the community and satisfaction with the neighbourhood and environmental contexts.

Within this theoretical context, some authors have acknowledged the complexity of the relational network that affects well-being, integrating political and economic dimensions that impact each context in which children live (Ben-Arieh et al., 2014). In other words, new theoretical frameworks have developed perspectives of well-being in which well-being is understood as a social phenomenon, studying broad social dynamics in which the subjective experience of life satisfaction arises, as well as the agency of the children and their interplay with cultural references of childhood present in these contexts (Ben-Arieh et al., 2014). These new approaches present a challenge to traditional concepts of well-being that emphasise individual choices and ignore the social and cultural contexts of daily life, as well as the ways in which the evaluative and subjective dimensions of well-being are situated and influenced by the context.

Such theoretical and analytical approaches have located the experiences of well-being as subjective and situated in relational contexts of childhood, which include families, peers and communities, amongst others. These lines of research have placed special emphasis on the relationships of familiarity, trust, autonomy and respect, integrating into the analysis structural issues of the relationship of childhood with the adult world, in the different socialisation processes in which children are involved (Fattore & Mason, 2017). Fattore and colleagues (2019) propose that the study of well-being in childhood be first based on the understandings of well-being derived from the opinions and representations of the children themselves, mainly accounting for the contexts in which constructions are produced. In other words, the understanding of well-being is one of a subjective experience of children as individuals positioned in various social orders. Within these social orders, issues such as power relations with adults, and naturalised ways of understanding and defining roles, rules and behaviours, are crucial determinants of their well-being (Fattore et al., 2019). These approaches provide a notion of well-being as a temporally and territorially located construct, highlighting its contextual and local singularity, and assuming it as a non–generalisable experience.

Along this same line, Community Psychology authors have proposed the incorporation of collective dimensions of well-being, defining well-being as a positive state of satisfaction that jointly integrates both individual and community levels. This state of satisfaction refers to personal needs and aspirations, as well as relational and collective ones. Through these inclusions of different levels of well-being, experiences of self-determination, social participation and community competences, as well as social justice, have gained relevance as determinants of well-being (Evans & Prilleltensky, 2007). From this perspective, well-being is shaped as inseparably connected to relational patterns of social class and/or gender (Evans, 2014). Within this analytical framework, social justice has become a main determinant of experience and of differences and inequalities of promoting personal and community well-being (Malpert et al., 2017).

Along the same lines, Camfield and Tafere (2009) understand well-being in childhood as a subjective experience, closely connected to the social relationships in which it arises, and inevitably linked to what happens in the specific and unique communities in which it is present. Thus, the relevance of the location, in a particular historical time and under certain conditions and economic strategies of the community and family of belonging, is added. In this way the authors have also incorporated into the analysis the relevance of inequality in the distribution of opportunities and in the agency patterns, as dimensions that affect the possibilities of experiencing well-being. In the same vein, the authors highlight that positive connections and interrelations with others are fundamental, as are the consistency, continuity and reciprocity in the networks and communities of belonging (Camfield, 2012).

Also, from this relational and community perspective of well-being, White (2017) questions the notion of the individual as a discrete, autonomous entity and a simple component of the collective. She highlights the inextricable and inseparable relationship between the individual and the collective and proposes what she calls a "relational ontology". In other words, she proposes a notion of well-being as emerging from everyday life, as the result of inherently shared processes with others in the community. Community interactions lived out in everyday life are understood as the means through which the goods that are necessary for well-being (psychological, symbolic, social and material) are distributed and exchanged. On the other hand, these relationships are also the space where the very experience of well-being is configured and where it emerges (White, 2017).

Well-being is then understood as a fundamentally relational phenomenon, where the experience of being well emerges, firstly, in an interactive way, inscribed in a dynamic of community and relational exchange, and then, secondly, as something internal whose meaning emerges in the experience of meeting with and relating to others. In consequence, well-being is produced by cultural and social practices (including the political, economic and environmental aspects), which are also singular and particular to specific contexts, and therefore impossible to standardise (White & Blackmore, 2015). Thus, well-being is always configured in a particular time and local context, as a result of the relationships with others, and therefore it cannot be generalised to other contexts (White, 2017).

Contributions of the New Sociology of Childhood to the study of well-being in childhood

Background of the New Sociology of Childhood

Since the mid-eighties, within the framework of the movements that support the rights of children, which culminated in the 1989 United Nations Convention, the New Sociology of Childhood (NSC) was born as a challenge to the mainstream way of studying and understanding the life and behaviour of children (Tisdall & Punch, 2012). Until then, modernist, biological and universalist views of childhood and children were predominant. Challenging these views gradually allowed sociology, and the social sciences in general, to develop a set of approaches to rethink the very idea of childhood and the notions related to it.

The NSC understands childhood as a social construction instead of a natural stage (Tisdall & Punch, 2012), and highlights the relevance of the voice of children, their specific and unique actions in their status as a minority group, excluded from the important topics of the adult world (Gaitán, 2006; Prout, 2011). Furthermore, the NSC understands childhood from a perspective that recognises its plurality and promotes the use of the term "childhood(s)" as a constant reminder of its heterogeneity (James & Prout, 1997). In addition, it highlights the impossibility of standardising childhoods and the importance of considering that their study must always respect the diversity that constitutes them (Prout, 2011). Moreover, they seek to shift the way and the methodologies through which the conditions, needs, problems and circumstances of children are addressed, including the research techniques used in their study (Gaitán, 2006).

Distinctions and theoretical considerations of the New Sociology of Childhood

The NSC and its theories and methods understand childhood as a complex phenomenon which requires an interdisciplinary approach for its study. First and foremost, it is emphasised that childhood is a social group that is part of, and inserted into, the social structure. Therefore, it must be conceived and studied as a social category, just like social class or gender. Thus, the phenomena linked to it must be understood and conceptualised as socio-historical constructions, intimately intertwined with the contexts of production (cultural, political, social and economic). In other words, childhood is not seen as a phenomenon derived from biological development. Rather, it is seen as a social construction delimited by social structure, and this structure in turn determines typical forms of behaviour related to a repertoire of cultural elements (Pascual, 2000).

According to Colángelo (2003), a central feature of this approach is the conceptualisation of childhood as a political phenomenon, which means that the way it is conceived and delimited as a studied object defines social limits, and produces a social order that each individual must occupy according to age, and centrally affected by the relationships between different groups in society. Therefore, the definition of what childhood "is", what is considered appropriate for this group, and its behaviours or characteristics are not data given by nature, or the result of only individual or simply micro-social processes. Rather, these are interpretations that always imply tensions of meaning aimed at giving legitimacy or imposing a particular vision.

In other words, it has to do with the distribution of power in a particular social context. For example, what has been proposed as some kind of essence or "infantile nature" (ideas of fragility, innocence, purity, incompleteness) is necessarily the product of a particular historical process (Colángelo, 2003), which also places adults as superior to children in every way (Tisdall & Punch, 2012).

Secondly, from the NSC perspective, children are conceived as fully social and political actors with a capacity for agency. They produce and reproduce positions and relationships which express and materialise their capacity to modify the world they live in and produce shared notions and social practices (Vergara et al., 2017). From this perspective, as proposed by Matthews (2007), the study of childhood and its practices and needs, leads to the rethinking and criticising of notions that portray children as products of socialisation processes, in the sense of understanding them as a tabula rasa, or as passive receivers of cultural influences and as shaped by society.

In this way, children are conceived as active participants in the construction of knowledge and daily experience. Recognition is placed on the production of singular and autonomous understandings and meanings, which must be understood and taken into consideration from children's own perspectives, assigning, therefore, immense importance to their visions and voices, as well as the interaction with the social worlds which they inhabit (James & Prout, 1997). Childhood is understood within frames of social constructions that, far from being uniform, are dynamic processes, permanently in tensions and conflict, insofar as they are the object of disputes and struggles of interpretations, having to be fully analysed and critically problematised regarding their effect on the restriction or promotion of emancipatory actions that include children's voices and participation as effective social agents (Gaitán, 2006).

According to Prout (2011), childhood phenomena should be understood as a result of a dialectical dynamic of constant iterative interaction between agency and social construction, avoiding falling into the mistaken duality that contrasts childhood as structure with childhood as agency. However, as Carnevale (2020) points out, agency is a generally excluded aspect, in direct relation to the "epistemological oppression" that occurs with childhood. There is an inability to hear the voices of children, which is reflected in the important knowledge gaps regarding childhood as a social group (Carnevale, 2020).

In this regard, Carnevale (2020) proposes transformations of the designs and methods of listening to these voices, recognising them as forms of expression of agency. Both researchers and professionals may have difficulties to achieve this task when handling universal and caricatured images of childhood. This makes necessary a deep analysis of the voices of children, through an intensive search for relational, social, cultural and political wholeness (Carnevale, 2020).

Thirdly, from the NSC perspective, the specific generational structures in which children live and in which their daily lives are played out, are fundamental within the study of childhood (Gaitán, 2006; Matthews, 2007). These are understood as a system of relationships between social positions that consider both the personal and the collective levels, emphasising (i) the connections between the positions; (ii) how these relationships causally affect the actions of those who hold these positions; (iii) where a structure is also causally affected by the actions of others, considering the complex set of relational social processes through which some people become children (they are ideologically constructed as children) while others become adults, such as in the case of relationships in which one position cannot exist without the other position (Gaitán, 2006).

Fourthly, from the methodological point of view, Gaitán (2006) has identified three aspects that challenge the study and research methods of childhood and the phenomena related to it: (i) childhood research should focus directly on their living conditions, activities and relationships, highlighting their conceptions, knowledge and experiences. In other words, children should study themselves from their own perspectives, as participant agents in the co-creation of knowledge and daily experience; (ii) constructionist perspectives must be assumed for social research, which implies the deconstruction of childhood and its main notions. Childhood should be addressed as formations, stories, meanings and discursive representations, which are socially constructed, and that simultaneously reflect and configure social orders, communicating ideas, images and knowledge about childhood. The methodological task, therefore, should be oriented towards contextualising, historicising and relativising (deconstructing) these notions, aiming at dismantling the discursive power of childhood representations in social life; (iii) the objective of the research should be to link the relevant facts observed in the living standards of the children (socio-economic conditions, sense of identity, subjectivity, comprehension) with the social structures and mechanisms that operate on macro levels and generate effects at the level of children as a social group.

Derived from these approaches, there is a demand for coherence in the epistemology and methodology of the study of childhood as a component of the social structure. At the same time, these approaches consider children as social actors that generate changes in the contexts in which they live and highlight the nature of the social construction of childhood.

Contributions of the intersectional perspective to the study of well-being in childhood

Background to intersectionality

Fundamentally, intersectionality is a theoretical approach that contributes to the task of making visible, analysing and understanding the existing relationships between different forms of oppression based on social categories such as gender, race, sexuality, class and age, among others (Goñalons & Ferree, 2014). A fundamental distinction is that thinking based on a single axis, which does not integrate the multidimensional analysis of social categories, limits and reduces the understanding of the human and undermines the fight for social justice (Cho et al., 2013).

Moreover, it is proposed to remain open-minded to the emergence of new differences that may generate inequalities and domination within different spheres of social life (Viveros, 2016). Since these developments, the concept of intersectionality has been integrated into various disciplines, in the same way that it has been used for the analysis of feminist research, for example in ethnic studies or also in legal studies (Cho et al., 2013); however, it has hardly been extended to the analysis of childhood (Harrison, 2017).

Distinctions and theoretical considerations of the intersectional perspective

Intersectionality, as a theoretical and methodological approach, has placed at the centre of contemporary social analysis the consideration that different social positions that people occupy in the world are the result of a multiplicity of factors (or social identities) that intersect with one another, shaping the dynamic determinants of oppression, exclusion, privilege and inequity (Hancock, 2016; Hill Collins & Bilge, 2016). These conditions are conceived as the result of an indivisible fabric – rather than a simple addition of different identities – that should be understood using a "nodal approach" (May, 2015). From this approach, the experiences of individuals must be understood as the result of a matrix of factors, which are not arranged linearly or hierarchically, but rather as a whole, as is the case in real life.

The intersectional perspective goes beyond merely describing forms of discrimination and adding them one on top of another, as an endless list of inequalities faced by individuals (Platero, 2014). Instead, this approach delves into how each person's experience is the result of the dynamic and multidimensional interrelation of many socially constructed structures. In this way, binarism and linear views are dismantled, in order to introduce the intricacies necessary to understand identities and privileges (Platero, 2014).

Intersectionality offers a perspective of the human experience that centres the analysis on the way in which people position themselves and operate in the world, highlighting the multiple, diverse and indivisible dynamics of power in which it is contextualised (Carastathis, 2016; Hill Collins & Bilge, 2016). Accordingly, the analysis of multiple systemic levels is favoured, challenging reductionist approaches to the study of asymmetrical distribution of opportunities. The analysis of groups that experience disproportionate levels of suffering, is also challenged. In such a way, as Moradi (2017) points out, the intersectional perspective presents us with a central question of "Whose experience is at the centre of the analysis?" With this question a move is made in the direction of making visible the experiences of certain social groups, and the study of how these experiences are affected by the experiences of the dominant group (adult, white, male, cis gender, middle class), which have been constituted as the norm (Igarashi, 2015).

This perspective has allowed us to see how the experience of certain groups is described as a deviation, an anomaly. They have become increasingly invisible and distant from the experiences reported by the dominant group. Thus, this perspective emphasises the study and permanent recognition of invisible groups and also invisible experiences, conceived as qualitatively different from those reported by the dominant population.

In this way, the intersectional perspective distinguishes basic assumptions such as: (i) more than one category of differentiation is involved in all social problems and processes; (ii) in their analysis, attention should be paid to all relevant categories, considering that the relationships between categories are variable and remain a permanently open empirical question; (iii) each category is internally diverse and their differences must be conceptualised as dynamic productions of individual and institutional factors; (iv) intersectional research must therefore examine the categories at various levels of analysis and question the interactions between them; (v) the perspective of intersectionality as an analytical paradigm requires both theoretical and empirical developments (Hancock, 2016).

Reflections for a community and relational notion of well-being in childhood

Criticism of the homogenisation of well-being

Firstly, both the NSC and the intersectional approach emphasise that there are many forms of childhood, placing age within a framework that includes at least distinctions of gender, race and ethnicity, class, nationality, culture and ability. These are intertwined with particular socio-historical aspects in which intergenerational relationships are framed and that function as components of the subjective experience of children. Thus, since there is a multiplicity of childhoods, it is impossible to think about universal experiences of children, or understandings of well-being that can be generalised to childhood. Experiences and representations of well-being are always rooted in the relational context in which they emerge.

In addition, time is also considered in the analysis, describing changes in the nature of intergenerational relationships and allowing for a more complex and diverse understanding of well-being. This is done in such a way that it is presumed that culture, ethnicity, class, gender and any other dimension of social belonging have a significant and profound impact on the way in which individuals understand, represent and act in the world.

According to NSC, there is a socio-historical plurality and a heterogeneity of experiences and understandings of well-being. These experiences are understood here as products of the intersection of social identities, embedded in a changing nature of relationships between adults and children, forming a social structure that allows unique ways of conceptualising well-being. Therefore, in order to study well-being, it is fundamental to pay attention to the presence, relevance and effect of the context in which the children live. Whilst doing so, it is assumed that well-being cannot be a universal experience but one of the many ways of experiencing the world, being the result of the intersection of factors that determine the way in which individuals as agents position themselves in it. This recognition of the plurality and heterogeneity of the notion of well-being constitutes a fundamental critique of universal approaches to well-being, whose starting point is usually found in the experience and cultural values of the dominant groups.

In this way, as proposed by Community Psychology, it must be taken into consideration that well-being is not distributed equitably in society. Instead, it is the result of the interaction between individuals and communities, with systems that determine patterns of social relationship based on economic, class and gender factors (Evans, 2014). Along the same lines, it is recognised that by not occupying a dominant social position, some specific groups of children, particularly those where the conjunction of marginalised social positions occurs, have become invisible (Buchanan & Wiklund, 2020), leaving their understandings and perspectives ignored and excluded from the study of children's well-being.

Consequently, special attention should be paid to differentiate the position of marginalised communities and social groups, giving priority to knowing, making visible and understanding the subjectivity of communities that are at a constant disadvantage with respect to others. Disadvantaged communities exposed to higher levels of stress and environmental hostility based on how they are perceived and how they perceive their environment, experience tangible consequences to their well-being. In this way, patterns are determined that are often inherited by several generations and that are multiplied by the conjunction of these exclusive spaces. This has a detrimental impact on the psychological experience of the individuals (Moradi, 2017). An example of this are the constant micro aggressions and their corrosive effects that negatively and systematically affect the daily lives of minority group members, limiting their possibilities to function and feel satisfied in the various dimensions of their lives.

Well-being as a socially constructed experience

The contributions of the NSC to the study of well-being in childhood highlights that childhood is a socially constructed phenomenon. It integrates the historical and cultural variations in which well-being emerges. It also recognises the influence of a set of mandates, guidelines and norms of conduct that match the way of being a child in a particular historical moment. Therefore, childhood and the particularities of the experiences of children are affected by political and cultural forces, as well as by the vicissitudes of social change.

From the perspective of the NSC, research on children's well-being should analyse the dynamics of power distribution and disputes of meaning about what is proper to childhood, as well as about the conditions that affect and constitute their satisfaction, well-being and quality of life. The intersectional approach provides a fundamental perspective to add complexity to the understanding of these dynamics. From this approach, dynamics are reinterpreted not as independent vectors of causal and linear impact on understandings of well-being in childhood, but as a complex and indivisible relational framework. In this way, constructions of meaning about well-being in childhood are positioned in different quadrants of relative social influence, depending on the actors and communities in which they emerge.

Also from this perspective, it is important to understand the effects on well-being of ideological formations and prevailing constructions of meaning in a given social context. These ideological formations and discourses performatively structure social and community practices that affect the circulation and communication of ideas, images and knowledge about children. Accordingly, the study of well-being in childhood should analyse and deconstruct these discursive, narrative and representational formations.

In this analytical framework, the contribution of Community Psychology is also relevant, by linking well-being, in this case of children, with issues of social justice, allowing the inclusion of analysis of how social structures operate and influence the experiences of well-being, as well as how they affect its distribution. The interface of well-being with the community is expressed in conditions of access to privileges, poverty, the intensity of the experienced deprivation, and oppression, all of them key determinants of children's experiences.

Similarly, Camfield (2012) highlights the link between the experience of well-being and what happens in the specific and unique community dynamics in which people live and where this experience emerges. The following are included in the analysis: (i) economic conditions and strategies of the community and the family, (ii) the distribution of opportunities, and (iii) the recognised and legitimised agency patterns in these communities. Intersectional explanations can be added to these ideas, contributing to the understanding of the formation of intergenerational patterns as a product of the conjunction of social positions. In turn, these intergenerational patterns determine within the communities' particular strategies that impact well-being, such as expectations about quality of life, about the positive nature of social and family dynamics, or about the set of socially shared meanings about leading a good life.

Finally, in the approach to well-being in childhood as a socially constructed experience, the developments of White (2017) have a very relevant contribution. Especially important is the notion of the "relational ontology" of well-being, and the importance and meaning that they assign to daily community interactions as a means and space where the experience of well-being itself is configured and emerges. Moreover, relevance is also assigned to cultural and social practices located in a particular time and local context.

Relevance of the agency and the voice of children in the construction of well-being and the methodological challenges of studying them

The contributions of the NSC to the research of well-being support the relevance of studying the understanding, representations and experiences of well-being of children. They do so from a focus in which the intersection of these with the social worlds which they inhabit is integrated as a central aspect, especially considering that these understandings and representations express and carry agency.

In this way, a relational understanding of childhood well-being must place children centrally as protagonists. That is, to see them as individuals with the capacity to produce and express positions, and participate in each context, space or social institution relevant to their living conditions and the phenomena that affect them. Furthermore, the children are considered valid and competent interpreters of their environment, whose opinions, representations, insights and critical analysis are recognised, and where they take the position of leading agents and experts in their own lives. This is a direct challenge to the traditional approach where the adult tends to have a privileged place in the analysis, interpretation and generation of conclusions regarding the well-being of children.

Furthermore, resorting to the contributions of the intersectional approach, these understandings must be conceptually analysed as portraying and expressing a particular social and community history. This history carries within itself collective learning, social memory and shared interpretations, transferred intergenerationally, and it plays a determining role in the nature and the singularities of the voices and the agency of children. The aforementioned understandings are also especially important to consider from an analysis aimed at making visible those groups in which the dynamics of marginalisation and oppression exert their impact from multiple positions, which may result in this memory and accumulated culture and community possibly being invisible.

In this analytical context, developing a programme to study children's well-being is highly demanding at the level of research methods, since on the one hand it must conceptualise well-being as a substantially relational phenomenon, intertwined and in connection with the social contexts in which it emerges. On the other hand, it seeks to listen to the voices of the individuals as protagonists, especially those whose opinions have not been taken into account, and their needs and subjectivity have been made invisible.

New methodological frameworks are therefore needed, which must be capable of assuming the complexity of understanding well-being as a process full of tensions, as a product of contextual and holistic relationships which express conflict dynamics, as well as social and individual changes. Analytical approaches are also needed for contextualising, deconstructing and dismantling socially produced constructions of childhood, which allow making visible the effects that these have on the experiences of well-being. These methodological and analytical approaches contribute to understanding how social and community practices, that is, ways of communicating ideas, images and knowledge about children, and about childhood, are performatively structured. They also contribute to understanding children as active individuals and social agents capable of transforming their reality.

In responding to these challenges, special relevance and value are given to social research tools that are aimed at understanding the production of knowledge and meanings within a socially constructed reality (Denzin & Lincoln, 2000), as well as understanding the way in which individuals experience the world, the way in which they interpret it, think about it and process it (Given, 2008).

Participatory methodologies (for example, photo-voice) may make a privileged contribution, as a necessary resource to ensure strategies that address and allow reflections on the differences of power in research processes, advocating for children to exercise their capacity for agency, critically reformulating research practices to position children at the centre of the process. The use of participatory methodologies for the study of well-being allows children to observe their daily context and identify the different forms of oppression they face within it, generating awareness that may eventually favour the process of social change.

It should be noted that in these processes, the participation of children is a fundamental aspect of successfully carrying out this task. Within it one must be especially careful not to invade with an external narrative, as this would imply reproducing the dynamics of power and oppression. Instead, one should listen, recover and deconstruct the meanings assigned by the children themselves to their own well-being, positioning them within the social structure in order to give contextual meaning to their particular discourse.

Related to this, it should be noted that participatory methodologies imply the development of specific languages to work with children, data collection, and analysis activities that force researchers to think outside the box and position the children's world and the specific context of the sample as the main reference for the research design. Active methodologies, which recognise that research participants are not only mere recipients of information but also co-creators of knowledge, are interesting alternatives to develop research processes and give meaning to the analysis, remembering that participants are agents in every moment, including when being silent or when deciding not to participate. A methodological design that recognises agency is one that provides concrete spaces and multiple opportunities to invite participants to make decisions in the different stages of research, as well as one whose motives are transparent, subjecting the researcher's wishes to a consensus and dialogue with the participants.

In conclusion, it is proposed that a programme to study children's well-being, from a community and relational perspective, requires methodological frameworks and research tools that allow for the study of the living conditions, as well as the conceptions, representations and experiences, of children from the perspective of the children themselves. At the same time, it is emphasised that children have a role as participating agents in the co-creation of knowledge and daily experience.

Moreover, we suggest considering an orientation to deconstruct stories, meanings and discursive representations about well-being, as proposed by Gaitán (2006). It is assumed that the complexity of the experience and understanding of well-being of children is the result of a dialectical dynamic of constant iterative interaction between agency and social construction, overcoming binary perspectives that contrast childhood as a framework with children as agents (Prout, 2011). Based on the notion of "relational ontology" (White, 2017), it is also essential to include, as we gather from White and Blackmore (2015), the particular daily community interactions, located in a specific time, place and community context.

Note

1 This work was developed within a FONDECYT REGULAR Project No.1180607 which is sponsored by the National Commission for Scientific and Technological Research (CONICYT-Chile).

References

Ben-Arieh, A., Casas, F., Frønes, I., & Korbin, J.E. (2014). *Handbook of child well-being: Theories, methods and policies in global perspective.* (Springer Reference). Springer. https://doi.org/10.1007/978-90-481-9063-8

Buchanan, N.T., & Wiklund, L.O. (2020). Why clinical science must change or die: Integrating intersectionality and social justice. *Women and Therapy*, *43*(3–4), 309–29. https://doi.org/10.1080/02703149.2020.1729470

Camfield, L. (2012). Resilience and well-being among urban Ethiopian children: What role do social resources and competencies play? *Social Indicators Research*, *107*(3), 393–410. https://doi.org/10.1007/s11205-011-9860-3

Camfield, L., & Tafere, Y. (2009). "No, living well does not mean being rich": Diverse understandings of well-being among 11–13-year-old children in three Ethiopian communities. *Journal of Children and Poverty*, *15*(2), 119–38. https://doi.org/10.1080/1079612090331088

Carastathis, A. (2016). *Intersectionality: Origins, constelations, horizons.* University of Nebraska Press.

Carnevale, F.A. (2020). A "thick" conception of children's voices: A hermeneutical framework for childhood research. *International Journal of Qualitative Methods*, *19*, 1–9. https://doi.org/10.1177/1609406920933767

Casas, F., Figuer, C., González, M., Malo, S., Alsinet, C., & Subarroca, S. (2007). The well-being of 12 to 16 year old adolescents and their parents: Results from 1999 to 2003 Spanish samples. *Social Indicators Research*, *83*, 87–115. https://doi.org/10.1007/s11205-006-9059-1

Casas, F., Sarriera, J.C., Alfaro, J., Figuer, C., Cruz, D.A. da, Bedin, L., Valdenegro, B., González, M., & Oyarzún, D. (2014). Satisfacción escolar y bienestar subjetivo en la adolescencia: poniendo a prueba indicadores para su medición comparativa en Brasil, Chile y España. *Suma Psicológica*, *21*(2), 70–80.

Cho, S., Crenshaw, K.W., & McCall, L. (2013). Toward a field of intersectionality studies: Theory, application, and praxis. *Signs: Journal of Women in Culture and Society*, *3 8*(4), 785–810.

Colángelo, M.A. (2003). La mirada antropológica sobre la infancia. Reflexiones y perspectivas de abordaje. *Infancias y Juventudes. Pedagogia y Formacion*, 1–8.

Denzin, N.K., & Lincoln, Y.S. (2000). The discipline and practice of qualitative research. In N.K. Denzin & Y.S. Lincoln (Eds.), *The SAGE handbook of qualitative research* (pp. 1–32). SAGE. www.sagepub.com/upm-data/40425_Chapter1.pdf

Dockett, S., & Perry, B. (2011). Researching with young children: Seeking assent. *Child Indicators Research*, *4*(2), 231–47.

Earls, F. (2011). Children: From rights to citizenship. *Annals of the American Academy of Political and Social Science*, *633*, 6–16.

Evans, S.D., (2014) Well-being. In T. Teo (Ed.), *Encyclopedia of critical psychology*. Springer. https://doi.org/10.1007/978-1-4614-5583-7

Evans, S.D., & Prilleltensky, I. (2007). Youth and democracy: Participation for personal, relational, and collective well-being. *Journal of Community Psychology*, *35*(6), 681–92. https://doi.org/10.1002/jcop.20172

Fattore, T., Fegter, S., & Hunner-Kreisel, C. (2019). Children's understandings of well-being in global and local contexts: Theoretical and methodological considerations for a multinational qualitative study. *Child Indicators Research*, 12(2), 385–407. https://doi.org/10.1007/s12187-018-9594-8

Fattore, T., & Mason, J. (2017). The significance of the social for child well-being. *Children & Society*, 31(4), 276–89. https://doi.org/10.1111/chso.12205

Fegter, S., Machold, C., & Richter, M. (2010). Children and the good life: Theoretical challenges. *Children and the Good Life*, 4, 7–13.

Gaitán, L. (2010). Ser niño en el siglo XXI. *Cuadernos de pedagogía*, 407, 12–17.

Given, L.M. (2008). Introduction. In L. Given (Ed.), *The SAGE encyclopedia of qualitative research methods* (Vol. 1–2). SAGE. https://dx.doi.org/10.4135/9781412963909

Gómez-Mendoza, M.Á., & Alzate-Piedrahíta, M.V. (2014). La infancia contemporánea. *Revista Latinoamericana de Ciencias Sociales, Niñez y Juventud*, 12(1), 77–89.

Goñalons, P., & Ferree, M. (2014). Practicing intersectionality in Spain. *Quaderns de Psicologia*, 16(1), pp. 85–95. https://doi.org/10.5565/rev/qpsicologia.1216

Hancock, A.-M. (2016). *Intersectionality: An intellectual history*. Oxford University Press.

Harrison, L. (2017). Redefining intersectionality theory through the lens of African American young adolescent girls' racialised experiences. *Youth and Society*, 49(8), 1023–39. https://doi.org/10.1177/0044118X15569216

Hill Collins, P., & Bilge, S. (2016). *Intersectionality*. Wiley.

Igarashi, Y. (2015) Health psychology. Towards critical psychologies for well-being and social justice. In I. Parker (Ed.), *Handbook of critical psychology*. Routledge. https://doi.org/10.1590/1807-03102015v27n3p569

James, A., & Prout, A. (Eds.). (1997). *Constructing and reconstructing childhood: Contemporary issues in the sociological study of childhood*. Falmer Press. https://doi.org/10.4324/9781315745008

Malpert, A.V., Suiter, S.V., Kivell, N.M., Perkins, D.D., Bess, K., Evans, S.D., Hanlin, C.E., Conway, P., McCown, D., & Prilleltensky, I. (2017). Community psychology. In C. Willig (Ed.), *The SAGE handbook of qualitative research in psychology* (pp. 318–35). SAGE. https://doi.org/10.4135/9781848607927

Matthews, S.H. (2007). Teaching and learning guide for: A window on the "new" sociology of childhood. *Sociology Compass*, 1(2), 832–9. https://doi.org/10.1111/j.1751-9020.2007.00044.x

May, V.M. (2015). *Pursuing intersectionality: Unsettling dominant imaginaries*. Routledge.

Moradi, B. (2017). (Re)focusing intersectionality: From social identities back to systems of oppression and privilege. In K. Debord, A. Fischer, K. Bieschke, & R. Perez (Eds.), *Handbook of sexual orientation and gender diversity in counseling and psychotherapy*. (pp. 105–27). American Psychological Association. https://doi.org/10.1037/15959-005

Muñoz Gaitán, L. (2006). La nueva sociología de la infancia. Aportaciones de una mirada distinta. *Política y Sociedad*, 43(1), 9–26.

Newton, J., & Ponting, C. (2013). Eliciting young people's views on wellbeing through contemporary science debates in Wales. *Child Indicators Research*, 6(1), 71–95. https://doi.org/10.1007/s12187-012-9159-1

OMS. (2013). Salud mental un estado de bienestar. Organización Mundial de la Salud. www.who.int/features/factfiles/mental_health/es/

OECD. (Organization for Economic Cooperation and Development). (2013). *Guidelines on measuring subjective well-being*. Paris. www.oecd.org/statistics/Guidelines%20on%20Measuring%20Subjective%20Well-being.pdf

Platero, R. (L.). (2014). Metáforas y articulaciones para una pedagogía crítica sobre la interseccionalidad. *Quaderns de Psicologia*, 16(1), pp. 55–72. https://doi.org/10.5565/rev/qpsicologia.1219

Proctor, C.L., Linley, P.A., & Maltby, J. (2009). Youth life satisfaction: A review of the literature. *Journal of Happiness Studies*, 10(5), 583–630. https://doi.org/10.1007/s10902-008-9110-9

Prout, A. (2011). Taking a step away from modernity: Reconsidering the new sociology of childhood. *Global Studies of Childhood*, 1(1), 4–14. https://doi.org/10.2304/gsch.2011.1.1.4

Rodríguez Pascual, I. (2000). ¿Sociología de la infancia? Aproximaciones a un campo de estudio difuso. *Revista Internacional de Sociología*, 58(26), 99. https://doi.org/10.3989/ris.2000.i26.796

Sarriera, J.C., & Bedin, L. (2015). Towards a socio-community model: A well-being approach. *Universitas Psychologica*, 14(4), 1387–98.

Tisdall, E.K.M., & Punch, S. (2012). Not so "new"? Looking critically at childhood studies. *Children's Geographies*, 10(3), 249–64. https://doi.org/10.1080/14733285.2012.693376

Vergara, A., Peña, M., Chávez, P., & Vergara, E. (2017). Los niños como sujetos sociales: El aporte de los Nuevos Estudios Sociales de la infancia y el Análisis Crítico del Discurso. *Psicoperspectivas. Individuo y Sociedad*, *14*(1), 55–65. https://doi.org/10.5027/psicoperspectivas-vol14-issue1-fulltext-544

Viveros Vigoya, M. (2016). La interseccionalidad: una aproximación situada a la dominación. *Debate Feminista*, *52*, 1–17. https://doi.org/10.1016/j.df.2016.09.005

White, S.C. (2017). Relational wellbeing: Re-centring the politics of happiness, policy and the self. *Policy & Politics*, *45*(2), 121–36. https://doi.org/10.1332/030557317X14866576265970

White, S.C., & Blackmore, C. (Eds.) (2015). *Cultures of wellbeing: Method, place, policy*. Palgrave Macmillan UK. https://link.springer.com/book/10.1057%2F9781137536457

13

DISASTER AND COMMUNITY PSYCHOLOGY

Focusing on the power of youth and children and their peer effects in disaster prevention and community empowerment

Mari Yoshinaga and Takehito Hagiwara

Abstract

After the Great East Japan Earthquake of 2011, there were reports of children and young people participating in reconstruction activities, giving adults in the affected areas the courage to do the same. The process of evacuation and reconstruction can be an opportunity for them to participate in community development. Through case studies, this chapter discusses: the peer effect of interactions between young people living in disaster areas and those living outside the disaster area; the importance of community workers with expertise in reaching out to children and young people in the disaster area; and the impact of young people's participation in disaster management activities on their sense of community empowerment.

Resumen

Cada año, el mundo es golpeado por una serie de desastres naturales. Tras el terremoto del Gran Este de Japón de 2011, hubo informes de niños y jóvenes que participaron en actividades de reconstrucción y dieron a los adultos de las zonas afectadas el valor de hacer lo mismo. El proceso de evacuación y reconstrucción puede ser una oportunidad para que participen en el desarrollo de la comunidad. Mediante estudios de casos, en este capítulo se examina el efecto de las interacciones entre los jóvenes que viven en la zona del desastre y los que viven fuera de ella, la importancia de los trabajadores comunitarios con conocimientos especializados para llegar a los niños y jóvenes de la zona del desastre, y los efectos de la participación de los jóvenes en las actividades de gestión de desastres en su sentido de empoderamiento de la comunidad.

Introduction

This chapter approaches disaster and Community Psychology with a focus on the role of children and youth in disaster management and recovery processes. Using case studies, we will

DOI: 10.4324/9780429325663-16

examine the process of empowering children and youth through the narratives of survivors, especially in terms of increased self-efficacy and participation in disaster management.

In 2011, the United Nations estimated that 100 million young people, including children, are affected by disasters each year. The NPRSB-NACCD Joint Youth Leadership Report (United States Department of Health and Human Services, Office of the Assistant Secretary for Preparedness and Response, 2017) discusses the importance of involving children and youth themselves in disaster management, evacuation and recovery processes. Specific methodologies are introduced in the report, but particular attention is given to developing youth as role models and encouraging a legacy of mentoring. While adults who listen to young people and engage them as equal partners can be models and mentors for young people, the report points to the fact that young people themselves can be models and mentors for the next generation of young people and children.

Disasters are a complex global problem and are inevitable occurrences in the lives of many (Makwana, 2019). Disasters can be divided into three categories: natural disasters, "man-made" disasters and combined phenomena (Shaluf, 2007). Natural disasters are those caused by subsurface, surface, climate-related and biological phenomena. The massive earthquake and tsunami that hit the Pacific coast of East Japan ten years ago can be considered a natural disaster. However, the subsequent explosion of the nuclear power plant in Fukushima resulting from the tsunami, which caused extensive damage, makes the Great East Japan Earthquake a complex disaster. Disasters as "accidental crises", sometimes called "situational crises", as Caplan described them (Caplan, 1964), have serious consequences for people's physical and mental health: widespread man-made disasters, such as the 9/11 terrorist attacks in the US in 1997, the 1995 sarin gas attack in Japan, the 2020 explosion in Lebanon, and the 2020 bushfires that destroyed 3% of Australia's land are blamed on human mismanagement. Natural disasters are usually more damaging in terms of the area affected and the number of people killed or injured. For example, since 1970, there have been 28 natural disasters that have caused more than 10,000 deaths, including six earthquakes and one flood (cyclone) since 2001 (International Fire Service Information Centre, 2018).

Natural disasters occur frequently in most regions of the planet, threatening the socio-economic development of many countries and regions and affecting people's physical and mental health (Kreimer, 2001). As human activity increases, climate change influences the frequency and magnitude of natural disasters, and economic factors have been shown to play a role in the magnitude of the damage (Padli et al., 2018). In other words, it is the poor people and communities that suffer the most, and because of this, they are also left behind in poverty (Hallegatte et al., 2018). Math et al. (2015) show that in developing countries, disaster damage tends to be greater due to factors such as poverty, lack of resources, lack of educational opportunities, inadequate infrastructure, lack of human resources and lack of knowledge. Mental health is an issue that is often neglected. However, this trend is also true for developed countries.

There are two main reasons why mental health may not be prioritised after a disaster. First, in the immediate aftermath of a disaster, the focus is first on life, and then on rebuilding lives and society, so people's mental health tends to get neglected. Second, methodologies such as psychological first aid (see Vernberg et al., 2008) have been developed, and specialist teams have been formed immediately after the disaster. However, as many trauma studies have shown, it is particularly difficult to articulate traumatic experiences in the immediate aftermath of a disaster for a variety of reasons, making it difficult to identify the target of support.

Trauma research is increasingly recognising that "talking" is an important therapeutic process, expressed by the word "narrative". Narrative refers to the narrator evoking the listener's emotions by re-enacting events or telling the listener how he or she felt at the time. However, creating a narrative is not an easy process for those who have been affected. Van der Kolk (2014) carefully reports on the ways in which trauma aims to overcome its effects through the embodiment of the state of mind suffered in trauma. Trauma is a state that is recoverable through clinical care attuned to each individual's experience of disaster and supports recovery.

Given that disasters affect many people at once, it is important that along with clinical care, there is a concurrent community approach that targets the health of all people. For example, using crisis intervention theory, there are well-documented examples of school-as-community approaches being attempted in the aftermath of an incident or accident (Nickerman & Zhe, 2004). In the aftermath of a major natural disaster, a similar community approach is used in schools, but where parents and teachers are also affected in the areas suffering the worst impact, children and young people may be cared for by people from outside the community. First aid methods have been proposed for various communities and, for example in some organisations, such as the Federal Emergency Management Agency (FEMA) in the United States. After a bit of time and after the emergency is dealt with, help will be provided for recovery. Madsen and O'Mullan (2016), in a qualitative study of community resilience, refer to social connectedness, optimistic acceptance, learning tolerance and patience, and learning from the past for the future as factors related to resilience. Particular attention has been paid to social connections, but when all communities (and all of the community) are caught up in the damage, connections become severed. Special methods are required to repair this.

In this chapter, we will discuss through case studies how to rebuild broken social ties in Japan, a volcanic island nation surrounded by the sea that is often struck by earthquakes and tsunamis. In doing so, we will focus on the aspects of mutual aid functioning in affected communities that are beyond the reach of public assistance. We would like to discuss how to regain the ability to help each other in vulnerable communities after the disaster, including suggestions for the future.

Mutual aid in Japan, a country prone to natural disasters

The oldest record of natural disasters in Japan describes an earthquake that struck the northern part of Nara Prefecture in 599 BCE. By the ninth century, records of disasters north of the Kanto region began to emerge, and the lack of records of major earthquakes for that century, with house collapses and tsunamis occurring at intervals of about every ten years, make it difficult to determine the extent of the damage. This indicates that there may have been a period when the occurrence of earthquakes was rare. In addition to earthquakes, there are many records of wind and flood damage, flooding caused by heavy rainfall from the rainy season fronts, and frequent typhoon storms and floods. In addition, the 1938 a cliff collapse in Kobe, Japan, caused by land development, is the first example of urban flooding.

The establishment of the Disaster Science Research Institute in 1937, the planning of Kobe's reconstruction of the city after urban flooding in 1938, and the implementation of the Urban Area Building Law are the earliest examples of community revitalisation activities after the disaster. Since then, wind and flood damage and landslides have occurred almost every year, and the Comprehensive National Land Development Law, the Coastal Law, regulatory provisions in the Building Standards Law, and the Basic Act on Disaster Countermeasures have been enacted, which have helped shape disaster prevention measures, mainly in terms of hardware. A major turning point was the court ruling in 1992 that warned against the "natural disaster theory of flooding" when the Tama River, which runs along the border of Tokyo and Kanagawa Prefecture, experienced a major flood that allowed residents to argue that the local government's management of the river was flawed, leading to the creation of a natural disaster prevention system. Since then, emphasis has been placed on activities that consider disaster prevention from the perspective of the residents. A major driving force behind this was the Great Hanshin-Awaji Earthquake of 1995, when it was revealed that communities that had been actively engaged in community development activities through the residents, prior to the disaster, were more likely to reduce the number of deaths and injuries through mutual aid.

It was in the aftermath of the Great East Japan Earthquake, in 2011, that the power of young people came into focus. In this disaster, large areas of eastern Japan were severely damaged, and it took a long time for lifelines to be restored. In addition to the disasters of the earthquake and tsunami, the Fukushima nuclear power plant explosion and subsequent radiation leaks were so severe that it took months or years for communities in each area to regain their minimum level of functioning. The magnitude of the earthquake was 9.0 on the Richter scale, and as of March 2021, the death toll was estimated at 24,582, with 2,525 missing and 6,157 injured. As of September 2020, the number of earthquake-related deaths over the past nine years was 3,767. Many houses were swept away by the tsunami, and the number of houses destroyed or washed away reached 117,948 in three prefectures in the Tohoku region.

Especially in the first month after the disaster, the young people and children were the "light" in exhausted and damaged communities. Teenagers were a great support to the people around them and helped the society to regain functioning. They also empowered the adults around them by communicating the situation in Japan to the rest of the world and making suggestions on how to rebuild their communities.

The power of youth and children: a case study approach

Methods and subjects in case studies

This section describes three case studies collected by the authors through two studies. For each case study, the research framework, details of the target population and key concepts related to youth and children from a Community Psychology perspective are summarised in Table 13.1.

Study 1: Peer Effects

Case 1: The importance of narratives in interactions between young people from affected and unaffected areas

In Case 1, we would like to share three stories about the significance of interactions between young people from the disaster area and those from other parts of Japan. The interactions between young people in different areas have had a significant impact on both sides, which we have termed the "peer effect". We use three examples to illustrate this in detail.

The first story concerns a project in which junior high school students from the Tokyo metropolitan area, far away from the disaster-hit areas of the Great East Japan Earthquake, travelled to the devastated town of Minamisanriku in the fall of 2015, four years after the disaster occurred. The purpose of this project was to investigate what young people and children feel when a disaster occurs, to understand the needs of this generation at the time of the disaster and to consider what mechanisms are needed to reflect their views in the subsequent recovery process. By sharing their experiences, survivors can gain empathy and improve their resilience and stress management skills. Those who have not experienced disasters can think about disasters imaginatively, and through empathy, increase their own ability to cope with disasters and contribute to recovery. For example, Rahiem et al. (2018) mentioning the same tsunami disaster in Aceh, Indonesia, suggested that children can overcome the crisis with the support of others and their own inner strength. It is also reported that children do not remain passive victims of

Table 13.1 Study framework

	Study 1: Interaction and peer effect	*Study 2: Role of play*
Time	2013.4–2016.3	2011.8–2016.8 2011.7–2017.2
Location	Minamisanriku, Miyagi Setagaya, Tokyo (visit to disaster areas for mutual exchange)	Kesennuma, Iwate Kazo, Saitama (evacuation site) Ishinomaki, Miyagi. Minamisanriku, Miyagi. Kooriyama, Fukushima.
Subjects	Case 1: Junior high school students & Highschool students Case 2: Junior high school students	Community workers supporting infants accompanied by parents, children and youth
Data	Case 1: Story 1: Interview and participant observation through workshop activities. Case 1: Story 2: Interview Case 1: Story 3: Interview & questionnaire inquiry Case 2: Questionnaire inquiry & participant observation through workshop activities.	Case 3: Interviews Case 4: Participant observation through Play Delivery Activities
Researcher	Yoshinaga and colleges	Case 3: Yoshinaga Case 4: Hagiwara and members of NPO Shari
Key concepts from community psychological perspectives	Case 1: Peer effects to strengthen resilience and to cope with stress of disaster among children and youth Case 2: Community empowerment by children and youth	Social support provided by community workers for children without sufficient care in community after disaster

the disaster but participate in the recovery process, thereby building social capital and enhancing disaster preparedness (Pfefferbaum et al., 2018).

The young people, who had just met for the first time, gradually became more open to each other and were able to have honest discussions. Box 13.1 summarises the narratives of junior high school students from the town of Minamisanriku, the disaster area. Box 13.2 summarises the impressions of both groups about the project, which brought them together to talk with each other. Figure 13.1 shows the author's photo of the young people in Story 1 and Figure 13.3 all the members involved lined up in front of the junior high school which had been affected by the tsunami.

Box 13.1 The interaction of narratives between youths in the disaster area and an unaffected area

- *We all covered ourselves with the blankets we had taken with us when we escaped from the school, but they were wet and cold. The shrine was filled with children in the fourth grade and younger, with adults around them. Figure 13.2 shows the inside of the shrine itself. Figure 13.3 shows some more of those young people* participating in the project. Some of them were older children who had escaped. It was also very cold inside the shrine. ★ I think there was a fire outside and it was warmer than inside, which was warmed only by candles

★ Shrines are ritual facilities where gods and spirits are believed to reside, and there are many of them throughout Japan. There is an old saying that it is good to run to a shrine in case of a tsunami. The shrine mentioned in this case is a small shrine called Isuzu Shrine, which was located at the place where the children, accompanied by their schoolteacher, ran to evacuate with the neighbouring nursery school children.

- *I turned around and saw the tsunami. There was a black wall coming. The shaking lasted so long that*
- *I couldn't even stand. I couldn't even stand up. I got under my desk, but I had to hold it down. It shook up and down and sideways. There were tiles falling around the shrine. We all picked them up because they were dangerous.*

- *Even after I escaped, I was scared because I heard a noise. It was a horrible sound. Three of my brothers were in this shrine. The older one was outside and two were inside. But I wasn't with my sister because we were stuck together by grade level. At first, we were at the entrance to the shrine. But the waves kept coming, so we went up the stairs. The bottom of the stairs have been scraped away and are now difficult to climb, but before, there were all these stone steps.*

- *The next day, I got to see my family, and as we were moving to the shelter, I found my dog's body on the railroad tracks. I was sad, but everyone told me that my friends and family had been saved. I couldn't say anything else because I thought that meant that it was good for us.*

- *It was hard to escape to the shelter. There was a lot of debris and water. We walked to the river, but an adult carried us on his back because it was dangerous. About two kilometres away, but it felt very far away. There were a lot of trees and other debris with nails sticking out of them, and my friend who stepped over them got injured.*

- *I was just worried about what would happen to me. When school started in May, I was really happy.*

- *The three of us shared one of the rice balls that our dad and his friends had brought from a neighbouring town where there was no damage, and we ate it together.*

- *The shelters were divided into three locations: the Nature House, the Togura Centre and the Oriental Factory. Even though the factory was right there, we walked up the cliffs on the opposite side of the cliffs and followed the cliffs through the woods. It was quite far.*

- *I panicked and lost track of my surroundings. We were turned into a black mass, and the car, the house, everything was swept away. I was so taken aback that I didn't know what to think about.*

- *All I could think about was getting away. All I could think about was getting to higher ground. We couldn't imagine that the tsunami wouldn't come because of that tremor.*

- *I couldn't sleep peacefully for a while. I couldn't sleep for days, wondering where I was going to go when it was dark and shaky with so many aftershocks.*

Box 13.2 The impressions of mutual talking

Young people of Minamisanriku:

- *I'm glad I had the opportunity to talk about it. I hope you'll pass it on to those around you.*

- *You never know when a disaster will strike, so it's important to have this opportunity to interact and think with people of my own generation. Talking about things that I had forgotten as the months have passed since the disaster has helped me to remember things again. I don't want it to happen again, but there is a possibility that it will happen again. I want to survive together with the people around me, and that's why I want to continue to tell others about it. I want many people to think about it with me.*

Young People from the Tokyo area:

- *The story I heard at the shrine on the mountain was the most memorable. He told me a very sad story. The fact that he could tell me his sad story made me feel like he was being positive.*

- *It was a painful experience for me, but I was happy to hear that he was able to talk about it.*

- *What I thought the most was how strong he was. If it were me, a big earthquake would be scary enough, but a tsunami would hit and I wouldn't be able to move.*

- *Water is amazing. Water is amazing. Steel bends. Concrete can be washed away.*

- *I've only seen it on TV, so listening to people of my generation, I feel like I can picture the scene in my mind's eye. I've learned to think more strongly about disaster prevention after seeing various places.*

- *I've learned to think more about disaster prevention by seeing various places. The stories I heard about those difficult times made me think about it.*

- *We live in the centre of the city and there are many buildings, so it may be difficult to escape from the broken glass.*

- *We would like to escape to a wide-open area, to a place where there are people, and to help people who need help.*

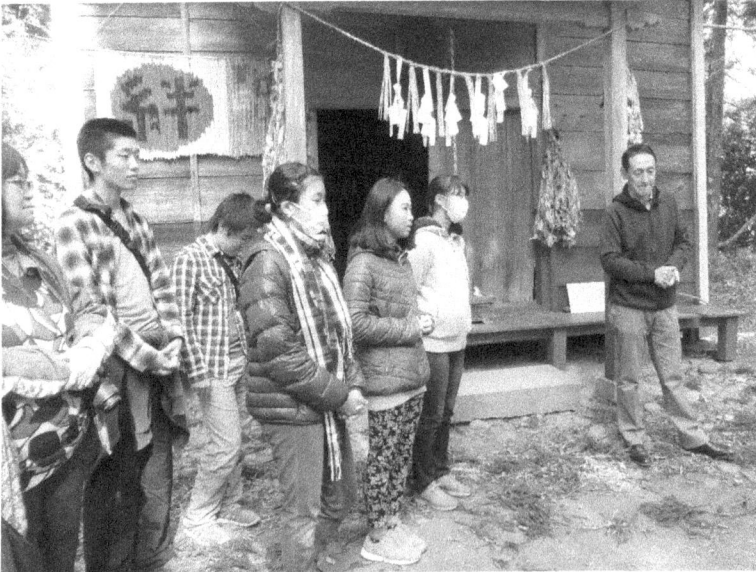

Figure 13.1 Young survivors share their experiences in front of the Shrine where they took refuge the night the tsunami hit the area

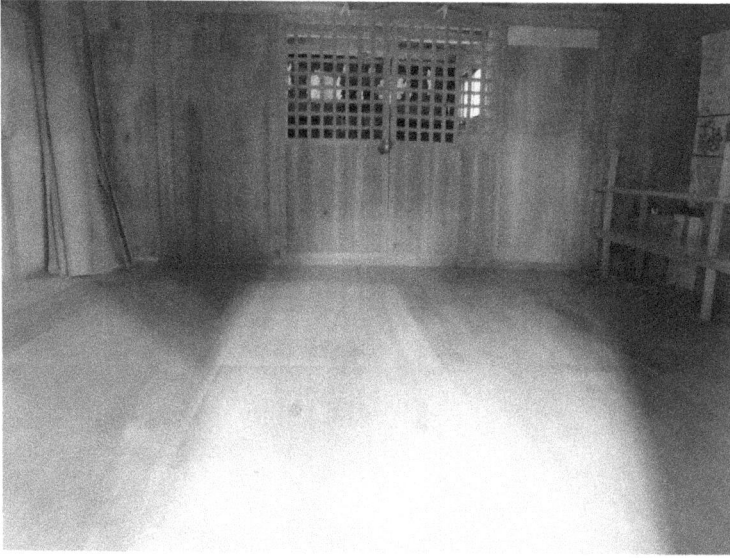

Figure 13.2   The inside of the shrine where the younger children spent the night

Box 13.1 shows the young people's own narratives of their experiences of the disaster and the narratives of those who heard them, even those who were not victims of the disaster. From the narratives of both young people, it is clear that the fear, anxiety and sadness that accompanied the disaster and its loss were described in concrete terms and made a strong impression on those who had not actually experienced it. In addition to the experience of pain, the author also mentions the pain of not being able to express one's emotions, suggesting that even a ten-year-old child at the time was unable to swallow and express his feelings in consideration of the disaster situation around him.

The experience of the disaster was shown to be just as unsettling for children as it was for adults, leading to problems such as insomnia, indicating the importance of paying attention to children's mental health. The event of reopening school was described in terms of "I was happy to see my friends", indicating that the rushed start to ensure academic continuity ultimately brought the children "the joy of getting back to their daily lives".

In Boxes 13.1 and 13.2, references to the meaning of telling, and feelings about telling, are made from the perspectives of both survivors and non-affected people. The expression that it was like seeing a scene was noteworthy, as was the listener's impression that it was a sign of the speaker's positivity that he or she was willing to talk about it. Some young people spoke directly about the benefits of interacting with their peers, which shows the significance of mutual interaction. In addition, the storytelling of their own roles in saving others by communicating, as well as of the increased sense of self-efficacy from being on the side of help by listening, were also evident.

The second story is of a high school girl (see Figure 13.4) who has begun to take on the role of telling the legends of her village. As one of the young people affected by the disaster, she expressed her determination to pass on local lore. She noted that even if traces of the lore are washed away, the narratives of the lore will remain, and it is striking that she explained the future possibilities of being able to pass on the narratives even if something tangible in a community is lost.

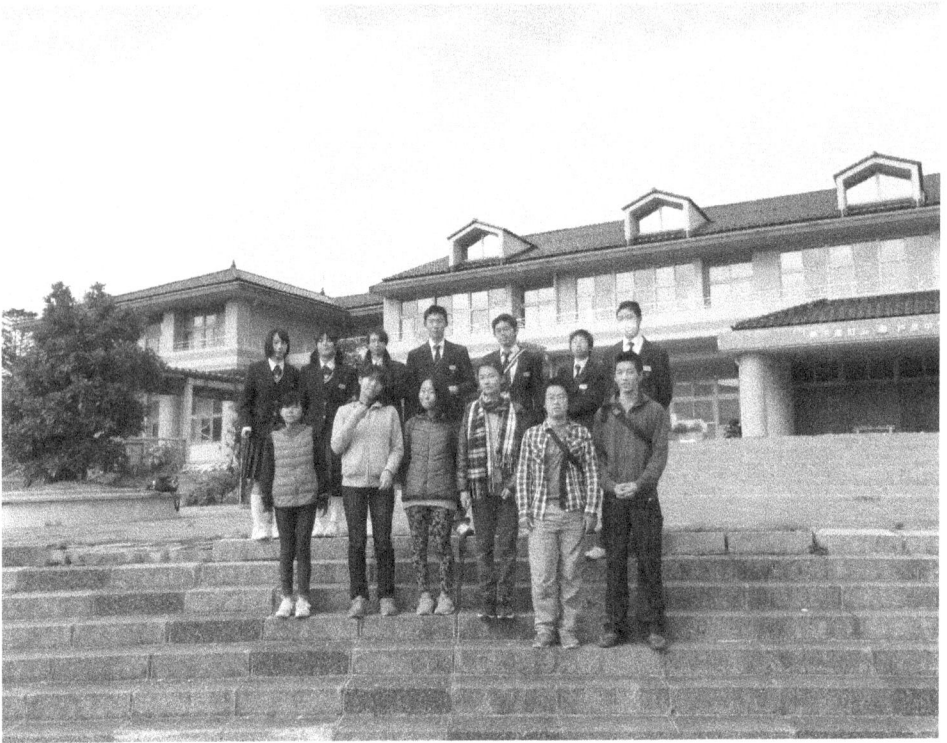

Figure 13.3 Young people from both groups who participated in the project standing in front of Togura Junior High School, which was affected by the earthquake and tsunami

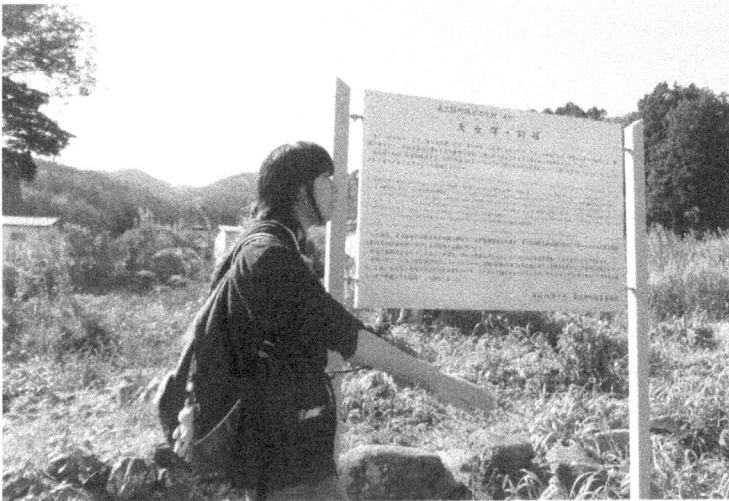

Figure 13.4 A young girl talking about the village legends

She was one of the young people who fled to a shrine on high ground with the young people in the first story, though they were in different grades at the time of the disaster. Her house, which was close to the beach, had been completely washed away except for the foundation, and she and her family had taken refuge on the slightly inland side of the house. She was not able to do this when she had to take classes at the high school, but when she had time, she was responsible for telling visitors from outside the disaster area about the legend of the Tennyo Mound that was located near her home . Box 13.3 shows the details of the legend.

Box 13.3 The story of the legend

- *There is a legend that my grandparents told me since I was little. On one of the small islands lined up across the sea, a heavenly maiden landed with her dog long ago. When she was hungry, she came to this beach and asked my ancestor, a fisherman, for help. She lived for a while in a remote part of the man's house, but the food was unpalatable, and she gradually wasted away and eventually died. There was a large stone in my house that marked the spot where the goddess was buried, and I was told since I was a child not to play on the stone.*

- *There was a mound on the beach dedicated to this legendary maiden, but it was washed away by the tsunami and all that remains is a sign. <u>Although the tsunami has destroyed the traces of the legend, the story can still be passed on, so I want to pass it on to those who visit.</u>*

The third story concerns a high school student, Mr O., shown in Figure 13.5, who left the disaster area to visit a junior high school in the Tokyo area and gave a lecture to 250 junior high school students.

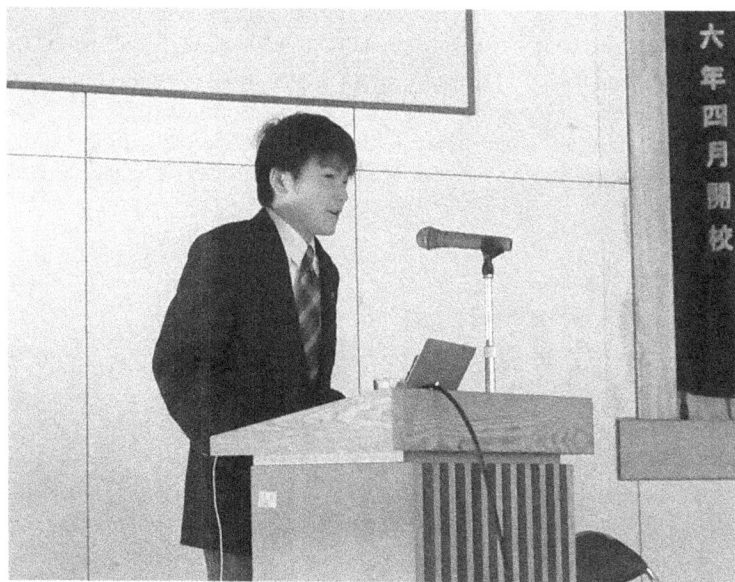

Figure 13.5   A young man who gave a memorable talk to the students

The scene is a lecture by Mr. O regarding the recovery process of his town destroyed by tsunami. Over 250 junior high school students listened to his narratives, which had a peer effect on them.

Mr. O (Figure 13.5) experienced the Great East Japan Earthquake when he was in his first year of junior high school. In his speech, he spoke about his experiences in the disaster and how the younger generation thought and acted during the recovery process. "But I would like you to remember, even if only once in a while", he began. Using maps and photos, he began by explaining how the rias (or indented, saw-toothed) coastline, which provides us with so many blessings, amplified the height of the tsunami many times over and caused extensive damage. After that, he projected photos of the town after the disaster to show how the environment and their lives have changed over time. In this area, there is a traditional dance called the "Deer Dance" that has been passed down from generation to generation. With the support of their teacher and the local people, they practiced and learned to be the bearers of the "deer dance" and were invited to perform overseas in France. The local people, who had lost their traditional performing arts equipment in the disaster and were in despair, were encouraged by the fact that these young people were successfully carrying on the precious traditional performing arts.

Mr. O also told us a story about how they overcame their fear of the "ocean" by learning the skill of catching fish and seaweed in the sea under the guidance of the classmates' parents who were fishermen. Mr. O urged the audience of his peers to start preparing for what they can do, because the unexpected disaster will always happen. Subsequent surveys showed that junior high school students' self-efficacy regarding disaster preparedness improved significantly after listening to Mr. O's story (Yoshinaga, 2021). Self-efficacy for disaster prevention was measured using a four-point scale ranging from "True", "Fairly True", "Not really True" and "Not at all True", for the following three items: "Junior high school students can play a role in disaster prevention", "I feel uneasy about junior high school students being responsible for disaster prevention", and "Junior high school students are more likely to be the ones rescued in a disaster". In conventional disaster education programmes, disaster prevention experts or adults from the disaster area usually give lectures for children. In this case, a survivor of the same generation as the students shared his or her experience, which is thought to have had a peer effect and improved the self-efficacy of the junior high school students who listened to the lecture. It is thought that the improvement of self-efficacy will lead to junior high school students, who are the leaders of local disaster prevention, playing an active role in the community at the time of a disaster, and that the concept of the peer effect should be emphasised in community empowerment.

Case 2: The link between the practice of continuous disaster management training activities and young people's sense of community empowerment

We have been conducting action research on community development activities conducted by residents in this area for many years, and every year we participate in a local disaster drill to observe the relationship between children and the community. In Case 2, we describe the case of junior high school students who participated in activities to experience various disaster drills while spending the night in gymnasiums and classrooms on the assumption that an elementary school would become an evacuation centre. Not only the school's teachers and staff, but also many community members and parents participated in these activities. In addition to the activities at the elementary school, the junior high school students participated

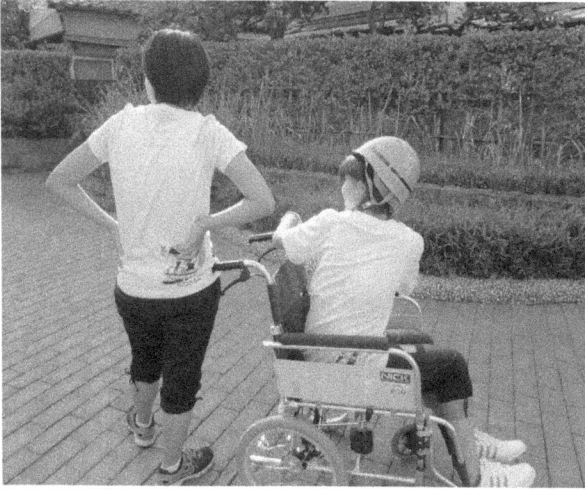

Figure 13.6   Experience of using a wheelchair

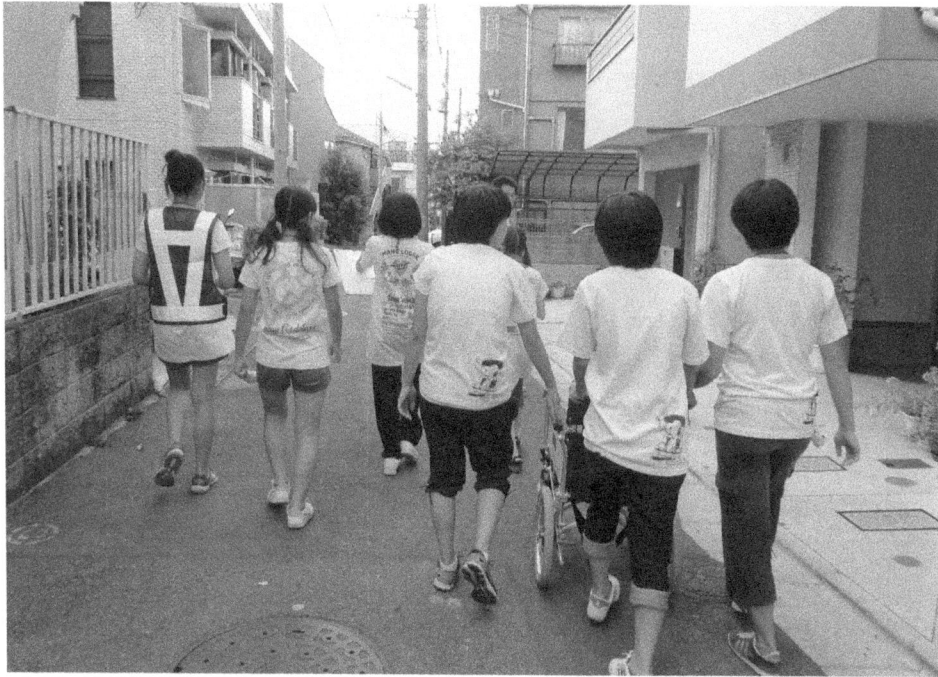

Figure 13.7   Students following the obstacle route

in an evacuation training that simulated the use of a wheelchair to help a person in need of assistance. The participants were divided into five groups. One person, playing the role of a disabled person, was placed in a wheelchair (see Figure 13.6), and the other members of each group pushed the wheelchair towards the goal (see Figure 13.7). The map they were handed showed collapsed buildings and fires, and some areas were impassable, so they had to make detours. The students aimed to reach the goal as quickly as possible. In addition, there were some sudden obstacles that were not clearly marked on the map, and these had to be avoided as well.

After reaching the goal, they went back to the elementary school and held a workshop to share their impressions. Figure 13.8 shows the scene at that time of the workshop. Box 13.4 shows the participants' comments after the workshop, where they were instructed to write about what they thought was important.

Box 13.4 Important thoughts of junior high school students after the disaster prevention training programme

- *Think and act for yourself.*

- *Water and food security.*

- *It's important to be prepared as a junior high school student.*

- *When a disaster strikes, I don't have to act alone, but we have to work together.*

- *I think it's important to be prepared to be a leader in disaster prevention. It's also important for us to work together, not just by ourselves.*

- *No matter what is happening, we should act calmly. I thought that junior high school students were able to help a lot of people.*

- *Make sure the people around you are safe. Be proactive in your actions.*

- *I think we need to say (and tell others), "I couldn't get through ahead of you", or "It was a close call".*

- *A sense of responsibility.*

- *Compassion.*

- *Know in advance what needs to be done.*

- *The first thing to do is to ensure your own safety*

- *Don't act apart on your own, but follow the instructions of adults.*

- *I knew that if he was truly crippled, he wouldn't be able to do what he did today.*

Figure 13.9 shows how community empowerment attitudes changed before and after the activity. This figure is a modified version of Yoshinaga's (2021) table. Scores increased on all items after the activity. In particular, the scores for "My opinion was reflected" and "It was an opportunity for community members to help each other" increased significantly. These two items did not score very high before the activity, indicating that the experience of having a large number of community members participating and supporting each other had an effect, even if their attitudes were not affected by the daily activities. In addition, the process of exchanging opinions at the workshop and presenting them in front of adults to make suggestions for future disaster prevention plans must have stimulated the awareness that "My opinion was reflected".

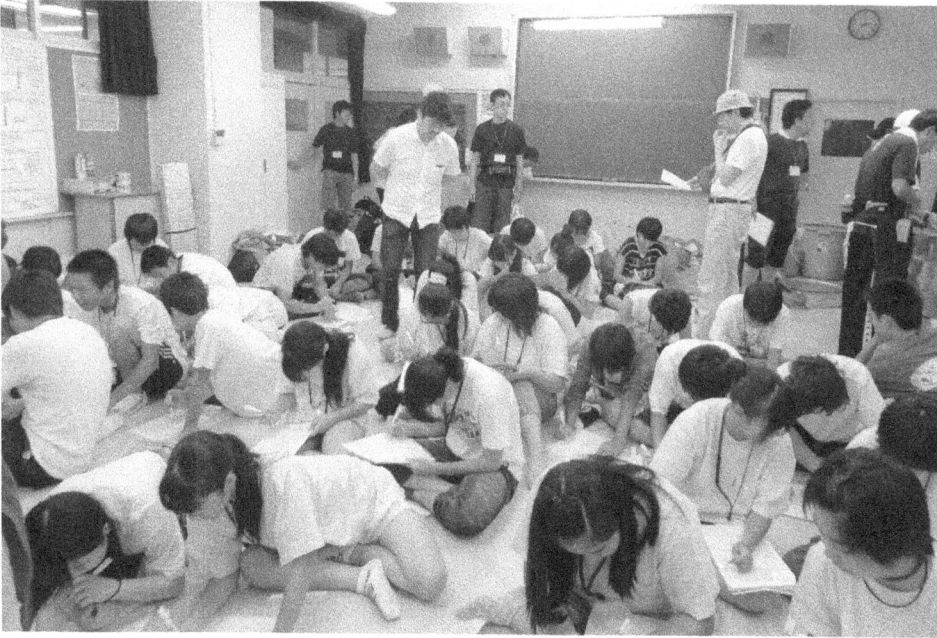

Figure 13.8　The participants exchanging opinions

The impact of disasters on children and young people through the eyes of community workers: the role of play

Case 3: Play work to build a community-based playground

Five years after the disaster, Mr. N lived in the affected area and was responsible for managing a playground for children. Initially, an NGO was responsible for the management of the playground, but eventually the residents became proactively involved. At the playground, the NGO staff sometimes encountered situations that differed from those of ordinary children and young people who had been affected by the disaster. For example, a girl's brother was playing with fire at the playground during the day, and when Mr. N went to check on him, he looked at him suspiciously at first, but then became friendly with him, saying that his sister was indebted to him. Those somewhat rambunctious youngsters said,

> *I'm glad there was a tsunami. Before the disaster, adults looked at us with a disapproving look on their faces. We did not go to school and stayed indoors, but thanks to the tsunami, we were able to go outside. Those annoying people who were watching our every move stopped looking at me and I felt comfortable.*

They said that they had been saved. The playground also attracted young people looking for a different kind of company than the school or the workplace, people they could really talk to. This generation of young people, who are often treated as persons that are often dealt with disapprovingly and side-lined by the public, feel a sense of liberation since the communities with old values were broken up by the tsunami.

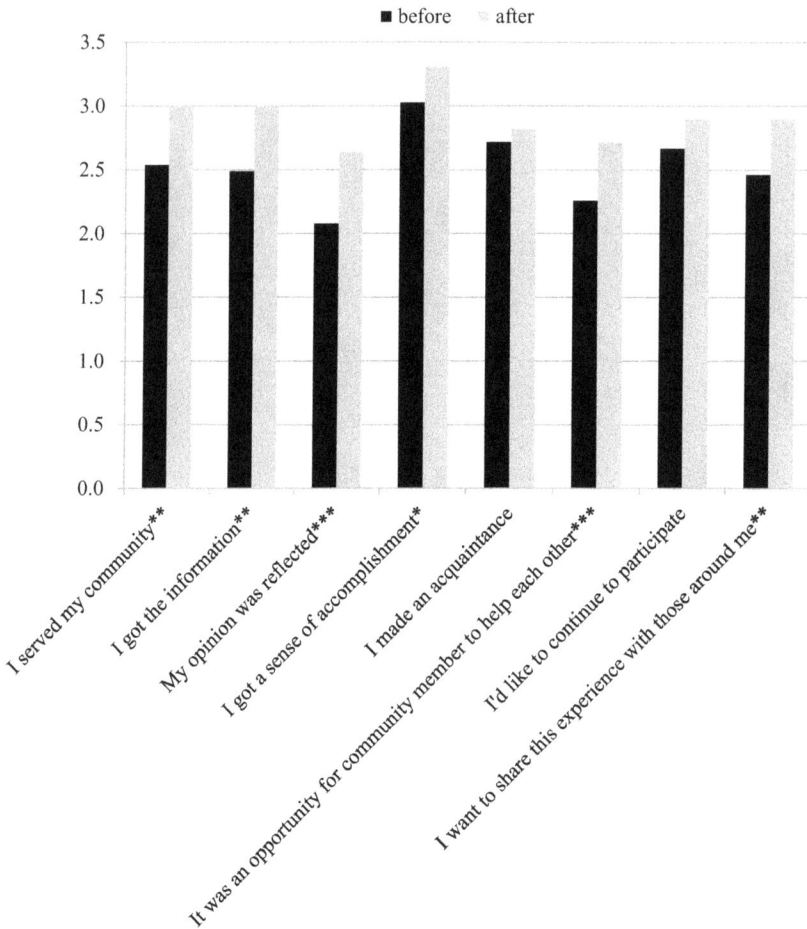

Figure 13.9 How community empowerment attitudes changed before and after the activity

Case 4: Play delivery activities

Hagiwara et al. (2015) described the support activities at a playground set up in an evacuation centre in the city of Fukushima, the site of the nuclear accident. They did not bring in large pieces of playground equipment, but they did play many games with clay and small toys. There were many toys, but they were just piled up, and although there was a play area, there was no one to play with them. It was difficult to obtain volunteers, as people were afraid of radiation. One of the most memorable scenes was when a child who had made a robot out of clay who held a shield in one of his hands, was apparently getting ready to make a sword to hold in the other, but changed his mind and made a shield for the robot's other hand as well. The children seemed to be trying their best to protect themselves from enemies attacking them, such as a tsunami and radiation. The robot would fall over because its hands were too heavy, but the child was still determined it should be so, and took it home. The robot with armour on both hands could be seen as an expression of the child's desire to protect himself under stress. Even if the work was such that it fell over under the weight, its construction was still valuable for the child. Hagiwara also volunteered during the 1995 Hanshin-Awaji earthquake, and he remembered the children's stress very strongly at that time as well. Themes related to the suffering experienced appear in their play, such as a child murmuring "the colour of suffering" when that child saw the colour black when there was a lot of fire damage. After the tsunami caused by the Great East Japan Earthquake, he also felt that tsunami-related themes appeared in children's play. Hagiwara et al. (2015) also carried out support activities at a playground set up in a large evacuation centre, housing 2,000 people who had escaped from the Tohoku region to the Tokyo metropolitan area because they could no longer live in their original location. Many of the evacuees were from areas affected by the nuclear power plant disaster. Some of the children were playing a game called "moving game", in which they repeatedly moved from one place to another. There were also many games in which food was served. The volunteer staff, including Hagiwara, strongly felt that the children had to endure and fight for survival in their own way, as the inconveniences and hardships of evacuation life were evident in these games.

Discussion

We have presented four case studies to illustrate different ways in which children and young people respond to disasters. Anselma et al. (2019), who conducted action research with children on disasters and recovery from them, point to the importance of working with individuals and organisations that know the community well and have diverse expertise, as well as trusting relationships with schools, as keys to success. In order to reach a level of awareness among children/youth, parents and community members that will improve the local disaster management system, it is important to conduct ongoing practical activities for disaster education, verify the effectiveness of such activities and share the results with collaborators, participants and investigators (researchers) in the process. There are three main things that we can draw from the case studies.

The first is the peer effect. There has been much discussion of the negative impact of peer influence on young people's tendencies to choose risky behaviours. In terms of more positive effects, for example, it has been reported that the university students easily accepted being taught about mental health literacy education by peers (Patalay et al., 2017). Through extracurricular activities, prosocial friendships have also been shown to play a developmentally regulating role (Fredricks & Eccles, 2005). Children who were affected by the disaster received and expressed in their own words an age-appropriate sense and understanding of the situation and their own feelings about the disaster, which differed from an adult's perspective on the disaster. It can be assumed that the stories of their peers acted as a surrogate experience and increased their self-efficacy in disaster-related actions. Peek et al. (2018) noted the resilience, strength and competence of children. They also stated that it is important to look at children's "voices", "perspectives" and "actions". These views of children's perspectives can transform society. The case studies also showed that the experience of the younger generation of disaster victims can have a significant impact on their peers and cause a change in attitudes. In the recovery process, it is necessary to strengthen the commitment of children and young people and ensure that they have opportunities to overcome the challenges brought by a disaster by interacting with their peers, enhancing their self-efficacy and communicating their experiences through narratives and other forms of interaction.

The second is the importance of adults during the crisis, in children's minds and lives. The direct safeguarders and protectors of children and young people may also have become victims, and they may be so concerned with basic survival and their own coping that there is less opportunity to focus on the children. The examples of young people who spoke with a sense of liberation about the lack of attention they received, show that today's society can be a difficult environment for young people to live in if they are unable to adjust to school and the workplace. They could not speak to adults who were also hurting from the disaster, but they could speak to community workers who are not just temporary volunteers but are rooted in society and responsible for the relief efforts. Those workers also played a role in "taking" young people's voices and speaking for them to the adults in the community.

Where there is invisible environmental pollution, following events such as nuclear accidents, a shortage of temporary volunteers may exist in those areas where people cannot get together. These volunteers play an important role. Many supplies are gathered in the disaster area, but even if there is material support, without human support, it is impossible to help those in need. Volunteer activities such as providing play for children can support adults as well as children. There are two types of support: direct support, where adults can do other things by taking care of children, and indirect support, where children's smiles and energy through play positively affect the adults around them. In this case the background of the volunteers was not as community workers but as community psychologists. They used their expertise to find the trauma expressed in children's play and get close to them in order to help the children express themselves and support them in releasing the stresses of their highly mobile lives through play. The importance of psychological first aid for children has become widely known, and the Red Cross and international NGOs have established methodologies and are working to spread the word. In the case of a disaster with large-scale damage, it is worthwhile to have not only large aid groups but also a small but highly specialised group to provide support, especially for children's play.

Finally, what can be noted, based on the results of these case studies is the importance of disaster prevention activities as town planning activities, in which adults and children participate on an equal basis. Feeling attached to where they live has been shown to help people become more resilient and active in post-disaster recovery, not only adults but also children and adolescents (Scannell et al., 2017). The experience of participating in disaster reduction activities enhances the community empowerment of children and young people and helps them grow as leaders of the next generation. A large body of literature on youth participation in disaster management activities is accumulating in diverse disaster-prone areas around the world, like Tanner (2010). Emphasis is placed on the importance of trusting relationships with adults and on methodological innovations such as the introduction of scientific learning methods. Osofsky et al. (2018) showed that through university student-led programme practices, post-disaster community cohesion and recovery are strengthened. As shown in Case 3, the youth-led simulations training programme led to an increased awareness of community empowerment among the participating youth. Strengthening awareness of community empowerment fosters a sense of community in the children and youth who are the future leaders of a community. Disaster prevention and recovery practices from the perspective of children and youth will enhance cooperation and mutual support among them, resulting in the formation of resilient communities.

To summarise this process from the perspective of Community Psychology, the spontaneous participation of children and youth in community development during the recovery period after a disaster can strengthen their sense of community empowerment, foster their sense of community and nurture them to be the next generation who are responsible for the construction of a community. Practising disaster prevention and recovery from the perspective of children and youth will enhance cooperation and mutual support, which will ultimately lead to the formation of resilient communities.

References

Anselma, M., Altenburg, T.M., Emke, H., van Nassau, F., Jurg, M., Ruiter, R.A.C., Jurkowski, J.M., & Chinapaw, M.J.M. (2019). Co-designing obesity prevention interventions together with children: intervention mapping meets youth-led participatory action research. *International Journal of Behavioral Nutritional and Physical Activity*, *16*, 1–15.

Caplan, G. (1964). *Principles of preventive psychiatry.* Basic Books.

Fredricks, J.A., & Eccles, J.S. (2005). Developmental benefits of extracurricular involvement: Do peer characteristics mediate the link between activities and youth outcomes? *Journal of Youth and Adolescence, 34*(6), 507–20.

Hagiwara, T., Okamoto, A., Fujii, Y., & Hisata, M. (2015). Psychological support to the children suffering from Great East Japan Earthquake: "Delivery of playing" activities to the children in shelter. *Japanese Journal of Community Psychology, 15*(2), 74–84.

Hallegatte, S., Fay, M., & Barbier E.D. (2018). Poverty and climate change: introduction. *Environment and Development Economics, 23*, 217–33.

International Fire Service Information Center. (2018). Natural disasters in the world. www.kaigai-shobo.jp/files/worldoffire/Disasters_2.pdf (in Japanese)

Kreimer, A. (2001). Social and economic impacts of natural disasters. *International Geology Review, 43*(5), 401–5. https://doi.org/10.1080/00206810109465021

Madsen, W., & O'Mullan, C. (2016). Perceptions of community resilience after natural disaster in a rural Australian town. *Journal of Community Psychology, 44*(3), 277–92.

Makwana, N. (2019). Disaster and its impact on mental health: A narrative review. *Journal of Family Medicine and Primary Care, 8*(10), 3090–3095.

Math, S.B., Nirmala, M.C., Moirangthem, S., & Kumar, N.C. (2015). Disaster management: Mental health perspective. *Indian Journal of Psychological Medicine, 37*(3), 261–71. https://doi.org/10.4103/0253-7176.162915

Nickerson, A.B., & Zhe, E. (2004). Crisis prevention and intervention: A survey of school psychologist. *Psychology in the School, 41*(7), 777–88.

Osofsky, H., Osofsky, J., Hansel, T., Lawrason, B., & Speier, A. (2018). Building resilience after disasters through the youth leadership program: The importance of community and academic partnerships on youth outcomes. *Progress in Community Health Partnerships: Research, Education, and Action, 12*, Special Issue: 11–21.

Padli, J., Habibullah, M.S., & Bahram, A.H., (2018). The impact of human development on natural disaster fatalities and damage: panel data evidence. *Economic Research, 31*(1): 1557–73.

Patalay, P., Anis, J., Sharpe, H., Newman, R., Main, D., Ragunathan, T., Parkes, M., & Claeke, K. (2017). A pre-post evaluation of Open Minds: a sustainable, peer-led mental health literacy programme in Universities and Secondary Schools. *Preventive Science, 18*, 995–1005.

Peek, L., Abraham, D.M., Cox, R.S., Fothergill, A., & Tobin, J. (2018). Children and disasters. In H. Rodriguez, W. Donner, & J.E. Trainor (Eds.), *Handbook of disaster research* (pp. 243–62). Springer.

Pfefferbaum, B., Pfefferbaum, R.L., & Van Horn, R.L. Involving children in disaster risk reduction: The importance of participation. *European Journal of Psychotraumatology, 9*, 1–6.

Rahiema, M.D.H., Kraussb, S.E., & Rahima, H. (2018). The child victims of the Aceh tsunami: Stories of resilience, coping and moving on with life. *Procedia Engineering, 212*, 1303–10.

Scannell, L., Cox, R.S., & Fletcher, S. (2017). Place-based loss and resilience among disaster-affected youth. *Journal of Community Psychology, 45*(7), 859–76.

Shaluf, I.M. (2007). An overview on disasters. *Disaster Prevention and Management: An International Journal, 16*(5): 687–703.

Tanner, T. (2010). Shifting the narrative: Child-led responses to climate change and disasters in El Salvador and the Philippines. *Children & Society, 24*(4), 339–51.

United States Department of Health and Human Services, Office of the Assistant Secretary for Preparedness and Response. (2017). *NPRSB-NACCD joint youth leadership report.* Author. www.phe.gov/Preparedness/legal/boards/nprsb/meetings/Documents/joint-youth-ldrshp-rpt.pdf

van der Kolk, B. (2014). *The body keeps the score: Brain, mind, and body in the healing of trauma.* Penguin Books.

Vernberg, E.M., Steinberg, A.M., Jacobs, A.K., Brymer, M.J., Watson, P.J., Osofsky, J.D., Layne, C.M., Pynoos, R.S., & Ruzek, J.I. (2008). Innovations in disaster mental health: Psychological first aid. *Professional Psychology: Research and Practice, 39*(4), 381–8. https://doi.org/10.1037/a0012663

Yoshinaga, M. (2021). Disaster prevention education with the participation of children and young people: Focusing on community empowerment awareness and self-efficacy. *Japanese Journal of Community Psychology, 24*(2) 95–113.

14

COMMUNITY ARTS FOR CRITICAL COMMUNITY PSYCHOLOGY PRAXIS

Towards decolonisation and Aboriginal self-determination

Christopher C. Sonn, Amy F. Quayle and Paola Balla

Abstract

This chapter describes community arts practice as decolonial aesthetics that can foster cultural strengthening, as well as counter storytelling for transformative witnessing to develop empathy. The first project is a testimonio of the creative work of Wemba Wemba Gundijmara artist Paola Balla who produced "healing cloths" to capture everyday acts of survival as part of the process of documenting matriarchy, resistance and Aboriginal Healing. The second project focuses on the Bush Babies portraiture project and exhibition(s) which in providing opportunities for Aboriginal counter storytelling in public settings created possibilities for transformative witnessing. These examples are both concerned with Aboriginal self-determination and provide insight into the potential of community arts when connected with a decolonial approach to contribute to personal and collective change. We suggest that arts are a powerful medium that invokes various senses and challenge people in deep and unsettling ways, opening spaces to bear witness, with effects that last beyond the arts encounters.

Resumen

Este capítulo describe la práctica del arte comunitario desde un enfoque de descolonización, haciendo énfasis en el potencial que el arte ofrece de generar cambios positivos a nivel individual, colectivo, y el fortalecimiento cultural. Similarmente, el arte comunitario brinda una contra narrativa testimonial que intenta desarrollar una perspectiva de empatía y transformación. El primer proyecto es un testimonio del trabajo creativo de la artista Wemba Gundijmara Paola Balla, quien produjo *"healing cloths"* (pañossanadores) para capturar los actos cotidianos de supervivencia como parte del proceso de documentación del matriarcado, la resistencia y el sanar Aborigen. El segundo proyecto describe *"Rekindling on Country"* (reconectando con la tierra madre), una iniciativa que involucra la colaboración entre una agencia de arte comunitario

DOI: 10.4324/9780429325663-17

de Western Australia y la comunidad Aborígen de Noongar. Estos ejemplos se centran entorno a la autonomía Aborígen y ofrecen una mirada que realza el potencial del arte comunitario desde un enfoque de descolonización. Esta perspectiva presenta al arte como un medio efectivo que desafía al público de manera profunda e inquietante, involucrando todos los sentidos para generar espacios testimoniales con efectos que perduran más allá de los encuentros artísticos.

In this chapter we draw on different community arts projects that were developed for and in support of Aboriginal self-determination and decolonial racial justice. Our ongoing efforts to develop and mobilise theories, methodologies, and methods are situated within the context of social relations within Australia. These relations are inherently racialised and premised on the dispossession of First Nations people, ongoing oppression and forms of violence, and its deleterious impacts witnessed in the present time. Resurgent social movements, such as those organised around indigenous sovereignty and Black Lives Matter, have elevated again the residue of colonialism, global capitalism, the ecological crises and its continuities and sequelae in the so-called post-colonial and post-colonising contexts around the world. These movements have brought into sharp focus the persistent and widening social inequalities that are produced and maintained through the resistant structures of white supremacy, heteronormativity, patriarchy, racism, capitalism and their intersections. In Australia, the ongoing struggles of Aboriginal and Torres Strait Islander people and other racialised communities for equity, justice and dignity in the face of this reality have also been met with and brought to the fore strategies of survival, resistance and activism that point to pathways and possibilities for community, liberation and well-being.

Within the Community, Identity, Displacement Research Network (CIDRN) in collaboration with Moondani Balluk Indigenous Academic Unit at Victoria University, Australia, the three authors have worked together on different projects that have used arts and cultural practices to foster voice, sense of community and place identity, and social justice consciousness in support of Aboriginal self-determination. Paola is a Koorie woman, and her Peoples are Wemba-Wemba and Gunditjmara. Her dominant matriarchal and Day family lineage of her mother and all her grandmothers makes her a Wemba-Wemba woman first. She is also a member of the Egan family and Gunditjmara woman through her patriarchal line of her great-grandfather. Amy is a non-indigenous, white settler Australian woman who through her research has come to recognise the taken-for-granted power, privilege and normativity that come with whiteness. Her research has examined racialised oppression, its impacts, how communities respond and resist, and how (counter-)storytelling through community arts and cultural practice can contribute to empowerment and self-determination, and challenge wilful ignorance of an ongoing history of dispossession. Christopher is a South African immigrant to Australia. Drawing on his own experiences and social and cultural locations, his research, informed by community and liberation psychology has focused on documenting the psychosocial effects of various systems of oppression, such as apartheid in South Africa and settler colonialism in Australia, along with elevating knowledge of the multiple, complex and creative ways people and communities resist, survive and enact liberation. CIDRN is the setting where we come together for dialogue around matters of race and whiteness, displacement, indigenous sovereignty, coloniality, memory and for collaboratively creating liberation-oriented praxis and methods.

We focus on how community arts and cultural development framed within the decolonial approaches of liberation and Critical Community Psychology can contribute to racial justice and Aboriginal self-determination. We contextualise the ongoing iterative generative reflexive practice within the ongoing dynamics and tensions of knowledge construction and the longer histories of colonialism. We outline key features of the frameworks that we draw from to craft Critical Community Psychology praxis for empowerment and liberation. Paola shares her practice-led inquiry "Disrupting Artistic Terra Nullius" as a testimonio highlighting the significance and meaning of the arts processes and practices for counter-storytelling for Aboriginal self-determination. Christopher and Amy then describe work that served as counter-storytelling rooted in and affirming of Aboriginal Elders' stories and experiences (see Quayle & Sonn, 2019).

Towards decoloniality: liberation, indigenous and critical community psychologies

There is ample writing in critical, cultural, community and liberation psychologies that have critiqued Eurocentric psychology for its complicity with colonialism, imperialism and in terms of its continuities through the colonial matrix of power/knowledge. Peruvian scholar Anibal Quijano (2000) referred to the continuity of dynamics of dominance and subjugation as the coloniality of power, noting that the notion "names the continuities in the so-called 'post-colonial era' of the social hierarchical relationships of exploitation and domination between Europeans and non-Europeans built during centuries of European colonial expansion emphasising cultural and social power relations" (p. 95). In Australia, this coloniality is reflected in racialised violence that has its roots in colonialism and the violent dispossession of land from indigenous people, denial of culture, removal of children from families, and various symbolic and material practices of control and domination that continue. Moreton-Robinson (2015) suggests that Australia was founded as a settler-colonial nation on the theft of land, the dehumanisation of a racialised "other", and simultaneous construction of the myth of a national white identity that has become ingrained and reproduced institutionally and culturally. She wrote:

> belonging to the new nation [...] was racialized and inextricably tied to the accumulation of capital and the social worth, authority, and ownership that this conferred. The Indigenous were excluded from this condition of belonging [...] The white body was the norm and measure for identifying who could belong.
>
> *(Moreton Robinson, 2015, p. 7)*

The ideologies of race, gender and culture are central pillars of Eurocentrism and the imposition of structures of domination in countries in the Global South and East, and through which social relations, experiences and subjectivities have been framed (Maldonado Torres, 2016). According to Grosfoguel (2016), "Racism is a global hierarchy of superiority and inferiority [...] that have been politically, culturally and economically produced and reproduced for centuries by the institutions of the capitalist/patriarchal western-centric/Christian-centric modern/colonial world system" (p. 10). Grosfoguel (2016) draws on Frantz Fanon's "line of the human", which divides those people above the line as "recognised socially in their humanity as human beings and, thus, [enjoying] access to rights (human rights, civil rights, women's rights, and/or labour rights), material resources, and social recognition to their subjectivities, identities, epistemologies and spiritualities" (p. 10). Those people who are relegated to below the line are constructed as subhuman, and thus as undeserving of the same rights, material resources, social recognition and dignity. The ongoing urgent project for Critical Community Psychology is the radical project of theorising from below. This is captured in how Ndluvo-Gathseni (2020) describes decoloniality as "a planetary liberation project dealing with the questions of life chances, life futures, and rehumanising particularly for those people who have been degraded into the zone of non-being" (no page number).

Liberation, Indigenous, Critical Community Psychologies

Researchers have pointed out that these critiques of psychology are not new, and that current archival retrieval provides ample evidence of knowledge that shows dissident, silenced, omitted knowledge (e.g. Adams et al., 2015; Stevens et al., 2013). As noted by Suffla and Seedat (2021), the quest for liberatory and decolonial community psychologies requires engagement with various knowledge traditions. This process, they suggest, unsettles and counters the persistence of Eurocentric assumptions that continue to frame psychological research and practice. It is also a pathway to reclaim and mobilise diverse traditions and archives to construct knowledge and practices that can support the aspirations, desires and futures of diverse peoples marginalised by colonising psychologies (see also Fine, 2018; Torre et al., 2017).

The liberation paradigm (see Freire, 1972; Martín-Baró, 1994; Montero & Sonn, 2009; Montero et al., 2017) is also an important resource for decolonial pathways grounded in different visions, methodologies and practices needed to counter systems of domination and their effects on the psychosocial functioning of people and communities. As summarised by Osorio (2009), praxis is a foundation stone for Latin American liberation practitioners and researchers who are compelled to explain the "history of successive modes of colonization, and constructing cultural identity as a principle to transcend the present, to leave behind the dominant rationality and to integrate reason, emotion and ethic values" (p. 32).

In Australia and Aotearoa/New Zealand there are also several examples of critical scholarship that have been developed in the pursuit of decolonisation and the creation of institutions, cultures and settings that can promote human and non-human well-being. Linda Smith's (1999) influential text *Decolonising Methodologies* continues to provide a significant resource reflecting resistance, unlinking and reconstituting ways of knowing, doing and being in Aotearoa/New Zealand. Kuapapa Māori theory and research have been developed to counter the effects of dispossession and dehumanisation that have resulted from Eurocentic research (Nikora, 2007; Smith, 1999). In Australia, Aboriginal and Torres Strait Islander scholars, activists and academics have also articulated decolonising and anti-colonial work, expressed in Aboriginal ways of knowing, doing and being. For example, Rigney (1999) wrote about principles of indigenist research that privilege indigenous voices, has political integrity and is aimed at resistance as central to emancipation. Martin and Mirraboopa (2003) have also outlined principles that are anchored in Aboriginal peoples' worldviews, knowledge and realities, and emphasise the need to privilege Aboriginal peoples' realities, honour social mores and practices on country and lands, and understand context in shaping experiences.

Within psychology, Glover et al. (2010; see also Dudgeon & Walker, 2015) have provided some direction for psychologists and psychology, which they argue has its roots in the global colonial framework and played a pivotal role in legitimising Eurocentrism. For these authors, key roles, functions and practices of psychology, and allied disciplines, should enact epistemic disobedience that includes deconstructing dominance and white supremacy, and elevating and affirming indigenous people and cultures. For Dudgeon and Walker (2015), a decolonised psychology would mean adopting a determinants approach, recognising and supporting indigenous spirituality, promoting cultural resilience, developing cultural awareness and respect, aspiring to cultural competence and defining/decolonising ourselves. Elsewhere, Thompson Guerin and Mohatt's (2019) special issue highlighted the various ways both indigenous and non-indigenous researchers, educators and practitioners "navigate discipline-dominated structures to incorporate Indigeneity in various forms" (p. 7), and how Community Psychology values are integrated with indigenous ways of knowing.

Finding our way: community arts and cultural practice for liberation

These various lines of decolonial work are concerned with the critique of coloniality and building knowledge with and from the standpoints of those who have been excluded. There are diverse approaches to decolonising praxis. From a liberation frame, research can be mobilised to "nurture community understanding" and "preserve community and cultural practice" (Watkins & Shulman, 2008, p. 276). For Watkins and Shulman (2008), decolonising praxis involves: "claiming resources, testimonies, storytelling, and remembering to claim and speak about extremely painful events and histories; and research that celebrates survival and resilience and that revitalises language arts, and cultural practices"(p. 276). As an intentional practice that involves partnerships between communities and artists, community arts and cultural practice is a key methodology through which social and cultural transformation can be achieved. As noted by the Australia Council for the Arts (2017), in community arts and cultural development (CACD) work, it is "the creative processes and relationships developed with the community to make the art that defines it, not the art form or genre" (para. 4). Goldbard (2006) suggested that it is a creative and collaborative approach to inspire individuals and communities to explore and express their own unique culture. CACD practice has been an effective vehicle for more responsive and sensitive ways to deconstruct dominant narratives, recover historical memory and create counter-stories. This approach shares with Community Psychology principles of participation, inclusion, and it embraces creative methods that are key to dialogue and processes of deconstruction and reconstruction. Different arts modalities are used to create settings and encounter spaces where differently positioned people can come together intentionally to participate in individual and collective change-focused action (Torre et al., 2017).

Watkins and Shulman (2008) place community arts and cultural practice within a liberation framework and suggest that the goal of liberation arts projects "is to resurrect resources to transform structures of language and society, and to de-ideologise understandings. They make space for remobilizing and resignifying the world, enlarging possibilities for restructuring economic, social and personal realities" (p. 234). Arts and cultural practice are also central to the recovery of historical memory, cultural reclamation and counter-storytelling (Watkins & Shulman, 2008), and as activism, it is:

> about creating a new culture rooted in the struggles against patriarchal capitalism from time-immemorial. It is where the interconnection between the rejection of the oppressors' mores meets with the quest to construct a new being and a new way of being.
>
> *(Barson & Rodriguez, 2019)*

In their article on creating inclusive knowledge framed by community and liberation psychology, and public pedagogy, Sonn and Baker (2016) documented the various critical theories, methodologies and practices scholar-activists mobilise across diverse settings and in the service of varied social change agendas. They suggested that creating inclusive knowledges through community pedagogies is necessarily an unsettling and disruptive project that blurs the boundaries between arts/cultural practice and knowledge production, researcher and researched, theory and practice, and centres praxis, that is, the theory and practice cycle (Lykes, 2013).

Furthermore, arts and cultural practice are framed within critical traditions of inquiry that advance a social and relational epistemology and ethics – it is dialogical. Dialogue invites collaboration and poly-vocality, embracing multiple voices and ways of knowing that unsettle the normativity and tunnel vision of dominant ways of knowing and being (Montero & Sonn, 2009). Importantly, the various modalities of arts allow for diverse ways of experiencing and expressing oneself in and imagining the world. In this way, oppressed groups can claim, name and externalise their social realities and produce counter-stories that contest dominant group narratives through which violence is enacted and systems of power and privilege maintained.

Over the years, different members of our group have collaborated to document and examine community arts and cultural practice in the context of migrant settlement and race relations, and to support indigenous self-determination. Through our process and practices, we continue to blur disciplinary boundaries as we transgress and move beyond the strictures of discipline-based conventions to imagine new horizons and practices needed to expand ecologies of knowledge (Santos, 2016). In the next section, we present a vignette informed by the methodology of *testimonio* to provide a snapshot of practice-led inquiry and visual arts that was developed by Paola in response to erasure and the need to honour Aboriginal matriarchs. The methodology of *testimonio* has its roots in the critical scholarship of Latina/o and Chicana/o critical theory, critical race and feminist theory (Delgado Bernal et al., 2012; Flores & Garcia, 2009) and also indigenous and indigenist approaches that highlight the importance of storytelling as a means to reclaim, own and validate experiences on their terms (e.g. Smith, 1999). As noted by Flores and Garcia (2009), "We understand the importance of testimonio and the power of telling others, especially other mujeres, about our experiences – thus recognizing that all experiences and voices and truths matter, none are more valuable than the other" (p. 157). Elevating voices and witnessing stories is central to the liberation project and opens to Community Psychology new pathways and approaches to enact emancipatory agendas.

Practice-led inquiry as *testimonio*: "Disrupting Artistic Terra Nullius"

The notion of an artistic terra nullius refers to the violent erasure of Aboriginal peoples and to First Nations women and builds from the historic notion of Aboriginal Peoples as "absent". I set out to document and respond to the work of Aboriginal women in art and community. In my practice I used practice-led inquiry informed by my intersecting roles and social locations of artist, writer, curator, community researcher and as a Wemba-Wemba and Gunditjmara, matriarchal and sovereign woman. I practice community ways of "being, knowing and doing" to witness, participate in and respond to Aboriginal women's art making and activism in a series of essays and a new body of visual work which culminated in the exhibition "Disrupting Artistic Terra Nullius" at Footscray Community Arts Centre .

The exhibition has two distinct yet interrelated spaces and approaches. The installation of "healing cloths" was an ontological space of respite (see Figure 14.1), contemplation and listening, and has grown out of the epistemological space of photography, documentation and active research with family, the archive and the field of Aboriginal women's work and contributions. The ontological space attempts to replicate the sense of home from our Wemba-Wemba homelands, and Moonahcullah Mission where my Old People come from and where I spent significant time camping as a child. An excerpt of a Super-8 silent colour film featuring my great-grandmother Nanny Nancy Egan flickers behind the installation created from healing cloths. It emulates a "mission house", a tent, the homelands, a place of healing and respite. Through research with my mother and daughter at the Australian Institute for Aboriginal and Torres Strait Islander Studies (AIATSIS) we retrieved this footage, and family photographs,

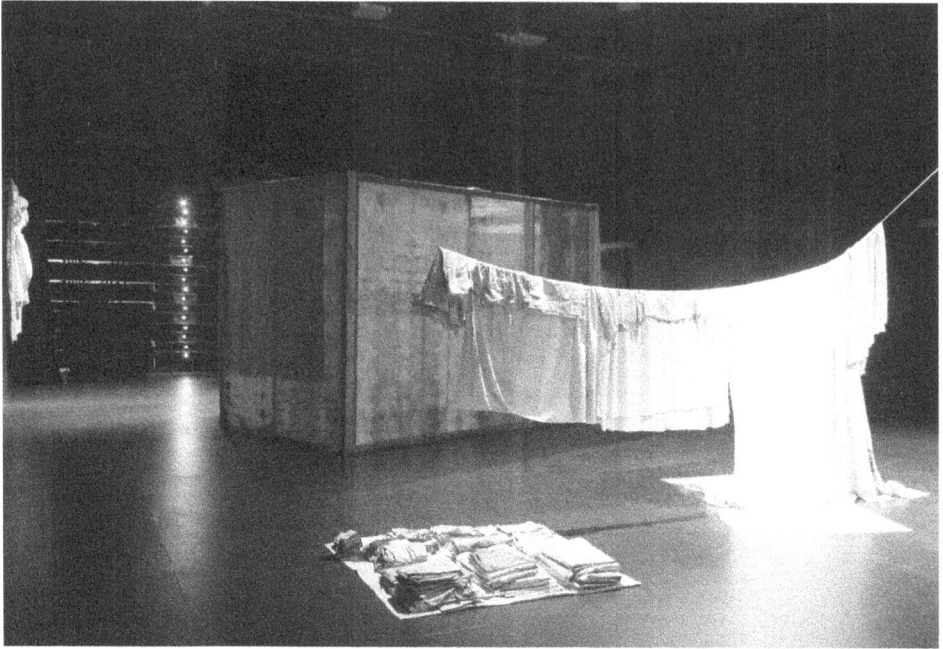

Figure 14.1 Healing space and cloths

stories and a highly significant collection of audio recordings of my great-grandmother and her brother, Uncle Stanley Day, which formed the Wemba-Wemba dictionary, authored by Dr Louise Hercus between 1961 and 1965.

The ontological space is a soft landscape of hundreds of hand-dyed cloths created with bush plants, flowers, fruits, barks and saps, all collected on Kulin Country and Yorta Yorta Country, and of family bush medicine, specifically *Old Man Weed* that my Aunties collected and prepared on our Wemba-Wemba homelands. My mother delivered this to me where I live on Kulin Country in Melbourne for my own healing and well-being to support my work on this project. I pay homage to all the Aunties who bush dye, make work for and with community in community settings, and work closely with Country to draw healing and well-being from plant knowledge. I pay respects to my mother and grandmother, who were artists and poets, fighters and storytellers and who showed me how to dye clothes and shoes to make do, "doll up", and how to make the best out of what you already have.

Creating multiple strands of art and cultural practice emerges from thousands of years of connected practice as sovereign people, and speaks back to an ongoing coloniality and responses aimed at healing and daily acts of resistance and repair. I have created new visual photographic works that honour matriarchal knowledge and ways of being and respond to the broad body of Aboriginal women's work. In development, Professor Tracey Bunda and I broadly named this creative project and process "ghost weaving", an attempt to weave key approaches and practices into a project that contains and holds the elements that are at the centre of how and why Aboriginal women resist and persist through art and story. Visually articulating the healing process; history, land, place, the body and politics of Aboriginal women's lived experiences of subjugation and violence, survivance, nurturance and healing that is ongoing and has been documented in various arts outputs.

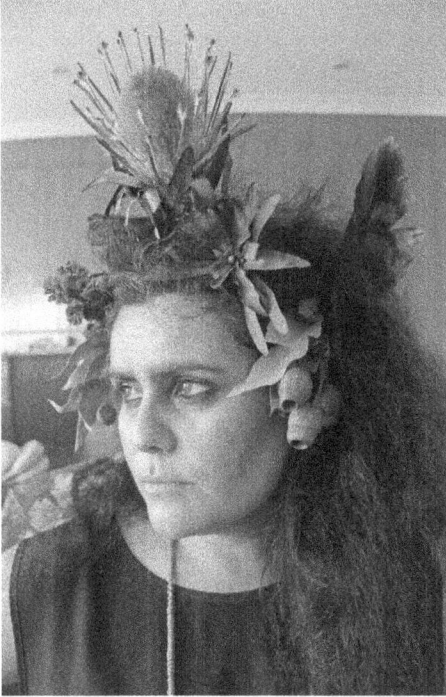

Figure 14.2 I woke up like

In 2016, I created a new body of photographic works, the *Mok Mok* series (see Figure 14.2) that celebrates the *Mok Mok* old woman/hag character written about by esteemed Elder Aunty Margaret Tucker in her 1977 biography, *If Everyone Cared*. Aunty Marge recounted a story about *Mok Mok*, one I had heard as a little girl from my matriarchs about a fearsome and fearless wild woman who lived in the bush with her huge hair, ugly features and red eyes. This story serves as an origin theory of why Aboriginal women in Victoria carried their babies on their backs, safely tucked into their possum skin cloaks, away from the danger of *Mok Mok* taking them. I loved *Mok Mok* and her wildness and wanted to bring a version of her into suburbia to speak back to the footy Mums, cult of motherhood and "domestic goddess", nonsense of gentrification and white, heteronormative cisgendered parenthood of the inner city. I posed as a *Mok Mok* in Footscray, mocking the process of "doing it all", and speaking back to my own anxieties about raising Black kids in the city away from the bush I grew up in, away from mobs of cousins and extended family. In urban spaces, without your family of origin, you have to work hard to maintain culture, story and connections to keep your children knowledgeable and strong away from your homelands. *Mok Mok* was also a way to resist racist and narrow white definitions of beauty and white feminism. *Mok Mok* was also for me a way to perform a liberated character that is fearless, healed and unapologetic.

I also created a series of works called *and the matriarchs sang*. This work was commissioned for an exhibition titled *Re-Centre Sisters* at City Gallery, 2016, a group show of Aboriginal and Torres Strait Islander women artists from around so-called Australia. The purpose of the work was to tell elements of stories told to me by my mother and grandmother, stories of my matriarchs from my mother, grandmother, great-grandmother and great-great-grandmother.

Their work struggles and resistance has inspired this series. I wanted to document this in a way that hinted at what is also not known, what is not told and what is kept secret. Aboriginal women in my family have suffered various forms of violence of the colony and state, patriarchal violence from their own men, white men and the colony itself. I wanted to speak to these stories without exploiting them and to honour their lives and to educate our family future generations. The work comprises 13 small white panels that I rubbed by hand with house paint mixed with ground bark from branches collected on Wurundjeri and Boon Wurrung Country on campus at Victoria University. Copies of photographic images sit with handwritten text in charcoal, a nod to the times my grandmother would take coal from the campfire and insist that I draw something. My grandmother was a self-taught visual artist and poet. The panels are accompanied by a poem of the same title, "and the matriarchs sang".

The creation of the healing cloths and installation became an urgent need at the end of the writing and photographic research and outcomes; I had an emotional and physical longing to learn and develop a new practice that would challenge me and push the research into a new realm. As soon as I moved into eco-dyeing of calico, clothing, bedding and rags, I realised a new release for the research that was immediate, ghostly, unpredictable and healing as I felt exhausted by the research and the academic processes it required from the university. The healing cloths reflected the healing of my own trauma within the historical setting of ongoing traumas and repressions. To provide a space that is at once dialectical; challenging to the settler and comforting to Aboriginal People, and perhaps other peoples who have experienced trauma and displacement. The space is also dialectical in the sense that it shows how two things can be true at once, in this case that healing can only be temporal whilst transgenerational historical traumas and injuries continue into the foreseeable future.

Narrating stories on country

Christopher started to collaborate with the Community Arts Network (CAN) Western Australia in the 1990s, initially at the invitation of the director. In earlier work alongside CAN, Green and Sonn (2008) highlighted the importance of dialogical approaches that are critical and responsive to indigenous ways of knowing, being and doing; examining standpoints and histories of colonialism, and the:

> need to move beyond a static and fixed understanding of self and other to engage conceptualisations of culture that is concerned with lived experiences and that focuses on the processes through which representations, cultural identities and lifeworlds are produced and reproduced.
>
> *(Green & Sonn, 2008, p. 62)*

Such priorities have been echoed by several authors advocating for Critical Community Psychology praxis (e.g. Kagan et al., 2019). Here we report on a CACD project undertaken by CAN that we examined using a decolonial lens and liberation paradigm. Through our engagement with research and evaluation alongside CAN, we have continued to push towards reflexive praxis that is attentive to and transformative of coloniality, which continues to shape subjectivities and interpersonal relationships.

The most recent project focussed on amplifying Aboriginal counter-stories in the context of CAN's "Rekindling Stories on Country" strategy and the Bush Babies project specifically. Smith (1999) has emphasised the importance of stories and storytelling, as part of the decolonial project:

To hold alternative histories is to hold alternative knowledges. The pedagogical implication of this access to alternative knowledges is that they can form the basis of alternative ways of doing things [...] Telling our stories from the past, reclaiming the past,
giving testimony to the injustices of the past are all strategies, which are commonly
employed by Indigenous peoples struggling for justice.

(p. 34)

In response to the expressed wishes of Noongar people, CAN partnered with Noongar
Communities on several projects including the Bush Babies project that would create opportunities for Noongar community Elders, all of whom grew up on missions or reserves on the
outskirts of towns, to share their "Bush Baby" stories and record their legacy. This project had
its beginnings in 2010 in Kellerberrin but was later delivered across several Wheatbelt towns.
In each of the towns, with the community, staff co-created a programme of activities with
the central thread being to create spaces for coming together, celebrate Noongar Elders and
produce an archive of stories for current and future generations. As part of the broader Bush
Babies project, the arts practices chosen by Noongar people included photography, print-
making, photography and hip-hop, textile craft, collage and Noongar language workshops,
oral history recordings, short film and portrait painting (Community Arts Network [CAN],
2014, 2017). As researchers, we had the role of documenting and theorising the overall programme in one of the Wheatbelt towns. In this town, the main component that emerged was
a portraiture project and exhibitions which involved both Aboriginal and non-Aboriginal
local artists (including students from an adult education institute) painting the portraits of
local Noongar Elders. It also included oral history collection and intergenerational storytelling workshops. An important part of CAN's broader "Rekindling Stories on Country"
strategy was to ensure that there were opportunities for these stories to be showcased in
public settings. The portraits, along with snippets of the Elders' stories and a soundscape of
digital storytelling created as part of intergenerational workshops with Noongar high school
students, and other cultural artefacts (such as woven baskets), were exhibited locally as well
as at the State Library in Perth, and later as part of the "Arts on the Move" travelling exhibition across the state.

Taking on what Chase (2005) described as the supportive voice, which "pushes the narrator's
voice into the limelight" (p. 665), elsewhere we reported on the narratives that were conveyed
by the Elders through the project and in conversational interviews (Quayle & Sonn, 2019).
While we were hesitant about how to represent the stories of the Elders as non-Aboriginal
outsiders to the community, we also realised the significance of creating space through the
research for the stories to be a central site for exposing the dynamics of privilege and disadvantage in the present (Fine & Ruglis, 2009). Hence, we brought community arts practice into
conversation with critical narrative inquiry to elevate the Elders' stories of oppression, psychosocial suffering and resistance through a process of mutuality implicated witnessing (Quayle &
Sonn, 2019). The storytelling through arts and research both serve to witness and contribute to
individual and collective memory. Sonn et al. (2013; Stevens et al., 2013) referred to this process
as psychosocial mnemonics, which entails the recollection of memories of lived experiences
and what these mean in the present. These memories provide insight into the continuity of the
past in the present, and the various constraints on subjectivities and identities, and the different
strategies of resistance and survivance (Vizenor, 2008). Quayle (2017; see Quayle et al., 2016b)
reported memories of dispossession that were shared as part of the project. The excerpt below
was shared by an Elder during an intergenerational storytelling workshop with local Aboriginal
high school students:

"they made to be as a different type of, as a different person to everyone else in society because of the colour of our skin and 'cause how, who we are, Aboriginal people. [...] We were taken away from our parents and put in the missions [...] reserves outside of towns, near dumps, near the bush where they segregate Aboriginal people away, out of sight because of their status in life, being a lower-class people. But it's not right really".

(Caroline)

Caroline wanted to emphasise that they are not less than, that they are not "a lower-class people". Another excerpt relayed the deleterious effects, the psychic harm, of dehumanisation: "It wouldn't even enter their brains like its locked in our brains you know, it got burnt in our brain, you might say, we got branded on our brains, how we was treated like animals you might say". Yet, while these forms of oppression structured everyday life, the Elders also spoke of the ways in which they survived and their ongoing connections with culture and country:

"to me going back to those places today, and taking my family back you know it makes you feel good because it's your country, you feel like you haven't lost it. It's still Noongar country and there's a lot of stories relating to all those countries".

(Janet)

The elevation of these stories is vital to displacing narratives of damage and to relaying the ways in which people have continued to struggle for land rights, recognition and survival. The stories reveal the mechanisms of oppression, while also showing Aboriginal conceptions of selfhood rooted in relationality and land, which entails respect for all living things on Country.

Elevating stories to the public sphere: "The exhibition provided an opportunity to connect heart to heart"

The elevation of the many stories of Aboriginal people, stories of dispossession, but also stories of resistance, survival and resilience, is important not only for Aboriginal people but for all Australians. In order to get a better understanding of people's encounters with the public exhibition of Elders' stories, we collected audience surveys and speech notes, examined visitor book entries from the local exhibition and conducted interviews with Elders, artists and facilitators involved in the project. We were interested in how different audiences witnessed the stories of the Elders. We have previously reported on Aboriginal participants' reflections on their participation and the meanings of the project, and argued that community arts as public pedagogy provides opportunities for disruptions into public memory (Quayle et al., 2016a). Specifically, we highlighted the significance of the project for Aboriginal people in terms of the opportunities for cultural continuity and for recognition and acknowledgement of Aboriginal people, culture and the history of dispossession.

It was also clear from our critical narrative analysis that arts practice as process and product and the new settings created engendered opportunities for witnessing that are transformative for audiences and that translate into action beyond the created setting (Sajnani, 2010). Here we draw on data collected from non-Aboriginal people involved in the project as well as survey respondents. The comments convey how through reconfigured relationships, with the Elders stories centred, the arts process created opportunities for dialogue, conscientisation and intersubjectivity within the longer racialised history that continues in the present.

In the excerpts below, both non-Aboriginal narrators commented on the significance of the intentional coming together in terms of it "opening up relationships" and this happening between "community that normally would never get together". Geoff (non-indigenous artist) noted, "this was a fantastic opportunity to actually paint people, who for one reason or another are not accessible in a lot of ways […] so it's opened up gates, it's opened up relationships". For him, this project provided a "non-threatening way of being in relation". Similarly, for Kathy,

> *really complex breakthroughs and profound breakthroughs have happened, and I can't speak for the other artists completely but I, I know seeing the care and the effort and the re-doing and re-doing to get it right, and haven't quite got the essence of them yet kind of you know and […] how people were moved by those stories […] there was a thread then that could connect between those two parts of the community that normally would never get together.*

Kathy's comments refer to the care and effort required to know another and represent "*the essence of them*", a comment that echoes the reality of building relations between separated communities. Kathy continued to name the barriers to coming together, that keep people apart, and what it meant to her and others to listen to the stories overshadowed, drowned out, by dominant cultural stories:

> *[…] I'm sure that the Noongar people in our community are subjected to our stories all the time, they're in the media, they are on the television, they're on the radio, they're in our history books but we don't get to hear them and that's, that was a very great privilege for me and I know that everybody, that, when I was on duty at the gallery, everyone that came in, stood and listened to those stories.*
>
> *(Kathy)*

Other survey respondents also emphasised the connections that were created between people who they "might not otherwise come to know".

> *The exhibition provided an opportunity to connect heart to heart with people who we might not otherwise come to know […] I think this was so important for building relationships; it was wonderful to feel the warmth in response from Aboriginal people who brought their families to join with those involved in the project and others who supported it.*
>
> *(67, female, non-indigenous)*

This respondent continued, stating:

> *We can't undo past wrongs, but we can make sure we don't repeat them by being in relationship – walking together. Education should not equate to assimilation to dominant culture. There is so much to learn from Aboriginal people and in my experience, they are only too willing to teach anyone who wants to listen. Art is a great meeting place.*

As highlighted in the above excerpt, across participants' responses there was an emphasis on the unique power of the arts to "connect heart to heart". The capacity for portraiture to build connections between artist and subject, is further reflected in the excerpt below, taken from the speech notes of the lead artist, who was deeply moved by his involvement in the project.

> we have been moved as we made some sort of connection with the Elders as the painting progressed. It is a kind of spiritual process, I can't think of any other way of describing it. Portraits are a way of directly connecting to the soul, bypassing all

the intellectual baggage of prejudice, attitude and fear. It is our hope that people viewing these portraits absorb this connection and respect. We have all been on a journey and seen how reconciliation can grow from this process of honouring and respecting the people who have gone before us, and for those living with us now. I hope that this exhibition provides the impetus for a ground swell of similar collaborations all over the country. It is one way for us to start communicating through our skins, a kind of osmosis, instead of relying on our preconceived and outdated ideas and attitude.

(Community Arts Network Western Australia, 2014, p. 3)

The aim of this project was to honour Noongar Elders, affectionately referred to as "Bush Babies" in the project. That the Elders felt honoured through this process was evident in the way some of the Elders spoke about the person who painted their portrait and/or the process. For example, Caroline said: "*could never get over what she done, she made my spirit my soul better since she drawed that. It can never come from a photo, another spirit doing it for you*".

Summary and conclusion

Our ongoing efforts to develop Critical Community Psychology praxis are situated within the context of social relations within Australia, and benefit from local and global critical scholarship. We have connected our effort at mobilising the theoretical and conceptual tools of Critical Community Psychology praxis with the broader movement of decoloniality with its roots in the Global South. Our own focus is on disrupting racism and white supremacy through our various projects of work in collaboration with not-for-profit and community groups. The chapter provided two examples of various methods through which community groups can document, assert their experiences and effect change. The methods used in these examples include narrative collection, intergenerational storytelling, portraiture, photography and oral histories as well as community exhibitions. The methods are examples of how to widen the scope of who can contribute to knowledge production. Importantly, in addition to expanding the scope of methods, the methods move beyond cognitive knowing to invite aesthetic knowing as a means to open to the voices of different groups, to value their lived experiences, and ways in which we perceive, experience, know and act in the world.

Reflexive cultural and arts practice can be central to creating settings for interculturality, where differently positioned people come together, contest discourse that limit subjectivities and create new insights about self and other. Community arts and cultural practice mobilised within and reconnected to critical and liberatory paradigms is an important avenue of counter-storytelling, remembering and cultural reclamation. The practice also provides an avenue to unsettle dominant narratives through which Eurocentrism, white supremacy and other structures of power are maintained. In these contested spaces fissures are created for transformative witnessing, for deconstruction and reimaging identities, subjectivities and relationships from below. Both projects provide powerful examples of arts-based interventions as a form of unsettling aesthetics. Through situated cultural and arts practice, indigenous artists/activists are documenting the legacy of coloniality, structural violence, resistance and survival. By crossing borders in the flesh into communities and symbolically through and across areas of inquiry, we have engaged in a form of bricolage, a process of harvesting conceptual resources for critical reflexive praxis that disrupts structural and epistemic violence as central to decolonial critical community praxis.

References

Adams, G., Dobles, I., Gómez, L.H., Kurtiş, T., & Molina, L.E. (2015). Decolonizing psychological science: Introduction to the Special Thematic Section. *Journal of Social and Political Psychology*, *3*(1), 213–38. https://doi.org/10.5964/jspp.v3i1.564

Australia Council for the Arts. (2017). *Community arts and cultural development*. www.australiacouncil.gov.au/artforms/community-arts-and-cultural-development/

Barson, B., & Rodriguez, G. (2019, September). *Artivism and decolonization: A brief theory, history and practice of cultural production as political activism*. New Music USA. https://nmbx.newmusicusa.org/artivism-and-decolonization-a-brief-theory-history-and-practice-of-cultural-production-as-political-activism/

Chase, S. (2005). Narrative inquiry: Multiple lenses, approaches, voices. In N.K. Denzin & Y.S. Lincoln (Eds.), *The SAGE handbook of qualitative research methods* (3rd ed.) (pp. 651–80). SAGE.

Community Arts Network Western Australia. (2014). *The Bush Babies Elders portrait exhibition: Honouring our Elders born in the bush*. https://www.can.org.au/community/bush-babies/narrogin

Community Arts Network Western Australia. (2017). *Bush Babies: Narrogin*. www.canwa.com.au/project/bush-babies/

Delgado Bernal, D., Burciaga, R., & Flores Carmona, J. (2012). Chicana/Latina testimonios: Mapping the methodological, pedagogical, and political. *Equity & Excellence In Education*, *45*(3), 363–72. https://doi.org/10.1080/10665684.2012.698149

Dudgeon, P., & Walker, R. (2015). Decolonising Australian psychology: Discourses, strategies, and practice. *Journal of Social and Political Psychology*, *3*(1), 276–97. https://doi.org/10.5964/jspp.v3i1.126

Fine, M. (2018). *Just research in contentious times: Widening the methodological imagination*. Teachers College Press.

Fine, M., & Ruglis, J. (2009). Circuits and consequences of dispossession: The racialized realignment of the public sphere for U.S. youth. *Transforming Anthropology*, *17*(1), 20–33. https://doi.org/10.1111/j.1548-7466.2009.01037.x

Flores, J., & Garcia, S. (2009) Latina testimonios: A reflexive, critical analysis of a "Latina space" at a predominantly White campus. *Race Ethnicity and Education*, *12*(2), 155–72. https://doi.org/10.1080/13613320902995434

Freire, P. (1972). *Pedagogy of the oppressed*. Penguin Books.

Glover, M., Dudgeon, P., & Huygens, I. (2010). Colonization and racism. In G. Nelson & I. Prilleltensky (Eds.), *Community psychology: In pursuit of liberation and well-being* (2nd ed.) (pp. 353–70). Palgrave Macmillan.

Goldbard, A. (2006). *New creative community: The art of cultural development*. New Village Press.

Green, M.J., & Sonn, C.C. (2008). Drawing out community empowerment through arts and cultural practice. Community Arts Network Western Australia.

Grosfoguel, R. (2016). What is racism? *Journal of World-Systems Research*, *22*(1), 9–15. https://doi.org/10.5195/jwsr.2016.609

Kagan, C., Burton, M., Duckett, P., Lawthom, R., & Siddique, A. (2019). *Critical community psychology* (2nd ed). Taylor and Francis.

Lykes, M.B. (2013). Participatory and action research as a transformative praxis: Responding to humanitarian crises from the margins. *American Psychologist*, *68*(8), 772–83. https://doi.org/10.1037/a0034360

Maldonado Torres, N. (2016). Outline of ten theses on coloniality and decoloniality. Foundation Frantz Fanon: http://frantzfanonfoundation-fondationfrantzfanon.com/article2360.html

Martin, K., & Mirraboopa, B. (2003). Ways of knowing, being and doing: A theoretical framework and methods for indigenous and indigenist re-search. *Journal of Australian Studies*, *27*(76), 203–14. https://doi.org/10.1080/14443050309387838

Martín-Baró, I. (1994). Towards a liberation psychology. In A. Aron & S. Corne (Eds.), *Writings for a liberation psychology: Ignacio Martín-Baró* (pp. 17–32). Harvard University Press.

Montero, M., & Sonn, C. (2009). About liberation and psychology: An introduction. In M. Montero & C.C. Sonn (Eds.), *Psychology of liberation: Theory and applications* (pp. 1–10). Springer.

Montero, M., Sonn, C. C., & Burton, M. (2017). Community psychology and liberation psychology: A creative synergy for an ethical and transformative praxis. In M.A. Bond, I. Serrano-García, & C.B. Keys (Eds.), *APA Handbook of Community Psychology*. (Vol. 1: *Theoretical foundations, core concepts, and emerging challenges*) (pp. 149–67). American Psychological Association.

Moreton-Robinson, A. (2015). *The White possessive: Property, power, and indigenous sovereignty*. University of Minnesota Press.

Ndluvo-Gathseni, S.J. (2020, April 22). *Planetary human entanglement and the crises of living* together (Video File). YouTube. https://youtube/LgHxsXIMNRM

Nikora, L. W. (2007). Maori and psychology: Indigenous psychology in New Zealand. In A. Weatherall, M. Wilson, D. Harper, & J. McDowell (Eds.), *Psychology in Aotearoa/New Zealand* (pp. 80–5). Pearson Education.

Osorio, J.M. (2009). Praxis and liberation in the context of Latin American theory. In M. Montero & C.C. Sonn (Eds.), *Psychology of liberation: Theory and applications* (pp. 11–36). Springer.

Quayle, A. (2017). *Narrating oppression, psychosocial suffering and survival through the Bush Babies project.* [PhD thesis]. Victoria University.

Quayle, A., Sonn, C., & Kasat, P. (2016a). Community arts as public pedagogy: Disruptions into public memory through Aboriginal counter-storytelling. *International Journal of Inclusive Education*, *20*(3), 261–77. https://doi.org.10.1080/13603116.2015.1047662

Quayle, A., Sonn, C.C., & van den Eynde, J. (2016b). Narrating the accumulation of dispossession: Stories of Aboriginal Elders. *Community Psychology in Global Perspective*, *2*(2), 79–96.

Quayle, A.F., & Sonn, C.C. (2019). Amplifying the voices of indigenous elders through community arts and narrative inquiry: Stories of oppression, psychosocial suffering, and survival. *American Journal of Community Psychology*, *64*(1–2), 46–58. https://doi.org/10.1002/ajcp.12367

Quijano, A. (2000). Coloniality of power and Eurocentrism in Latin America. *International Sociology*, *15*(2), 215–32. https://doi.org/10.1177/0268580900015002005

Rigney, L. (1999). Internationalization of an indigenous anticolonial cultural critique of research methodologies: A guide to indigenist research methodology and its principles. *Wicazo Sa Review*, *14*(2), 109–21. https://doi.org.10.2307/1409555

Sajnani, N. (2010). Mind the gap: Facilitating transformative witnessing amongst audiences. In P. Jones (Ed.), *Drama as therapy* (Vol. 2). Routledge.

Santos, B. de Sousa. (1026). *Epistemologies of the South: Justice against epistemicide.* Routledge.http://unes cochair-cbrsr.org/pdf/resource/Epistemologies_of_the_South.pdf.

Smith, L.T. (1999). *Decolonizing methodologies: Research and indigenous peoples.* Zed Books.

Sonn, C., & Baker, A. (2016). Creating inclusive knowledges: Exploring the transformative potential of arts and cultural practice. *International Journal of Inclusive Education*, *20*(3), 215–28. https://doi.org/10.1080/13603116.2015.1047663

Sonn, C.C. (2018). Mobilising decolonial approaches for community-engaged research for racial justice. *The Australian Community Psychologist*, *29*(1), 8–21. www.psychology.org.au/for-members/publications/journals/Australian-Community-Psychologist/ACP-Issues/Volume-30,-No-1,-January-2020

Sonn, C.C., Stevens, G., & Duncan, N. (2013). Decolonisation, critical methodologies and why stories matter. In G. Stevens, N. Duncan, & D. Hook (Eds.), *Race, memory and the Apartheid Archive: Towards a transformative psychosocial praxis* (pp. 295–314). Palgrave Macmillan.

Stevens, G., Duncan, N., & Sonn, C. (2013). Memory, narrative and voice as liberatory praxis in the apartheid archive. In G. Stevens, N. Duncan, & D. Hook (Eds.), *Race, memory and the Apartheid Archive: Towards a transformative psychosocial praxis* (pp. 25–44). Palgrave Macmillan.

Suffla, S., & Seedat, M. (2021). Africa's knowledge archives, Black consciousness and reimagining community psychology. In G. Stevens & C.C. Sonn (Eds.), *Decoloniality, knowledge production and epistemic justice in contemporary community psychology* (pp. 21–35). Springer.

Thompson-Guerin, P., & Mohatt, N.V. (2019). Community Psychology and Indigenous Peoples. *American Journal of Community Psychology*, *64*(1–2), 3–8. https://doi.org/10.1002/ajcp.12383

Torre, M.E., Stoudt, B., Manoff, E., & Fine, M. (2017). Critical participatory action research on state violence: Bearing wit(h)ness across fault lines of power, privilege and dispossession. In N. Denzin & Y. Lincoln (Eds.), *The SAGE handbook of qualitative research* (pp. 492–515). SAGE.

Vizenor, G.R. (Ed.). (2008). *Survivance: Narratives of native presence.* University of Nebraska Press.

Watkins, M., & Shulman, H. (2008). *Toward psychologies of liberation.* Palgrave Macmillan.

PART III

Community Psychology through an ecological lens

15

CLIMATE JUSTICE

In pursuit of a practical utopia: transitioning towards climate justice

Carlie D. Trott, Kai Reimer-Watts and Manuel Riemer

Abstract

The evolving climate crisis is demonstrating with unequivocal clarity that the dream of unlimited economic growth driven by ever-increasing material consumption is, in fact, ensuring a living nightmare for the human species. In this chapter, we will argue that as citizens of this planet, we need to collectively and quickly pursue a new pragmatic ideal: climate justice (CJ). We will draw on social and environmental justice frameworks and indigenous perspectives to describe key aspects of CJ. Next, we will provide a critical analysis of some key issues, barriers and potential leverage points to be considered in the pursuit of CJ. For this, we will place strong emphasis on the analysis of neoliberalism and the need for transformative social change. The final section of the chapter will feature concrete approaches for working towards CJ, including those that community psychologists have been or could be involved in. In this section, strong emphasis will be placed on the role of visioning, the arts and prefigurative practice in societal transformation, and how we can facilitate these processes as community psychologists. Finally, we will argue that CJ is the logical response to the climate crisis for Community Psychology.

' Resumen

La evolutiva crisis climática demuestra con claridad inequívoca que el sueño de un crecimiento económico ilimitado impulsado por el aumento des mesurado en el consumo de materiales es, de hecho, garantizar una pesadilla viviente para la raza humana. En este capítulo, argumentaremos, como ciudadanos de este planeta, que necesitamos de manera colectiva y rápida seguir un nuevo ideal pragmático: justicia climática (JC). Haremos uso de marcos de referencia sociales y de justicia ambiental, así como de perspectivas Indígenas para describir aspectos clave de la JC. Posteriormente proveeremos un análisis crítico sobre puntos clave, barreras, así como puntos influyentes a ser considerados en la búsqueda de la JC. Para esto pondremos un fuerte énfasis en el análisis del neoliberalismo y en la necesidad de un cambio social transformador. La sección final del capítulo presentará enfoques concretos para trabajar hacia la JC, incluyendo aquellos en que los psicólogos comunitarios han estado o podrían estar involucrados. En esta sección se le dará un importante énfasis al rol de visionar, las artes, y la prefiguración práctica en la

DOI: 10.4324/9780429325663-19

transformación social, y cómo podemos facilitar esos procesos como psicólogos comunitarios. Finalmente, argumentaremos que, para la psicología comunitaria, la JC es la respuesta lógica a la crisis climática.

Introduction

In Albuquerque, New Mexico, in 1998, participants in the "Circles of Wisdom" Native Peoples-Native Homelands Climate Change Workshop came together to express their "profound concern for the well-being of our sacred Mother Earth and Father Sky and the potential consequences of climate imbalance for our Indigenous Peoples" (Maynard, 1998, p. 71) as well as its consequences at environmental, economic and community levels.

> Indigenous prophecy meets scientific prediction. What we have known and believed, you also now know: The Earth is out of balance. The plants are disappearing, the animals are dying, and the very weather – rain, wind, fire itself – reacts against the actions of the human being. For the future of the children, for the health of our Mother Earth, Father Sky, and the rest of Creation, we call upon the people of the world to hold your leaders accountable.
>
> *(Maynard, 1998, p. 71)*

For the purpose of ensuring harmony between the needs of individuals and communities, the sacred tree teachings of the Anishinaabe, an indigenous people in the Northern part of Turtle Island known to most as Canada and the USA, emphasise the spiritual and visionary aspect of individuals based on four principles.

> First, the capacity to have and to respond to realities that exist in a non-material way such as dreams, visions, ideals, spiritual teachings, goals and theories. Second, the capacity to accept those realities as a reflection (in the form of symbolic representation) of unknown or unrealised potential to do or to be something more or different than we are now. Third, the capacity to express non-material realities using symbols such as speech, art, or mathematics. Fourth, the capacity to use this symbolic expression to guide future action – action directed toward making what was only seen as possibility into a living reality.
>
> *(Bopp et al., 1984, p. 30)*

As climate change is increasingly recognised as a profoundly human problem whose devastating shocks are being felt – with greater frequency and intensity – in the here and now, it is essential that we draw upon such principles to develop compelling visions of a better future and take steps to make those a living reality (Foran et al., 2017). We argue in this chapter that the possibilities ahead are broad and the outcomes are not fixed. Climate activists in unprecedented numbers have succeeded in pressuring political leaders in at least 34 countries and more cities worldwide, representing over 820 million citizens, to formally declare climate emergencies (Climate Emergency Declaration, 2021). There is widespread recognition that without rapid and comprehensive action at every level of society, the consequences of climate change could be irreparable, foreclosing the possibility of widespread human and ecosystem flourishing. As a significant and growing global injustice, the consequences of climate disruption are already falling disproportionately on those who are most marginalised in societies around the globe and who have often done the least to contribute to climate change (Wuebbles et al., 2017). Urgent action is needed to reverse this trend and build a future based on climate justice. Community Psychology, with its strong values for social justice and well-being, and its tools and ability to span the boundaries of disciplines and sectors, as well as theory, research and action, has an important role to play in this movement (Riemer & Harré, 2016; Riemer et al., 2020).

Before us is a fleeting window of opportunity that must be used not for power consolidation among the already privileged few (Klein, 2007), but for people-powered transformative change in order to benefit the many – particularly society's most vulnerable. Through the lens of climate justice, this chapter attempts to envision what a more just, equitable and sustainable world might look like – one that centres the voices and actions of those most affected by the climate crisis. We then attempt to chart a way forward, anticipating barriers and potential leverage points as well as the role of community psychologists on the path towards climate justice.

Climate justice as a pragmatic ideal

One of the most glaring injustices of climate change is that those who have historically contributed the least to the problem often experience its impacts first and worst. In the 25 years between 1990 and 2015, the world's richest 10% (approximately 630 million people) were responsible for over half (52%) of cumulative carbon emissions, whereas the poorest half of the population (approximately 3.1 billion people) – who do not have access to affordable fossil fuels – were responsible for just 7% (Gore, 2020). Despite this inequity, these same three billion people, which include the poorest nations and the poorest and most marginalised groups within nations, suffer the most from climate disruption due to numerous factors, including poorer access to quality healthcare, greater risk exposure and limited adaptive capacity (Wuebbles et al., 2017). In addition, equity-deserving groups also tend to benefit less from local climate actions and, in fact, may experience exacerbated levels of inequality as a result of climate actions (Agyeman, 2013; Rice et al., 2019; Schrock et al., 2015). A climate justice perspective recognises that climate risks and vulnerabilities, as well as the benefits and burdens of climate actions, are anything but equally distributed, and that climate shocks often exacerbate existing inequalities. Further, enacting climate justice means working with communities on the frontlines of extreme climate impacts to reverse these trends. As we have argued elsewhere (Unanue et al., 2020; Riemer & Harré, 2016; Riemer et al., 2020; Riemer & Van Voorhees, 2014; Trott, 2021; Trott, Rockett, Gray, Lam, Even, & Frame, 2020), community psychologists interested in working towards social justice and community well-being are well placed to pay close attention to these complex but critical intersections of social and environmental challenges and recognise them as possibly the most pressing global threats to social justice and well-being.

The global climate justice movement, with ongoing leadership by young people and Black, Indigenous and People of Color (BIPOC) communities, calls to address both the climate crisis and social injustice as intersecting symptoms of deeper systems-wide issues that can only be solved through systemic, justice-based changes (see for example 350.org, n.d.; Indigenous Climate Action, n.d.). By defining the problem not merely as climate change but also as climate injustice – a many-layered global, social and deeply human problem – community psychologists may begin to envision what a path forward might look like, and work towards achieving the 'pragmatic ideal' (Thiele, 2016, p. 9) of climate justice. Where ideals urge us to aim high and aspire to a desirable future outcome, pragmatism anchors us in the practical and strategic considerations of the present moment. Moreover, where idealism deals mostly in dreams, visions and theoretical possibilities, being pragmatic means keeping focused on the actual doing–or practice–of things. For community psychologists working for climate justice, this means being anchored in the field's core principles while working in solidarity with marginalised communities for transformative change. As we move in that direction, Riemer and Van Voorhees (2014, p. 61) argue that critical work is needed "on how to create a shared vision that presents a joined orientation towards a true alternative to current societal models that are not sustainable and just."

Finding the levers for change

In "Dancing with Systems," Donella Meadows (2001) said "the future can't be predicted, but it can be envisioned and brought lovingly into being" (p. 58). To move towards the pragmatic ideal of climate justice, it is crucial to recognise that we are not destined to live within fixed economic, political and social realities, but that instead there are viable alternatives to these human-made systems in which we are embedded. A number of destructive, though not inevitable systems and ideologies frame many people's existence, including those of neoliberalism, capitalism, white supremacy, hetero-patriarchy, imperialism and colonialism. For transformative change to happen, it is necessary for us, as individuals and collectives, to believe that we have agency to act on these human-made and socially enforced systems, and in doing so help to push them toward preferable alternatives. Yet, in order to know in which direction to push and how, we must have (i) some idea of what we are pushing against (i.e. systems as they exist now); and (ii) what we – as social movements for change and society more generally – might hope to move towards (i.e. visions of alternative systems) (Riemer & Van Voorhees, 2014).

Systems thinking is a useful tool for understanding these system-wide forces, how they operate and how they might best be disrupted and shifted to alternative, preferable systems within specific contexts. Systems are dynamic, with systems components connected through reinforcing and balancing feedback loops; hence, addressing a specific 'high impact' leverage point in a system can ripple through the system to create significant changes (Meadows, 1997). Following this insight, we believe that a strategic way forward would be to place the lever for change at one specific core ideology that has accelerated the drive into the interconnected climate and social justice crises being faced– namely neoliberal capitalism, *or more specifically the ideology of* neoliberalism. Neoliberalism is one of the major, contemporary forces that dominates not only the global economic system but also many aspects of day-to-day life for billions of people. Whilst there are many ideological systemic forces that predate neoliberalism, including white supremacy, colonisation, the genocide of indigenous peoples and capitalistic exploitation of people and planetary resources, neoliberalism dominates much of the world. Challenging neoliberal ideology and practice with the pragmatic ideal of climate justice would be one powerful way to begin to holistically address climate change and related societal crises, as we argue in the next section.

Transcending neoliberalism

In his book *Utopia for Realists*, Rutger Bregman (2014) reminded us that "Ideas, however outrageous, have changed the world, and they will again. 'Indeed,' wrote Keynes, 'the world is ruled by little else'" (p. 207). Neoliberalism is both a political ideology and economic policy framework, profoundly shaping people's lives across nearly all levels of society. Advocates of neoliberalism promote an ideology focused on individualism, shrinking government and elevating the private sector and free market. Thus, policies of deregulation, globalisation, open markets, free trade, the removal of license and quota systems, and the withdrawal of the state from many areas of social provision are seen as solutions to the challenges created or faced by capitalism (Liboro, 2015).

Neoliberalism's embrace of the free market and simultaneous gutting of many social and environmental protections in societies worldwide has led directly to the accelerated plundering of Earth's resources and an unhinged exploitation of people, contributing greatly to the climate, ecological and social emergencies we are facing today (Monbiot, 2020). As the dominant global, social and economic paradigm, neoliberal ideology has had profound implications for how we perceive and frame ourselves, society and the world, as well as the specific policies that societies around the globe consider in response to the major challenges of our times. One example of this is the typical municipal-level approach to climate action planning in North American cities. Typically, the municipal-level approach is guided by technological, individualistic and market-driven approaches to climate change adaptation and mitigation, which has resulted in a critical equity deficit that is further marginalising equity-deserving groups through otherwise well-intended policies and investments (Agyeman, 2013; Rice et al., 2019). Community Psychology (CP) has a great deal to offer in shifting these realities. The Climate Justice Partnership, for example, led by the Viessmann Centre for Engagement and Research in Sustainability (VERiS), is working with municipalities and equity-deserving groups to challenge those very mental models and cultural myths shaped by neoliberal and colonial ideologies (VERiS, n.d.). CP approaches to social change, along with systems and leverage theories are used to raise the critical consciousness of municipal leaders about how these ideologies shape their day-to-day approaches to planning and engagement of community stakeholders. CP practitioners then work with leaders and local equity-deserving groups in challenging and shifting these mental models towards systems thinking and climate justice.

The dominance of neoliberalism, which is often taken for granted as if the free market system simply "always was and always will be", must be challenged. As it is, it places a massive restriction on society's social imagination that leaves us ill-prepared to imagine and fight for viable alternatives (Foster, 2015). Climate justice requires a paradigm shift driven by alternative visions of what is possible, themselves underpinned by people's sense of agency for change and thorough understanding of the inequitable causes and consequences of climate change. As Haiven and Khasnabish, (2014, p. 61 [emphasis added]) have said,

> what seems to be lacking today, in social movements and in society at large [...] is *the ability to envision and work towards better futures based on an analysis of the root causes of social problems.*

CP can help achieve these changes through community-led actions.

Alternative paradigms

Imagining the "beyond" can be a powerful and motivating exercise. Strong visions – led by justice-informed social movements – are critical for knowing where we wish to go and considering how best to get there, while remaining iterative and adaptable as situations change. For these movements to capture a majority of public support, they must do more than simply communicate a *NO* to systemic harms; they must also facilitate a bold *YES* to alternative stories and visions that will help guide us forward (Klein, 2017). To envision radically different systems based on alternative core purpose(s) and value(s) is to nurture a collective "radical imagination" (Haiven & Khasnabish, 2014), enabling communities to see beyond what is, to what could be.

The ability to "convoke" (that is, call into being as part of a collaborative praxis) radical imagination within a community via the sharing of stories about potential alternative futures, opens the possibilities that these stories themselves can become sites of imagining and prefiguring not only possible futures but also active resistance (Haiven & Khasnabish, 2014). Radical imagination can also be used to convoke the pragmatic ideal of climate justice and what this might mean within different contexts.

Indigenous worldviews and ontologies embody ecological and spiritual traditions that recognise the deep interdependence human beings have with life on Earth and natural systems. These stand in sharp contrast to the dominant Western, neoliberal worldview of individual autonomy and separateness from nature (Kimmerer, 2013; Latulippe & Klenk, 2020). This insight reminds us that climate justice work including social transformation is not only about changing our system's hardware, but also about *cultural transformations* affecting our ways of knowing, learning, valuing and acting together" (Kagan, 2012, p. 10; emphasis in original). In a time when one's lived reality is increasingly connected to and influenced by larger realities and globalised systems, a deep sense of interconnectedness is an increasingly vital quality to better navigate, influence and respond to these systems (Ehrenfeld & Hoffman, 2013). This sense is at the core of the four Anishinaabe principles shared at the beginning of this chapter, and other indigenous teachings. For example, "Two-Eyed Seeing", or *Etuaptmumk* in Mi'kmaw, encourages all peoples to bring together indigenous and Western perspectives on an equal basis, recognising each of their inherent values when approaching a topic or issue, and hence learning to see that topic through "both eyes" (Iwama et al., 2009). This approach has been shown to enhance the effectiveness of environmental action, social justice work and community health outcomes, among other benefits, and can be applied collaboratively by indigenous communities alongside non-indigenous ally partners (Abu et al., 2020; Cyr & Riediger, 2021). CP practitioners could usefully embrace "Two-Eyed Seeing" when partnering with indigenous communities to help inform collective strategies for climate justice – or indeed any other purpose.

Indigenous teachings that remind us of the interconnectedness of all life, and that humans are deeply connected to and dependent upon larger ecosystems and even larger Earth systems, should give us humility as we seek to change those destructive human-made systems that have undermined natural Earth systems along with other harms, instead striving to build systems grounded in natural limits and climate justice. By connecting individuals to their community, region, nation state or beyond, all the way up to global systems and realities such as climate change, nurturing the collective radical imagination may also serve to increase consciousness of individual connections to larger system-wide structures and forces (Christens et al., 2007), and hence ground our work in the need for systems-level changes. Here, community psychologists can play unique roles including as researchers or evaluators; programme innovators; public intellectuals; policy advisers; allies to progressive social movements; and boundary spanners, among other possibilities (Nelson, 2013).

Envisioning climate justice

So, what does moving towards climate justice look like? Though defined in different ways by different groups, the meaning of climate justice is often best captured by its shared aims and principles, which can be usefully summarised as follows:

1. Working towards this vision should be a collaborative, creative, life-affirming endeavour.
2. Recognition of the fundamental injustices of climate change that require justice- and equity-based responses, including recognising the imbalance that exists between historical responsibilities and present-to-future harms as a way to guide climate change mitigation and adaptation strategies and the "common but differentiated" responsibilities between nations (United Nations Framework Convention on Climate Change [UNFCCC], n.d.).
3. Attending to the specific needs of vulnerable communities in transitioning to a post-carbon economy.
4. Attending to process by balancing the need for collective visioning and democratic participation with respecting the need for self-sufficiency and autonomy in the process of transitioning to a post-carbon, more sustainable economy. This includes prioritising land and food sovereignty for vulnerable communities and especially indigenous peoples; honouring the rights of BIPOC communities, labour, women, and nature; and attending to local impacts and experiences in the process.
5. Attending to power imbalances means doing so at multiple levels – across trans-localised networks as well as within any collaborative group working towards a just transition. This also means working through a decolonial framework to disrupt the ongoing colonial project of Western countries that frequently denies indigenous title and sovereignty, working in solidarity with indigenous communities striving towards greater self-determination. It is worth reflecting that, despite comprising less than 5% of the global population and residing on just 20% of Earth's land surface, indigenous peoples reside on lands that support as much as 80% of global biodiversity including wide swaths of Earth's forests, vital regulators of the Earth's climate (Gurria, 2017; Raygorodetsky, 2018). Hence, indigenous peoples' role as land, water and climate protectors worldwide is critical, and one that non-indigenous people should also be learning from and defending in solidarity in any efforts towards climate justice (for example, Indigenous Climate Action, 2020; Etchart, 2017). Yet perversely, indigenous people remain among those most marginalised worldwide, and are frequently subjected to colonial violence for their vital roles as Earth protectors. Climate justice requires decolonisation in theory and in practice, which can begin by working in meaningful solidarity with and following the lead of affected communities working for liberation from colonial oppression (Adams et al., 2017).
6. In addition to the necessary "top-down" policy changes that reflect the scale and urgency of the need for transformation, "bottom-up" transition planning led by community members is also crucial as the impacts of climate change vary greatly from place to place, as do the strengths and needs of specific communities. At the grassroots level, advocates of climate justice are building trans-local solidarity through global networks of place-based actors who are attending to the specific features of their communities, while remaining connected with each other to share resources, information and support (Featherstone, 2013).
7. Supporting democratic participation and front-line leadership means that communities most impacted by climate change and decisions responding to it should have a leading voice in designing appropriate, locally relevant, just climate solutions.

The art of visioning

"The role of the artist," said writer, documentarian and political activist Toni Cade Bambarayou, "is to make the revolution irresistible" (brown, 2017, p. 36). It is clearly difficult, if not impossible, to fight for deep systemic changes if we cannot first imagine them – and the larger the systems-level change required, the more critical it is to engage society's full collective radical imagination to envision it. The arts can play a vital role in such vision creation, catalysing the imagination of alternative stories and futures worth fighting for, while articulating a layered, evolving meaning of "climate justice" to better inform and sustain ongoing social transformation. When done well, artistic visions and stories can make one stop and think broadly about what is truly possible beyond the current system, disrupting the status quo and opening up possibilities, while serving as powerful living symbols for actions forward. Art and vision creation can offer powerful metaphors, embodying the very idea that alternative futures are both desirable and possible – and can help in catalysing systems change, particularly when designed strategically to intervene in and challenge existing systems (Galafassi et al., 2018; Kagan, 2012).

Radical imagination also encourages a great tradition of activist scholarship that strives to work in solidarity with progressive social movements and serve their interests (Trott, 2016). While the future may be full of uncertainty, dramatic change is clearly inevitable – and CP scholars have an obligation like all others to situate our work on the "right side of history" aligned with the field's core values. Considering CP's value of social justice, it is sobering to realise that in the midst of a climate and ecological crisis, a just future is far from guaranteed. It is clear that if we wish to have any chance at enacting a critical call for climate justice, supporting powerful grassroots social movements to push back against the neoliberal agenda remains critical. One way we can do that is by supporting the development of place-based collective visions of climate justice, as critical visioning remains an important strategy for effective social movements. In the next section, we present three case studies that used art to push back, creating collective visions for climate justice as alternatives to the dominant social paradigm.

Images of possibility

The Climate is Life *mural, Wilfrid Laurier University (2018–2019)*

As discussed above, it is difficult to address a problem if you cannot first "see it" – a challenge frequently recognised as a barrier to action on climate change, which given its diffusion can still feel like an "invisible" crisis to some. Visual symbols such as murals can play a powerful role in framing and "seeing" an issue, to tell its story, remember its importance in our day-to-day lives and move more people from concern to action. Far from being aesthetic "add-ons", intentional visual symbols designed to help increase community engagement can be crucial pathways for changing individual/collective mindsets and cultural myths – as Meadows (1997) argues, the highest leverage point for effectively changing a system.

The *Climate is Life* mural (see Figure 15.1) – designed to connect viewers both to a local/global climate movement and to the life-giving climate system – is one example of such a visualisation, installed on Laurier's Waterloo campus in the Fall of 2019 (see www.wlu.ca/news/news-releases/2019/sept/laurier-marks-global-climate-strike-week-with-events-and-climate-mural.html). It is also a mural clearly integrating a deeper concern for social justice, with visual representation of a diverse intergenerational social movement rising to confront the climate crisis, being led by frontline BIPOC communities with the support of a broader community. In addition, the design process that led to the final mural design integrated a diversity of voices including from front-line communities, directly shaping the final image (discussed more below).

The idea for a permanent on-campus mural installation to honour climate action and justice was proposed by Wilfrid Laurier University CP PhD student, artist and co-author to this chapter Kai Reimer-Watts, and supported in part through Laurier's Sustainability Office. To reach the point of physical mural creation in September was a long and in-depth process involving the collaboration of dozens of people campus-wide; the creation of a diverse "mural

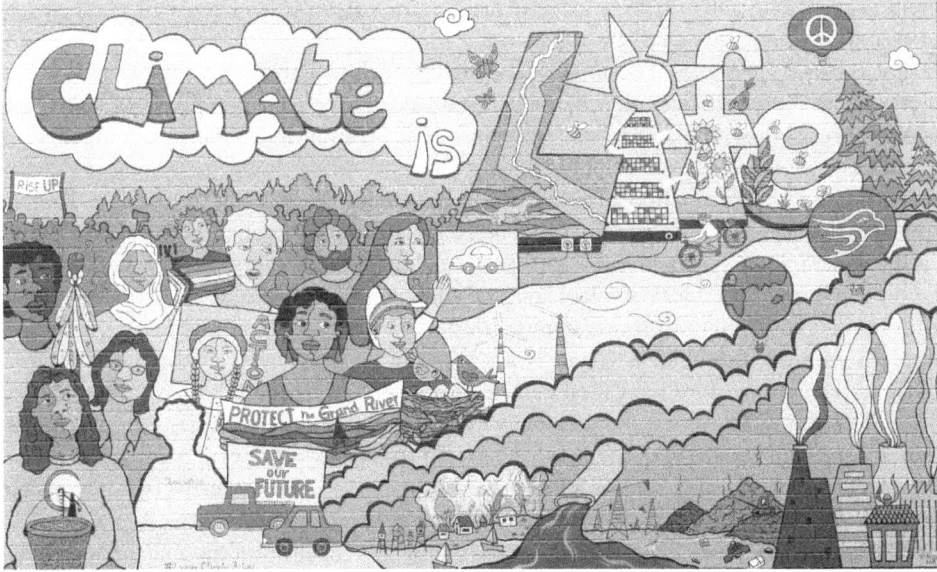

Figure 15.1 The *Climate is Life* mural, Wilfrid Laurier University (2018–2019). Painted by Pamela Rojas with the support of several hundred volunteers

planning committee" that met regularly over many months; consultation with community leaders; permissions from across multiple levels and authorities within the institution; and the recruitment of a skilled community mural artist, Pamela Rojas, to lead the participatory design and final painting process (among others).

The final artistic co-creation of the mural took place strategically over 10 days in Fall 2019 to draw attention to the Global Climate Strike Week happening at the same time, led by the international youth-led climate movement Fridays for Future (350.org, 2019). Over 200 Laurier students, staff, faculty and community members contributed to painting the mural over this 10-day period, under the skilled leadership of Pamela and her team – a significant community-building exercise that also attracted local media attention. Now a 15'×9' permanent installation on an exterior wall at the heart of Laurier's Waterloo campus, the *Climate is Life* mural sends a clear, enduring message for the Laurier community and institution to commit to climate justice, continuing to share this message with many thousands of people. In addition, the mural has helped spark numerous related actions and collaborations for climate justice that are each ongoing as of this writing, demonstrating their current sustainability – including the launch of Climate Justice Laurier, a student-led research and action group; the creation of a faculty-led climate committee; the passing of department resolutions at Laurier for climate action; the providing of a venue for community climate and indigenous justice actions, and more.

Visual symbols like the *Climate is Life* mural can act as powerful openings into further conversations and action on the issues being centred, supporting movement-building processes and giving the broader community the courage to face tough issues together and work towards meaningful solutions. While there was no direct opposition to creating the mural in principle, arriving at its final design and approval did require a many months-long process "pitching" the concept to numerous key university stakeholders involved. Here, the skill sets (see below) of CP practitioners including Kai along with other Laurier CP students and faculty supporting the project went a long way in helping navigate these systems of university bureaucracy and power, to eventually secure the mural's final approval.

Just as climate justice itself is complex and multilayered, to arrive at the final *Climate is Life* mural design took time, intentionally listening to and actively seeking input from a diversity of key voices both within and outside of the university. This included but was not limited to consultation with key university staff including through Laurier's Indigenous Student Centre; the Centre for Student Equity, Diversity and Inclusion; the Sustainability Office; the Robert Langen Art Gallery; Communications, Public Relations and Marketing; the Faculty of Music (as the mural is located on a music department building); Grounds Services; and the Executive Leadership Team (ELT, for final mural approval), among others. This also included consulting with relevant community members outside Laurier, including indigenous knowledge holders involved with the Anishinaabe Grand River Water Walk represented in the mural; Pamela Rojas as the lead mural painter; local climate justice organisers, and others. Securing buy-in from these many diverse stakeholders both for a permanent public mural centring climate justice along with broad consensus on what it should look like was not easy. Many CP skill sets, including hosting complex and multilayered dialogues, employing collective vision creation processes and engaging in consensus-building amongst diverse actors, were essential to the success of this project. Taking the time to talk through the nuances of the mural design with key stakeholders from the beginning also helped in securing higher-level support for the project down the road from Laurier's ELT, while emphasizing a shared vision for climate justice helped achieve a broad level of buy-in across the Laurier community and celebration of the mural's core message that many involved felt they could also believe in.

The *Climate is Life* mural visually honours the broad diversity of people who make up the global climate movement and local Laurier community, in particular honouring the indigenous peoples whose stolen land the mural is painted on, recognising Laurier's location on the Haldimand Tract of the Six Nations. It thereby centres the "justice" component of climate justice. The mural honours the ongoing land, water and climate stewardship of indigenous peoples, giving thanks to local water walkers and all land and water protectors – with a commitment from the broader climate movement following to "back them up" in their ongoing struggles for justice. An empty human silhouette at the centre of the image invites viewers to step in, and "join the movement".

The *Climate is Life* mural lives on today as a clear symbol and message of hope through action, in solidarity with all people who continue to RISE for climate – and illustrates the powerful role that artistic co-creation and symbolism can have in supporting climate justice movement-building efforts. It is also a powerful beacon of active hope, inviting viewers to engage in meaningful climate justice work in their communities. For community psychologists pursuing the "pragmatic ideal" of climate justice, participatory arts-based co-creation is a powerful option for community engagement and mapping the vision forwards.

Christi Belcourt: Indigenous art creation for social, environmental and climate justice

Christi Belcourt is an internationally acclaimed Métis visual artist with Mânitow Sâkahikan roots based in Ontario, Canada, whose work honours the traditions and knowledge of her people while also showcasing a uniquely personal style and artistic approach. Among other themes, her work draws attention to the rich complexity of the natural world and broader conversations on social, environmental, climate and indigenous justice, with all their interconnections. Much of the artist's most iconic work, co-created with fellow indigenous artist Isaac Murdoch, remains available online for free. This series of black-and-white prints with bold red accents has been generously gifted to and taken up by a broad global activist community, as powerful symbols of indigenous solidarity and resistance to resource extraction projects around the world. In Belcourt's words: "Every good revolution has good revolutionary art" (Anderson, 2020, p. 1). The pair began this series of work in 2016 in support of the Standing Rock protests against the Dakota Access Pipeline, USA, blending traditional indigenous imagery with anti-pipeline protest imagery and the maxim "Water is Life". Their imagery was soon printed on posters featured across the camp. In 2018, Belcourt was one of six artists from six continents commissioned by international climate organisation and movement 350.org to create an original piece for the *Rise for Climate* global day of protest happening that year (Rise for Climate, 2018a). Her piece features an indigenous woman with her hands held high, a feather in one hand and a lightning bolt in the other, and the words "Rise for Climate to Build a Fossil Free World" emblazoned in bold black text across the top (see Figure 15.2).

The final *Rise for Climate* day of action on September 18, 2018, drew participation from hundreds of thousands of people across 95 countries worldwide, many of whom were doubtless inspired by Belcourt's work (Rise for Climate, 2018b).

As an indigenous woman, Belcourt's work also regularly centres the stories and concerns of other indigenous women, without presuming to speak on others' behalf. For instance, in the profound group exhibit *Walking with Our Sisters,* Belcourt invited "caring souls" worldwide to contribute beaded moccasin "vamps" (tops) to honour the estimated 600 missing and murdered indigenous women across Canada, drawing international support

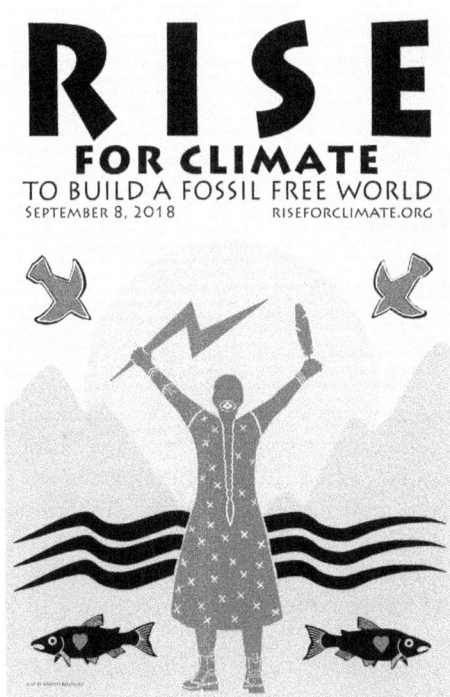

Figure 15.2   A climate justice poster designed by Métis artist Christi Belcourt for the global *Rise for Climate* day of action on September 8, 2018 (see www.riseforclimate.org)

and contributions (Nahwegahbow, 2013). This work can also be understood as a form of climate justice, as it is clear that indigenous people and women worldwide are both on the frontlines of the climate crisis, and those with intersections of these identities (indigenous women) are even more so. In addition to the deep pain of lives lost, the loss of indigenous women is often the loss of vital guardians of the land, water, climate and other people, who are urgently needed today. Recognising the deep intersections and inseparability of climate justice and indigenous justice, we wish to honour Belcourt's work, and the work of all land, water and climate defenders in their ongoing struggles for justice – work that as community psychologists, we must also *rise* to support. While Belcourt is not a trained community psychologist, her work fills a gap left unfilled by many CP practitioners: the need for far greater solidarity with indigenous communities, as this work aligns with so many core CP values, and is clearly a central component of meaningful climate justice. It also links to calls within CP for engaging in our own decolonisation process as an academic discipline (Dutta, 2018).

Art–science integration for youth-led climate justice action (2016–present)

Climate justice is deeply connected with the concept of intergenerational justice – the notion that current generations have obligations towards future generations, namely protecting the habitability of the planet (Foran et al., 2017). Young people alive today are key stakeholders in efforts to address the climate crisis not only because they will face intensifying risk exposure over the duration of their lives, but also because children are among the groups most physically vulnerable to climate impacts (Menke & Schleussner, 2019). Despite this, young people are often not invited to participate in climate decision-making or action in their communities, perhaps because they are considered "adults in waiting". The climate justice goal of centring the perspectives and experiences of those most vulnerable to climate disruption means recognising that children and youth have a critical role to play in voicing their concerns and taking action to avoid climate catastrophe.

Opening up alternative futures fuelled by young people's "democratic imaginations" needs pedagogies that invite youths' active and substantive participation (Hayward, 2012). Research by Carlie Trott explores how to cultivate empowering spaces for children and young people – particularly low-income and youth of colour – to learn about and actively address the climate crisis according to their own interests and visions for a more just and sustainable future. In doing so, she uses youth-led participatory action research methods to engage children as co-researchers and critical actors for societal transformation. In one study, she designed and implemented a 15-week after-school climate change education and action programme for 10- to 12-year-olds, which combined emancipatory and place-based educational techniques with arts-based and participatory methodologies. These culminated in youth-led action projects (see Figure 15.3), including a city council presentation, a tree-planting campaign and establishing a community garden (Trott, 2019). Building on this research, Trott has been collaborating with a community arts centre in Jacmel, Haiti, on a multicycle youth-centred programme that combines the arts and sciences to position youth as change agents for climate justice through water quality testing, community asset mapping and arts-powered advocacy – see Figure 15.4 (Trott, Even, & Frame, 2020).

Findings from both partnerships emphasize the critical importance of participatory process and collaborative action in strengthening children's sense of agency (Trott, 2019; Trott, Rockett, Gray, Lam, Even, & Frame, 2020) as well as the importance of informal learning environments for children's intergenerational and policy influence (Trott, 2020).

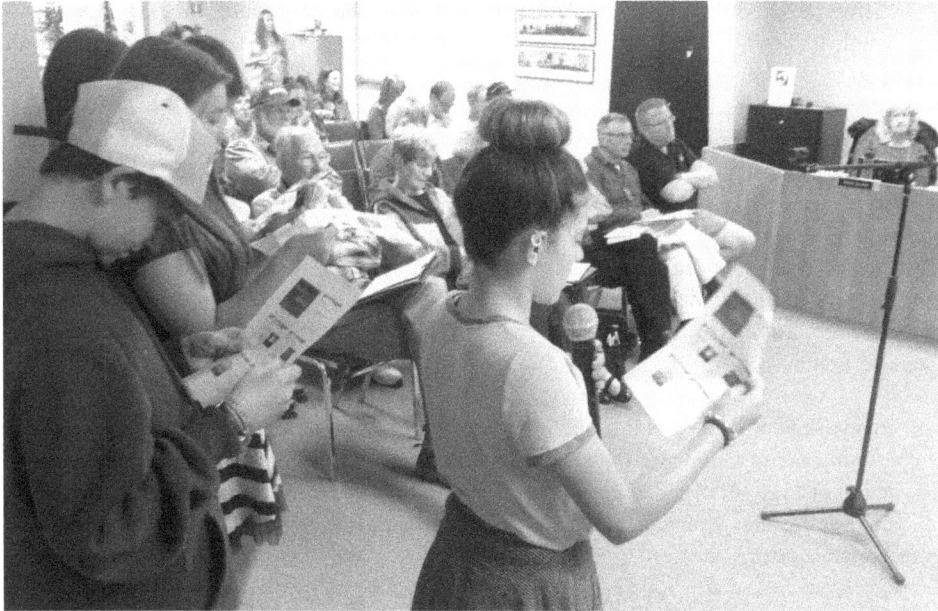

Figure 15.3 Children address city council members in rural Colorado. Presentation titled "Climate Change: OPERATION DO SOMETHING!" (see www.sciencecameraaction.com)

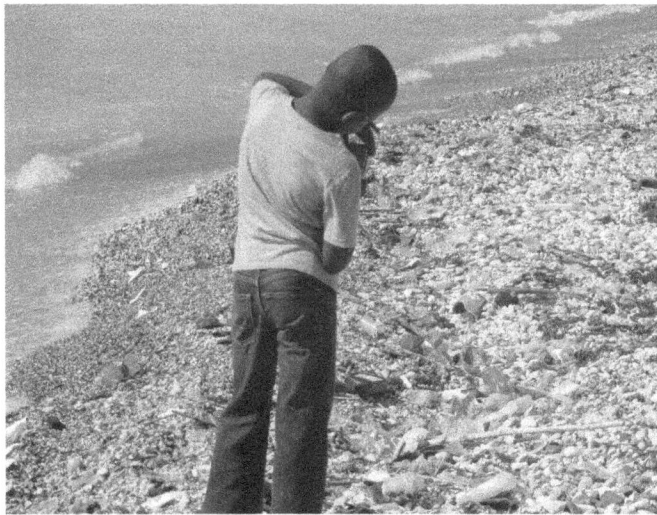

Figure 15.4 A child takes a photograph capturing his environmental concerns, Jacmel, Haiti (see http://je.atisjakmel.org/)

Together, these projects respond to a need for methods that invite marginalised groups, especially young people, to critically engage with the present, imagine a better future and collaboratively act for sustainability today (Trott, 2021). Art can be a powerful way to facilitate young people's meaning-making, self-expression and agency in the context of the climate crisis (Trott, Even, & Frame, 2020). By experimenting with art–science integration to facilitate youth-led collaborative action, Trott's research engages with "prefigurative" research methodologies and practices (e.g. Kagan & Burton, 2000; Haiven & Khasnabish, 2014), and offers alternatives to classroom-based learning about climate change (Trott & Weinberg, 2020). Prefigurative research practices seek to enact, in the present, the types of relationships and forms of exchange that are envisioned as part of a not-yet-existent, but aspirational, future society (Trott, 2016). Prefigurative action research pays simultaneous attention to research and experiments in social change, and shares many commonalities with other action-research approaches, such as community-based participatory action research (e.g. Kindon et al., 2007), transdisciplinary action research (e.g. Stokols, 2006), critical utopian action research and systemic action research (Gayá & Brydon-Miller, 2017). Prefigurative action research is characterised by:

> Analysis of both the structural and ideological dimensions of oppression; Emphasis on creating and sustaining examples of alternative forms of social relations that provide a vision of a just society; Participation of less powerful people; Multiple cycles of reflection, doing, and knowing; and simultaneous attention to both agency and structure in emancipatory practice.
>
> *(Kagan & Burton, 2000, p. 73)*

Prefigurative methodologies, then, embody alternative university–community relations and societal conditions in ways that instantiate, in the present, a more just and sustainable future (Trott et al., 2018). As a form of experimentation in conducting research "otherwise", the case studies presented here represent "images of possibility" (Kagan & Burton, 2000, p. 73) – or, in this case, examples of alternative future-making methodologies that demonstrate another way of conducting research is possible. They also show ways in which community psychologists can partner with marginalised groups in researching climate justice, whilst simultaneously standing in solidarity with those groups.

Conclusion

Given the scale and impenetrability of the climate crisis, deciding where and how to enter the fight for alternatives is a challenge. The enormity of the problem can make it feel as if truly meaningful action at the scope and scale necessary is beyond reach, and that local-scale action is not enough. Achieving climate justice requires transformative change. Because the drivers of climate chaos are built into the very systems – social, political, economic – and the neoliberal imaginaries that shape our everyday lives, one place to start is to reimagine our structures and institutions, with a view to transforming them with human and ecological flourishing in mind. Community psychologists are well positioned to facilitate transformative change across sectors and scales. We have argued that developing strong senses of agency and a radical collective imagination through envisioning alternative futures is a good pathway into climate justice work. Envisioning alternative futures through decolonial ways of working can reveal the space for collective action. We should be in no doubt, though, that climate justice requires "repertoires of action" at all levels of the system and through every means possible, including "legislative, judicial, advocacy, direct action, and community work" (Chatterton et al., 2013, p. 617). Climate justice will require collective action across sectors, including all levels of government, the private sector, international organisations, faith-based institutions, non-profits, universities and community groups of all kinds. While the scale of the problem is significant and no single solution is sufficient, this should not be a barrier to action. On the contrary, the fact that the climate crisis touches everyone where they are means there is ample work to be done – and community psychologists need not look far to find it.

From a climate justice perspective, addressing climate change is not just a matter of restoring ecosystem stability to sustain human life in our inequitable, unjust and at times uninhabitable societies as they exist today. Rather, climate justice anchors us in a vision committed to the equitable flourishing of human communities and ecosystems everywhere, while transforming those unjust systems that prevent this flourishing, starting now. Situated at the intersections of the local and the global as well as of injustices both social and environmental, climate justice solidarities can "bring together geographically, culturally, economically and politically different and distant peoples and enable connections and alliances to be drawn that extend beyond the local and particular" (Chatterton et al., 2013, p. 614). As a unifying force that can build momentum for transformative change, the pragmatic ideal of climate justice is not only the moral decision but also an astutely strategic one. In a time of crisis, the seemingly radical *is* the realistic basis for hope, and the contributions of community psychologists can be integral to facilitating such a transformation.

References

350.org. (n.d.). *Stop fossil fuels: Build 100% renewables.* https://350.org/

350.org. (2019, September 28). *7.6 million people demand action after week of climate strikes.* Global Climate Strike. https://globalclimatestrike.net/7-million-people-demand-action-after-week-of-climate-strikes/

Abu, R., Reed, M.G., & Jardine, T.D. (2020). Using two-eyed seeing to bridge Western science and Indigenous knowledge systems and understand long-term change in the Saskatchewan River Delta, Canada. *International Journal of Water Resources Development, 36*(5), 757–76.

Adams, G., Gomez Ordonez, L., Kurtis, T., Molina, L.E., & Dobles, I. (2017). Notes on decolonising psychology: From one special issue to another. *South African Journal of Psychology, 47*(4), 531–41.

Agyeman, J. (2013). *Introducing just sustainabilities policy, planning, and practice.* Zed Books.

Anderson, C. (2020). Christi Belcourt, Nimkii Aazhibikong (near Elliot Lake, Ont.). *Chatelaine, 93*(2), 66–7.

Bopp, J., Bopp, M., Brown, L., & Lane, P. (1984). *The sacred tree.* Guilford.

Bregman, R. (2014). *Utopia for realists.* Back Bay Books.

brown, a.m. (2017). *Emergent strategy.* AK Press.

Chatterton, P., Featherstone, D., & Routledge, P. (2013). Articulating climate justice in Copenhagen: Antagonism, the commons, and solidarity. *Antipode, 45*(3), 602–20. https://doi.org/10.1111/j.1467-8330.2012.01025.x

Christens, B.D., Hanlin, C.E., & Speer, P.W. (2007). Getting the social organism thinking: Strategy for systems change. *American Journal of Community Psychology, 39*, 229–38.

Climate Emergency Declaration. (2021, April 5). *Climate emergency declarations in 1,921 jurisdictions and local governments cover 826 million citizens.* https://climateemergencydeclaration.org/climate-emergency-declarations-cover-15-million-citizens/

Cyr, M., & Riediger, N. (2021). (Re)claiming our bodies using a Two-Eyed Seeing approach: Health-At-Every-Size (HAES®) and Indigenous knowledge. *Canadian Journal of Public Health, 112*(3), 493–7.

Dutta, U. (2018). Decolonizing "community" in community psychology. *American Journal of Community Psychology, 62*, 272–82.

Ehrenfeld, J.R., & Hoffman, A.J. (2013). *Flourishing: A frank conversation about sustainability.* Stanford University Press.

Etchart, L. (2017). The role of indigenous peoples in combating climate change. *Palgrave Communications*, 1–4. https://doi.org/10.1057/palcomms.2017.85

Featherstone, D. (2013). The contested politics of climate change and the crisis of neo-liberalism. *ACME: An International Journal for Critical Geographies, 12*(1), 44–64.

Foran, J., Gray, S., & Grosse, C. (2017). "Not yet the end of the world": Political cultures of opposition and creation in the global youth climate justice movement. *Interface: A Journal for and About Social Movements, 9*(2), 353–79.

Foster, J.B. (2015). The great capitalist climacteric: Marxism and "system change not climate change". *Monthly Review, 67*(6), 1–18.

Galafassi, D., Tàbara, J.D., & Heras, M. (2018). Restoring our senses, restoring the Earth: Fostering imaginative capacities through the arts for envisioning climate transformations. *Elementa: Science of the Anthropocene, 6*(69), 1–14.

Gayá, P., & Brydon-Miller, M. (2017). Carpe the academy: Dismantling higher education and prefiguring critical utopias through action research. *Futures, 94*, 34–44.

Gore, T. (2020). *Confronting carbon inequality: Putting climate justice at the heart of the COVID-19 recovery.* [Oxfam Report]. https://oxfamilibrary.openrepository.com/bitstream/handle/10546/621052/mb-confronting-carbon-inequality-210920-en.pdf

Gurria, E. (2017, May 2). *Celebrating indigenous peoples as nature's stewards.* United Nations Development Programme. www.undp.org/content/undp/en/home/blog/2017/5/2/Celebrating-Indigenous-Peoples-as-nature-s-stewards-.html

Haiven, M., & Khasnabish, D.A. (2014*). The radical imagination: Social movement research in the age of austerity.* Zed Books.

Hayward, B. (2012). *Children, citizenship and environment: Nurturing democratic imagination in a changing world.* Routledge.

Indigenous Climate Action. (n.d.). *Climate justice: Indigenous-led.* www.indigenousclimateaction.com/

Indigenous Climate Action. (2020). *2020 annual report.* www.IndigenousClimateAction.com

Iwama, M., Marshall, M., Marshall, A., & Bartlett, C. (2009). Two-eyed seeing and the language of healing in community-based research. *Canadian Journal of Native Education, 32*(2), 3–23.

Kagan, C., & Burton, M. (2000). Prefigurative action research: An alternative basis for critical psychology. *Annual Review of Critical Psychology, 2*, 73–87.

Kagan, S. (2012). *Toward global (environ)mental change: Transformative art and cultures of sustainability.* Heinrich-Böll-Stiftung.

Kimmerer, R.W. (2013). *Braiding sweetgrass: Indigenous wisdom, scientific knowledge and the teachings of plants.* Milkweed Editions.

Kindon, S., Pain, R., & Kesby, M. (Eds.). (2007). *Participatory action research approaches and methods: Connecting people, participation and place.* Routledge.

Klein, N. (2007). *The shock doctrine: The rise of disaster capitalism.* Macmillan.

Klein, N. (2017). *No is not enough: Resisting the new shock politics and winning the world we need.* Alfred A. Knopf Canada.

Latulippe, N., & Klenk, N. (2020). Making room and moving over: Knowledge co-production, Indigenous knowledge sovereignty and the politics of global environmental change decision-making. *Current Opinion in Environmental Sustainability, 42*, 7–14.

Liboro, R.M. (2015). Forging political will from a shared vision: A critical social justice agenda against neoliberalism and other systems of domination. *Social Justice Research, 28*, 207–28.

Maynard, N.G. (1998). *Circles of Wisdom: Native Peoples-Native Homelands Climate Change workshop: Final Report.* US Global Change Research Program, October 28–November 1, 1998, Albuquerque Convention Center, Albuquerque, New Mexico. NASA Goddard Space Flight Center.

Meadows, D. (1997). Places to intervene in a system. *Whole Earth, 91*(1), 78–84.

Meadows, D. (2001). Dancing with systems. *Whole Earth, 106*, 58–63.

Menke, I. & Schleussner, C.F. (2019). Climate analytics: Global climate change impacts on children. https://climateanalytics.org/media/report_cc_impacts_on_children_2019.pdf

Monbiot, G. (2020). *Out of the wreckage: A new politics for an age of crisis.* Verso.

Nahwegahbow, B. (2013, August). Belcourt project paying tribute to 600 souls. AMMSA.com. *Windspeaker, 31*(5).

Nelson, G. (2013). Community psychology and transformative policy change in the neo-liberal era. *American Journal of Community Psychology, 52*(3–4), 211–23.

Raygorodetsky, G. (2018, November). Indigenous peoples defend Earth's biodiversity – but they're in danger. *National Geographic.*

Rice, J.L., Cohen, D.A., Long, J., & Jurjevich, J.R. (2019). Contradictions of the climate-friendly city: New perspectives on eco-gentrification and housing justice. *International Journal of Urban and Regional Research, 44*(1), 145–65. https://doi.org/10.1111/1468-2427.12740

Riemer, M., & Harré, N. (2016). Environmental degradation and sustainability: A community psychology perspective. In M.A. Bond, C. Keys, & I. Serrano-García (Eds.), *APA handbook of community psychology* (Vol. 2) (pp. 441–55). American Psychological Association.

Riemer, M. & Van Voorhees, C.W. (2014). Psychology, sustainability, and environmental justice. In C. Johnson, H. Friedman, J. Diaz, B. Nastasi, & Z. Franco (Eds.), *Praeger handbook of social justice and psychology* (pp. 49–66). Praeger.

Riemer, M., Reich, S.M., Evans, S., Nelson, G., & Prilleltensky, I. (2020). *Community psychology: In pursuit of liberation and well-being* (3rd ed.). Palgrave-Macmillan.

Rise for Climate. (2018a, September 8). *ART FOR RISE.* https://riseforclimate.org/rise-art/

Rise for Climate. (2018b, September 8). *RISE FOR CLIMATE.* https://riseforclimate.org/

Schrock, G., Bassett, E.M., & Green, J. (2015). Pursuing equity and justice in a changing climate: Assessing equity in local climate and sustainability plans in U.S. cities. *Journal of Planning Education and Research, 35*(3), 282–95. https://doi.org/10.1177/0739456X15580022

Stokols, D. (2006). Toward a science of transdisciplinary action research. *American Journal of Community Psychology, 38*(1–2), 63–77.

Thiele, L.P. (2016). *Sustainability* (2nd ed.). Polity Press.

Trott, C.D. (2016). Constructing alternatives: Envisioning a critical psychology of prefigurative politics. *Journal of Social and Political Psychology, 4*(1), 266–85. https://doi.org/10.5964/jspp.v4i1.520

Trott, C.D. (2019). Reshaping our world: Collaborating with children for community-based climate change action. *Action Research, 17*(1), 42–62. https://doi.org/10.1177/1476750319829209

Trott, C.D. (2020). Children's constructive climate change engagement: Empowering awareness, agency, and action. *Environmental Education Research, 26*(4), 532–54. https://doi.org/10.1080/13504622.2019.1675594

Trott, C.D. (2021). What difference does it make? Exploring the transformative potential of everyday climate crisis activism by children and youth. *Children's Geographies.* Advance online publication. https://doi.org/10.1080/14733285.2020.1870663

Trott, C.D. & Weinberg, A.E. (2020). Science education for sustainability: Strengthening children's science engagement through climate change learning and action. *Sustainability, 12*(16), 6400. https://doi.org/10.3390/su12166400

Trott, C.D., Even, T.L., & Frame, S. (2020). Merging the arts and sciences for collaborative sustainability action: A methodological framework. *Sustainability Science, 15*(4), 1067–85. https://doi.org/10.1007/s11625-020-00798-7

Trott, C.D., Rockett, M.L., Gray, E., Lam, S., Even, T.L., & Frame, S.M. (2020). "Another Haiti starting from the youth": Integrating the arts and sciences for empowering youth climate justice action in Jacmel, Haiti. *Community Psychology in Global Perspective, 6*(2/2), 48–70.

Trott, C.D., Weinberg, A.E., & Sample McMeeking, L.B. (2018). Prefiguring sustainability through participatory action research experiences for undergraduates: Reflections and recommendations for student development. *Sustainability, 10*, 1–21. https://doi.org/10.3390/su10093332

Unanue, I., Patel, S.G., Tormala, T.T., Trott, C.D., Piazza Rodríguez, A., Méndez Serrano, K., & Brown, L.M. (2020). Seeing more clearly: Communities transforming towards justice in post-Hurricane Puerto Rico. *Community Psychology in Global Perspective, 6*(2), 22–47.

United Nations Framework Convention on Climate Change (UNFCCC). (n.d.). *Introduction to Climate Finance.* https://unfccc.int/topics/climate-finance/the-big-picture/introduction-to-climate-finance/introduction-to-climate-finance

VERiS. (n.d.). *Viessmann Centre for Engagement and Research in Sustainability.* https://researchcentres.wlu.ca/viessmann-centre-for-engagement-and-research-in-sustainability/

Wuebbles, D.J., Fahey, D.W., & Hibbard, K.A. (2017). *Climate science special report: fourth national climate assessment* (Vol. 1). https://nca2018.globalchange.gov/chapter/14/

16

PARTICIPATION FOR A BETTER FUTURE

Communities of action for the environment in Aotearoa New Zealand[1]

Niki Harré, Sally Birdsall, Daniel Hikuroa, Daniel Kelly, Karen Nairn and Te Kerekere Roycroft

Abstract

Global systems of production and consumption are damaging the biosphere on which human life depends. We offer four vignettes from a variety of allied disciplines aimed at understanding vibrant "communities of action" for the environment in Aotearoa New Zealand. We outline how they help build, and build on, policies and institutions that regenerate people's relationship to the land and protect natural ecosystems; and their struggles to create resilient, reliable social networks in the fractured, mobile world of an industrialised society. Finally, we reflect on the insights the vignettes offer for a Community Psychology that extends its purview to the biosphere.

Resumen

Los sistemas globales de producción y consumo están dañando la biosfera, de la que depende la vida humana. Ofrecemos cuatro viñetas de disciplinas afines con el propósito de entender las vibrantes "comunidades de acción" por el medio ambiente presentes en Aotearoa/Nueva Zelandia. Describimos como éstas ayudan a construir y a fortalecer políticas e instituciones que buscan regenerar la relación de las personas con la tierra y proteger los ecosistemas naturales, además de los desafíos que enfrentan para crear redes sociales resistentes y fiables en el mundo móvil y fracturado de la sociedad industrializada. Finalmente, reflexionamos sobre las perspectivas que las viñetas le ofrecen a una psicología comunitaria que extiende su ámbito de influencia a la biosfera.

Introduction

Community Psychology is an applied discipline that focuses on well-being in context (see Gridley & Breen, 2007; Nelson, Lavoie, & Mitchell, 2007). To date, the emphasis has been on human contexts; primarily "communities". Traditionally, these are disadvantaged communities that hold a common identity and often the core consideration is social justice (see Harré,

DOI: 10.4324/9780429325663-20

2019). Some community psychologists have, however, proposed a broader approach that takes account of the larger biosphere and the way in which people affect and are affected by it (e.g. Moskell & Allred, 2013; Riemer & Harré, 2017), and we take that approach here. This broader understanding is also consistent with indigenous knowledge systems including *Te Ao* Māori, the worldview of the indigenous people of Aotearoa New Zealand (Marsden, 2003; Roberts, Norman, Minhinnick, Wihongi, & Kirkwood, 1995; Williams, 2019), the country from which we write this chapter.

We have four core assumptions. First, that global systems of production and consumption are damaging the biosphere on which our well-being depends. For example, in a review article, Sandra Díaz and colleagues (2019) discuss how 72% of the natural elements identified as important by indigenous people and communities are in decline, largely due to human activity. This includes reduced biodiversity, a decrease in fish stocks, damage to coastal ecosystems, deteriorating air quality, climate change and contamination of freshwater.

Second, we assume a world made up of complex systems that are networked rather than hierarchically nested (see Hawe, 2017; Neal & Neal, 2013), consistent with an Earth Systems science approach (see Bretherton, 1988). We consider these systems, and their problems, to be "messy". As Chapman (2004) has noted, messy problems "are unbounded in scope, time and resources, and enjoy no clear agreement about what a solution would even look like, let alone how it could be achieved" (p. 19). This means that attempts to change a system are subject to *inherent* risk (Capra & Luisi, 2014), and experimentation, observation and flexibility are more suitable than detailed plans (Hassan, 2014). It also means that both change and resistance can come from any part of the social system (see Harré, 2019).

The third assumption is that the natural world is of intrinsic value (Harré, Madden, Brooks, & Goodman, 2017).This, we argue, is an obvious extension for a discipline that values life, diversity, caring for those who are vulnerable, and multiple forms of knowing. For practical purposes we are drawn to meaning frameworks that emphasise the relations between people and the rest of nature (see Chan et al., 2016; Coope, 2019). *Mātauranga* Māori (Māori knowledge, values, culture and worldview), which is a relational tradition in this sense, emphasises *whakapapa* (ancestral lineage) that connects people to both the human and more-than-human ancestors of their place. Thus all are kin, have *mauri* (holistic health, life force), and are part of the community (Marsden, 2003). Within psychology, the relatively new subdiscipline of ecopsychology is similarly focused on human–nature relationships (Doherty, 2009; Fisher, 2002; Riemer & Harré, 2017).

Finally, we assume that real-world action is essential to restoring the natural world and reintegrating a relational perspective to contemporary worldviews. Action has long been recognised as critical to all forms of social change in Community Psychology and beyond (e.g. Freire, 1970/1996; Krause & Montenegro, 2017). Here we discuss four "communities of action" for the environment, some of which are local, and others global, in orientation. They all involve the work of creating community; skills that can be developed through Community Psychology practice.

We come from different academic orientations: two community psychologists (Niki and Daniel Kelly), an Earth scientist located in a Department of Māori Studies (Daniel Hikuroa), a student of landscape architecture (Te Kerekere), and two educators with backgrounds in science and geography respectively (Sally and Karen). We take an interdisciplinary approach here, because, in the words of Perkins and Schensul, we want to "solve a shared problem" (2017, p. 91). Two of us identify as Māori (Te Kerekere and Daniel Hikuroa) and the other four as Pākehā (non-indigenous New Zealanders). Importantly, as researchers in the communities we discuss, we have "skin in the game [...] a compelling sense of personal recognition rather than just wanting to help [a community] with their problems" (Harré, 2019, p. 84). We are participants, allies, supporters, documenters, storytellers; this work matters to us.

Each vignette is written by a different author or authors who position themselves at the beginning of their piece. They therefore reflect that author's voice and disciplinary perspective. At the end of each vignette we use a collective voice to reflect on the insights and questions raised for a Community Psychology that extends its concerns to the biosphere. In light of the vignettes, the discussion reflects on how Community Psychology can contribute more fully to work in this sphere. Writing this chapter has given each of us valuable insight into allied disciplines and deepened our understanding of the human/nature interface; we hope other readers are similarly enriched by what we offer.

Note that consistent with the important role of *te reo Māori* (Māori language) in Aotearoa New Zealand, we use a number of Māori terms, especially in the first vignette. These are italicised and are translated (with the exception of the traditional *pepeha* – recitations – at the start of the vignette to follow) the first time they are used in a new section.

Restoring the *mauri of place*
Te Kerekere Roycroft and Daniel Hikuroa

As Māori, we start with our *pepeha* (recitation of connections to place and people) that speak of where, and who, we are from and allow others to orient themselves in relation to us. We each refer to key elements relevant to our connections, for example *maunga* (mountains), *waka* (canoe/s our ancestors arrived on), and *iwi* (our tribal affiliations).

> *Ko Te Ramaroa te maunga, Ko Matariki te rere, Ko Rāhiri te tangata, Ko Whiria te pā*
> *Ko Matahaorua raua ko Ngatokimatawhaorua te waka, Ko Ngāpuhi nui tonu te iwi,*
> *Ko Ngāti Korokoro, Ko Ngāti Whārara, Ko Te Poukā ngā hapū, o te wahapu o Hokianga nui*
>   *a Kupe, Hokianga whakapau karakia e, Ko Maraeroa te marae, Ko Ro Iho te urupa, Ko Te*
>   *Kerekere Louise Verneē Roycroft toku ingoa*

> *Ko Owhawhe te maunga, Ko Waitomo te awa, Ko Maniapoto te tangata, Ko Pohatuiri te pā*
> *Ko Tainui raua ko Te Arawa ngā waka, Ko Ngāti Uehaka, ko Ngāti Ruapuha ngā hapū*
> *Ko Ngāti Maniapoto te iwi, Ko Tokikapu te marae, Ko Tionui te urupa, Ko Daniel Carl*
>   *Henare Hikuroa toku ingoa*

Te Kerekere Roycroft is currently studying landscape design at UNITEC in Auckland. Daniel Hikuroa uses earth systems science and environmental humanities approaches and methods, and is based in Te Wānanga o Waipapa, at the University of Auckland.

In the Māori worldview, people are an interconnected element in a larger ancestral schema that includes natural entities. We draw identity from the landmarks of our *rohe* (tribal area); and are linked to our *whenua* (land) by *whakapapa* (ancestral lineage) through the primal parents Ranginui (Sky-father) and Papatūānuku (Earth-mother). We are the younger siblings of *maunga* (mountains), *awa* (rivers), *ngahere* (forests), and *moana* (seas). It is our responsibility to care for our elders as they care for us, and to offer respect to our *uri* (descendants). *Tikanga* (protocols) have been developed over centuries of layered connections with our *whenua*. One example is *kaitiakitanga* (guardianship responsibility), the practices undertaken to achieve intergenerational sustainability. Flexible refinement of our *tikanga* means that the relationship we have with our place evolves with each generation.

In 1975, the government of Aotearoa New Zealand passed the Treaty of Waitangi Act and established the Waitangi Tribunal to address historical injustices. The tribunal negotiates settlements between *iwi* and the crown, and to date has entered into negotiations for 117 settlements with 73 of these passed into law (Te Arawhiti, 2020). Many of these settlements reflect the relational values described earlier, and acknowledge the importance of people as place, and place as people. For example, the 2014 Te Urewera Act covers 594 hectares of Tūhoe land and gives it legal personhood, acknowledging that "Te Urewera has an identity in and of itself, inspiring people to commit to its care". Similarly, the Te Awa Tupua (Whanganui River Claims Settlement) Act 2017 gives customary rights and responsibilities to local *iwi* and declares the river to be "a legal person [with] all the rights, powers, duties and liabilities of a legal person".

These settlements have helped *iwi* restore the *mauri* (holistic health or life force) of local land and waterscapes. As part of a 2019/20 Ngā Pae o te Māramatanga (Aotearoa New Zealand's Māori Centre of Research Excellence) internship, Te Kerekere interviewed leaders of restoration projects. One example is Pūniu River Care, a project started in 2015 with a grant funded by Te Puni Kōkiri (The Ministry of Māori Development). The Pūniu River is located in the central North Island, beginning in the Pureora Forest and meeting the Waipā River at Pirongia. The main *Kaupapa* (purpose) of the project is to enable local *hapū* (kinship groups/sub-tribes) to be involved in improving water quality within the Pūniu River Catchment. This includes propagating and planting 500,000 native trees each year. In an interview with CEO Shannon Te Huia, he described the project as "*an opportunity for the* whanau *[extended family] to participate in the restoration of the* awa", and that "*many people wanted to become involved, we didn't anticipate it getting so big so fast*". Shannon further explained that its success involved forming partnerships and understanding the connection between people and place. As he said, "*The goal of the project is to restore the* mauri *of the* awa *[…] but there is a lot of* whanaungatanga *(kinship or a sense of family connection) and strengthening of relationships with people and organisations who have similar goals*".

Pūniu River Care pays the core people involved in restoration (these are members of the local *hapū*), which Shannon described as a "sustainable" model. Nevertheless, the vision, he said, is something you "*constantly have to work at. By holding fast to the* whakataukī *(proverbs encapsulating ancestral wisdom) of our* tupuna *(ancestors) and evolving in an ever changing world we are able to provide fruits for our people through employment*". The project's experience with volunteers from the *hapū* has been variable, as they do not live on the land and are often drawn away by other commitments. This echoes issues raised by Daniel Kelly in his piece on urban food production to follow.

Summary and reflection

In the Māori world view people and place are entwined. Consistent with this worldview, recent legislation has acknowledged large areas of *iwi* land, and provided financial settlements that enable restoration projects. Pūniu River Care is one such project run by the local *hapū*. The project must nevertheless constantly work to keep people involved and reassert its underlying purpose and associated practices. This raises two key questions. Can we tell stories of relationship between people and place that generate restorative, sustainable practices? How does a historically continuous and localised approach to environmental protection sit within a fractured, contemporary world where land is privately owned and people are mobile?

Urban food production

Daniel Kelly

My gardening interests (and history of volunteering) inform my PhD research in Community Psychology: working as a researcher-participant within Auckland's urban agriculture movement, collaborating across diverse projects to try to increase volunteer participation.

Much like the Māori groups discussed in the previous vignette, urban residents are seeking to connect with and care for the places in which they live, starting not with ancestral connection but the food they eat. Participation in this space is inescapably collaborative, catalysing the cooperation at the heart of community transformation, sketching new, solidarity-based worlds amidst a mainstream of social decay. In the following vignette, I explore issues with contemporary food production and the transformative potential of community gardening.

For urban residents, food is ubiquitous: from greasy take-outs to stacked supermarket shelves, nature's bounty is never far away. However, this proximity masks a hugely fragile, globalised network (Steel, 2008), dependent on fossil fuels and implicated in a number of interlinked social, economic and environmental issues. These include biodiversity loss (Martin, 2019), the decimation of local economies (Patel & Moore, 2018), and the food insecurity experienced by our most vulnerable (Robson, 2019). In the words of Rose (2013), the rise of this global food system supports an "ontology of alienation" (p. 2) in which urban consumers are disconnected from the source of their food.

In response, advocates for food system change utilise a variety of framings from food justice to food sovereignty (Swords, Frith, & Lap, 2018), prioritising locally owned, environmentally sustainable and socially just forms of production (Patel, 2009). In contrast to the alienation of industrial food systems, Rose (2013) describes these approaches as supporting an "ontology of connectedness" (p. 2), providing the means for people to connect with both the source of their food and each other.

One way in which this connection is facilitated in an urban setting is via community gardening. Community gardening encompasses "a variety of horticultural activities that either have a community component or are located on public land" (Earle, 2011, p. iii). Like projects overseas (e.g., Pudup, 2008), community gardens in New Zealand are diverse and include individual allotments, communal growing spaces and *marae* gardens (gardens located on Māori land; Earle, 2011). Despite the historical decline in gardening associated with urbanisation, community gardens have been increasing since the 1980s, with their rise linked to the environmental movement, rising food prices and economic precarity (Dawson, 2010).

As a result of this diversity, different community gardens in New Zealand emphasise different, often overlapping, objectives. For example, while Auckland's Kelmarna City Organic Gardens promotes educational outreach and organic farming (Little, 2010), Wellington's Operation Green Thumb sets up gardens so people "can grow low-cost food" (Earle, 2011, p. 22). More recent projects expand this scope, with the central Auckland *OMG* – Organic Market Garden forming part of a nascent Urban Farmers' Alliance that aims to deliver 11 key outcomes from carbon sequestration to food security, local jobs and increased community (Urban Farmers' Alliance, 2020).

While such "silver bullet" claims have their critics (e.g. Daftary-Steel, Herrera, & Porter, 2015), the international literature is replete with research linking community gardening to a range of positive outcomes (Porter, 2018). These include improvements in physical and mental health (Soga, Gaston, & Yamaura, 2017), community cohesion (Alaimo et al., 2010), increased biodiversity (Taylor & Lovell, 2014), and economic revival (Kaufman & Bailkey, 2000). Viability, however, is often tenuous. Security of tenure (Fox-Kämper et al., 2018), funding (Firth, Maye, & Pearson, 2011), community buy-in and volunteer support (Earle, 2011) are among the issues gardens struggle with. While research by Fox-Kämper et al. (2018) suggests that help from paid professionals is a key enabler, many projects exist outside the formal economy and must do without (Drake & Lawson, 2015).

For gardens that do succeed, a common outcome is increased community cohesion (Alaimo et al., 2010). Firth et al. (2011) link this cohesion to community gardens' status as "third spaces" distinct from work and home, in which participants can interact on a regular basis, contribute to shared projects and engage in networks of mutual aid. Such relationship building is central to the success of Auckland's *OMG* with semi-regular social gatherings helping support the 70–100 hours of volunteer participation recorded each week (Urban Farmers' Alliance, 2020).

Other research emphasises how the relationships nurtured by urban food production can catalyse deeper shifts amongst the wider community (Armstrong, 2000). For example, a study of food sovereignty initiatives in Whaingaroa (a coastal town in Aotearoa New Zealand) shows how community gardening can build shared identity and support a network of active, mutually supportive citizens participating in other community work (Ritchie, 2016).

Summary and reflection

As a site of community action, urban agriculture has the potential to create productive zones where values are lived, social bonds forged and further change is ignited; all core features of vibrant communities. As we saw with Pūniu River Care, funding is extremely helpful, as is access to land. Volunteers come and go; indeed, how to recruit and retain volunteers in this space is a central question of Daniel Kelly's PhD research. Along similar lines to the previous vignette, we are left wondering about how to encourage commitment to local food production in the geographically mobile world in which we live.

A secondary (high) school with a sustainability culture
Niki Harré

Before beginning a PhD in 1993, I was a secondary school teacher and I am still drawn to working along-side young people to promote flourishing people and thriving ecosystems. I identify as a community psych-ologist and teach both psychology and sustainability courses at the University of Auckland.

Both the preceding vignettes discuss people working directly with the land. For many participants in these projects, they are a relatively small part of their daily lives, and sit within a "third space" as Daniel Kelly described. Here I discuss a community of action for the environment located within a secondary school, and hence a place that participants occupy on a daily basis (see Harré, Blythe, McLean, & Khan, 2021).

Western Springs College/Ngā Puna O Waiōrea (WSCW) is located in central Auckland, a city of 1.6 million people. WSCW has a co-governance model, with a larger English-medium college (Western Springs College) and a smaller Māori-medium college (Ngā Puna O Waiōrea) working in partnership. In 2008, the school's governance board invited me, as an outgoing member of the board and parent at the school, to establish and chair a sustainability panel that would "work towards environmental sustainability in all areas of school life". The panel acted as a "bridging" structure (Lawlor & Neal, 2016; Todd, 2012) that brought together members of the school community interested in environmental sustainability. It is still in operation and its members include student leaders with sustainability-related portfolios and their liaison teachers, a representative of the school's governance board, and external advisers from Auckland City Council and the nationwide Enviroschools programme (see Eames, Cowie, & Bolstad, 2008). I chaired the panel for 11 years; during this time it included graduate students in psychology who worked on an action research project to support and document the school's progress towards sustainability.

The project was based on three theoretical frameworks. One was complex soft systems theory (Chapman, 2004; Checkland & Scholes, 1990). This has the assumptions of complex systems thinking outlined in the introduction to this chapter, including the importance of experimentation and flexibility. Second, it drew on core principles of Community Psychology, such as empowerment and focusing on strengths, to help panel members, particularly the students, identify and manage initiatives (Blythe et al., 2013); and third it incorporated action competence and the iterative, collective, learning cycles that are part of environmental educa-tion (Wals & Dillon, 2013).

Since 2008, sustainability has increasingly become part of how WSCW operates. The school now has a fully separated waste system and a large worm farm, and a recent building project has several green features. There are several sustainability-related student leader-ship roles with four associated student teams. These teams lead regular sustainability events including eco-weeks, clothes swaps, bike expos, riparian planting and an interschool Green Jam. Environmental science is offered to senior students and involves practical projects as well as theory; junior students create and sell products in a biannual sustainability market and help maintain the local streams (these teaching initiatives are enabled by the principles of the national curriculum, discussed further in the next vignette); and there have been sev-eral school-wide fundraising efforts to preserve endangered species (e.g. Townrow, Laurence, Blythe, Long, & Harré, 2016). WSCW students were also amongst the leaders of School Strike 4 Climate in Auckland.

WSCW is by no means "sustainable" in an objective sense. It still uses more resources than is feasible long-term and progress towards sustainability is often compromised by com-peting values. However, it has something resembling a sustainability culture. As a student leader, interviewed as part of the research component of the project, said, "[there is] this *personality* for our school that we are sustainable" (Harré et al., 2021). As with any complex system, this culture appears to have *emerged* from the interaction of numerous elements, including those outlined in the previous paragraph, that have amplified each other in positive feedback loops. The presence of the Māori-medium college that enacts the language and practices of *Te Ao* Māori, was also described in the research interviews as a key contributor to the growth of envir-onmental sustainability at WSWC.

Summary and reflection

WSCW shows the transformative potential of communities for the environment situated within sites inhabited by the participants as part of their everyday lives, in this case within a school. A soft systems approach combined with Community Psychology and environmental education principles helped build a community of action which has become more elaborated and resilient over time. We ask: what does this project teach us about working in partnership with commu-nities located inside schools and other organisations?

Young people's action for climate change
Sally Birdsall and Karen Nairn

Sally Birdsall

After teaching in primary schools, I now educate teachers how to teach science and sustainability in their classrooms. My research focuses on pedagogy; exploring ways of learning that lead to both people and other living organisms thriving together.

Karen Nairn

I worked with rangatahi *(young people) as a high school geography teacher. Now, as an academic in the College of Education at the University of Otago, my curiosity about young people's activism for the environment has led to research with Generation Zero whose vision is a carbon-neutral Aotearoa NZ. Here I'm reporting research done in collaboration with Carisa Showden, Kyle Matthews, Judith Sligo and Amee Parker.*

Thanks to Greta Thunberg and School Strike 4 Climate, youth are now associated with climate action worldwide. Aotearoa New Zealand youth are no exception. Not only did our *rangatahi* (young people) organise three school strikes (SS4C NZ), but Generation Zero, a youth-led climate action group, were a driving force behind the country's 2019 Zero Carbon Act legislation. In this vignette we briefly describe the achievements of each movement, and then focus on the collective emotional landscape that underpins them. We ask if, and how, such movements can be supported by teachers, community psychologists and other adult allies.

Generation Zero was established in 2011 and most members are in their twenties. Their aim is a "zero carbon Aotearoa" (www.generationzero.org) and they have been remarkably successful. They have pushed for policy change through producing and promoting a blueprint for the Zero Carbon Act, creating communities of action in local centres, and developing their skills for navigating and influencing politics within central and local government. In Auckland, Generation Zero is well known for its scorecards rating political candidates based on their policies for addressing climate change.

School Strike 4 Climate New Zealand (SS4C NZ) is led by high school students. They have organised three national strikes; the third attracted 170,000 people in over 40 events (RNZ, 2020). SS4C NZ's vision includes "plentiful native forests, clean rivers and thriving ecosystems" along with acknowledging that people's "wellbeing is inextricably linked" to that of their environment (https://our.actionstation.org.nz/petitions/climate-declaration-from-the-youth-of-aotearoa). Like Generation Zero, SS4C have a strong focus on legislation that aligns with a zero-carbon future and the Paris Agreement 1.5. Both groups, then, are focused primarily on macro-level change. And both groups are embedded in the complex, shared emotions that have been shown to accompany the climate catastrophe and climate activism (Bryan, 2020; Holmberg & Alvinius, 2020; Nairn, 2019).

Karen's research asked Generation Zero activists in Auckland to reflect on their experiences and how hopeful they were that the Zero Carbon Act (ZCA) would make a difference. What sustained many was their sense of being part of a community concerned about urgently addressing climate change. Olivia explained how *"shared experiences and solidarity and also shared emotions [and] [...] understanding"* were *"key to keeping us moving forward together"* and at the same time, helped her cope with the distress of reading the Intergovernmental Panel on Climate Change (IPCC) report about what a climate-altered future will look like. *"[I knew] if I went to people in Generation Zero and said I had to read the IPCC 2018 Report, they'd be like, 'oh, man, are you OK? Can I buy you a coffee? How are you feeling?'"* (interview, 2019).

Despite the emotional support provided by Generation Zero, members found it an ongoing challenge to sustain community. A number of people left after the ZCA was passed, which they called "ageing out". The ZCA was described as carrying Generation Zero's "organisational energy for so long" (Avery, interview, 2019), and while its passing was considered a significant achievement, some participants expressed disappointment and anger because politicians "water[ed] down some of the most important parts of the Act" (Dewy, interview, 2019). The ZCA work was described by many as all-consuming, and although some were focused on the next steps, others were relieved it was over: *"I am looking forward to not having to lobby for the ZCA anymore"* (Jai, interview, 2019).

Youth leaders of the Auckland SS4C articulated their educational needs during a panel discussion with teachers organised by the NZ Association for Environmental Education and documented by Sally. The leaders focused largely on accessible resources that would help them, and their teachers, learn about climate change and develop action-taking skills (Birdsall, 2019). They also discussed their anxiety and despair at the lack of progress on climate change, echoing the distress and plea for action articulated by some of Karen's Generation Zero interviewees (see also Nairn, 2019). As Steven, one of Karen's participants, said, the zero carbon goal actually belongs to *"the larger community […] who are part of this broader movement […] towards […] a more progressive and just society"* (interview, 2019). So how can we, as teachers and allies, support young people's climate activism?

The New Zealand Curriculum (Ministry of Education, 2007) directs learning in the nation's schools and reveals opportunities for classroom teaching. For example, the document provides a set of principles to underpin curriculum decision-making, one of which is "Future Focus". This principle encourages students to look to the future through the lenses of sustainability, citizenship and globalisation. There is even a mandate for students to work alongside people in their community aiming to ensure sustainable "social, cultural, physical and economic environments" (Ministry of Education, 2007, p. 13).

A scant handful of formal resources are available, such as the *Climate Change Learning Programme*, where students learn about the science of climate change and explore ways of taking action and preserving well-being (Ministry of Education, 2020a; 2020b). While these resources have been welcomed by educators, they have a strong emphasis on individual responses, like choosing to walk or ride a bike, and eating less meat.

They also fail to address the emotional landscape that accompanies climate politics. As well as despair and anxiety, this includes the hostility and anger directed at activists such as Greta Thunberg, along with ecological guilt about one's impact on the planet (Bryan, 2020; Holmberg & Alvinius, 2020; Nairn, 2019). If teachers and students explore this emotional landscape, they may be able to see a way forward that works with people's feelings, concerns and contexts rather than overlooking or judging them. Such a process also builds solidarity as articulated in Olivia's earlier quotation (see also Bryan, 2020).Schools are in many ways ideal sites for the extended learning needed, as students and teachers meet regularly and over long periods.

A core part of this process should be the fostering of hope. As we imagine possible futures, hope, as both a cognitive and affective construct (Snyder, 1995), enables people to plan and motivate themselves to take appropriate action (Li & Monroe, 2017). Action also fosters hope in a cycle articulated by Generation Zero interviewees. For Rhys: "if you're in a wider community that's working together then it can build that sense of hope or that sense of optimism, and a vision for the future that is achievable" (interview, 2018; see also Nairn, 2019).

The educative approach briefly outlined here is built from listening to young climate activists, and could be a valuable part of society's response to the climate emergency. Schools serve *all* young people and so have considerable reach, providing a training ground for active citizenship. Groups comprised largely of young adults, such as Generation Zero, may then be more readily refreshed by new members. However, the international call of SS4C remains: adults must take decisive, legislative action.

Summary and reflection

As educational scholars, Sally and Karen show how the formal NZ school curriculum can help create solidarity for collective action and be a training ground for active citizenship, as demonstrated by Generation Zero. Moving into the discussion, we take with us this question: as a discipline focused on understanding and working with people in their full psychological depth, what can Community Psychology contribute to, and learn from, research on youth activism from allied disciplines?[2]

Discussion

The four vignettes offered here showcase work based in Aotearoa New Zealand from a variety of disciplines, each aimed at understanding and facilitating vibrant "communities of action" for the environment. All are experimenting with, and advocating for, different ways of living that must be negotiated alongside the myriad of other values, assumptions and practices that underpin contemporary life. Success is unpredictable and always partial. For example, Pūniu River Care saw an explosion of interest but struggles with volunteer commitment (as do many community gardens, see also Drake & Lawson, 2015); Generation Zero helped achieve Aotearoa New Zealand's Zero Carbon Act but some members were disappointed with the compromises involved.

In one sense these communities are driven from the bottom by people committed to action for the environment. But they have also been supported by high-level structures including a mandate from the school's governance board in the case of WSCW's sustainability culture, and government legislation that has enabled environmental restoration driven by Māori. The opportunities Sally and Karen outlined for teachers to support young climate activists through the formal school curriculum also provide an intriguing example of working with macro-level structures to change the priorities of the system as a whole.

Community psychologists are experienced at drawing from all levels of the social-ecological system to facilitate the well-being of the communities they serve (e.g. Christens & Perkins, 2008; Riemer et al., 2016) and place considerable emphasis on power. However, the communities of action discussed here go beyond a focus on human power relations and insist on coming back to the tangible and shared foundation of all life. For some the importance of nature is explicitly woven into the community's story of itself, for example in Te Kerekere and Daniel Hikuroa's vignette on the work of Māori to restore the *mauri* (holistic health, life force) of their ancestral places. But no matter their foundational narrative, all the vignettes reflect that Papatūānuku (Earth-mother) responds only to how we as people interact with her, not to how we interact with each other.

Having said that, the communities discussed recognise both the importance of robust human relationships to effective action *and* that action for the environment builds relationships. In relation to the first two vignettes, we ended by asking how to encourage commitment to environmental protection and/or food production in a fractured, contemporary world. Can Community Psychology help with this process of engagement?

By using and sharing our skills, values and experience as people who pay close attention to community building (see Krause & Montenegro, 2017; Lazarus, Seedat, & Naidoo, 2017), the answer may be a tentative yes. This work is not intuitive or straightforward and activist groups often implode due to destructive interpersonal dynamics (see Harré, Tepavac, & Bullen, 2009; Smucker, 2017). Community building is assisted by semi-formal practices that consciously shape these processes (Block, 2008; Harré, 2018). Notably, collective practices of welcoming new people and ideas, holding regular meetings, and providing food, listening and support were a key part of the WSCW project and may have contributed to its resilience (Blythe et al., 2013; Harré et al., 2021).

But no matter how good communities of action for the environment are at managing interpersonal dynamics (or community psychologists are at assisting with this), voluntary work with the land is always accompanied by issues of mobility and ownership. The WSCW project overcame this to some extent by focusing on a locality the students and staff inhabit daily. Many successful community gardens are also tended by local residents (Fox-Kämper et al., 2018; Ritchie, 2017; Firth et al., 2011).

The Māori world view encourages commitment to collectively owned land that is storied with ancestral links, in keeping with the relational stories of place common to indigenous people (Coope, 2019; Marsden, 2003; Williams, 2019). However, these stories do not easily align with most people's lives in industrialised societies. In their emphasis on historical continuity of kinship with a particular place, these stories also cannot work in their original form for non-indigenous people who are more recent arrivals (see e.g. Roberts et al., 1995). We are, then, left with the possibility of an ethic that calls us all to be guardians of the land *we occupy* and to recognise the interconnection between *all* living systems on Earth. This ethic is already at the heart of ecopsychology (Fisher, 2002) and, we argue, could help inform a Community Psychology that extends to the biosphere. It is also an ethic that makes sense of nationally and globally focused climate activism.

The final insight from our communities of action that we wish to draw attention to, is the deeply psychological nature of this work, shown especially in the intense emotionality outlined in the vignette on youth climate activism(see also Clayton & Karazsia, 2020). Disappointment, anger, despair, guilt and distress are some of the emotions described. Generation Zero, while highly focused on legislative change, was also recognised by participants as a space in which they could express these feelings and be understood. In this way the community is therapeutic, helping members make collective sense of the threatened world they inhabit. "Hope" was described as a key motivator for continued climate change action, due to its link to the future (Hicks, 2014; Nairn, 2019), and we add, to the human story more generally. That communities all over the world are doing this work is in large part what makes local efforts worthwhile, especially in relation to global issues. Community Psychology as a discipline that aims to understand and work alongside people in context, must surely pay attention to the struggle for hope in communities focused on protecting the biosphere.

In closing, we see this work as based on identifying and working with possibilities throughout the social system, rather than emphasising resistance and critique. While the particulars of our communities are specific to Aotearoa Zealand, we suggest their struggles and successes resonate with similarly focused communities in other parts of the globe; and that Community Psychology's values and skills in supporting people and community building have much to contribute. Ultimately, we offer our chapter as a contribution to the global effort to protect and regenerate the natural world and hence ourselves as part of it.

Notes

1 Aotearoa was originally used by some Māori to refer to New Zealand's North Island. Aotearoa New Zealand is now commonly used to refer to the whole country; this is how we use it here.
2 Some participants' real names are used (with their permission) while others have code names or are not named if there is a risk of identification; we do not distinguish between these approaches to ensure confidentiality of those who chose the latter option.

References

Alaimo, K., Reischl, T.M., & Allen, J.O. (2010). Community gardening, neighborhood meetings, and social capital. *Journal of Community Psychology, 38*(4), 497–514. https://doi.org/10.1002/jcop.20378

Armstrong, D. (2000). A survey of community gardens in upstate New York: Implications for health promotion and community development. *Health & Place, 6*(4), 319–27. https://doi.org/10.1016/S1353-8292(00)00013-7

Birdsall, S. (2019). *What do our student climate strikers want?* https://naaee.org/eepro/blog/what-do-our-student-climate-strikers

Block, P. (2008). *Community: The structure of belonging.* Berrett-Koehler Publishers.

Blythe, C., Harré, N., Sharma, S., Dillon, V., Douglas, B., & Didsbury, A. (2013). Guiding principles for community engagement: Reflections on a school-based sustainability project. *Journal of Social Action in Counselling and Psychology, 5*(3), 44–69.

Bretherton, F. (1988). *Earth system science: A closer view. A program for global change.* The Committee on Earth System Science, National Aeronautics and Space Administration.

Bryan, A. (2020). Affective pedagogies: Foregrounding emotion in climate change education. *Policy and Practice: A Development Education Review, 30*, 8–30. www.developmenteducationreview.com/issue/issue-30/affective-pedagogies-foregrounding-emotion-climate-change-education

Capra, F., & Luisi, P.L. (2014). *The systems view of life: A unifying vision.* Cambridge University Press.

Chan, K.M.A., Balvanera, P., Benessaiah, K., Chapman, M., Díaz, S., Gómez-Baggethun, E., … Turner, N. (2016). Opinion: Why protect nature? Rethinking values and the environment. *Proceedings of the National Academy of Sciences, 113*(6), 1462–5. https://doi.org/10.1073/pnas.1525002113

Chapman, J. (2004). *System failure: Why governments must learn to think differently* (2nd ed.). Demos.

Checkland, P., & Scholes, J. (1990). *Soft systems methodology in action.* John Wiley.

Christens, B., & Perkins, D.D. (2008). Transdisciplinary, multilevel action research to enhance ecological and psychopolitical validity. *Journal of Community Psychology, 36*(2), 214–31.

Clayton, S., &Karazsia, B.T. (2020). Development and validation of a measure of climate change anxiety. *Journal of Environmental Psychology, 69*, 101434. https://doi.org/10.1016/j.jenvp.2020.101434

Coope, J. (2019). How might Indigenous traditional ecological knowledge (ITEK) inform ecopsychology? *Ecopsychology, 11*(3), 156–61. https://doi.org/10.1089/eco.2019.0005

Daftary-Steel, S., Herrera, H., & Porter, C.M. (2015). The unattainable trifecta of urban agriculture. *Journal of Agriculture, Food Systems, and Community Development, 6*(1), 19–32. https://doi.org/10.5304/jafscd.2015.061.014

Dawson, B. (2010). *A history of gardening in New Zealand.* Random House.

Díaz, S., Settele, J., Brondízio, E.S., Ngo, H.T., Agard, J., Arneth, A., … Zayas, C.N. (2019). Pervasive human-driven decline of life on Earth points to the need for transformative change. *Science, 366*(6471), eaax3100. https://doi.org/10.1126/science.aax3100

Doherty, T.J. (2009). A peer reviewed journal for ecopsychology. *Ecopsychology, 1*(1), 1–7.

Drake, L., & Lawson, L.J. (2015). Results of a US and Canada community garden survey: Shared challenges in garden management amid diverse geographical and organizational contexts. *Agriculture and Human Values, 32*(2), 241–54. https://doi.org/10.1007/s10460-014-9558-7

Eames, C., Cowie, B., & Bolstad, R. (2008). An evaluation of characteristics of environmental education practice in New Zealand schools. *Environmental Education Research, 14*, 35–51.

Earle, M. (2011). *Cultivating health: Community gardening as a public health intervention* [Unpublished master's thesis]. Wellington School of Medicine and Health Sciences, University of Otago.

Firth, C., Maye, D., & Pearson, D. (2011). Developing "community" in community gardens. *Local Environment, 16*(6), 555–68. https://doi.org/10.1080/13549839.2011.586025

Fisher, A. (2002). *Radical ecopsychology: Psychology in the service of life.* State University of New York Press.

Fox-Kämper, R., Wesener, A., Münderlein, D., Sondermann, M., McWilliam, W., & Kirk, N. (2018). Urban community gardens: An evaluation of governance approaches and related enablers and barriers at different development stages. *Landscape and Urban Planning, 170*, 59–68. https://doi.org/10.1016/j.landurbplan.2017.06.023

Freire, P. (1970/1996). *Pedagogy of the oppressed*. Penguin Books.

Gridley, H., & Breen, L.J. (2007). So far and yet so near? Community psychology in Australia. In S.M. Reich, M. Riemer, I. Prilleltensky, & M. Montero (Eds.), *International community psychology: History and theories* (pp. 119–63). Springer.

Harré, N. (2018). *Psychology for a better world: Working with people to save the planet*. Auckland University Press.

Harré, N. (2019). Let's assume people are good: Rethinking research in community psychology. *The Australian Community Psychologist, 30*(1), 81–91.

Harré, N., Blythe, C., McLean, L., & Khan, S. (2021). A people-focused systems approach to sustainability. *American Journal of Community Psychology*. https://doi.org/10.1002/ajcp.12550

Harré, N., Madden, H., Brooks, R., & Goodman, J. (2017). Sharing values as a foundation for collective hope. *Journal of Social and Political Psychology, 5*(2), 342–66. https://doi.org/10.5964/jspp.v5i2.742

Harré, N., Tepavac, S., & Bullen, P. (2009). Integrity, efficacy and community in the stories of political activists. *Qualitative Research in Psychology, 6*(4), 330–45.

Hassan, Z. (2014). *The social labs revolution*. Berrett-Koehler Publishers.

Hawe, P. (2017). The contribution of social ecological thinking to community psychology: Origins, practice, and research. In M.A. Bond, I.E. Serrano-García, C.B. Keys, & M.E. Shinn (Eds.), *APA handbook of community psychology: Theoretical foundations, core concepts, and emerging challenges* (Vol. 1) (pp. 87–105). American Psychological Association.

Hicks, D. (2014). *Educating for hope in troubled times: Climate change and the transition to a post-carbon future*. Institute of Education Press.

Holmberg, A., & Alvinius, A. (2020). Children's protest in relation to the climate emergency: A qualitative study on a new form of resistance promoting political and social change. *Childhood*. https://doi.org/10.1177/0907568219879970

Kaufman, J., & Bailkey, M. (2000). *Farming inside cities: Entrepreneurial urban agriculture in the United States*. Lincoln Institute of Land Policy.

Krause, M., & Montenegro, C. R. (2017). Community as a multifaceted concept. In M.A. Bond, I.E. Serrano-García, C.B. Keys, & M.E. Shinn (Eds.), *APA handbook of community psychology: Theoretical foundations, core concepts, and emerging challenges* (Vol. 1) (pp. 275–94). American Psychological Association.

Lawlor, J.A., & Neal, Z.P. (2016). Networked community change: Understanding community systems change through the lens of social network analysis. *Journal of Community Psychology, 57*(3/4), 426–36.

Lazarus, S., Seedat, M., & Naidoo, T. (2017). Community building: Challenges of constructing community. In M.A. Bond, I.E. Serrano-García, C.B. Keys, & M.E. Shinn (Eds.), *APA handbook of community psychology: Methods for community research and action for diverse groups and issues* (Vol. 2) (pp. 215–34). American Psychological Association.

Li, C.J., & Monroe, M. (2017). Exploring the essential psychological factors in fostering hope concerning climate change. *Environmental Education Research*. https://doi.org/10.1080/13504622.2017.136916

Little, P. (2010). Common ground. *New Zealand Gardener, 66*(January), 15–21.

Marsden, R.M. (2003). *The woven universe*. Te Wānanga-o-Raukawa.

IPBES. (2019, May 6). *UN Report: Nature's dangerous decline "unprecedented"; species extinction rates "accelerating."* United Nations Sustainable Development. www.un.org/sustainabledevelopment/blog/2019/05/nature-decline-unprecedented-report

Ministry of Education. (2007). *The New Zealand curriculum*. Ministry of Education.

Ministry of Education. (2020a). *Climate change learning programme – Teacher resource*. https://nzcurriculum.tki.org.nz/Curriculum-resources/Education-for-sustainability/Tools-and-resources

Ministry of Education. (2020b). *Climate change learning programme – Wellbeing guide*. https://nzcurriculum.tki.org.nz/Curriculum-resources/Education-for-sustainability/Tools-and-resources

Moskell, C., & Allred, S.B. (2013). Integrating human and natural systems in community psychology: An ecological model of stewardship behavior. *American Journal of Community Psychology, 51*(1–2), 1–14. https://doi.org/10.1007/s10464-012-9532-8

Nairn, K. (2019) Learning from young people engaged in climate activism: The potential of collectivizing despair and hope. *Young, 27*(5), 435–50. https://doi.org/10.1177/1103308818817603

Neal, J.W., & Neal, Z.P. (2013). Nested or networked? Future directions for ecological systems theory. *Social Development, 22*(4), 722–37. https://doi.org/10.1111/sode.12018

Nelson, G., Lavoie, F., & Mitchell, T. (2007). The histories and theories of community psychology in Canada. In S.M. Reich, M. Riemer, I. Prilleltensky & M. Montero (Eds.), *International community psychology: History and theories* (pp. 13–36). Springer.

Patel, R. (2009). Food sovereignty. *The Journal of Peasant Studies, 36*(3), 663–706. https://doi.org/10.1080/03066150903143079

Patel, R., & Moore, J.W. (2018). *A history of the world in seven cheap things: A guide to capitalism, nature, and the future of the planet.* University of California Press.

Perkins, D.D., & Schensul, J.J. (2017). Interdisciplinary contributions to community psychology and transdisciplinary promise. In M.A. Bond, I.E. Serrano-García, C.B. Keys, & M.E. Shinn (Eds.), *APA handbook of community psychology: Theoretical foundations, core concepts, and emerging challenges* (Vol. 1, pp. 189–209). American Psychological Association.

Porter, C.M. (2018). What gardens grow: Outcomes from home and community gardens supported by community-based food justice organizations. *Journal of Agriculture, Food Systems, and Community Development, 8*(Suppl 1), 187–205. https://doi.org/10.5304/jafscd.2018.08A.002

Pudup, M.B. (2008). It takes a garden: Cultivating citizen-subjects in organized garden projects. *Geoforum, 39*(3), 1228–40. https://doi.org/10.1016/j.geoforum.2007.06.012

Riemer, M., & Harré, N. (2017). Environmental degradation and sustainability: A community psychology perspective. In M.A. Bond, I. Serrano-García, C.B. Keys & M.Shinn (Eds.), *APA handbook of community psychology: Methods for community research and action for diverse groups and issues* (Vol. 2, pp. 441–55). American Psychological Association.

Riemer, M., Voorhees, C., Dittmer, L., Alisat, S., Alam, N., Sayal, R., … Schweizer-Ries, P. (2016). The Youth Leading Environmental Change project: A mixed-method longitudinal study across six countries. *Ecopsychology, 8*, 174–87. https://doi.org/10.1089/eco.2016.0025

Ritchie, I.P. (2016). *Shared lunch: An ethnography of food sovereignty in Whaingaroa and beyond* [Unpublished PhD dissertation]. University of Waikato.

RNZ. (2020). Students call for climate action restart after COVID-19. www.rnz.co.nz/news/environment/422063/students-call-for-climate-action-restart-after-covid-19

Roberts, M., Norman, W., Minhinnick, N., Wihongi, D., & Kirkwood, C. (1995). Kaitiakitanga: Maori perspectives on conservation. *Pacific Conservation Biology, 2*, 7–20.

Robson, S. (2019, October 16). *Auckland City Mission: 10% of Kiwis experiencing food insecurity.* RNZ. www.rnz.co.nz/news/national/401082/auckland-city-mission-10-percent-of-kiwis-experiencing-food-insecurity

Rose, N. (2013). *Optimism of the will: Food sovereignty as transformative counter-hegemony in the 21st century* [Unpublished PhD dissertation]. College of Design and Social Context, Royal Melbourne Institute of Technology.

Smucker, J M. (2017). *Hegemony how-to: A roadmap for radicals.* AK Press.

Snyder, C.R. (1995). Conceptualizing, measuring, and nurturing hope. *Journal of Counseling & Development, 73*, 355–60.

Soga, M., Gaston, K.J., & Yamaura, Y. (2017). Gardening is beneficial for health: A meta-analysis. *Preventive Medicine Reports, 5*, 92–9. https://doi.org/10.1016/j.pmedr.2016.11.007

Steel, C. (2008). *The hungry city: How food shapes our lives.* Vintage Books.

Swords, A., Frith, A., & Lapp, J. (2018). Community-campus collaborations for food justice. *Journal of Agriculture, Food Systems, and Community Development, 8*(A), 261–77. https://doi.org/10.5304/jafscd.2018.08A.009

Taylor, J.R., & Lovell, S.T. (2014). Urban home food gardens in the Global North: Research traditions and future directions. *Agriculture and Human Values, 31*(2), 285–305. https://doi.org/10.1007/s10460-013-9475-1

Te Arawhiti. (2020). *Treaty Settlements Quarterly Report 1 July 2019–30 June 2020.* Te Kāhui Whakatau (Treaty Settlements), Te Arawhiti. www.govt.nz//assets/Documents/OTS/Quarterly-reports/Quarterly-report-to-30-Jun-2020.pdf

Todd, N.R. (2012). Religious networking organizations and social justice: An ethnographic case study. *American Journal of Community Psychology, 50*(1–2), 229–45. https://doi.org/10.1007/s10464-012-9493-y

Townrow, C., Laurence, N., Blythe, C., Long, J., & Harré, N. (2016). The Maui's Dolphin Challenge: Lessons from a school-based litter reduction project. *Australasian Journal of Environmental Education, 32*(3), 288–308.

Urban Farmers' Alliance. (2020). *Our 11 key outcomes.* www.urbanfarmersalliance.org.nz/11-key-outcomes

Wals, A.E.J., & Dillon, J. (2013). Conventional and emerging learning theories: Implications and choices for educational researchers with a planetary consciousness. In R.B. Stevenson, M. Brody, J. Dillon &A.E.J. Wals (Eds.), *International handbook of environmental education research* (pp. 253–61). Routledge.

Williams, L. (2019). Reshaping colonial subjectivities through the language of the land. *Ecopsychology, 11*(3), 174–81. https://doi.org/10.1007/s10464-012-9493-y 10.1089/eco.2018.0077

17

EXPLORING THE ECOTONE OF CRITICAL FOOD STUDIES IN COMMUNITY PSYCHOLOGY

A framework for addressing well-being through food system transformation

Mirella L. Stroink, Charles Z. Levkoe and B. Mackenzie Barnett

Abstract

The acquisition and consumption of food plays a major role in human well-being. It shapes culturally significant symbols, social ties and practices, and relationships with natural environments. The dominant food system is global, and capitalist in nature, and has led to many challenges in respect to equity and sustainability. In this chapter, we introduce the interdisciplinary and emerging field of food studies and put it into conversation with Community Psychology to surface a framework that leverages the areas of intersection between these fields of scholarship (i.e., ecotone) for examining psycho-social-ecological well-being through food, emphasising a systems perspective, critical scholarship and action-oriented engagement in place.

Resumen

La adquisición y el consumo de alimentos juega un papel importante en el bienestar humano y da forma a los símbolos, lazos y prácticas sociales de importancia cultural y a las relaciones con los entornos naturales. El sistema alimentario dominante es global y de naturaleza capitalista, y ha dado lugar a muchos desafíos entorno a la equidad y la sostenibilidad. En este capítulo, presentamos el campo interdisciinario y emergente de los estudios alimentarios y lo ponemos en conversación con la psicología comunitaria para sacar a la luz un marco que aproveche las áreas de intersección entre estos campos de investigación (es decir, el ecotono) para examinar el bienestar psico-social-ecológico a través de la comida, que enfatiza las perspectivas de los sistemas, la erudición crítica y el compromiso orientado a la acción.

Food links individual bodies to the earth itself and is essential to physical, psychological and social health. The ways we acquire, prepare, consume and dispose of food are inherently social processes, connecting individuals to social groups and cultures, and to economic and political

DOI: 10.4324/9780429325663-21

systems that facilitate and constrain these processes. In Community Psychology (CP), research relating to food has focused largely on individual health, such as disordered eating and nutrition, as well as on community-level processes such as food insecurity, poverty and psychological sense of community. There has been relatively little research from CP that critically examines or addresses the larger crises in the numerous linked systems and processes, from the ecological to the economic, that bring food to people's plates.

Food systems refer to the collective processes and interactions involved in the production/harvesting, processing, distribution, consumption, and disposal of food. Critical scholars refer to the dominant food system as global, capitalist and corporate in nature (Holt-Giménez, 2017). While able to provide plentiful food in some places and to some people, this system is a cause for growing concern for the health and well-being of people, communities, and the earth. Crises of the dominant food system include deep social inequities, soil degradation, agrarian distress, contamination of the oceans and depleting fish populations, highly dangerous agricultural occupations, diet-related disease, and inequities in terms of access to safe and nutritious food (Koç et al., 2016; De Schutter, 2017).

CP has the potential to play a larger role in understanding and critically questioning the dominant food system and its impact on people and communities. The acquisition and consumption of food drives human behaviour, from individual beliefs and behaviour to socially coordinated behaviour in families, organisations and communities spanning to the global scale. Food behaviour shapes culture, and food is rooted in culture. Food systems reflect unique histories, places and sociopolitical systems, and are shaped by historic and recent events including conflict, geopolitical agreements and trade routes. Food systems are also impacted by social systems of racialisation, gender, class and other social locations, and are a key mediator of our relationships with and impact on our ecological systems (Tansey & Worsley, 2014). Food is also deeply personal; food preferences develop with family history, personality and early childhood experiences, as well as with genetics, allergies and intolerances (Beckerman et al., 2017).

The purpose of this chapter is to establish a framework to support research on the role of community psychological factors in the emergence of food systems and to mobilise the praxis of CP towards empowering community-level transformative change in relation to food systems. We argue that to critically study and address well-being and the multiscale nature of food systems, a more expansive and interdisciplinary framework is required. To do so, we draw upon the concept of ecotone, which describes the area of transition or the edges between ecosystems (Kagan, 2007). Specifically, we explore the edges between CP and the field of food studies (FS) to propose a framework to better study and address psycho-social-ecological well-being through food systems scholarship. This framework interweaves the strengths of both CP and FS to identify novel insights and approaches. It also draws from our own work as a network of researchers and community organisations in Northwestern Ontario, Canada, and our decades of partnerships and projects. The ecotone framework for addressing well-being through food includes three interrelated themes: (1) a systems perspective, (2) a critical approach and (3) a commitment to place-based engagement and action.

We begin by introducing our network of community organisations and multidisciplinary researchers, grounded in place. We then introduce the fields of CP and FS and explore their edges through the three themes that support the ecotone framework. These themes are then explored along with their applications in our own research. We conclude with opportunities for future exploration.

Nourishing communities: the Northwestern Ontario Network

Our work is grounded in the people and places of Northwestern Ontario, Canada – signatory to the Robinson Superior Treaty of 1850, Treaty #3, Treaty #5 and Treaty #9. Ontario is a centrally located province which is home to the highest number of inhabitants of any in Canada (~14.7 million, Statistics Canada, n.d.). Northwestern Ontario is one region within this province, comprising nearly 60% of its area while home to less than 2% of its human population (~231,000, Statistics Canada, 2017). Considering square kilometres, Northwestern Ontario is roughly the size of Thailand, Yemen or Spain. Ecologically, the region includes a portion of the world's largest, intact boreal forest, and borders the world's largest freshwater lake, Lake Superior. It is also home to tens of thousands of other lakes, rivers, and streams, and many non-human animals such wolves, bears and lynx. In addition, there is an abundance of wild or country foods, such as native fish and wild meats (e.g. moose, grouse), mushrooms, rice and berries (Nelson et al., 2019). These foods may be challenging to access given competing land uses (e.g. mining, logging), potential contamination of sources of wild foods, and loss of traditional skills related to hunting, fishing and gathering (Stroink & Nelson, 2012).

Nourishing Communities was established in 2007 by a group of university faculty, students, and community-based practitioners across Canada that came together to collaborate on research related to equitable and sustainable food systems (see http://nourishingontario.ca; this network evolved into a larger research partnership called Food: Locally Embedded, Globally Engaged, see https://fledgeresearch.ca/). Within the network, a group of scholars based at Lakehead University and a range of community partners (some recent and some continuing from an earlier network; see www.fsrn.ca) made up the Northwestern Ontario Node and have engaged in a range of food systems projects for many years using various methods (see Table 17.1 for a summary of selected research projects and partnerships). As researchers, one recurring theme in our approach to partnerships has been taking the stance of "being in community," embracing our multiple roles as community members, activists and academics (Harrison et al., 2013).

The authors of this paper have been involved in various ways with the network. We engage in this work as scholar-activists (two faculty – Mirella Stroink and Charles Levkoe – and one graduate student of clinical psychology – Mackenzie Barnett) at a midsize university. We worked together to write and muse about the intersections between human (internal psychological processes, those of communities and social systems) and planetary health. We next introduce the fields of CP and FS and bring them together to explore their ecotone.

Community Psychology

In Canada, Community Psychology (CP) emerged from the Psychology Department at the University of Toronto with the work of its first chair, Edward Bott, in the 1920s and developed across Canada along the same lines as in other Western countries, with a particular emphasis on various forms of oppression, including sexism, homophobia, the processes of colonization in Canada and treatment of its indigenous peoples (Nelson et al., 2007). Along with other Western community psychologists, we study people in interaction with the layered systems of their context and do so with an action orientation and an ecological systems approach. By focusing on the interdependency of individuals and their social and societal settings, we draw on knowledge of psychological processes within and between people, and on knowledge of community and societal processes through an inherently interdisciplinary perspective. Our CP is a scholarship of community-based action, aiming to understand and improve the well-being of individuals by building empowerment, engaging participation and by targeting preventative

Table 17.1 Selected projects from the Northwestern Node of Nourishing Communities

Project and Date	Description	Source
Five case studies of food hub projects in northern Ontario: complex systems theory and the adaptive cycle as a lens (2011–2013)	Case studies of five local food hub initiatives that included a greenhouse, two food co-operatives, a community service-learning research network and the region's district health units. It explored the development of each hub and their interactions with the capitalist food system and policy environment through the lens of CAS theory, drawing on the concept of the adaptive cycle.	Stroink & Nelson (2013)
Social Economy of Food (2016–2019)	This partnership project examined social economy initiatives across Canada. Three case studies were examined in Northwestern Ontario including a local food co-operative, a social enterprise promoting growth through creative expression, and a set of four case studies of blueberry foraging initiatives. Analysis of unique northern aspects of these social economy initiatives and in the lens of CAS theory were provided.	Kakegamic, R. , Nelson, C., Levkoe, C.Z. (2017). Nelson, Stroink, Levkoe, Kakagemic, McKay, Streutker, & Stolz (2019) Nelson &Stroink (2020) Stephens, Nelson, Levkoe, Mount, Knezevic, Blay-Palmer, Martin (2019). Social Economy of Food: Cloverbelt Local Food Coop (2019). Social Economy of Food: Aroland Blueberry Initiative (2019). Social Economy of Food: Willow Springs Creative Centre (2019). Social Economy of Food: Nipigon Blueberry Blast (2019). Stolz, W., Levkoe, C.Z., & Nelson, C. (2017, September). Streutker, A., Levkoe, C.Z., & Nelson, C. (2017).
An investigation into the local and traditional ecological knowledge of the Saugeen Ojibway Nation regarding the status of ciscoes in Lake Huron (2018–2020)	This partnership project with the Saugeen Ojibway Nation (SON) and researchers at Lakehead University and Queens University explored the contributions of indigenous ecological knowledge to fisheries governance and social-ecological relationships through community-based research with fishers and knowledge keepers.	Duncan (2020). Lowitt, et al. (2019).

Table 17.1 Cont.

Project and Date	Description	Source
Confronting settler colonialism in food movements (2018–2020)	This collaborative community-engaged research project involved scholars from Lakehead University and William Angliss Institute in Australia concerned about the limited studies of settler colonialism within food movements. The project involved individuals working in settler-led food movement organisations in Northwestern Ontario and in Southern Australia.	Bohunicky, Levkoe & Rose (2021). Bohunicky, M. (2020).
Agroecology and seed sovereignty in Northern Ontario (2018–2021)	This partnership project was led by Lakehead University's Sustainable Food System Lab and worked with local and national non-profit organisations including Roots to Harvest, the Superior Seed Producers, Root Cellar Gardens, the Bauta Family Initiative on Seed Security and the Lake Superior Living Labs Network. The project aimed to improve knowledge, skills and capacity to produce healthy and sustainable food in Northwestern Ontario. A series of ecological seed trials were established, research with local seed savers was conducted, and a series of virtual workshops on planting, cultivation, harvesting, preserving and seed saving were offered.	Laforge, Dale, Levkoe, & Ahmed (2021). Levkoe, Portinga, Van Blyderveen, & McIllfaterick (2021) Levkoe, Van Blyderveen, & Stephens (2019). Seed Saving and Agroecology (2020).

and transformative social change efforts at multiple levels of community and society (Kagan et al., 2020).

In this context of Canadian CP, we seek to address psychological, social and ecological health in examining and reimagining contemporary food systems. To do so we build upon the interdisciplinarity of CP and open a conversation with the interdisciplinary field of FS.

Food studies

FS is an emerging field of scholarship that explores the social and ecological relationships as well as the processes and structures that bring food from the fields, forests and watersheds to our plates. The study of food-related issues in academia is not new; however, it is only in the past two decades that FS has been identified as a comprehensive area of study (Koç et al., 2016).

FS is an eclectic field of study with an expanding range of issues and viewpoints being brought to the table. Common elements that characterise FS are:

i. the use of food as a lens to interrogate social and ecological phenomena across scales, from the individual and the household levels to the community, region and beyond. Here, food is often used as a tool to connect various elements that operate in isolation such as historical and anthropological aspects of food and eating (Murcott et al., 2013), identity and culture (Counihan & Van Esterik, 2012), food provisioning (Morgan et al., 2008), consumption and health (Mason & Lang, 2017), and governance, policy and regulation (Andrée et al., 2019). In this way, FS aims to "read the world" through food (Sumner, 2013).
ii. bringing together a wide range of interdisciplinary approaches across the social sciences, arts and humanities, health sciences, and increasingly the natural sciences (Albala, 2013). Beyond simply combining approaches, FS has benefited from an analysis that integrates multiple ways of knowing to derive new insights and approaches.
iii. the evolution of FS as an engaged approach to scholarship that integrates theory and practice, articulates distinct research methods and advocates engaged teaching and learning (e.g. Levkoe, Brem-Wilson, & Anderson, 2019).

CP and FS: an emerging ecotone framework

In order to strengthen CP action research on food system issues, we bring CP together with the field of FS and explore their ecotone. We highlight three themes for addressing well-being through a food systems lens that includes (1) a systems perspective; (2) critical scholarship; and (3) commitment to place-based engagement and action.

For each of these themes, CP and FS offers unique perspectives, and at the edges where these perspectives meet there are novel insights and opportunities. It should be noted that while we address CP and FS separately in this chapter for the heuristic purpose of exploring their conceptual ecotone, in practice the two disciplines are already intertwined, with food studies research published in Community Psychology journals and community psychologists conducting food studies research (e.g. Freedman & Bess, 2011). Similarly, the three themes intersect and support one another, but are described separately to highlight their essence and application.

Systems perspective

The first theme at the ecotone of CP and FS is a shared tendency to adopt a systems perspective. In our own work, we explicitly draw upon complex adaptive systems (CAS) theory as a theoretical lens (Goldstein, 2008; Gunderson & Holling, 2001; Mitchell, 2011). CAS theory originated from the ecological sciences, rooted in non-linear and dynamic systems theories, and is associated with social-ecological systems theory. Our proposed framework draws explicitly on CAS theory.

Systems perspectives in CP

Systems perspectives are fundamental to CP, as individuals and organisations comprise interdependent and adaptive agents in many nested and interacting community systems. Indeed, the very focus of the discipline is on understanding the person as interdependent within a wider context of layered social systems, unique in this way from its parent discipline of psychology (Riemer et al., 2020). Systems theory principles, in particular soft systems methodologies (Checkland & Scholes, 1999), continue to shape CP research and practice (Kelly, 2006). However, in many CP interventions the focus remains on single issues operating at one or two system levels (e.g. family and local community), and systems perspectives remain largely theoretical in the discipline. There is also a tendency to neglect the ecological level in systems analyses of human and community well-being, with notable exceptions (e.g. Moskell & Allred, 2013).

Systems perspectives in FS

FS scholars often critique research for studying individual elements of the food system (e.g. farming, hunger, health etc.) without recognising the relationships and interconnections between them (Levkoe, 2011). FS scholars that take a more critical approach consider the various elements that bring food to our plates and the many forces impacting activities across the food chain as an interactive and interdependent web (Tansey and Worsley, 2014). The food system is composed of multiple actors at many different scales interacting with each other in non-linear ways that influence the overall behaviour of the system. To understand the inner workings of a food system, we must also look to influencing factors such as ecosystems (e.g. water, soil, energy), policy and governance (e.g. rules, laws, and regulations), and culture and identity. Although the components are important to identify and explore, it is the relationships among the various components that make the food system function. Furthermore, food is embedded within multiple and overlapping systems that are also interconnected and interdependent.

Critical scholarship

A second theme found at the ecotone of CP and FS is the centring of critical perspectives. Critical scholarship builds on a range of theoretical approaches that describe the ways that power flows through and controls systems and impacts social and environmental well-being. A commonality among these approaches is that they go beyond abstract theoretical insights and have an explicit goal of social and environmental transformation. For the purposes of our framework, critical scholarship is considered a form of resistance against dominant modes of power that are predicated on injustice, exploitation and oppression and draw on political economy, political ecology, anti-colonialism and feminism.

Critical scholarship in CP

Being critical as a community psychologist is understood to be an engaged process, undertaken by both researchers and professional bodies (Montero, 2011). Critical CP attempts to address the causes of human suffering through liberatory means, and recognises that "people are the agents of their own liberation" (Kagan et al., 2020, p. 31). Liberation in this sense is not limited to individual freedoms, and instead refers to a movement of collective societal change. In this way criticality involves an adherence to certain morals and social aims and cannot be conceptualised as merely any psychological work done in consideration of community.

A critical lens also shifts the focus of CP from the local community to global systems of both oppression and social movements for liberation. Without this perspective, uncoordinated actions at the local scale risk remaining isolated and incapable of addressing systems issues. This does not negate the need for local action. However, critical community psychologists should engage in place-based projects while remaining conscious of the broader systems within which communities are embedded, and the power relations within and between these systems. For example, Bell (2016) describes how colonialism and white supremacy have led to ongoing police violence, crime and segregation of those of African descent in modern-day Jamaica. Their team developed a reggae opera which might enhance the critical consciousness of its audience. Thus, being critical involves recognising and attending to these larger patterns of power and oppression and adopting a decolonial stance. As community psychologists, it is imperative that we continue to question our own approaches to criticality and to infuse critic-ality into the practice of CP itself (Montero, 2011).

Critical scholarship in FS

Beyond simply explaining the elements of the food system, many FS scholars have adopted critical analytical tools to understand how power and control permeate the systems that bring food to our plates. Much of this work is premised on the fact that there is more than enough food produced and harvested to feed the world's current population, yet more than two billion people continue to have insufficient access to safe, nutritious food (FAO et al., 2019). This means that solutions do not need to find ways to increase production but must address inequi-ties and power dynamics underlying who has access to food and who does not. Moreover, it demands a critical look at the structures underlying the dominant food system that promote business as usual.

Building on traditional academic approaches, FS brings insights from social movement theory and practice to inform evolving critical scholarship. For example, investigations into the flows of power have played a role in shaping FS by examining the ways that race, gender, capit-alism and settler colonialism have shaped food systems over time and in particular places (Alkon & Agyeman, 2011). These critical lenses have been applied to a range of elements within food systems to address the underlying and systemic causes of inequity that lead to corporate con-centration, poverty and food insecurity, and the climate crisis (Koç et al., 2016). In the vein of critical reflexivity, these questions have been asked not only of food systems but also of FS scholars themselves (Bellows et al., 2018).

Place-based action and engagement

The third theme at the ecotone between CP and FS is their mutual adoption of action-based research. Action-based research refers to an orientation as well as a set of practices which involve ongoing cycles of reflection, data collection and action in pursuit of producing knowledge which is practical for people in their everyday lives and/or addresses critical social issues (Kagan et al., 2010). It challenges a positivist philosophy, favouring a worldview which underscores that we are all participants, "part-of, rather than apart from" our reality (Reason & Bradbury, 2008, p. 10).

Action research then has the potential to be enacted as a liberatory practice, one which strives for improving human flourishing and challenging systems of inequity. Action-based research avoids mechanically following a particular methodology. In its ideal form it disrupts notions of who is capable of producing and using knowledge, challenging conventional paradigms that relegate participation of certain groups to being subjects of research or recipients of services (Gaventa & Cornwall, 2008), instead placing the involvement of those impacted by the research at its core. It also involves embracing complexity and community-specific nuances on what might be larger, systemic problems. While action-research teams may look to broader trends, findings or methods, engaging with place-specific social and ecological realities is essential (Montero, 2011).

Action-based research in CP

Action-based research is close to the very essence of CP as a discipline and draws directly from its values and commitment to social change. The approach taken to action research in CP is participatory and emphasises empowerment with careful attention to the particular place or context of the work. Indeed, CP has made many contributions to the evolution of community-based participatory (action) research as a multidisciplinary research method (e.g. Lazarus et al., 2015). To this effort to study and address the conditions of well-being at the level of social, community and institutional processes, CP contributes numerous models, approaches and theories of social change.

Action-based research in FS

Many food studies scholars have adopted an action-based approach as a core part of their practice. Reynolds et al. (2018) have described these approaches as scholar-activism in an explicit attempt to blur the lines between academic research and being actively engaged in supporting community-based food movement struggles. Much of this work has been rooted in examples of and/or calls for scholars to act in solidarity with activists in resistance to dominant corporate industrial food systems (Alkon & Guthman, 2017). Wakefield (2007) writes about the opportunities for food movements combining theory and action to create more just and sustainable food systems. Food justice and food sovereignty are social movement discourses that have played a significant role in shaping the evolution of food systems scholarship. Food systems scholarship has incorporated practical and applied research that includes action-based methodologies which engage practitioners and activists and aim to have a real impact on food systems. For example, reflecting on their experiences of collaborative action-based food systems scholarship, Levkoe et al. (2019) propose a food sovereignty research praxis with three pillars – humanising research partnerships, upsetting unequal power relationships and seeking transformation of the food system.

Applying the ecotone framework

We have identified and introduced three themes at the ecotone between CP and FS. In this section we build on the strengths of both fields through these themes to provide a conceptual space at their ecotone. This analysis deepens critical understanding of pan-system processes and reveals systems variables that could be addressed through place-based and engaged action. We examine this ecotone through our reflections on our partnerships and our research projects on food systems in Northwestern Ontario within the Nourishing Communities Network, which involves scholars from both CP and FS. The examples provided in the following analysis draw from the sources listed above in Table 17.1.

Systems perspectives at the ecotone

CP and FS share a systems perspective, yet both are limited in the degree of elaboration of systems concepts. Thus, at their ecotone, our proposed framework draws out this perspective and incorporates CAS theory to provide a closer examination of the systems dynamics that impact well-being through food. Furthermore, CP and FS each tend to examine a limited range of systems involved, with CP focusing on community and social systems, and FS providing greater focus on macro social and ecological systems. At their ecotone, this framework leverages this combination and adds the systems processes operating within the individual as well (e.g. meaning-making processes etc.). The CAS concepts of the *adaptive cycle* and *panarchy* (Gunderson & Holling, 2001) have been particularly useful. The adaptive cycle describes four phases of change in CAS, from diverse *growth* through increasing structure and *conservation* of resources, through a *release* of system structure followed by a phase of *reorganisation* prior to new growth (Gunderson & Holling, 2001). These four phases have been evidenced in ecological and social systems including food systems (e.g. Walker et al., 2009; Stroink & Nelson, 2013), and suggested in psychological systems (Stroink, 2020).

The *panarchy* concept is useful in describing the processes that link systems across levels from the psychological (e.g. meaning system) and physical (e.g. digestive system) at the individual level outward through social and ecological systems (Stroink, 2020). These levels are nested within and mutually influence each other across scale through the adaptive cycle both by triggering cascading release phases (called *revolt*) and by constraining and shaping each other's growth (called *remembering*).

CAS theory has served as a lens to facilitate our observations, analysis and action in relation to the food system for many years. For example, Stroink and Nelson (2013) reviewed five case studies of community "hub" initiatives that sought to enhance availability or access to locally produced food in Northwestern Ontario. Among the insights of this work was that the development of each initiative could be tracked through the adaptive cycle and were interdependent with other systems. For example, one greenhouse initiative for growing vegetables formed out of the release of human and physical capital in a tree seedling business that did not survive the downturn in the forest product industry. There have also been many examples of small local food organisations struggling to grow within the constraints presented by the *remembering effect* of the surrounding systems in the panarchy, such as provincial food policies and regulations which suit the needs and interests of more populated areas in Southern Ontario. As an example of psychological systems and their interdependence with other social and ecological systems, in one set of case studies on the social economy of food we observed the particular role of people's attachment to the land as a driver of land-based food behaviour. The people involved, both indigenous and settlers, sought ways to support their own and others' emotional connection to the land through food activities including through blueberry festivals and horticultural therapy (Nelson & Stroink, 2020).

By specifying and articulating systems processes through CAS theory, this framework enables closer examination of the processes that link the level of psychological systems through to political, economic, and ecological systems. In this way we go beyond the mere use of systems language to examine the system as a whole. This is particularly essential in addressing food as an issue for CP because food weaves through all these levels and impacts well-being through processes that emerge at each level as well as through the interactions among different levels. A systems perspective also helps us see the work of the "node" itself not as a series of disconnected projects but as interdependent and nested within other systems, evolving dynamically over time in adaptive cycles as each project builds on previous relationships and findings.

Critical scholarship at the ecotone

Both CP and FS offer insight into critical perspectives. At their ecotone, the framework draws on their respective strengths and builds on the systems perspective to articulate how the dynamics of social power flow reciprocally through food between the level of individual thought and behaviour and the level of social and ecological systems. For community psychologists interested in engaging with food system issues, critical FS theory and research provide tools to critically address systemic social, political, economic and historical factors that result in inequity and harm to people and our planet. To this task, community psychologists bring their own tools for advancing liberation through engaged social change, as well as the tools of social psychology for examining processes that operate within and sustain systems of oppression, such as implicit prejudice, implicit theories and stigma. By imagining the entire system in the lens of CAS theory, we may be able to identify key leverage points towards altering the dynamics of power, loosening select structures to release resources from conservation and reorganise aspects of food systems for more equitable, just and healthy outcomes.

The critical scholarship theme also reminds us to turn the critical gaze back on both disciplines to encourage reflexivity, continual learning, and evolution in scholarship. In particular, we note the need to work together towards greater diversity and Black, indigenous, People of Color leadership in both FS and CP research and education. This includes the need to bring community-based learning (Hart & Akhurst, 2017) into the psychology curriculum to ensure that students are able to integrate their psychology training with a critical understanding of the wider context. The emerging framework at the ecotone of CP and FS encourages a systemic and critical approach to examining the many interacting factors that drive the dominant food system towards ill health and inequity for individuals and communities, and the possibilities for new approaches to emerge.

Our research projects have adopted a critical approach, moving beyond simple descriptors to explore underlying power relations. Much of our research in north-western Ontario has worked with indigenous people, or in solidarity with indigenous food sovereignty efforts, to focus on patterns of settler colonialism and extractive capitalism in understanding our unique local reality which removed indigenous peoples from their land and sought to eradicate their culture and their personhood (Truth and Reconciliation Commission of Canada, 2015). Such settler-colonial logics are rampant and evidenced by the systemic racism found in local police departments (OIPRD, 2019), and documented in health, justice and other social service systems, as well as between community members (Haiven, 2019). In recognising connections to broader social movements (such as food sovereignty, anti-colonialism, anti-racism, agroecology), and the particulars of living in this region, it becomes possible to conduct transformative work with and through our food systems. Indeed, the region is home to many folks dedicated to addressing systems challenges and bolstering psycho-social-ecological well-being through food systems work.

The Confronting Settler Colonialism in Food Movements project (Bohunicky, et al., 2021) is one example of critical scholarship at the ecotone. It was initiated from conversations with several settler-led food movement organisations in Northwestern Ontario and in Southern Australia that recognised the limited engagement of food movements with issues of settler colonialism. While the flows of power within food systems are being explored, there has been less work addressing the ways that the dominant food system has been built on the systematic erasure of indigenous peoples. While food movements aim to create more equitable and sustainable food systems, a failure to address issues of settler colonialism risks them being complicit in injustices of a food system built on capitalism and white supremacy. Through a community-engaged research project, conversations were held with individuals working in settler-led food movement organisations. Findings revealed three intersecting categories that synthesised participants' experiences and observations: (1) expressions of settler inaction; (2) mere inclusion of indigenous peoples and ideas; and (3) productive engagements and visions to confront settler colonialism. A continuum was proposed that explained the ways that organisations might address settler colonialism in their food systems work – from situating our(settler)selves within the framework of settler colonialism to (re)negotiating relationships with indigenous peoples to actualising productive positions of solidarity with indigenous struggles. From this study, the researchers argued that confronting settler colonialism demands "dynamic, place-based engagements through which settlers overcome fragility and inclusion of Indigenous Peoples that primarily benefits settlers and fails to redistribute power" (Bohunicky et al., 2021, p. 139).

In another example of the critical perspective in the ecotone framework, Nelson and Stroink (2019) report on the unique northern aspects of four social economy initiatives (reported more fully in Nelson et al., 2019). In these case studies the capitalist economy as an organising system for food was seen as particularly limited in the northern context, where the greater distance among communities and their remoteness from larger centres make people reluctant to count exclusively on the capitalist economy for food. The limitations of the provincial policy environment were again evident where, for example, blueberry foraging is constrained by legislation focusing on resource extraction (timber, mining), which makes even the application for permits difficult.

Place-based engagement and action at the ecotone

Given the centrality of place-based, participatory and engaged approaches to action research in both CP and FS, the proposed framework at their ecotone likewise emphasises this approach, drawing upon the many examples and tools available from both perspectives. For community psychologists seeking to address the health and well-being of people through food, we suggest critically identifying systemic interactions within and across scales and targeting these through interventions to maximise system level change, incorporating reflection and participatory evaluation and analysis.

The research projects from the Northern Node have all been action-based and/or engaged. Each project evolved from the needs and interests of communities and was developed to support goals and objectives of the communities involved. For example, the SON fisheries project (Lowitt et al., 2019) was developed and conducted in partnership with members of the SON located in the Saugeen (Bruce) Peninsula (note: the SON is made up of two representative bands, the Chippewas of Nawash Unceded First Nation No. 27 and the Chippewas of Saugeen First Nation No. 29). The research team adopted a two-eyed seeing approach that embraces both Western science and indigenous ways of knowing, while also recognising and respecting the distinctions between them. Evolving from needs expressed by the SON fishing community, the research investigated how indigenous ecological knowledge could better inform fisheries governance and social-ecological relationships with ciscoes (a species of fish) in Lake Huron. Specifically, it focused on the cultural and socio-economic importance of ciscoes and involved one-on-one conversations with fishers along with interactive mapping activities to identify past and present harvest locations, movement and spawning locations. The findings enabled the research team to make connections between broader scholarly debates and place-based experiences of the SON fish harvesters. Beyond gaining a better understanding of ciscoes, the results contributed to: enhancing connection of the fisheries to Ojibway culture, ideology and spirituality; demonstrating the value of indigenous ecological knowledge to decision-making about the fisheries; SON's self-determination as a sovereign First Nation. Beyond the specific project, the research has already led to broader partnerships and the recent acquisition of a grant from the Great Lakes Fisheries Commission to continue this work.

The Agroecology and Seed Sovereignty in Northern Ontario project (e.g. Laforge et al., 2021) provides another example of place-based engagement and action at the ecotone. Working with multiple partners from Northwestern Ontario and from across Canada, the team conducted research focusing on ways to improve knowledge, skills and capacity to produce healthy and sustainable food in Northwestern Ontario. The participatory breeding project was originally established to conduct ecological seed trials in the region in connection with a national farmer-led research network to determine which vegetable varieties could be optimised for specific geographic locations and organic growing. The seeds were grown in three different locations and the data was analysed locally and in comparison to other trials across the country. Public tasting events were held to solicit feedback on the quality of the produce. The data was used to determine which seeds to save and plant in future years. The research team also worked with the partners to conduct interviews with seed savers in Northwestern Ontario to explore the direct and indirect health benefits related to community seed saving. The research was used to create a series of practical workshops on issues of interest to the community. These included a range of topics such as planting, cultivation, harvesting, preserving and seed saving. The team also worked with the indigenous Food Circle (a network of indigenous-led and indigenous-serving organisations in the Thunder Bay region) to offer a workshop and share heritage seeds with First Nations.

Conclusion – future possibilities

In this chapter, we have presented a framework at the ecotone of CP and FS that brings a critical systems perspective and a commitment to action research and engagement to the study of the psycho-social-ecological dimensions of well-being through food. With its aim of understanding and addressing well-being at the level of community and social systems, CP integrates well with FS and is well positioned for impact in this area. Indeed, while we have presented the two fields as separate, they are already enmeshed with each other as both emphasise interdisciplinarity and many FS scholars come from a CP background.

There are numerous opportunities for future research to make use of the ecotone framework, drawing upon a systemic, critical and action-based approach. Food systems have a substantial impact on the physical and social settings of communities, and this impacts the formation of social ties and relationships. Furthermore, these ties will differ depending on social location. For example, while alternative food systems initiatives can offer local and sustainable food options, as well as social settings that support community engagement, access to these initiatives often have significant barriers (e.g. location, price). This can render such options ineffective at addressing underlying social inequities and may have an impact on community development and well-being. Thus, one line of research could examine and support a range of initiatives in generating social settings that raise awareness of the flows of power and oppression within food systems while providing spaces that enhance both physical access to nutritious food and opportunities to form social ties and linkages. In addition, further research might continue to develop the ecotone framework by exploring additional applications. This work might extend beyond northern Ontario and North America to include community food systems initiatives in different geographies and at different scales. We recognise that our lens represents one of many that are necessary to address psycho-social-ecological change through food systems, and we look forward to this work adding to a body of complexity and interdisciplinary scholarship in both the Global North and South.

References

Albala, K. (Ed.). (2013). *Routledge international handbook of food studies*. Routledge.
Alkon, A., & Agyeman, J. (Eds.). (2011). *Cultivating food justice: Race, class, and sustainability*. MIT Press.

Alkon, A., & Guthman, J. (Eds.). (2017). *The new food activism: Opposition, cooperation, and collective action.* University of California Press.

Andrée, P., Clark, J.K., Levkoe, C.Z., & Lowitt, K. (2019). *Civil society and social movements in food system governance.* Taylor & Francis.

Beckerman, J.P., Alike, Q., Lovin, E., Tamez, M., & Mattei, J. (2017). The development and public health implications of food preferences in children. *Frontiers in Nutrition, 4*, 66. https://doi.org/10.3389/fnut.2017.00066

Bell, D. (2016). A raison d'être for making a reggae opera as a pedagogical tool for psychic emancipation in (post)colonial Jamaica. *International Journal of Inclusive Education, 20*(3), 278–91. https://doi.org/10.1080/13603116.2015.1047657

Bellows, A., Welsh, R., Ludden, M., & Alfaro, B.(2018). *Promotion and tenure, journals and impact factor in the field of food studies.* A Report to the Professional Societies: Agriculture Food and Human Values. Association of Food and Society, Canadian Association for Food Studies.

Bohunicky, M. (2020). *Confronting settler colonialism in food movements.* [Master's thesis]. Lakehead University, Thunder Bay, Ontario.

Bohunicky, M., Levkoe, C.Z., & Rose, N. (2021).Working for justice in food systems on stolen land? Interrogating food movements confronting settler colonialism. *Canadian Food Studies/La Revue canadienne des études sur l'alimentation, 8*(2), 137–165.

Checkland, P., & Scholes, J. (1999). *Soft systems methodology in action.* John Wiley.

Counihan, C., &Van Esterik, P. (Eds.). (2012). *Food and culture: A reader.* Routledge.

De Schutter, O. (2017). The political economy of food systems reform. *European Review of Agricultural Economics, 44*(4), 705–31. https://doi.org/10.1093/erae/jbx009

Duncan, A.T. 2020. An investigation into the local and traditional knowledge of the Saugeen Ojibway Nation regarding the status of ciscoes (*Coregonus* spp.) in Lake Huron. [Master's thesis]. Lakehead University, Thunder Bay, Ontario.

FAO, IFAD, UNICEF, WFP &WHO. 2019. *The state of food security and nutrition in the world 2019. Safeguarding against economic slowdowns and downturns.* FAO.

Freedman, D., & Bess, K. (2011). Food systems change and the environment: Local and global connections. *American Journal of Community Psychology, 47*(3), 397–409. https://doi.org/10.1007/s10464-010-9392-z

Gaventa, J., & Cornwall, A. (2008). Power and knowledge. In P. Reason, & H. Bradbury (Eds.), *The SAGE handbook of action research* (pp. 172–89). Sage. www.doi.org/10.4135/9781848607934

Goldstein, J. (2008). Conceptual foundations of complexity science: Development and main constructs. In M. Uhl-Bien and R. Marion (Eds.). *Complexity Leadership Part 1: Conceptual Foundations.* (pp. 17–48). Information Age Publishing.

Gunderson, L., & Holling, C.S. (Eds.). (2001). *Panarchy: understanding transformations in human and natural systems.* Island Press.

Haiven, M. (2019, February 13). The colonial secrets of Canada's most racist city. *ROAR magazine.* https://roarmag.org/essays/colonial-secrets-canadas-racist-city/

Harrison, B., Nelson, C.H., & Stroink, M.L. (2013). Being in community: A food security themed approach to public scholarship. *Journal of Public Scholarship in Higher Education, 3*, 91–110.

Hart, A., & Akhurst, J. (2017). Community-based learning and critical community psychology practice: Conducive and corrosive aspects. *Journal of Community & Applied Social Psychology, 27*(1), 3–15. https://doi.org/10.1002/casp.2287

Holt-Giménez, E. (2017). *A foodie's guide to capitalism.* Monthly Review Press.

Kagan, C. (2007).Working at the edge: Making use of psychological resources through collaboration. *The Psychologist, 20*(4), 224–7.

Kagan, C., Burton, M., & Siddiquee, A. (2010). Action research. In S. Willig (Ed.), *The SAGE handbook of qualitative research in psychology* (pp. 32–53). Sage.

Kagan, C., Burton, M., Duckett, P., Lawthom, R., & Siddiquee, A. (2020). *Critical community psychology: Critical action and social change.* Routledge.

Kakegamic, R., Nelson, C., Levkoe, C.Z. (2017). Willow Springs Case Study. (2017). http://nourishingontario.ca/willow-springs-creative-centre

Kelly, J. (2006). *Being ecological. An expedition into community psychology.* Oxford University Press.

Koç, M., Sumner, J., & Winson, A. (2016). *Critical perspectives in food studies.* Oxford University Press.

Laforge, J., Dale, B., Levkoe, C.Z., & Ahmed, F. (2021). The future of agroecology in Canada: Embracing the politics of food sovereignty. *Journal of Rural Studies, 81*, 194–202.

Lazarus, S., Bulbulia, S., Taliep, N., & Naidoo, A.V. (2015). Community-based participatory research as a critical enactment of community psychology. *Journal of Community Psychology, 43*(1), 87–98.

Levkoe, C.Z. (2011). Towards a transformative food politics. *Local Environment, 16*(7), 687–705.

Levkoe, C.Z., Brem-Wilson, J., & Anderson, C.R. (2019). People, power, change: Three pillars of a food sovereignty research praxis. *Journal of Peasant Studies, 46*(7), 1389–412.

Levkoe, C.Z., Portinga, R.L.W., Van Blyderveen, J., & McIllfaterick, E. (2021). *Agroecology and seed sovereignty in Northern Ontario, 2019–2020.* The Lakehead University Agricultural Research Capacity Development Program. Thunder Bay, Ontario. https://livinglabs.lakeheadu.ca/partner-organizations/https-livinglabs-lakeheadu-ca-partner-organizations-lakehead-university-labyrinth-learning-community/lakehead-university-agricultural-research-station/

Levkoe, C.Z., Van Blyderveen, J., & Stephens, A. (2019). *Ecological agriculture, food security and economic prosperity in Northern Ontario, year one report, 2018–2019.* The Lakehead University Agricultural Research Capacity Development Program. https://livinglabs.lakeheadu.ca/partner-organizations/https-livinglabs-lakeheadu-ca-partner-organizations-lakehead-university-labyrinth-learning-community/lakehead-university-agricultural-research-station/

Lowitt, K., Levkoe C.Z., Lauzon, R., Ryan, K., & Seyers, D. (2019). Indigenous self-determination and food sovereignty through fisheries governance in the Great Lakes Region. In P. Andrée, J.K. Clark, C.Z. Levkoe, & K. Lowitt (Eds.), *Civil society and social movements in food system governance* (pp. 145–163). Routledge.

Mason, P., & Lang, T. (2017). *Sustainable diets: How ecological nutrition can transform consumption and the food system.* Taylor & Francis.

Mitchell, M. (2011). *Complexity: A guided tour.* Oxford University Press.

Montero, M. (2011). A critical look at critical community psychology. *Social and Personality Psychology Compass, 5*(12), 950–9. https://doi.org/10.1111/j.1751-9004.2011.00403.x

Morgan, K., Marsden, T., & Murdoch, J. (2008). *Worlds of food: Place, power, and provenance in the food chain.* Oxford University Press on Demand.

Moskell, C., & Allred, S.B. (2013). Integrating human and natural systems in community psychology: An ecological model of stewardship behavior. *American Journal of Community Psychology, 51*(1), 1–14. https://doi.org/10.1007/s10464-012-9532-8

Murcott, A., Belasco, W., & Jackson, P. (Eds.). (2013). *The handbook of food research.* Bloomsbury Publishing.

Nelson, C., Stroink, M., Levkoe, C.Z., Kakagemic, R., McKay, E., Streutker, A., & Stolz, W. (2019). Understanding social economy through a complexity lens: Four case studies in Northwestern Ontario. *Canadian Food Studies/La Revue canadienne des études sur l'alimentation, 6*(3), 33–59.

Nelson, C.H., & Stroink, M.L. (2020). Exploring the unique aspects of the northern social economy of food through a complexity lens. *Northern Review, 49*, 7–38. http://doi.org/10.22584/nr49.2019.007.

Nelson, G., Lavoie, F., & Mitchell, T. (2007). The history and theories of community psychology in Canada. In S.M. Reich, M. Riemer, I. Prilleltensky, & M. Montero (Eds.), *International community psychology* (pp. 13–36). Springer US.

Office of the Independent Police Review Director (OIPRD). (2019). *Broken trust: Indigenous people and the Thunder Bay Police Service.*

Reason, P., & Bradbury, H. (2008). *The SAGE handbook of action research participative inquiry and practice* (2nd ed.). Sage.

Reynolds, K., Block, D., & Bradley. K. (2018). Food justice scholar-activism and activist-scholarship: Working beyond dichotomies to deepen social justice praxis. *ACME: An International E-Journal for Critical Geographies, 17*(4), 988–98.

Riemer, M., Reich, S.M., Evans, S.D., Nelson, G., & Prilleltensky, I. (2020). *Community Psychology: In pursuit of liberation and wellbeing.* Red Globe Press.

Seed Saving and Agroecology. (2020). Lake Superior Living Labs Network Sustainability Stories Video Series. https://livinglabs.lakeheadu.ca/partner-organizations/https-livinglabs-lakeheadu-ca-partner-organizations-lakehead-university-labyrinth-learning-community/sustainability-stories-video-series/

Social Economy of Food: Cloverbelt Local Food Coop. (2019). Social Economy of Food. Nourishing Communities. [Video]. YouTube. Sheba Films. www.youtube.com/watch?v=O3Jz6I6-pjI

Social Economy of Food: Aroland Blueberry Initiative. (2019). Social Economy of Food. Nourishing Communities. [Video]. YouTube. Sheba Films. https://www.youtube.com/watch?v=mtvB4uaWxxc

Social Economy of Food: Willow Springs Creative Centre. (2019). Social Economy of Food. Nourishing Communities. [Video]. YouTube. Sheba Films. www.youtube.com/watch?v=sjPX9G6XAzo

Social Economy of Food: Nipigon Blueberry Blast. (2019). Social Economy of Food. Nourishing Communities. [Video]. YouTube. Sheba Films. https://www.youtube.com/watch?v=iDeot4p8Ano

Statistics Canada. (n.d.). Table 17-10-0009-01Population estimates, quarterly. https://doi.org/10.25318/1710000901-eng

Statistics Canada. (2017). Northwest [Economic region], Ontario and Ontario [Province] (table). Census Profile. 2016 Census. Statistics Canada Catalogue no. 98-316-X2016001. Ottawa. Released November 29, 2017. www12.statcan.gc.ca/census-recensement/2016/dp-pd/prof/index.cfm?Lang=E

Stephens, P., Nelson, C., Levkoe, C.Z., Mount, P., Knezevic, I., Blay-Palmer, A., & Martin, M.A. (2019). A perspective on social economy and food systems: Key insights and thoughts on future research. *Canadian Food Studies/La Revue canadienne des études sur l'alimentation, 6*(3), 5–17.

Stolz, W., Levkoe, C.Z., & Nelson, C. (2017, September). Blueberry foraging as a social economy in Northern Ontario. A case study of Aroland First Nation, Arthur Shupe Wild Foods, Nipigon Blueberry Blast Festival, and the Algoma Highlands Wild Blueberry Farm and Winery. (2017). Centre for Sustainable Food Systems. http://nourishingontario.ca/blueberry-foraging-as-a-social-economy-in-northern-ontario

Streutker, A., Levkoe, C.Z., & Nelson, C. (2017). The Cloverbelt Local Food Co-op Case Study. (2017). http://nourishingontario.ca/the-cloverbelt-local-food-co-op

Stroink, M. (2020). The dynamics of psycho-social-ecological resilience in the urban environment: A complex adaptive systems theory perspective. *Frontiers in Sustainable Cities.* https://doi.org/10.3389/frsc.2020.00031

Stroink, M.L., & Nelson, C.H. (2012). Understanding local food behaviour and food security in rural First Nation communities: Implications for food policy. *The Journal of Rural and Community Development, 7*(4),24–41.

Stroink, M.L., & Nelson, C.H. (2013). Complexity and food hubs: Five case studies from Northern Ontario. *Local Environment, 18*(5), 620–35. http://dx.doi.org/10.1080/13549839.2013.798635.

Sumner, J. (2013). Food literacy and adult education: Learning to read the world by eating. *Canadian Journal for the Study of Adult Education, 25*(2), 79–92.

Tansey, G., & Worsley, A. (2014). *The food system.* Routledge.

Truth and Reconciliation Commission of Canada. (2015). The survivors speak. http://nctr.ca/assets/reports/Final%20Reports/Survivors_Speak_English_Web.pdf

Wakefield SEL. (2007).Reflective action in the academy: Exploring praxis in critical geography using a "food movement" case study. *Antipode, 39*(2), 331–54.

Walker, B. H., Abel, N., Anderies, J. M., & Ryan, P. (2009). Resilience, adaptability, and transformability in the Goulburn-Broken Catchment, Australia. *Ecology and Society, 14*(1), 12. http://www.ecologyandsociety.org/vol14/iss1/art12/

18

COMMUNITY SOCIAL PSYCHOLOGY AND NATURE CONSERVATION

Alejandra Olivera-Méndez and Marcelo Calegare

Abstract

Natural protected areas (NPAs) are an expression of the dichotomy in modern society in which nature is both exploited as a merchandise and preserved untouched. People living nearby or within NPAs are facing the challenge of surviving modern demands, while keeping their traditions. The ecological crisis involves a transdisciplinary effort, and community social psychology (CSP) can contribute by aiding conservation whilst improving the communities' quality of life. This chapter focuses on the contributions of CSP to nature conservation in Brazil's and Mexico's NPAs, which involves local individuals and communities as well as their non-human inhabitants. Rural communities lose their resilience capabilities when they no longer have control of the decisions taken. The challenge is to give them back their voices so they can participate in the management of the NPAs in which they live. Examples of CSP's contribution to participatory processes and governance endeavours in the Brazilian Amazon region are provided. At the same time, CSP can contribute to stopping biodiversity loss by working with the community members in understanding the interaction between wildlife and humans, and finding ways for both to coexist in the same regions. We will illustrate this with examples of studies in Mexico. Life on this planet depends upon a complex and integrated balance of human well-being and nature conservation. Local communities have the right to govern their own territories, and CSP has several tools and methods that can be useful to make this happen, whilst conserving our planet's resources.

Resumen

Las áreas naturales protegidas (ANPs) son una expresión de la dicotomía en la sociedad moderna, donde la naturaleza es tanto explotada, como preservada. La gente viviendo cerca o dentro de las ANPs está enfrentando el reto de las demandas modernas de supervivencia, al mismo tiempo que mantienen sus tradiciones. La crisis ecológica implica un esfuerzo transdisciplinario, y la psicología social comunitaria (PSC) puede contribuir apoyando a la conservación y mejorando la calidad de vida de las comunidades. Este capítulo se enfoca en las contribuciones de la PSC a la conservación de la naturaleza en ANPs de Brasil y México, involucrando a individuos y comunidades locales, así como a los habitantes no humanos. Las comunidades rurales pierden

DOI: 10.4324/9780429325663-22

sus capacidades de resiliencia cuando pierden el control de las decisiones que se toman. El reto es regresarles su voz para que puedan participar en el manejo de las ANPs en las que viven. Se proporcionan ejemplos de la contribución de la PSC en procesos participativos y de gobernanza en la amazona brasileña. Asimismo, la PSC puede contribuir a detener la pérdida de biodiversidad, trabajando con los miembros de las comunidades para entender la interacción entre fauna silvestre y humanos, y buscando formas para que ambos coexistan. Esto se ilustra con ejemplos de estudios en México. La vida en este planeta depende de un balance complejo e integrado entre el bienestar de los seres humanos y la conservación de la naturaleza. Las comunidades locales tienen el derecho de gobernar sus propios territorios, y la PSC cuenta con varias herramientas y métodos que pueden ser útiles para lograrlo, al mismo tiempo que se conserven los recursos del planeta.

Introduction

This chapter focuses on the contributions of Community Social Psychology (CSP) to nature conservation in Brazil and Mexico's natural protected areas (NPAs), which involves the voice of local individuals and communities as well as its non-human inhabitants. Each of us authors worked on NPAs in his/her respective country, having met at the 5th International Conference on Community Psychology, in 2014. Since then, we have been interacting through the Latin American Rural Psychology network and exchanging experiences. This chapter is the result of this interaction and expresses our joint reflections on the theme of nature conservation using the work we have done in our countries as examples.

First, we need to understand what we mean by nature conservation and why it is important that community social psychologists participate in it. When we talk about nature, we are referring to the biological diversity that underpins it. The term "biological diversity", better known as biodiversity, according to the UN Convention on Biological Diversity (CBD), is defined as "the variability among living organisms from all sources including, inter alia, terrestrial, marine and other aquatic ecosystems and the ecological complexes of which they are part; this includes diversity within species, between species and of ecosystems" (CBD, 2020). Basically, we are talking about all life on Earth.

Biodiversity is vital for many reasons. It provides humans with several benefits obtained from its ecosystem services. Stolton et al. (2015) synthesise these services into four types: supporting, provisioning, regulating and cultural (see Figure 18.1). Supporting services are those required for the maintenance of all others, such as soil formation, nutrient cycling, species interactions, seed dispersal and the maintenance of genetic, species and habitat diversity. Provisioning services encompass the provision of resources such as food, water, raw material, medicinal and biochemical resources, ornamental, and genetic resources. Regulating services include air, water and soil purification, pollination, and the regulation of climate, natural hazards, water availability and flow, erosion and soil fertility, and pests and diseases. Finally, cultural services refer to all non-material benefits obtained from the ecosystem like recreation and tourism opportunities, inspiration, aesthetics, spiritual/religious experience, cultural identity and heritage, mental well-being and information for education and research.

Biodiversity varies from ecosystem to ecosystem, making the resources limited and not evenly distributed (Bertzky et al., 2015). Around the world, the threats to biodiversity are growing, mostly due to human-related activities. Among the efforts to prevent biodiversity loss, the establishment of NPAs is the most commonly implemented worldwide.

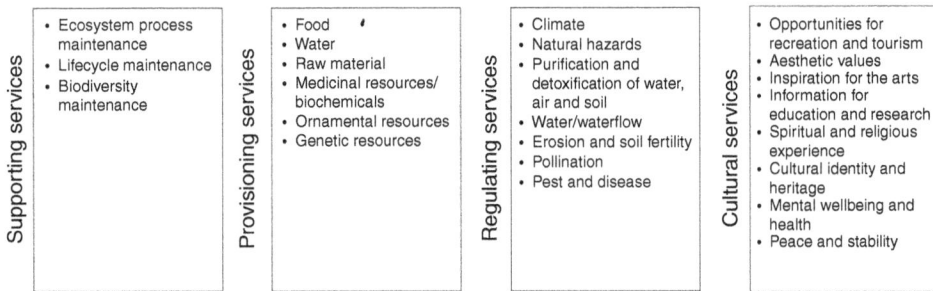

Supporting services	Provisioning services	Regulating services	Cultural services
• Ecosystem process maintenance • Lifecycle maintenance • Biodiversity maintenance	• Food • Water • Raw material • Medicinal resources/ biochemicals • Ornamental resources • Genetic resources	• Climate • Natural hazards • Purification and detoxification of water, air and soil • Water/waterflow • Erosion and soil fertility • Pollination • Pest and disease	• Opportunities for recreation and tourism • Aesthetic values • Inspiration for the arts • Information for education and research • Spiritual and religious experience • Cultural identity and heritage • Mental wellbeing and health • Peace and stability

Figure 18.1 Ecosystem services and related goods from protected areas

Note: Adapted from Stolton et al. (2015)

Natural protected areas

According to the definition of the International Union for Conservation of Nature (IUCN), an NPA is "a clearly defined geographical space, recognised, dedicated and managed, through legal or other effective means, to achieve the long-term conservation of nature with associated ecosystem services and cultural values" (IUCN, 2020). This modern concept of protected areas developed in the late 19th century following a heightened concern over the exponentially growing change of land use, environment deterioration and extinction of wild species, and a longing to retain natural landscapes (Calegare & Higuchi, 2013; Diegues, 2008; Worboys, 2015a).

NPAs are the main instruments for nature conservation, providing a wide range of environmental services for the benefit of humans and other life beings. Protected areas support human livelihoods, allow people to connect with nature, support life and healthy environments, protect culture and heritage, bring sustainable development benefits through tourism and are critical for mitigating climate change, among other direct and indirect benefits provided (Sandwith, MacKinnon, & Hoeflich, 2015; Worboys, 2015a; Worboys, 2015b).

Although the establishment, governmental regulations and professional management of protected areas is a fairly recent phenomenon, its concept has existed long before (Worboys, 2015a). Some of the earliest locally based environmental protection efforts were based on the spiritual association with the natural world represented in sacred cultural places (Feary et al., 2015). Recently, there has been a recognition that the cultural heritage and social value of nature has to be considered in the management of NPAs. To truly achieve this, we need to include local people in the organisation and governance of protected areas.

Rural communities lose their resilience capabilities when they no longer have control of the decisions taken. The challenge is to give them back their voices so they can participate in the management of the NPAs in which they live. Examples of CSP's contribution to local organisation and governance endeavours in the Brazilian Amazon region are provided. At the same time, CSP can contribute to stopping biodiversity loss by working along with the community members in understanding the interaction between wildlife and humans, and finding way for both to coexist in the same regions. We will illustrate this with examples of studies in Mexico. But first, we need to briefly understand the history of protected areas in both Brazil and Mexico.

Protected areas in Brazil

Between the 16th and 18th centuries, the Portuguese crown established very few initiatives aimed at the Brazilian colony for the protection of nature, carrying them out only with isolated and vertical actions to protect renewable resources of economic value. In the 19th century, with the change of the Portuguese court to the Americas and later with the establishment of the Empire of Brazil, the crown ordered the creation of some protected forest spaces, but without there being an imperial policy for the protection of nature. Only from the 1930s, in the Republican period, was there a delimitation of parts of the national territory for nature conservation, by the establishment of the Constitution and the Forest Code of 1934. From that moment on, nature gained national heritage and protected status, initially with the creation of the Itatiaia National Park in 1937 (Rios, 2004; Medeiros, 2006; Medeiros, Irving, & Garay, 2006).

The NPA model adopted in Brazil followed that of North American national parks, whose central idea was to keep pieces of the natural, pure and primitive world free from human presence, to inspire and entertain visitors with great scenic beauty (Diegues, 2008). However, the adoption of this model has undergone reconfigurations in Brazil due to the historical processes related to the continental, megadiverse and pluricultural dimension of the country; the legal-normative instruments adopted in the creation of the different areas; and the disputes between strict preservationists and conservationists (Calegare, Higuchi, & Bruno, 2014). This resulted in the creation of different types of protected areas, configured according to a typology that had an influence on the international model as well. Until the 1980s, most of the NPAs created were strictly preservationist, which resulted in the expulsion of the inhabitants that traditionally occupied these territories and generated many socio-environmental conflicts. In the state of Amazonas, in northern Brazil, there were many cases of expulsion from communities after the creation of an NPA, and we had the opportunity to talk to people who, even after years in a new community, were still resentful of the forced displacement. After the appeals for sustainable development from the 1990s onwards, NPAs started to be created that integrated resident populations with conservationist objectives, but always under pressure that they did not destroy nature too much (Calegare & Higuchi, 2018).

Currently, there are three legal-normative forms that configure NPAs in Brazil. The first is in the Forest Code of 2012 (law number 12.727/2012), with the Permanent Preservation Areas (PPA) and Legal Reserves (LR), that defined which places and percentages of land cannot be degraded or must be restored. The second form is provided in the National System of Conservation Units (Law number 9.985 of 18th July, 2000), with two types of "Conservation Unit" (CU): (a) full protection, allowing only the indirect use of natural resources, but without authorising human presence (Ecological Station; Biological Reserve; National Park; Natural Monument; Wildlife Refuge);(b) sustainable use, which allows the use of natural resources under particular conditions by the traditional peoples and communities residing in these CUs (Environmental Protection Area; Area of Relevant Ecological Interest; National Forest; Extractive Reserve; Fauna Reserve; Sustainable Development Reserve; Private Reserve of Natural Heritage). The third way is through the indigenous lands (IL) and territories with remnants of *quilombo*[1] communities, both territorial modalities established by the 1988 Constitution (Art. 231 and Art. 68, respectively), which have inhabitants with sustainable practices of use of natural resources (Calegare & Higuchi, 2013).

According to data from the Instituto Socioambiental ([ISA], 2020) – a highly respected Brazilian environmental NGO – until early 2020, Brazil had approximately 33.32% of its continental area as NPAs: 19.52% as CUs (2,201 CUs, 777 of which are fully protected and 1,669 of sustainable use) and 13.8% as IL (7,103) – the vast majority of both located in the Amazon. There is no precise information to reveal the percentage of PPA and LR in the national territory. The CU management can be federal, state or municipal and, if the CU modality provides for the existence of a Management Council or Advisory Council (in the case of a sustainable use CU, provision in its type of modality and prescription in law), people or organisations from civil society, including psychologists in multidisciplinary teams, can participate.

Protected areas in Mexico

Nature conservation in Mexico has a complex origin. In his paper, Castañeda Rincón (2006) states that the Mayas and the Mexica (also known as Aztecs) implemented various actions to conserve relevant natural areas. Not only did they protect forests with bans and regulations, but they also established botanical gardens and parks (De la Maza Elvira, 1999). Afterwards, at the beginning of the colonial period, there was mass deforestation for construction and fuel. The Spanish crown became worried and protected some of the natural resources considered vital for the economy (Castañeda Rincón, 2006). The Chapultepec Forest became the first protected forest and also the first recreational park of Mexico City (De la Maza Elvira, 1999). Despite some efforts (especially the establishment of some national forests and private protected areas, felling regulations and the creation of the Forestry, Hunting and Fisheries Department in the early 20th century), the colonial period and the first century after the Mexican independence in 1821 were detrimental to conservation.

At the end of the Mexican Revolution, President Venustiano Carranza decreed the first national park in 1917, but it was not until the 1930s with the creation of the National System of Forest Reserves and National Parks that conservation actions were seriously undertaken. Several of the existing national parks were decreed during this period, as well as more than 30 forest reserves (Castañeda Rincón, 2006; González Ocampo et al., 2014). Between 1940 and 1970, the government concentrated more on the agriculture and industrial sectors than on the conservation of natural areas. In the 1970s, new conceptual and management elements were introduced, such as biosphere reserves. In 1982, the Ministry of Urban Development and Ecology (SEDUE) was created, and a new boost was given to the natural protected areas. In 1988, the current General Law of Ecological Balance and Environmental Protection (LGEEPA) was established, and six years later the Ministry of Environment, Natural Resources and Fisheries (now Ministry of Environment and Natural Resources –SEMARNAT) was founded (González Ocampo et al., 2014).

NPAs in Mexico are those in which the original environments have not been significantly altered by human activities or that require to be preserved and restored (LGEEPA, 2018). Currently, the National Commission of Natural Protected Areas (CONANP) manages 182 federal NPAs, representing close to 91 million hectares (including both terrestrial and marine areas), and supports 354 voluntarily designated areas for conservation, covering around 550,000 hectares (CONANP, 2019). These NPAs comprise around 11% of the national land area. There are several types of federal NPAs: national parks, biosphere reserves, protected areas of flora and fauna, sanctuaries, natural resources protected areas, and national monuments (LGEEPA, 2018; CONANP, 2019). In addition, there are state parks and reserves, municipal ecological conservation zones and voluntarily destined areas for conservation (LGEEPA, 2018). However, in our experience, some of the NPAs are just registered and do not have any type of management. We have even found people who are not aware they live within one.

Community social psychology contributions to nature conservation
Organisation and local governance in Brazil

The creation of a CU requires first that studies be carried out regarding both the biodiversity of fauna and flora and the way of life of the communities living in a given area. Assessment research is carried out by teams from different areas of knowledge, especially those related to biological and forest sciences, whose information serves to delimit the areas of use of natural resources. Socio-environmental research is carried out by teams of researchers from the human and social sciences, where there may be a psychologist. Based on all the data collected, a management plan is constructed, and the rules of coexistence are elaborated, both are official documents containing possibilities, permissions and prohibitions on the use of the territory.

A first valuable contribution that we have developed (the Brazilian author along with his team), from the perspective of the CSP, is to broaden and qualify the socio-environmental assessment to comprehensively and completely address the way of life of the Amazonian rural communities of the NPAs in the Amazon. Many surveys previously carried only economic data, without considering a series of dimensions of community life. Based on our expertise, we were able to suggest other dimensions for the socio-environmental surveys, revised and expanded by Calegare and Higuchi (2013):

- Geo-referencing: location of the community, houses and other buildings.
- Demography: number of inhabitants, age, sex, size of families; schooling; infrastructure of the houses.
- Access to social goods and services (social rights): social security; social assistance; payment for environmental services; basic sanitation (water, sanitary sewage and waste disposal); conditions of education provision; health care.
- Productive practices: agriculture; fishing; hunting; extractivism; collect; manufacture; animal breeding; management of renewable resources; services; trade; use of wood and non-wood products; income.
- Living conditions: use of energy; media; transport; recreation; parties; nutrition; expectations of change or permanence in the community; land tenure and ownership; use of medicinal plants and herbs; conceptions of health/illness.
- Sociopolitical organisation: formal and informal community forms of organisation; formal and informal leadership; intra- and intercommunity networks; community activities; community struggles; collective identities; difficulties and conflict resolution strategies; community potential.
- Environmental perception: meaning attributed to the place; feeling of belonging and ownership of the place; attachment to the place (satisfaction and dissatisfaction); perception of the Amazon rainforest; knowledge of environmental laws and regulations; perception of climate change.

Another important element is the realisation of the socio-environmental survey, which requires the participation of PA managers and community leaders in the choice of categories to be surveyed. Once agreements with these social actors have been made on which categories to raise together, the other step is to reach communities – that were previously advised by general leaders – and involve the leaders and local inhabitants in the survey. We always seek to hold community meetings to share all the work to be done and to involve as many local actors as possible in this task. In this way, we seek to get as close as possible to a true participatory approach.

We had the opportunity to participate in the socio-environmental assessment in two areas. In the first one, the population had been claiming the creation of an NPA since 2001. After a series of conflicts between them and the local government preventing the creation of the NPA, between 2007 and 2009 partnerships were established with universities and national and international NGOs, which financed the assessment surveys – including the socio-environmental survey we carried out in 2008 and which we subsequently published (Chaves et al., 2017). Only after changes in government and new political guidelines, the Baixo Rio Branco-Jauaperi Extractive Reserve (Resex) was created in 2018 (decree n° 9.401 of 05/06/2018). This Resex does not yet have a management plan.

In the second area, local communities started formal mobilisation to create a PA in 1997 and, in 2002, managed to create the Resex do Rio Jutaí (Decree [without number] of July 16, 2002). The construction of the management plan started in 2005. Only in 2011 were we invited to carry out a socio-environmental survey to provide support to this document (Higuchi et al., 2011). Finally, in 2012, the management plan for this Resex was published. On both areas instead of occasions occasions we were able to adopt these different dimensions of social life, not restricted only to the economic variable, as well as to use participatory ways of collecting data in communities. We did this by presenting the multiple dimensions to Resex managers and some leaders, showing the importance of approaching social life from different angles. We discussed each item with them and then approved the data collection instrument. When we started the field activities, we held meetings with the leaders and residents of each community to explain how the form had been built and to ask for any suggestions for changes or additions. We then asked some residents to help us, explaining in their words what the work was about to the other residents and helping us with data collection. Once the analysis was completed and the report was written, we held feedback meetings with Resex managers and leaders to present the work done.

These and other experiences in riverine Amazonian communities led us to develop a second contribution from CSP: the realisation of participatory action research (PAR) in rural Amazonian communities in NPAs (Calegare & Higuchi, 2018). In partnership with forest and biological sciences teams, we had the opportunity to develop sustainable development project that utilised fallen wood at the Resex Auati-Paraná, which involved several communities in this NPA and partner institutions. Based on a request from the residents, our plan was to have some families in this Resex produce wooden marquetry objects from trees which had already fallen in the forest, for sale and generation of income to these families. Teams of forestry engineers raised the potential for using fallen wood. Our team was responsible for involving the leaders and residents in all stages of the project's development, from its conception to production and trading of the marquetry objects. With this, we intended to strengthen their community networks and generate autonomy in conducting the project. Unfortunately, due to a series of factors external to the communities, the project was halted, gradually generating disengagement, and later abandoned by the residents. These factors were: (a) lack of people, structure and funding from the federal management institution to guarantee good conditions for the only two managers in the area; (b) difficulties in the control and execution of the conservation task by the managers, who visited the Resex a few times a year; (c) conflict and difficulty in interpersonal relationships between managers and residents, based on disagreements about the use of natural resources; and all of this resulted in (d) managers being discouraging and adopting a strictly preservationist stance on environmental laws, hampering the project. Only at the end of the project period (three years) were we able to sensitise managers, but it was too late. From this experience, we were able to learn that:

• Working with groups (group work) in communities, especially by those pre-existing the arrival of external agents, is a tool of fundamental importance for the community social psychologist. This helps create interpersonal and interinstitutional trust in cooperative behaviours and practices by sharing values and goals between those involved. In this work, it is necessary to know how to collectively create rules for the functioning of the group, to share problems, values and objectives, as well as to know how to deal with conflicts inherent to the group's dynamics, having confidence in the relationships between internal and external agents.

- The conflict between society with real autonomy, democracy, equality and sustainability (counter-hegemonic movement) versus the good intentions of participatory nature conservation (capitalism's green agenda) cannot be denied. Especially because of this conflict, which is expressed in disagreements between NPA managers and the needs of the communities' progress, it is common to have constant tensions between these social actors. Thus, there is great importance in the work of mediation, articulation and political negotiation that the community social psychologist can exercise between the different internal and external agents of a project, listening to each one of them, encouraging them to talk and also positioning themselves in favour of the common objective – leaving behind the mere neutral position typical of a clinical or mainstream investigative psychological bias. As an example, we note two meetings that we organised between scientists and the heads of the federal management institution, to pressure and negotiate in favour of Resex residents. We also mediated conversations between CU managers and residents, so that the latter could be heard.

Finally, more recently, we have been working in favour of strategies to tackle environmental issues in a different way. We partner with groups of organic farmers, whose production takes place through family farming in a model of agroecology and fair, collaborative and sustainable economy. There is a family or group of farming families that offer their products weekly to a number of loyal customers, who pay a monthly fee. The difference is that these customers are considered co-producers: they go to the market garden from time to time, establish a direct personal relationship with farmers, share production problems and consume the products that farmers have available that week. We have increased our awareness of socio-environmental issues, the strengthening of ties between farmers and clients, helped in solving some of the farmers' difficulties – when appropriate – and collaborated in the training of new psychologists who are sensitive to rural issues and to economic alternatives sustainable and humanised. In a schematic way, the activities undertaken were to:

- Broaden the awareness of community social psychologists about socio-environmental issues involving family farming, organic food production, agroecology and permaculture, fair, collaborative and sustainable economy. Participate in the work with the land.
- Encourage others in society to adhere to this form of economic production.
- Know the community networks involving farmers, customers ("co-producers") and other social actors, to enable them to insert themselves in these networks and strengthen them when necessary and if it is within the scope of psychosocial work.

Biodiversity conservation and human–wildlife coexistence in Mexico

As mentioned before, one of the main reasons for the creation of NPAs is biodiversity conservation. However, it is not sufficient to legally establish a protected area. Effective conservation requires an understanding and consideration of the factors that motivate human behaviour such as the motives, interests and values of all the stakeholders, as well as an interactive, reciprocal and continuous communication among them (Jacobson, McDuff, & Monroe, 2007; Bragagnolo et al., 2016). As Selinske et al. (2018) mention, despite the evident relevance of psychology for understanding and managing human behaviour for biodiversity conservation, there is still little research done in this area, especially in Latin America. We are certain that CSP can contribute to stopping biodiversity loss by working alongside the community members in understanding the interaction between wildlife and humans, and finding ways for both to coexist in the same regions. The examples presented in this section are part of an ongoing multidisciplinary jaguar conservation project in the Sierra Madre Oriental region in the northeast of Mexico. Specifically, we will focus on the work done in the surrounding communities of the Sierra del Abra Tanchipa Biosphere Reserve (RBSAT), in the state of San Luis Potosí, Mexico.

Many conservation studies have focused on the ecological aspects of conservation. The project we have collaborated on was initiated in 2006 by Rosas-Rosas, a colleague from the Colegio de Postgraduados, with research that provided evidence of jaguar presence in the area (Villordo-Galván et al., 2010). The ecological aspects of conservation are important, and in this case have been essential to the whole project. However, all conservation problems have ecological, economic and social aspects, and although the mix may vary, these three aspects should be included in problem solutions. Beadle de Palomo & Luna (2000) mention the importance of initiating multidisciplinary projects with a community needs assessment in order to determine community needs, the state of services, infrastructure and resources, as well as to understand their use and management of natural resources. Therefore, when the Mexican author began working in the Colegio de Postgraduados, and heard about the efforts towards jaguar conservation, she proposed including the socio-economic aspects. With the help of an expert in environmental education, we began with participatory rural appraisal (PRA) workshops in 14 communities (two of them in the aforementioned study area). The objective was to understand the state and usage of their natural resources, the main problems they faced and their perception of living in their community. The workshops had a strategic planning vision and consisted of four group activities and two individual ones. The group activities were designed to understand the interaction they had with their natural resources through the active participation of the community members. The individual activities were both voluntary and consisted of two different exercises to better understand the problems in their community. These workshops were the first meeting we had with the communities, and we were amazed by the quantity of natural resources described. Many of these were used for food, medicine, fuel, foraging, construction and ornamentation. However, there were several wild animals that did not have a use. The main problem mentioned was garbage disposal (with no public service available). Interestingly, in the two communities closer to RBSAT, there was no mention of having problems with jaguars.

We were particularly interested in the conflicts with predators (mainly jaguars and pumas) in communities surrounding RBSAT, so our next step was to survey three communities where we had done the PRA, which were closer to the reserve. A master's student did a socio-economic study (González-Sierra, 2011), similar to what has been previously described, in order to analyse the perceptions and attitudes towards jaguars while considering conservation and sustainable development actions in the communities. The survey included several elements: main demographics; access to basic services and available infrastructure; livelihoods; livestock production and predation, with an emphasis on jaguar predation, perceptions towards jaguars and conservation in general; tourism; what people liked about their communities, the problems they had and possible solutions; and alternative livelihood activities they would like to do. We found that predation by jaguars was attributed to just 2.47% of livestock loss, mainly of bull calves. Although some people considered jaguars to be a threat to humans and were afraid of them, the majority considered it important that jaguars exist. Considering these results along with other ecological ones, we organised a multidisciplinary training workshop for preventing and mitigating livestock predation, where we shared the results of the survey and gave some information about improving human–jaguar coexistence.

In addition, this information provided the basis for designing a model to understand and improve tolerance towards large carnivores (Olivera-Méndez et al., 2014). Tolerance towards large carnivores is the ability or willingness of humans to tolerate large carnivore presence and the risks involved in coexisting with them. The perceptions people have of the conflicts are critical to managing them (Sillero-Zubiri, 2007) for they can distort the scale of conflict (Inskip & Zimmermann, 2009). This model considers both tangible and intangible costs and benefits due to the presence of predators in the surrounding areas of a rural community. Tangible costs are those that can be observed, such as livestock and pet predation, loss of wild prey for human benefit, human injuries or fatalities, zoonosis, and losses in agricultural productivity. Intangible or indirect costs are loss of security, reduction in well-being and fear of carnivores. On the other hand, the direct benefits are those that provide the community with income generation or governmental subsidies due to the presence of the carnivores. Finally, indirect or intangible benefits are the intrinsic values associated with the species. The model proposes four strategies according to the existing balance of costs and benefits: (1) policies and regulations, (2) mitigation of predation and other losses, (3) environmental education and conscientisation, and (4) conservation and sustainable development projects, all of them through conflict resolution that considers good governance processes. As Decker et al. (2012) explain, tolerance increases when the balance between the positive and negative effects of the interaction with wildlife changes in a way that the positive aspects surpass the negative.

Using part of this model, we implemented a survey in some communities near the RBSAT where conflicts with jaguars and pumas had been reported, in order to understand the determinant factors that explain these conflicts (Olivera-Méndez & Utrera-Jiménez, 2020). The items focused on evaluative beliefs of both tangible and intangible costs using a Likert scale. We found the main problem was predation, as many authors have found (Amit & Jacobson, 2017; Palmeira et al., 2015). However, this predation was mainly referring to pet predation, a conflict that is not mentioned in scientific publications (we only found one publication: Linell et al., 2010). In addition, the conflict with predation was not the act itself but the losses generated as a result. Dickman and Hazzah (2016) agree that the amount of time, energy and money invested to prevent and mitigate predations can be an important motive for conflict. Moreover, we found that "fear of carnivores" had the highest variance in its related items. In two of the communities, it was the main factor explaining conflicts with large carnivores. Remarkably, one of the communities that had a high percentage of people afraid of jaguars in the first survey, had the lowest level in this factor 10 years later. This could be explained by all the other multidisciplinary actions that have been implemented in the area, such as environmental training workshops and better husbandry practices (Rosas-Rosas et al., 2020).

Finally, it is important to note that all the data and recommendations generated throughout the different activities have been shared with the stakeholders, mainly the RBSAT's manager, our colleagues, community leaders and relevant government agencies (local, state and federal). Some of the recommendations have been transformed by them into the other multidisciplinary actions mentioned above.

Final remarks

In Latin America, CSP contributions have been characterised by their attention to context, social transformation, conscientisation and liberation (Calegare & Higuchi, 2018). Through the cases in Brazil and Mexico that we have discussed, it is evident that we are aligned with this perspective and, further, we seek to demonstrate that it is possible to articulate CSP's ideals and perspectives to nature conservation. As Crawhall (2015) states, in order for conservation through NPAs to be effective, we need to understand human values, priorities and decision-making, and combine professionalised conservation with good governance. CSP can offer "insight into human cognition, value systems, costs and benefits, psychological biases, and conflict" to improve conservation practice (Clayton & Myers, 2009, p. 179).

More than that, as we have mentioned, there is a wide variety of tools, methods and expertise that our experiences from CSP can contribute for nature conservation, including:

- Assessing and identifying emotions, values, beliefs, social norms and attitudes that promote or obstruct conservation endeavours, in both quantitative and qualitative perspectives.
- Studying the way people interact with nature and its role in community life and social struggles in identity development, conscientisation and emancipation.
- Bringing a broader psychosocial perspective on life in rural communities to carry out socio-environmental surveys, involving variables that go beyond those that are merely economic.
- Encouraging and facilitating participation of community members in the governance process of the NPA. Actively engaging in the negotiations and political struggles of rural communities with NPA managers and other social actors in favour of the well-being and concerns of local residents.
- Using collaborative and participatory methodologies to work with groups in communities, respecting and strengthening existing community networks and formal and informal leaders.
- Promoting pro-environmental and sustainable behaviour by the integration of humans with non-humans. Designing and implementing environmental education and conscientisation processes.
- Broadening our own awareness as community social psychologists to see the relationships between nature conservation; organic food production by family farming; travel between the urban and rural worlds; and agroecology paradigms and patterns of conscious, responsible and sustainable consumption.

Life on this planet depends upon a complex and integrated balance of humans' well-being and nature conservation. Local communities have the right to govern their own territories, and CSP has several tools and methods that can be useful to make this happen, whilst conserving our planet's resources.

Note

1 A *quilombo* was a Brazilian settlement founded by people of African origin during the slavery period.

References

Amit, R., & Jacobson, S.K. (2017). Understanding rancher coexistence with jaguars and pumas: a typology for conservation practice. *Biodiversity Conservation, 26,* 1353–74. https://doi.org/10.1007/s10531-017-1304-1

Beadle de Palomo F., & Luna, E. (2000). *The needs assessment: Tools for long term planning, community-based health program tip sheet, conference follow-up tools.* Annie E. Cassey Foundation Conference-Neighbourhood Health Partnerships: Building a Strong Future. October 29–31, 1999. Washington, DC.

Bertzky, B., Bertzky, M., Worboys, G.L., & Hamilton, L.S. (2015). Earth's natural heritage. In G.L. Worboys, M. Lockwood, A. Kothari, S. Feary, & I. Pulsford (Eds.), *Protected area governance and management* (pp. 45–80). ANU Press. https://press.anu.edu.au/publications/protected-area-governance-and-management

Bragagnolo, C., Malhado, A.C.M., Jepson, P., & Ladle, R.J. (2016). *Conservation and Society, 14*(3), 163–82. www.jstor.org/stable/10.2307/26393240

Calegare, M.G.A., & Higuchi, M.I.G. (2013). Psicologia social e ambiental em Unidades de Conservação do Amazonas. In J.F. Leite, & M.Dimenstein (Eds.), *Psicologia e contextos rurais* (pp. 171–99). EDUFRN.

Calegare, M.G.A., & Higuchi, M.I.G. (2018). Participatory action research in an Amazon protected area: Lessons for community psychology in Northern Brazil. *Journal of Community & Applied Social Psychology, 28*(6), 460–70. https://doi.org/10.1002/casp.2379

Calegare, M.G.A., Higuchi, M.I.G., & Bruno, A.C.S. (2014). Traditional peoples and communities: from protected areas to the political visibility of social groups having ethnical and collective identity. *Ambiente & Sociedade, 17*(3), 115–34. https://doi.org/10.1590/S1414-753X2014000300008

Castañeda Rincón, J. (2006). Las áreas naturales protegidas de México: de su origen precoz a su consolidación tardía. *Scripta Nova. Revista electrónica de geografía y ciências sociales, X*(218), 13. www.ub.es/geocrit/sn/sn-218-13.htm

Chaves, M.P.S.R., Castilho, A.P., Souza, A.L., Araújo, C.N., Calegare, M.G.A., Costa, M.R.L., Lira, T.M., & Barroso, S.C. (2017). Organização sociocultural e gestão dos recursos naturais. In M.L. Oliveira (Eds.), *Mariuá: a flora, a fauna e o homem no maior arquipélago fluvial do planeta* (pp. 164–81). Editora INPA.

Clayton, S., & Myers, G. (2009). *Conservation psychology: Understanding and promoting human care for nature.* Wiley-Blackwell.

Comisión Nacional de Áreas Naturales Protegidas. (2019). *Áreas Naturales Protegidas decretadas.* http://sig.conanp.gob.mx/website/pagsig/datos_anp.htm

Convention on Biological Diversity. (2020). *Convention text.* www.cbd.int/convention/articles/?a=cbd-02

Crawhall, N. (2015). Social and economic influences shaping protected areas. In G.L. Worboys, M. Lockwood, A. Kothari, S. Feary, &I. Pulsford (Eds.), *Protected area governance and management* (pp. 119–44). ANU Press. https://press.anu.edu.au/publications/protected-area-governance-and-management

De la Maza Elvira, R. (1999). Una historia de las áreas naturales protegidas en México. *Gaceta Ecológica, 51*, 15–34. www.paot.org.mx/centro/ine-semarnat/gacetas/GE51.pdf

Decker, D.J., Riley, S.J., & Siemer, W.F. (2012). *Human dimensions of wildlife management.* The Johns Hopkins University Press.

Dickman A.J., & Hazzah, L. (2016). Money, myths and man-eaters: Complexities of human–wildlife conflict. In F.Angelici (Eds.), *Problematic wildlife* (pp. 339–56). Springer. https://doi.org/10.1007/978-3-319-22246-2_16

Diegues, C.A.S. (2008). *O mito moderno da natureza intocada* (6ª ed., rev. e ampl.). HUCITEC: NUPUAUB-USP.

Feary, S., Brown, S., Marshall, D., Lilley, I., McKinnon, R., Verschuuren, B., &Wild, R. (2015). Earth's cultural heritage. In G.L. Worboys, M. Lockwood, A. Kothari, S. Feary, & I. Pulsford (Eds.), *Protected area governance and management* (pp. 83–116). ANU Press. https://press.anu.edu.au/publications/protected-area-governance-and-management

González Ocampo, H.A., Cortés-Calva, P., Íñiguez Dávalos, L.I., & Ortega-Rubio, A. (2014). Las áreas naturales protegidas de México. *Investigación y Ciencia, 22*(60), 7–15. www.redalyc.org/articulo.oa?id=67431160002

González-Sierra, E.R. (2011). *Des arrollo sustentable y conservación del jaguar (Pantheraonca) entres comunidades de la Huasteca Potosina, S.L.P., México* [Master's thesis]. Colegio de Postgraduados, Campus Montecillo, Texcoco, Mexico.

Higuchi, M.I.G., Calegare, M.G.A., Porto, M.L.S.G., Lima, M.B.D.F., & Feitosa, R. M. (2011). *Vida social das comunidades da Resex do Rio Jutaí e uso dos recursos florestais* (Relatório Técnico). INPA, JICA, ICMBio.

Inskip, C., & Zimmermann, A. (2009). Human-felid conflict: A review of patterns and priorities world-wide. *Oryx, 43*(1), 18–34. https;//doi.org/10.1017/S003060530899030X

Instituto Socioambiental [ISA]. (2020). https://www.socioambiental.org/pt-br

International Union for Conservation of Nature. (2020). *About. What is a protected area.* www.iucn.org/theme/protected-areas/about

Jacobson, S.K., McDuff, M.D., & Monroe, M.C. (2007). *Conservation education and outreach techniques.* Oxford University Press.

Law nº 9.985, of 18 July 2000; Decree nº 4.340, 22 August2002; Decree nº 5.746,5 April 2006. *SNUC – Sistema Nacionalde Unidades de Conservação da Natureza.* Decree nº 5.758, 13 April 2006. *PNAP – Plano Estratégico Nacional de Áreas Protegidas* (2011). MMA/SBF.

Ley General del Equilibrio Ecológico y la Protección al Ambiente. (2018, June 5). Cámara de Diputadosdel H. Congreso de la Unión. www.diputados.gob.mx/LeyesBiblio/pdf/148_050618.pdf

Linell, J.D.C., Rondeau, D., Reed, D.H., Williams, R., Altwegg, R., Raxworthy, C.J., Austin, J.D., Hanley, N., Fritz, H., Evans, D.M., Gordon, I.J., Reyers, B., Redpath, S., & Pettorello, N. (2010). Confronting the costs and conflicts associated with biodiversity. *Animal Conservation, 13,* 429–31. https://doi.org/10.1111/j.1469-1795.2010.00393.x

Medeiros, R. (2006). Evolução das tipologias e categorias de áreas protegidas no Brasil. *Ambiente & Sociedade, 9*(1), 41–64. https://doi.org/10.1590/S1414-753X2006000100003

Medeiros, R., Irving, M.A., & Garay, I. (2006). Áreas Protegidas no Brasil: interpretando o contexto histórico para pensar a Inclusão Social. In M.A. Irving (Ed.), *Áreas protegidas e inclusão social: construindo novos significados* (pp. 15–40). Fundação Bio-Rio.

Olivera-Méndez, A., & Utrera-Jiménez, E. (2020). Factores de conflicto por la presencia de grandes felinos. In O.C. Rosas-Rosas, A. Silva-Caballero, & A. Durán-Fernández (Eds.), *Manejo y conservación del jaguar en la Reserva de la Biosfera Sierra del Abra Tanchipa* (pp. 127–39). Colegio de Postgraduados, SEMARNAT, CONANP, PNUD. www.mx.undp.org/content/mexico/es/home/library/environment_energy/manejo-y-conservacion-del-jaguar-en-la-reserva-de-la-biosfera-si.html

Olivera-Méndez, A., Palacio-Núñez, J., Martínez-Calderas, J.M., Morales-Flores, F. J., & Hernández-Saint Martín, A.D. (2014). Modelado del nivel de tolerancia a la presencia de grandes carnívoros en un área rural de México. *Agroproductividad, 7*(5), 24–31. https://revista-agroproductividad.org/index.php/agroproductividad/article/view/551/422

Palmeira, F.B.L., Trinca, C.T., & Haddad, C.M. (2015). Livestock predation by puma (Puma concolor) in the highlands of Southeastern Brazilian Atlantic forest. *Environmental Management, 56,* 903–15. https://doi.org/10.1007/s00267-015-0562-5

Rios, A.V.V. (2004). Populações tradicionais em áreas protegidas. In F. Ricardo (Ed.), *Terras indígenas & unidades de conservação da natureza: o desafio das sobreposições* (pp. 78–84). ISA.

Rosas-Rosas, O.C., Silva-Caballero, A., & Durán-Fernández, A. (Eds.). (2020). *Manejo y conservación del jaguar en la Reserva de la Biosfera Sierra del Abra Tanchipa.* Colegio de Postgraduados, SEMARNAT, CONANP, PNUD. www.mx.undp.org/content/mexico/es/home/library/environment_energy/manejo-y-conservacion-del-jaguar-en-la-reserva-de-la-biosfera-si.html

Sandwith, T.S., MacKinnon, K., & Hoelich, E.H. (2015). Foreword. In G.L. Worboys, M. Lockwood, A. Kothari, S. Feary, & I. Pulsford (Eds.), *Protected area governance and management* (pp. xxii–xxvi). ANU Press. https://press.anu.edu.au/publications/protected-area-governance-and-management

Selinske, M., Garrard, G., Bekessy, S., Gordon, A., Kusmanoff, A., & Fidler, F. (2018). Revisiting the promise of conservation psychology. *Conservation Biology, 32*(6), 1464–8. https://dx.doi.org/10.1111/cobi.13106

Sillero-Zubiri, C., Sukumar, R., & Treves, A. (2007). Living with wildlife: the roots of conflict and the solutions. In D. MacDonald & K. Service (Eds.), *Key topics in conservation biology* (pp. 255–72). Blackwell Publishing.

Stolton, S., Dudley, N., Çokçalışkan, B., Hunter, D., Ivanić, K.-Z., Kanga, E., Kettunen, M., Kumagai, Y., Maxted, N., Senior, J., Wong, M., Keenleyside, K., Mulrooney, D., & Waithaka, J. (2015). Values and benefits of protected areas. In G.L. Worboys, M. Lockwood, A. Kothari, S. Feary, & I. Pulsford (Eds.), *Protected area governance and management* (pp. 147–68). ANU Press. https://press.anu.edu.au/publications/protected-area-governance-and-management

Villordo-Galván, J.A., Rosas Rosas, O.C., Clemente Sánchez, F., Martínez Montoya, J.F., Tarango Arámbula, L.A., Mendoza Martínez, G., Sánchez Hermosillo, M.D., & Bender, L.C. (2010). The jaguar (Panthera onca) in San Luis Potosí, Mexico. *The Southwestern Naturalist, 55*(3), 394–402. www.jstor.org/stable/40801038

Worboys, G.L. (2015a). Concept, purpose and challenges. In G.L. Worboys, M. Lockwood, A. Kothari, S. Feary, & I. Pulsford (Eds.), *Protected area governance and management* (pp. 11–39). ANU Press. https://press.anu.edu.au/publications/protected-area-governance-and-management

Worboys, G.L. (2015b). Introduction. In G.L. Worboys, M. Lockwood, A. Kothari, S. Feary, & I. Pulsford (Eds.), *Protected area governance and management* (pp. 3–8). ANU Press. https://press.anu.edu.au/publications/protected-area-governance-and-management

PART IV

Community Psychology through a reflective lens

19

COMMUNITY PSYCHOLOGY AND THE LIBERATION PROCESS OF FIRST NATIONS IN GUATEMALA

Jorge Mario Flores Osorio and Mariola Elizabeth Vicente Xiloj

Abstract

We will use a knowledge dialogue (*diálogo de saberes*) to question the Eurocentric and American visions of Community Psychology based on the reality of exclusion-pauperisation suffered by the First Nations in Guatemala, as a consequence of the capitalist project, installed after the Peace Agreements (PA) signed by the Guatemalan National Revolutionary Unity (URNG) and the government presided over by Álvaro Arzú in 1996. We will also highlight the role of psychology in the Transitional Justice Project, promoted by the United Nations, and the options for psychologists to participate in the struggles of the Mayan people in defence of their lands and against the predatory extractivist project, as well as against the violation of human rights and the criminalisation of the population.

Chapter outline: a) historical contextualisation of the project of exclusion-pauperisation of First Nations; b) territorial dispossession as a justification for PA; c) struggle in Mayan territories; d) questioning of Eurocentric and American Community Psychology; e) conclusions.

Resumen

Con diálogo de saberes, cuestionaremos las visiones eurocéntricas y estadounidenses de la Psicología Comunitaria a partir de la realidad de exclusión-pauperización que sufren las Naciones Originarias en Guatemala, como consecuencia del proyecto capitalista, instalado tras los Acuerdos de Paz (AP) firmados por la Unidad Revolucionario Nacional Guatemalteca (URNG) y el gobierno que presidido porÁlvaro Arzú en 1996. Destacaremos también el papel de la psicología en el Proyecto de Justicia Transicional, impulsado por Naciones Unidas, y las opciones de participación de los psicólogos en las luchas del pueblo Maya en defensa de su territorio y contra el proyecto extractivista depredador, así como contra la violación de los derechos humanos y la criminalización de la población.

Esquema del capítulo: a) contextualización histórica del proyecto de exclusión-pauperización de las Naciones Originarias b) despojo territorial como justificación de la AP

DOI: 10.4324/9780429325663-24

c) lucha en territorios mayas y d) cuestionamiento de la psicología comunitaria eurocéntrica y norteamericana, e) conclusiones.

Introduction

Knowledge dialogues (or *diálogos de saberes*) are one of the critical communicative methodologies (Gómez et al., 2011) that open the way for integrating ancestral, metaphysical and holistic indigenous knowledge with scientific knowledge. Through this method, new epistemologies and practices, that are essentially anti-colonial emerge (see for example Gómez et al., 2011). A knowledge dialogue involves deep conversation about cultural beliefs and practices, and the ways in which indigenous knowledge differs from Western, scientific knowledge.

Knowledge dialogues ideally take place at the start of, or even before, a process of working with communities and continue throughout the work. This chapter invites you, the reader, to use the information here as if you were a part of this dialogue, to reflect upon your own praxis: your own training, assumptions and cultural values, and how they might differ from those of the Maya-K'iche' (one of the Mayan peoples, to which MEVX, one of the authors, belongs, and with whom the other author, JMFO, has worked).

In this chapter we present the results of a knowledge dialogue (Gómez et al, 2015), undertaken for a period of six months, between MEVX, a Maya-K'iche' psychologist and a ladino (JMFO), as the mestizo and de-cultured indigenous populations are called in Guatemala. Our dialogue concerned practising as a community psychologist with First Nation communities in Guatemala. The dialogue focused on thinking about European or North American Community Psychology (CP) from the reality of exclusion-pauperisation that the indigenous First Nations have historically suffered in Guatemala. As a result of talking about CP from a standpoint outside of Western thought, capital and capitalism, that is, from the position of the excluded-pauperised, the two participants in the dialogue postulated a way of redefining the work of CP that is coherent with the anti-colonial struggles and the defence of territory carried out by the Maya-K'iche' First Nation.

In the Maya-K'iche' and Ladino knowledge dialogue, we explore two major themes:

1. The genesis of the Exclusion-Pauperisation of the First Nations, their consolidation up until the 21st century, and the struggles of the Mayab' (or Mayan) collectives in defence of their territory and of Mother Nature threatened by the predatory project of neoliberalism and, in turn, by the criminalisation of the inhabitants by the government, which, in essence, means a project that tends towards the disappearance of the Guatemalan First Nations. In this we emphasise the recovery of historical and cultural memory.
2. American and dominant European Community Psychology (CP) as colonial expressions that adopt a homogeneous view of the person, denying and denigrating the non-European.

The results of the dialogue are organised as follows.

1. An analysis of the genesis of the ignominy experienced by the First Nations.
2. A section on the Peace Accords as a neoliberal strategy to dispossess the Maya-K'iche' communities of their lands, along with the actions carried out by the extractive industry, specifically the cultivation of oil palm and the construction of hydroelectric dams.
3. We document the significance of the 13th B'aktun which, according to Mayan prophecies, marks the end of the resistance carried out by the First Nations for more than 500 years and

the beginning of a new epoch, as a dynamic of organised rebellion to decolonise thought and life.

4. We then reflect the hegemonic views of psychological thinking, and the counter-hegemonic response, from the dynamics of exclusion-pauperisation, thus explaining the cosmogony of the Maya-K'iche' First Nation and their sense of community.

5. Finally, the possibility of CP in the Maya-K'iche' context is analysed. through intercultural or bilingual education programmes.

As a result of thinking about CP from outside Western capital, that is, from the excluded-impoverished, represented by the First Nations, we postulate a way to redefine the work of CP, in support of anti-colonial struggles and the defence of the territory liberated by the First Nation, Maya-K'iche', a rebellion guided by the predictions revealed at the end of the 13th B'aktun and at the beginning of the new epoch, which, as we will see, heralds the path of community-organised rebellion based on the teachings of the grandmothers and grandfathers and from these visions to defend Mother Nature, the land and the right to be recognised as nations.

Ignominious history of First Nations

The ignominy carried out by the colonisers towards the First Nations of the Americas began in 1492, with the supposed discovery and the subsequent invasion carried out by the Spanish and Portuguese in the 16th century. In the case of the Maya world, the invasion is recounted in the books of *Chilam Balam* (Anonymous, 1948), which contain a European language account, originally written in hieroglyphics, of a series of prophetic cylindrical wheels, or *Katuns*, each lasting a period of roughly 20 years (Taube, 1988).

The initial prophetic wheel of *Katun* ends with a prediction that "foreigners with ruddy beards, the sons of the sun, the light-coloured men will arrive", that is, the European invaders.

The *Chilam Balam* prophecy states that the original inhabitants of the Americas should be saddened by the arrival of "the bearded ones, the messengers of the sign of divinity, the foreigners of the earth" (Anonymous, 1948, p. 68), and that, with the arrival of the invaders, their own gods will lose their value, a prediction that was to be confirmed by the presence of the invaders in 1524, who imposed the God of the Christians through Catholic missionaries.

In the second prophetic wheel of *Katun,* it is written that the God of the invaders will only speak of sin, that the soldiers will be inhuman and their mastiffs cruel, "Woe to you my younger brothers that [by the end of this period] you will have excess of pain and excess of misery for the tribute gathered with violence and first of all delivered with haste" (Anonymous, 1948, p. 69), events that continue in spite of the community organisation in defence of Mother Nature and the land as fundamental principles of community life.

In 1524, with the Spanish invasion of the Mayab' lands, the prophecy related to the inhuman acts of the bearded men was fulfilled, as de las Casas (1958, p. 4) pointed out in 1516:

> They say that they make them work on holidays and Sundays, because on those days they send them loaded with tools to the mines, and that on the said days, which are for rest, because they do not give them anything to eat, the Indians go all night and all day to look for food in the fields, so that the day of rest is negated and they do not lose time on the days they have to work.

The prophecy points out that Christianity will bring the power to enslave the rightful owners of the American lands and, as Dussel points out, 1492 will mark the beginning of the negation of the non-European-other, wherein: Spain and Portugal

> are the first step towards Modernity itself. It was the first region in Europe to have the originating "experience" of constituting the Other as dominated under the control of the conqueror, of the domination of the centre over a periphery.
>
> *(Dussel, 1994, p. 11)*

After three centuries of Spanish colonialism, in 1821, the supposed independence from Spain took place in Guatemala, led by the Creoles (those of European descent, born in America), who, tired of paying tribute to the crown, rebelled and then, under the supposed independence, deepened the dynamics of discrimination and racism towards the First Nations, and in general, towards the non-European. In 1871, this liberal revolution was consolidated, and the Guatemalan nation state was configured under mono-ethnic and mono-cultural principles, making invisible the condition of a country with diverse cultures, under principles of cultural homogeneity, and strengthening discrimination and racism towards the First Nations (Casaus, 2009).

During the armed conflict that began in 1962, the Guatemalan government, advised and financed by the United States of America, implemented a project of extermination against Guatemalans, seeking to fracture the fabric of their community (Flores Osorio, 2017), using terror as a counterinsurgency strategy, arguing that it was necessary to "take the water from the fish", that is, to remove the communities' support for the revolutionary vanguard represented by the various rebel forces (Falla, 2006, p. 18).

The counter-insurgency strategy also involved a group of Protestant churches, which sought to consolidate individualistic rather than community behaviour in the population, and the Protestant churches also justified the ethnocide carried out by the Guatemalan army. The government created military-controlled model villages and the evangelical churches, sponsored by US neo-Pentecostal organisations, grew in the Mayab' communities and drew up a supposed humanitarian project, agro-villages (*agro-aldeas*), financed by businessmen and Guatemalan and US politicians affiliated with these churches.

The Protestant sects recruited new followers in the communities through home visits, promising eternal salvation; the purchase of land; the creation of irrigation systems for agriculture; and the technical supervision of community members who accepted belonging to these religious sects. They managed to recruit community groups who were persuaded to leave their communities to concentrate in the agro-villages and profess evangelical beliefs (Cantón, 2005).

Peace agreements as a neoliberal strategy

The consolidation of the neoliberal project in Guatemala was consolidated with the Peace Accords, signed in 1996 by the Guatemalan National Revolutionary Unity (URNG) and the government represented by Álvaro Arzú. With the signing of the Peace Accords, organisations were created such as the Commission for Historical Clarification (CEH), the Commission for the Recovery of Historical Memory (REMHI) and the Human Rights Office of the Archbishopric of Guatemala (ODHA), the latter presided over by Monsignor Juan Gerardi, who was assassinated on April 26, 1998, after presenting the report *Guatemala Nunca Más* (Guatemala never again).

This ODHA report (1998) accuses the Guatemalan state of 93 per cent of the acts of genocide, torture and forced disappearance. The massacres carried out by the Guatemalan state are classified as ethnocide and as crimes against humanity. The CEH (1999) documented that nearly 200,000 people were victims of state terrorism, including 45,000 disappeared, and forced displacements internally and to neighbouring Mexico.

In the north-western region of Guatemala, where most of the Mayab' population lives, the Guatemalan army carried out the most cruel acts; in this region, most of the massacres were conducted and entire towns and villages were razed to the ground, with greater emphasis on the department of El Quiché, where the highest rates of violence are documented. According to CEH (1999), there were 327 massacres of the Maya K'iche' and Ixhil population. Between 1978 and 1996, 626 massacres took place throughout Guatemala (CEH, 1999, p. 257).

As a result of the Peace Accords, the levels of exclusion-pauperisation of the Mayab' population worsened and, despite these agreements, in the 21st century (Flores Osorio, 2017) the Guatemalan state still denies the possibility of recognising the Maya-K'iche' as a First Nation, criminalises their leaders and attempts to halt the path towards the re-foundation of the state, ignoring the right of the First Nations to guide their lives by their ancestral culture, their cosmogony and the traditional teachings left by their grandmothers and grandfathers. However, despite the actions of the Guatemalan state to cover up for those who planned and executed the terrorist actions, the Maya-K'iche' First Nation is organising itself to recover the Maya-K'iche' historical memory and cosmogony, aligned with the end of the *13 B'aktun* epoch and the beginning of a new epoch. (Each *B'aktun* is an era of 20 *katun* cycles: *13 B'aktun* ended on December 21, 2012). In this struggle the utopian liberation imaginary of the Mayab' collectives is strengthened as they emerge in defence of Mother Nature, of the indigenous territory, and struggle to overcome the present reality of exclusion-pauperisation: this is understood as an anti-colonial expression in defence of life itself.

Land, racism and peace agreements

The dispossession of the lands of the Mayab' population is carried out by extractive companies, principally through the cultivation of the African oil palm, and the construction of hydroelectric dams. The Guatemalan government, taking the role of servant of global capital, protects the companies concerned, while imprisoning, criminalising and violating the human rights of community leaders (UDEFEGUA, 2009). It is ironic that despite the Peace Accords signed by the URNG and the Guatemalan government, which recognise racism and therefore assume the commitment to eliminate it, the First Nations continue to be excluded and impoverished. Racism is strengthened by a

> generalised and definitive valuation of biological or cultural differences, real or imaginary, to the benefit of one group and to the detriment of the Other, in order to justify aggression and a system of domination […] racism is […] the negation of the Other, as opposed to the affirmation of oneself, is a historical constant that survives in the Creole elite.
>
> *(Casaus, 1999, p. 64)*

From resistance to rebellion

For more than 500 years the First Nation Maya-K'iche' resisted the colonial attacks and preserved their cosmogony, language, customs and respect for Mother Nature; safeguarded the teachings of their grandmothers and grandfathers; and guided their lives according to the times defined in the Mayan calendar. This includes the convergence of space and time in one unique place (the *Najt*); when movement and speed is added, they combine to form "reality". Furthermore, the *Najt* refers to the fact that everything that exists in the universe is life, and the dynamics of life on earth is always in relation to that universe.

On December 21, 2012, the 13th *B'aktun* marked the end of a period of 5,200 years, an important date for the First Nation Maya-K'iche', heir to the lands of the Mayab' (Barrios, 2004; Hernández Ixcoy, 2020). This date marks the beginning of the new era. It marks the end of the resistance carried out for more than 500 years, and the beginning of the organised rebellion in defence of Mother Nature and the land; the beginning of the struggle for the refoundation of the Guatemalan state, which implies the achievement of cultural recognition of the Maya-K'iche' as a First Nation and respect for life in community.

Refounding the state is necessary for the liberation of the First Nations, because it would enable the reconstruction of historical memory, the challenge to the capitalist mode of production, the decolonisation of thought, the defence of Mother Nature (Hernández, 2020); and the defence of the land as the basis for the sustenance of community life. For the First Nation Mayab', the relationship with Mother Nature is synonymous with life; it represents a life that is green and full. The Mayabs' consider Mother Nature to be the mentor of life, so that through her the world is reflected as an expression of a bigger totality; the cycles of life are evidenced; respect, care and reciprocity or complementarity with the Different-Other are made concrete; and the community dimension is consolidated.

The Maya-K'iche' cosmogony

For the *Maya' na'oj*, or wisdom, the greening of life is the axis of community life that has as its centre of action respect for Mother Nature, in terms of totality, complementarity and symmetry. As we were able to confirm through our knowledge dialogue, in the Maya-K'iche' tradition, respect is shown for creation, be it visible or invisible to human eyes. As we have seen, *Najt* refers to the universal balance among the Maya-K'iche' and has an important presence in community life. In the life of the Maya, community implies balance among all those who make it up, since everything has life and its own *k'u'xaj*, spirit or heart (Par Sapón, 2009).

Cosmogony aims to establish a reality by helping to actively construct the perception or understanding of the universe (space), the origin of gods, the origin of humanity and the elements of nature; at the same time it gives the option of appreciating and conceiving the physical order; that which can be seen, touched and the metaphysical order, which refers to what is difficult to understand, which allows us to conjure or invoke chaos. That is, the state of confusion and disorder in which matter was until the moment of the creation of the cosmos, and uncertainty, which would be the doubt or perplexity born of astonishment or surprise, is known as cosmogony (Ak'abal, 2019, p. 21).

Our knowledge dialogue found that the cultural richness contained in the Maya-K'iche' cosmogony is an engine for the constitution of the *psychological*, and manifests itself as the future and as becoming. From that cosmogony, the history of the community is interpreted, and the reasons why the invaders tried to wipe the First Nations off the face of the earth are understood. In this way, cosmogony points to the path, the ethical-political praxis towards the liberation and/or decolonisation of the Maya-K'iche' Nation. Mayab' intellectuals point out that the worldview of the Maya-K'iche' Nation is contained in texts such as the *Pop Wuj*, known as *Popol Wuj*. According to Father Jiménez's translation, which refers to the idols destroyed by Spanish invaders, this text:

> recounts the destruction of the wooden beings whose utensils and animals rebelled against their poor treatment.
>
> *(Ak'abal, 2019, p. 21)*

The *Popol Wuj* augurs the liberation of the Original Maya-K'iche' Nation from the oppression suffered for more than 500 years, and, as we have seen, the 13th B'aktun marks the end of an epoch on December 21, 2012, known as Oxjajuj B'aktun. It is during the years of the following, 14th B'aktun, that the liberation of the Mayan people will come and the cultural heritage of the First Nations will be reasserted along with the defence of Mother Nature (Hernández Ixcoy, 2019; Flores Osorio, 2020.

In colonial-Western thought the Maya-K'iche' cosmogony is considered a set of beliefs, myths and rituals that do not correspond to instrumental, objective and neutral Eurocentric or Anglocentric rationality, derived from the fact that the invaders and/or colonisers could not or would not understand that the "world" inherited by the grandmothers and grandfathers, from the heart of the Maya-K'iche' world, is contained in the ancestral cosmogony. Westerners, however, needed to create artificial languages to understand the "world" and justify domination, racism and discrimination. This stands in stark contrast to the First Nations who possess an ancestral cosmogony, from which reality is explained as and by becoming.

The power of the knowledge dialogue is seen in the exposure of this clash of world views. Those who do not know the history of the Maya-K'iche' world, mistakenly think that the community members orientate their lives based on superstitions as an adjective to disqualify ancestral thought. The colonisers/invaders mistakenly believed that colonial thought is universal and true, so they disqualified any other way of explaining the world.

In addition to the above, the invaders and their heirs argued that myths do not reflect historical changes, and that myths are expressions outside of time and space. This has a degree of certainty, if considered only from the Western notion of time-space. Lopez (1997) puts the case for an alternative view:

> a human product that must be studied in its temporal development and in the context of the societies that produce it and act on the basis of it. Its historical character implies its dialectical link with the social whole and, therefore, also implies its permanent transformation. (Lopez, 1997, p. 472)

Myth is a fundamental category for understanding Maya thought. Ak'abal (2019) states that myth is a historical expression of the community, which refers to an ancestral belief system. For *Ak'abal* in the *Popol Wuj* and in the Book of the Books of *Chilam Balam* of *Chumayel*, different kinds of myths serve different purposes. Cosmogonic myths are analysed to explain the creation of the world; theogonic myths relate the origin and history of the gods; aetiological myths give reason for the existence of something; anthropogenic myths narrate the appearance of human beings; moral myths explain the existence of good and evil; myths narrate the foundation of cities; and eschatological myths prophesy the future of the Maya-K'iche' Nation.

In Maya-K'iche' cosmogony, ancestral history, then, constitutes the reference to the dynamic and living history that embodies the constitution of the Mayab' Self (Colop, 1999; Estrada, 2010).

Indeed, the *Popol Wuj* relates a transition between mythology and history which at no point can be conceived as a linear narrative, according to Ak'abal (2019). León Chic summarises these links:

> For the Mayab' cosmogony, a part of the world is inhabited by spiritual beings, spirits or presences with whom it is possible to communicate. All are important, but the time bearers, who are the caretakers, watch over and redeem over the face of the earth until the last days of humanity (León Chic, 2003, p. 42).

Sense of community in the Maya-K'iche' world

The universal balance in the Maya-K'iche' First Nation is manifested in community life defined as the *Najt,* the space-time where daily life takes place itself orientated by the cosmogony of life. Flores Osorio (2014) defines this notion of community as follows:

> The community is the space-time where community members converge to become interpellants; the community takes shape in the dynamics generated by difference and is characterised by being made up of oppressed people who, by becoming aware of their condition, start on the path towards liberation.

For the Original Nations, the *Najt* in its references to space-time has continuity in Heaven, Earth and the Underworld. Time is both historical and future becoming in this framework. The historical-cultural construction of the self, along with a future orientation, is central:

> the constitution of the Mayab' Self supposes that being with others and with the world is a present that becomes historical-cultural, with a projection towards the to-be, as a present that is denied. (Flores Osorio, 2020, p. 176)

Thus, life in community materialises within the spiritual-political-organisational, and is orientated by the ancestral cosmogony, transmitted by the teachings left by the grandmothers and grandfathers. Through this dynamic, the family-community balance is maintained.

> Among those who offer their Patan are the Kamalbe, the grandmothers and grandfathers, the Ajq'ijab, and the Iomatit. The Kamalbe – Principals or Elders – are the highest authority in a community, they are in charge of guiding and giving advice to the families. They are people who are distinguished by their impeccable conduct and the quality of their advice. (Vigor, 2020, p. 108)

In the life of the Maya-K'iche' it is not possible to separate one's gaze from the universal, since the times indicated in the Maya calendar delineate the path walked by community members in the company of metaphysical beings. Hence the importance for Western psychologists to understand that the spiritual space of the Mayab' world is shaped as a socio-political-organisational practice.

Within the community space-time, then, there are socio-political-organisational cosmogonic forms, delegated to the ancestral authorities who are designated by "call" the community. This happens in the same way with all the people who share the Maya-K'iche' tradition – the day of their birth defines the role they will play in the community.

In the Maya-K'iche' world, people recognise that their destiny is defined on the day of birth, according to the *Cholq'ij*; the destined person has a series of *achik'*, dreams, which indicate that they must present themselves to the World. The earth deity also experiences the lightening of the body, as if the air were passing rapidly through the flesh in the form of fluttering or rippling; then comes the *yab'il* or sickness that manifests itself in different forms, announcing that it is time to begin the destiny (Tedlock, 2011; Rupflin, 1999; Lucas, 2017).

In the Maya-K'iche' communities, community and ancestral authorities are designated by a set of gifts translated into the *Patan* or community service, legitimised by the community members. The Mayab' tradition states that when the *Patan* is fulfilled and the community member responds to the call of destiny to carry out tasks that help the community, he/she is fulfilled as a person, and that not fulfilling their destiny constitutes a denial of the self.

In the *Maya' na'oj* (philosophy), people are called from the moment of their birth, and then comes the time when *Ajaw*, God, reminds them of their destiny, a reminder to prepare, initiate and act accordingly all their lives. It is important to note that there are differences between the *Patan* and professional service. For example, in the *Patan,* people exercise their spiritual and material authority; they work physically and metaphysically; they do not receive financial remuneration; and they do require the support of the community members who pay them according to their means. However, the most important thing for the person is recognition by the community.

This is captured by the idea that in *Patan*, "I help the other because to that extent I help myself". Through our knowledge dialogue, we can see that relationships of are achieved with the other. This dynamic is *healing*, physically, emotionally and spiritually. This healing differs from that achieved through professional practice. Western thought has led to professional practices that are delineated by a certification granted because of the fulfilment of instrumental evaluation criteria, and thereafter a person is accredited to carry out his practice with the mediation of a salary, without commitment to transformation. Whilst psychological health is important to Western professionals, there is an emphasis on individual – at most family – health and their practices and techniques are not designed to shore up life as a fundamental principle of community relations.

In the Maya-K'iche' world every service or gift is considered a gift from *Ajaw*, God; the energies and knowledge that are given to the person have a protective guardian: each person must know, cultivate and take responsibility for their destiny. Community members must be willing to invest their time, creativity and strength to achieve the common good (Lucas, 2017).

In the Maya-K'iche' tradition, grandmothers and grandfathers are the living face of *Ajaw.* They are prepared to bear family and community problems; as well as being authorities prepared to deal with problems of the heart or of the spirit, they observe, analyse and propose possible solutions to personal and community problems.

Grandparents are the people who have lived, know and interpret the changes of Mother Nature's phenomena, have the intuitive ability to read and interpret the Mayan calendar, to understand the messages of *Ajaw* in the sky, in Mother Rain, in the stars, in the moon, in dreams, in the work and life of our animals and everything that is around us (León Chic, 2003, pp. 54–5).

Other community members, too, act as spiritual guides. The *Ajq'ijab* or *Chuchqajaw*, or Tellers of Time, are trained to interpret the Mayan calendar: they are responsible for guiding spirituality as the living representation of the ancestors, of the tradition and wisdom contained in the Maya-K'iche' world view. They are confidants in the family, in society and in the village. They communicate with nature and with *Ajaw*, God, through *Uk'u'x Q'aq* (Sacred Fire ceremonies) on the highest hills, asking for forgiveness, protection for families and the community.

The *Iomatit*, or midwife, is wise with regard to human reproduction; she takes care of women in the whole process: prenatal monitoring, pregnancy and delivery and even the restoration of the health of newborn children and other illnesses suffered by women and men. She is a counsellor and spiritual support in the family, and she brings together all the family members to advise on the situation of the pregnant woman or for the upbringing of the children (Camey, 2020).

The First Nation, then, builds knowledge based on wisdom and love taken from the beings that inhabit the sky, the earth and the underworld. This knowledge is passed down from the grandparents to their generations. In short, the cosmogony is based on love made tangible in the Mayan languages. The Mayab' or *Maya' na'oj* (thought or philosophy) comes from love, and it manifests itself in a way contrary to modern Western thought, which is based more on objective and neutral reason. The *Maya' na'oj* advises the community to seek balance in caring for both the Heart of Heaven (*Uwachulew* and *Uk'u'x Kaj*) and the Heart of the Earth(*Uk'u'x Ulew*).

From the individual to the community

Psychology as a scientist vision and as a professional practice in its various fields of application had its genesis in the second half of the 19th century, at crucial moments of European industrial capitalist development. The ideological underpinning is to be found in liberal philosophy, the focus of which is the individual within the relations of capital production and reproduction (Danziger, 1990), characterised by the image of whiteness as a referent of superiority.

According to MEVX, the training of psychologists in Guatemala is dissonant, because on the one hand, knowledge is transmitted that explains the Eurocentric or North American world, and on the other, professional practice is carried out in time-spaces which, although colonised, continue to organise life according to ancestral cosmogonies, contrary to those of colonial thought. MEVX reinforces the notion that colonial theories are based on liberal philosophy, which has the individual as its reference, while the cosmogony of the First Nation has the community as its reference.

This dissonance disadvantages and discriminates against young Maya-K'iche' in universities: they must confront, and reconcile in some way, ancestral thinking with colonial worldviews. For young Maya-K'iche', colonial thought represents a de-structuring mechanism because Eurocentric and Anglo-centric ideological-colonial visions are transmitted, which plant a racist spirit in the student's consciousness.

The Maya-K'iche' psychologists, after the 13th *B'aktun* and the beginning of the new epoch encompassing the decolonising struggle of thought, face a dilemma. They can accompany the ongoing colonial project of becoming ideologising instruments of the system, contributing to prolonging Eurocentrism or Anglo-centrism, doing research based on hegemonic Western thought that marginalises morality and ethics as lines of research (Flores Osorio, 2007, p. 40). Alternatively, they can assume their Mayab' identity and join the struggles for the defence of Mother Nature and land.

Tensions revealed through the knowledge dialogue

During our dialogue, the significance for MEVX of her training as a psychologist was highlighted. Her inclination to study psychology included the assumption that the training would provide her with elements to move towards the transformation of the racist Guatemalan reality and to exercise a professional practice, without harming ancestral wisdom. She also considered that her condition as a Maya-K'iche' woman could open the opportunity to understand the colonial dynamics. However, when she embarked on her professional path, she realised that what she had learned at the university was challenged by the Maya-K'iche' reality.

Through the dialogue, we came to the conclusion that in order to recover the *Maya' na'oj*, that is, Mayan thought or philosophy, and to carry out a community practice committed to anti-colonial struggles, it was necessary to: learn to respect Mother Nature, to put ancestral knowledge into dialogue with that learned at the university and to carry out a community praxis and ethics, orientated towards the production, reproduction and development of life (Dussel, 1998; Flores Osorio, 2018) as well as to fight to refound the state.

We came to the conclusion that in order to be both complementary to, and work on equal terms with the communities, it was fundamental to work for the liberation of the First Nations and the oppressed in general, as well as to act shoulder to shoulder with the community members to refound a plurinational state.

Only from this position is it possible to transcend the paternalistic and aid-orientated perspectives of the West and the belief in white supremacy that is brought to justify the exclusion and pauperisation of the K'iche' Mayan population.

Martinez Camarillo (2018) points out that in order for there to be symmetry between the communal and psychological, and an emergence of a decolonising practice, the contradictions posed by the division of labour between the physical and the intellectual must be overcome.

Through our dialogue, we agree with Martinez Camarillo (2018) when she suggests it is necessary to fight for the transformation of social structures and the construction of a different psychological practice, to trace a path of conscientisation – de-ideologisation – and reconstitution of the psychological. At its core, this demands, recovering historical-community memory (Flores Osorio, 2007), to assume a rebellious epistemology and a decolonising praxis, and "without pretending to be an agent of change and imposing beliefs and ways of life that do not coincide with the community's perspective of reality and the spatial-temporal dimension that becomes cultural-historical" (Flores Osorio, 2014, p. 71).

Conclusion

To summarise, Western psychologists must learn that when we work with First Nations we face a rationality different from ours. Understanding the "other" is to open the way to becoming aware that our praxis is full of contradiction. On the one hand we assume that we are researchers and, on the other, community members. Only then is it possible "to open up bonds of trust between the researcher and the key people. In the end, the community researcher is a tool of the community to systematise history and narratives" (Jerónimo, 2020, p. 19).

JMFO wants to emphasise that his work in Mayab' communities for more than 30 years has developed from a position of learning about the ancestral culture and working on the basis of the commissions that the community members assign him, all related to the anti-colonial struggles that they face. Consequently, he always works on the basis of the community projects undertaken by them, in the context of anti-colonial resistance and organised struggle in defence of their lands and Mother Nature, as fundamental principles of life.

Being Mayab' demands a particular way of life, a conception of the world and of being human that commits them to the *Patan* or community service, which implies carrying out the task beyond a simple labour compliance. We ladinos or colonised mestizos must face professional practice in these communities with the understanding that we will encounter different knowledge systems:

From the logic of the community, knowledge is common and is safeguarded orally, a long-standing tradition. The subjects do not blur; on the contrary, they reappear in moments of crisis to restore organisational practices and/or correct individualistic or unsupportive behaviours (Ochoa, 2020, p. 16).

Maya'no'oj, or Mayan thought, has spirituality and the cosmogony of life at its centre, always referring to the heart, the community and the mythical work of the ancestral authorities. In the Mayan tradition, the community members, by carrying out the *Patan* or community service, contribute to the collective balance, contrary to the Western vision centred on imposing ways of life through instrumentalised strategies and under the pretext of neutrality and scientific objectivity that deny the ethical-emotional and spiritual commitment proper to human experience.

Community Psychology from the Maya-K'iche' Nation

After learning about the importance of cosmogony in the Maya-K'iche' world, we consider that in order to promote a psycho-community project, it is necessary to start by questioning Eurocentric and Anglocentric thought, especially with regard to the notion of the individual and, consequently, individualism. The Maya-K'iche' conception is quite different, starting from the belief in the existence of ancestral authorities who fulfil various functions, including those corresponding to the maintenance of spiritual balance, or knowing that community work is a fundamental part of the service that each person has to perform in their community, which implies that there is no labour-salary relationship.

Community psychologists in Guatemala, and indeed elsewhere, must learn from the different-other through knowledge dialogues. In our case, this means seeking to understand the ancestral thought of the Maya-K'iche' First Nation, from the exteriority of Western rationalism. To understand the dynamics of exclusion-pauperisation, discrimination and racism that these nations have suffered since the Spanish invasion, we must question the philosophical, cultural, scientific and social foundations of hegemonic thought, a task that we need to carry out by working shoulder to shoulder in the struggles in defence of Mother Nature, the defence of territory and the bringing about of a plurinational state.

Despite the colonised views that we ladinos have of Mayab' knowledge, we need to realise that understanding of Maya-K'iche' cosmogony is open to all intellectuals who seek to decolonise their thinking, who are willing to dialogue with other-different people about community issues from within Maya-K'iche' life and not through the imposition of Western ways of life. The knowledge dialogue opens the way to share similarities and differences between ancestral Maya-K'iche' thought and Western thought, one focused on theoretical visions of the world, the other focused on its relationship with Mother Nature. In other words, we need to understand and transcend the Eurocentric and North American colonial perspectives and place at the centre the right of indigenous First Nations to education, health, work and economic wellbeing from their historical-cultural dimensions, specifically from their cosmovision.

References

Ak'abal, H. (2019). *Cosmogonía, la cruz maya*.Editorial Maya Wuj.

Anómimo. (1948). *El libro de los libros de Chilam Balam*. Fondo de Cultura Económica.

Barrios, C. (2004). *El libro del destino Kam Wuj*. Editorial Sudamericana.

Camey Huz, J.D. (2020).Terapeuta de la cultura Maya, Ajq´ij, medico epidemiologo. www.facebook. com/AEUoliverioCDL/

Cantón Delgado, M. (2005). *Echando fuera demonios, neo pentecostalismo, exclusión, étnica y violencia política en Guatemala. En protestantismo en el mundo Maya contemporáneo.*. Centro de Estudios Mayas, notebook 30. Universidad Nacional Autónoma de México y Universidad Autónoma Metropolitana.

Casaus, M.E. (1999). La metamorfosis del racismo en la elite de poder en Guatemala. In C. Arenas Bianchi, C.R. Hale, & G. Palma (Eds.), *¿Racismo en Guatemala?. Abriendo el debate sobre un tema Tabú*. Editorial AVANCSO.

Casaus, M.E. (2009). El racismo la discriminación en el lenguaje político de las élites intelectuales en Guatemala. *Discurso y Sociedad, 3*(4), 592–620.

CEH. (1999). Ed. *Guatemala, memoria del silencio: Informe*. Comisión Para El Esclarecimiento Histórico (Guatemala). https://digitallibrary.un.org/record/379513?ln=en

Colop, S. (1999). *Popol Wuj: Version poetica K'iche'*. Proyecto Maya de Educación Bilinguie Intercultural. PEMBI, GTZ.

Danziger, K. (1990).*Constructing the subject: Historical origins of psychological research*. Cambridge University Press.

de las Casas, B. (1958).Representatción a los Regentes Cisneros y Adriano – extracio. In B. de las Casas & T.B.J. Pérez (Eds.), *Obras escogidas de Fray Bartolomé de las Casas*(Vol. 5) . EdicionesAtlas. https://enriquedussel.com/txt/Textos_200_Obras/PyF_siglo_/Opusculos_cartas_memoriales-Bartolome_Casas.pdf

Dussel, E. (1994). *1492 el encubrimiento del otro. Hacia el origen del :mito de la Modernidad*. Plural Editores.

Dussel, E. (1998). *Ética de la liberación en la era de la globalización y la exclusión*. Editorial Trotta.

Estrada, A. (2010). *Popol Wuj: version actualizada basada en los textos Quiche con anotaciones del manuscrito de Fran Francisco Ximenez*. Editores Mexicanos Unidos, S.A.

Falla, R. (2006). *Historia de un gran amor, recuperación autobiográfica de experiencias con las comunidades de Poblacón en Resistencia, Ixcán, Guatemala*. Ediciones San Pablo.

Flores Osorio, J.M. (comp.) (2007). *Ciencia, ética y práctica psicológica en Psicología, globalización y desarrollo en América Latina*. Editorial Latinoamericana.

Flores Osorio, J.M. (2013). *De la intervención psicosocial a la praxis comunitaria en Psicología Social Comunitaria. Segunda Época, 2*(2), 40–55.

Flores Osorio, J.M. (coord.) (2014). *Repensar la psicología y lo comunitario en América Latina*. Universidad de Tijuana y Centro Latinoamericano de Investigación, Intervención y Atención Psicosocial.

Flores Osorio, J.M. (2017). Justicia transicional, acuerdos de paz en Guatemala y cosmovisión Maya-Quiché. In A.C. Castillejo Cuéllar (Ed.), *La ilusión de la justicia transicional:perspectivas críticas desde el Sur global*. Ediciones Uniandes. http://dx.doi.org/10.7440/2017.25

Flores Osorio, J.M. (2018). Martín-Baró descentrado de la psicología. *Teoría y Crítica de la Psicología, 11*, 23–43. http://teocripsi.com/ojs/index.php/TCP/article/view/266

Flores Osorio, J.M. (2020). Para comprender el mundo Maya después del 13 Baktún. *Teoría y Crítica de la Psicología,14*, 169–182. http://teocripsi.com/ojs/index.php/TCP/article/view/338

Gómez, A., Puigvert, L., & Flecha, R. (2011). Critical communicative methodology: Informing real social transformation through research. *Qualitative Inquiry, 17*(3), 235–45. https://doi.org/10.1177/1077800410397802

Gómez, H. et al. (2015). *Diálogo de saberes e interculturalidad: indígenas afrocolombianos y peasantry en la ciudad de Medellín*. University of Antioquia.

Hernández Ixcoy, D. (2020). *Nuevo B'aktun. Teoría y Crítica de la Psicología, 14*, 166–8. http://teocripsi.com/ojs/index.php/TCP/article/view/339

Hinkelammert, F.J. (1998). *El grito del sujeto. Del teatro-mundo del evangelio de Juan al perro mundo de la globalización*. Editorial DEI.

Jerónimo, L. (2020). *Metodologías comprometidas: La construcción de la investigación científica dentro del movimiento en defensa de los bosques de Cherán K'eri, Mkichoacán*. Asociación de Estudios Latinoamericanos, Universidad de Guadalajara.

León Chic, E. (2003). *El corazón de la sabiduría del pueblo Maya. Uk'ux'xal Ranima' ri Qano'jib'al*. Guatemala, editorial Maya´ Na´oj.

López Austin, A. (1997). La cosmovisión mesoamericana. In Enrique Nalda (coord.), Temas mesoamericanos. https://litmexicana.files.wordpress.com/2015/01/cosmovisic3b3n-en-pdf.pdf

Lucas, N. (2017). *May q'ij may saq, Filosofía del tiempo y de la claridad. Conocimientos y sabidurías ancestrales mayas*. Guatemala Ediciones Maya' Na'oj.

Martínez Camarillo, M. (2018). El mito de las relaciones simétricas entre miembros de la comunidad y psicólogos comunitarios. *Teoría y Crítica de la Psicología, 11*, 154–62. http://teocripsi.com/ojs/index.php/TCP/article/view/273

Ministry of Culture and Sports. (2014). *Nuevo Amanecer Maya*. Editorial Cultura.

Ochoa, Y. (2020). *Vicisitudes de los estudiantes investugadires Púrhepecha de Charapan Michoacán, la importancia de la red social*. Tesis de Grado, Universidad de Guadalajara.

ODHAG. (1988). *Guatemala, Nunca más*. Informe del Proyecto Interdiosesano de Recuperación de la Memoria Histórica.(REMHI). Guatemala.

ODHA. (1998). Guatemala Nunca Más. Impacts of violence. Oficina de Derechos Humanos de Apzobispado, Guatemala City.

Par Sapón, M.B. (2009). "El Kú´xa (corazón/espíritu) como base del sentir, penar y actuar de la cultura maya´K´iché. Una introducción a las raíces del conocimiento/práctica Maya K´iche´." Symposium on "Studies on the development of Indigenous American cultural traditions from precolonial times to the present". XV Congreso AHILA, Leiden. In Spanish. https://www.academia.edu/38862964/El_Mundo_Precolonial_y_sus_Transformaciones_a_partir_del_Contacto_con_los_Europeos.

Rupflin Alvarado, W. (1999). *El Tzolkin es más grande que un calendario*. CEDIM.

Taube, C.A. (1988). A prehispanic Maya Katun wheel. *Journal of Anthropological Research, 44*(2), 183–203.

Tedlock, B. (2011). Los sacradotes Mayas. in H. Ak'abal and R. Carmack (Eds.), *La Comunidad Maya K'iche' de Santiago Momostenango: su historia, cultura, lengua y arte* (pp. 51–80). Editorial Maya' Wuj.

UDEFEGUA. (2009). *Criminalisation of human rights defenders and defenders of human rights. Human. Reflexión sobre mecanismos de proección*. UDEFEGUA.

Velásquez Nimatuj, I. (2020). Colonialism and spiritual radicalism condemned to burn at the stake Domingo Choc Che. https://elperiodico.com.gt/opinion/opiniones-de-hoy/2020/06/13/el-colonialismo-y-radicalismo-espiritual-condeno-a-la-hoguera-a-domingo-choc-che/

Vigor, C. (2020). *Humberto Ak'abal, testimonio de un indio K'iche'*. Editorial Sophos.

20

SCHOLAR ACTIVISM

Mothering, disability and academic activism

Katherine Runswick-Cole, Andrea Ellwood,
Kerry Fox and Sara Ryan

Abstract

In this chapter, we explore the concept of scholar activism. We draw on our experiences as mothers of disabled children, activists and academics, and include case study examples to illustrate the ways in which we make sense of, and attempt to enact, scholar activism. We argue that:

The lines between what counts as "scholarship" and "activism" are inevitably blurred;
It is important to recognise the activisms of marginalised and minoritised groups that have, thus far, been overlooked as sites for the emergence of radical social movements;
Global crises have shone a spotlight on the bankruptcy of models of scholarship that seek to maintain a "respectable" distance between scholarship and activism.

Resumen

En este capítulo, exploramos el concepto del activismo erudico. Partimos desde nuestras experiencias como madres de niños discapacitados, y como activistas y académicas, e incluimos ejemplos de estudios de casos para ilustrar las formasen las que le damos sentido e intentamos poner en práctica el activismo académico. Argumentamos que:

Inevitablemente, las líneas entre lo que cuenta como "erudición" y "activismo" no son tan claras;
Es importante reconocer los activismos de grupos marginados y minorizados que, hasta ahora, hansido pasados por alto como lugares para el surgimiento de movimientos sociales radicales.
Las crisis globales han puesto de relieve la quiebra de modelos de estudios que buscan mantener una distancia "respetable" entre los estudios y el activismo.

Preface

We find ourselves, very unexpectedly, writing this chapter from England, in the midst of the global COVID-19 pandemic – a context that we simply cannot ignore. We hope that when this book is published, you will be reading this chapter in post-pandemic times. And yet, we are cautious about this "before" and "after" talk. Talk of "before" and "after" pandemic isolates

DOI: 10.4324/9780429325663-25

the pandemic as a single event, one to be overcome and moved on from in orderly fashion (Andermahr, 2015). To talk in these ways is to risk erasing long histories of inequality and social oppression which were there "pre-pandemic" as privilege (and lack of it) is shaping life and death as the pandemic unfolds. By positioning the pandemic as a temporally bounded event, it becomes possible to ignore the systems of oppression in place that made it possible for governments across the globe to deprioritise minoritised people during the pandemic (Altermark, 2020; Ktenidis, 2020; Runswick-Cole et al., 2020). At the time of writing from the UK, March 2021, and as we sit waiting for the second wave to wash over us, the Office for National Statistics (2020) has published figures that show 6 out of 10 COVID-related deaths since March 2020 are of disabled people.

These figures reveal the inadequacy of claims that "we are all in it together"; histories of oppression mean that the pandemic is disproportionately impacting upon people who are already marginalised through the workings of (hetero)sexism, racism, colonialism, poverty and disablism (Goodley, 2013). Across the globe, the pandemic has made it possible for human disposability to be openly referenced in public policy discourse as some bodies (and minds) are constructed as more "vulnerable" than others (Runswick-Cole et al., 2020). Discourses of "risk groups" have proliferated as a means of reassuring "normal" people that only "others" will die (Altermark, 2020). And yet, it is already clear that who lives and who dies in a pandemic is not simply a matter of biological "fact" but a matter of (bio)political choices (Ktenidis, 2020). As we write, we are beginning to glimpse some of the challenges that will face us post-pandemic, but we know that the shadows of the challenges that we faced before, and during the pandemic, will continue to shape all our lives in what comes "after". Scholar activists must have something to offer in these times of crisis and beyond.

Introduction

In this chapter, we reflect on the meaning of the term "scholar activism" and how this might be enacted in communities of practice, which include community psychologists, by reflecting on our experiences of mothering of disabled children, activism and scholarship. We hope that our reflections will offer something to activists and academics who care about scholarship and social justice. We begin with a discussion of the contested term "scholar activism", reflecting on our position in debates about its meaning, as academics and mothers of disabled children. We then describe some of the theoretical resources that inform our work, before describing three case study examples of the ways in which our scholarship and activism have been entwined. We conclude by reflecting on what can be learned from our experiences.

Scholar activism

Scholar activism is an umbrella term for the approach taken by academics who believe they have a role to play in creating social justice (Farnum, 2016). The place of social justice in Community Psychology has been the subject of continued debate (Prilleltensky & Nelson, 1997). Kagan et al. (2011) call for a Community Psychology which is embedded in local action and in wider movements for social justice. They draw on the Latin American Community Psychology concept of *incerción* to focus on the importance of "becoming one of the community, living there and experiencing life alongside other community members" (Kagan et al., 2011, p. 141). However, traditionally, academics, in psychology and elsewhere, have often sought to maintain a respectable distance between their political activism and their research publications and teaching (scholarship) (Kitchin & Hubbard, 1999), and have been positioned by others as "non-activists" (Taylor, 2014, p. 305). In the UK, the university system demands that academics promote their work so that it can be assessed for research quality and for the change, or "impact", it makes in the "real world" (REF, 2018). What counts as impact is driven by the demands of the UK's Research Excellence Framework (REF) criteria (REF, 2018). Subject-based units are assessed on the quality of outputs (e.g. publications, performances and exhibitions), the environment that supports research and their impact beyond academia (REF, 2018). This has led to a drive for academics to demonstrate their community-focused work, though what counts as "impact" is a highly contested topic, as we see below in the case study examples.

In the field of critical pedagogy, there have long been calls for educators to "reach beyond the boundaries of the classroom into communities, workplaces, and public arenas" (Darder, 2009, p. 158). The language of "reach" has drawn criticism. There is a danger that by reaching out, academics might simply reproduce the logics of the academy as they colonise community spaces (Webb, 2019). Webb (2019, p. 233) argues that social movements are not spaces which activist-scholars should be "reaching into"; rather, they are: "the primary sites in which activist-scholars collectively should be operating". Chomsky (2010) has argued that academics have a responsibility to use their privileges in the service of movements for social change (Webb, 2019), but Wark (2011, n.p.) stresses that the role of the academic is an "adjunct one", providing "a language for what the movement already knows".

It is clear from these discussions that scholar activists need to work in and with, not on, the communities they seek to serve; principles with which community psychologists can readily ally themselves. However, we notice that these debates are built on the assumption that the would-be scholar-activist is not already a member of the community into which they reach (Webb, 2019). We notice this assumption because of our own position in relation to scholarship and activism.

The authors of this chapter are all mothers of disabled children, and, like many mothers of disabled children, through our advocacy for our disabled children, we have become disability activists who have embraced scholarship as activism and activism as scholarship (Ryan & Runswick-Cole, 2008a). We first engaged with the academy in the hope that research and scholarship could shed light on the lives of children and their families that are too often ignored, and challenge the discrimination and oppression families face (Ryan & Runswick-Cole, 2008b). And yet, we discovered that the persistent inequalities in the lives of disabled children, young people and their families, have, too often, been ignored in studies of childhood while at the same time studies of disability have typically been an adult-centric field of inquiry (Curran & Runswick-Cole, 2014).

Our identity as mothers of disabled children has often been a contested one within disability activism and scholarship (Ryan & Runswick-Cole, 2008b). Our status as perceived to be "non-disabled mothers" of disabled children has raised questions from disability rights activists and academics about voice and power and our right to claim a place within disability studies scholarship and activism (Ryan & Runswick-Cole, 2008b). And yet while many mothers of disabled children are often perceived to be non-disabled and may, themselves, not identify as disabled people, we know that care work is associated with the acquisition of physical impairments over time. And many mothers live with mental health distress associated with the impact of engaging with a relentlessly disablist system in their advocacy for their child (Douglas et al., 2021). There is a blurring of the boundaries of dis/ability in the lives of mothers of disabled children who also experience disablism by virtue of their relationship to their disabled child (Goffman, 1963).

Both maternal scholarship and maternal activism have also struggled for recognition in the Global North. In neoliberal-ableist contexts (Goodley et al., 2014), disability and mothering are frequently constructed as private troubles for families and, as a result, they emerge as seemingly unlikely sites for the emergence of a radical new social movement. On the one hand, activism premised on mothers seeking a "cure" or rehabilitation for disabled children is validated as a "reasonable" response in neoliberal contexts where it has become the mother's duty to reduce her and her child's dependency on the state (Douglas et al., 2021; Jensen, 2012).On the other hand, maternal activism and scholarship, driven by the principles of social justice and a celebration of disability as part of the natural variation (Michalko, 2002), are invalidated as emotion-led (O'Reilly, 2016; Douglas et al., 2021).

And so, the scholar activism of mothers of disabled children is not, as Webb (2019) describes it, an attempt to reach into a community; rather, we are always and already members of that community. As mother-scholar-activists these roles are inseparable. We are not suggesting that this is the "right" way, or that there is only one way, to be a scholar-activist. Nor are we suggesting that only members of the community the academic seeks to serve can take the role of scholar-activists. Indeed, we would argue that we need academic-activist allies who are committed to social justice, as Chomsky (2010) suggests above, regardless of their personal positioning. However, we also need to resist the implicit, persistent assumption that it is always possible, and, perhaps by implication always desirable, to separate scholarship from activism. We must acknowledge our entanglements with others in our lives and resist "the artificial boundaries between spaces of scholarship and spaces of activism" (Routledge et al., 2015, p. 392).

Our academic work is about developing understanding and about making change. Over time, our academic activism has been driven by the persistent inequalities that remain entrenched in the lives of people with learning disabilities. The COVID-19 pandemic has shone a light on those inequalities and brought insidious practices around the discounting of particular lives to the surface.

Theoretical resources

In this section, we introduce some of the theoretical resources that are written through our scholar activism. We begin with the belief that disability is an opportunity. For readers more familiar with accounts of disability as a problem or a tragedy for unfortunate, isolated individuals (Oliver, 1990), this might seem a surprising place to start. But we have learned through our scholarship and activism that disability opens up opportunities to think differently (Goodley et al., 2017). The presence of our disabled children in our lives has disrupted many of the unspoken assumptions that circulate about "normal" family life.

It is important to remember that studies of disability and the discipline of psychology have an uneasy history (Goodley & Lawthom, 2005). As mothers of disabled children, we have experienced the legacies of the histories of psychologisation in our encounters with psy-professionals. Psychologists, psychiatrists, teachers and allied health and social care practitioners are often saturated in the view that mothers of disabled children must make a psychological adjustment to the trauma of becoming a parent of a disabled child (Bruce & Schulz, 2002). Mothers are made vulnerable to a diagnosis of post-traumatic stress disorder as a result of their child's diagnosis of disability (Roberts et al., 2014). And while we do not wish to deny that mothers of disabled children experience mental distress, we challenge the view that this is the inevitable consequence of grief or denial about our children's impairments (Lazarus &

Folkman, 1984). Rather, we seek to shift the focus of attention and to point to the impact of raising a child in a disabling world in which children who deviate from the mythical norms of child development are pushed to the margins of the category of child (Douglas et al., 2021; Goodley et al., 2015). Nonetheless, the dominant narrative, that disabled children are the cause of their mothers' distress, has proved difficult to disrupt (Douglas et al., 2021).

As a result, much of our scholarship and activism has sought to offer a more affirmative account of mothering disabled children (Darling, 1979; Douglas, 2014, 2014; Green, 2002; Ryan & Runswick-Cole, 2008b). In doing so, we have been drawn to emerging forms of activism and critique that consider what it might mean to reposition disability as something that we might desire precisely because it disrupts "normal" ways in which we live our lives (Goodley et al., 2017; McRuer, 2006).

Writing from the UK, our approach has been heavily influenced by the work of disabled scholars and activists who have called for a rejection of deficit models of disability that promote the pathologisation and exclusion of disabled people (Campbell & Oliver, 1996) and called instead for an understanding of disability as a form of social oppression; that is, a social model where disability is understood as the product of specific social and economic structures which cause institutional, cultural and psycho-emotional forms of discrimination and exclusion (Thomas, 1999). We follow Carol Thomas (2007, p. 73) in defining disablism as:

> a form of social oppression involving the social imposition of restrictions of activity on people with impairments and the socially engendered undermining of their psycho emotional well being.
>
> *(Thomas 2007, p. 73)*

We are particularly grateful for the contributions of feminist thinkers, like Thomas, to the development of critical disability studies. Feminists have demanded that gender be acknowledged in conceptualising disability (Thomas, 1999). Indeed, the social model has been criticised for privileging the concerns of "white, middle-class, professional, physically disabled men" (Lloyd, 2001, p. 726). Feminists, including Thomas (1999), Morris (1992) and Crow (1996), have challenged the assumption that disability studies must maintain a dignified distance between "public issues" and "private troubles" (Hanisch, 1970). By paying attention to the subjective experiences of disabled people, feminists have opened up the space for us to talk about disability, emotion and family life (Ryan & Runswick-Cole, 2008b).

We also recognise the importance of the theory and politics of postcolonial writing in critical disability studies and psychology (Nguyen, 2018; Fanon, 1986). We acknowledge the risks of appropriation, but as white, cisgender, activist-academics, we seek to ally ourselves to a commitment to expose and to challenge histories of oppression (Said, 1993). In particular, in postcolonial writing we have found critiques of models of trauma theory that: "adhere to the traditional event-based model of trauma, according to which trauma results from a single, extraordinary, catastrophic event" (Craps, 2013, p. 31 as cited in Andermahr, 2015). We agree that when trauma is framed as an historical event, as something to be worked through, this obscures the damage that continues to be inflicted on people who are expected to "come to terms with an event" and "move on" despite the failure to recognise or to address the persistence of the inequality and discrimination that caused the trauma in the first place (Andermahr, 2015; Douglas et al., 2021).

In the next section, we set out examples of what we are describing as case studies of scholar activism to illuminate the meanings and practices of scholar activism.

Scholar activism: three case studies

Case study one: Art as practice, art as activism – Kerry Fox

We as human beings do not operate within a social vacuum. Our assumptions, what we think and how we make sense of our world are part of our Dasein (Heidegger, 1962); our everyday being in the world is intrinsic to art and the work of art. The multiple variables that humans encounter and the entities that influence and impose themselves upon us are central to how we come to think about who and what we are and what things mean to us (Bolt, 2011).

My art practice navigates my motherhood as a carer, an ally and an activist and how materials tie these strands together like a lineage littered with emotion, twists and turns, and how a somewhat fraught and browbeaten narrative underpins the visual form. I seek to represent the strength of mother carers when faced with bureaucracy and the fragility of negotiating that journey. The rich tapestry of the materials and the underpinning of what they signify is complex and multi-layered, as is the navigation of the world from which they originate. I use documents that relate solely to my journey as a mother and carer from my son's birth to the present day. They document legal battles, his statementing of special educational needs,[1] his endless health assessments and diagnoses, his social care plans and SENDIST tribunals.[2] This is a charter of banal bureaucracy that follows a path of an officious system that has mapped our lives over 20 years.

I began my master's in fine art in 2018 when I was already involved in helping coordinate the SEND[3] Crisis March[4] for the Yorkshire Region as well as being an active member of SEND Action[5] and the founder of Save SEND Services North Yorkshire. I had been a regular sight at local council meetings, where provision for children with special educational needs was discussed, dressed as Madame Tricoteuse, sitting and knitting on the council building steps and in the chambers as cuts to Special Educational Needs services were voted upon and that I attended to speak on behalf of families opposing the cuts (see Figure 20.1). My life before

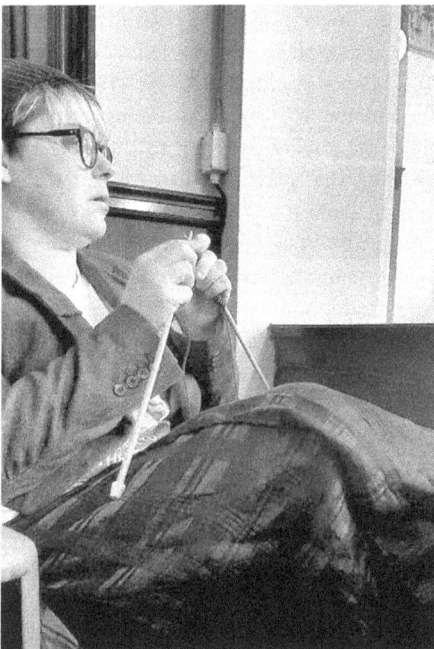

Figure 20.1   Mme Tricoteuse. Photograph credit, Andrea Ellwood (2018)

study was very much embedded in activism on a personal level, advocating for my son for over two decades and advocating for families. I have always considered myself a mother, a carer, an ally, an activist and an artist; they are the many roles I attribute to myself and see no separation between them. My work is autobiographical and the narratives experienced and journeys I take as a parent of a young person with disabilities weave through my art practice and inform my research.

As a researcher through art practice, scholar activism is embedded within my work as part of my "thrownness," the flux of my everyday life circumstances (Heidegger, 1962). The SEND Crisis Movement was planning a national march for May 2019. SEND Action were already in the process of bringing a National Judicial Review against the secretary of state and the children and families minister, and Save SEND Services had just campaigned locally on home school transport cuts and were also campaigning against the lack of social care for children on the autistic spectrum and closure of enhanced mainstream provision. While my research focused upon bureaucracy and how materials, namely Education, Health and Care plans and narratives give agency to the mother carer in the process of making, I was mindful that I was part of what was happening at this specific time, or as Tania Bruguera (2017) suggests, the "political timing specific" whereby the political conditions were such for the artwork or work to be necessary.

SEND Crisis

The SEND Crisis March was the first large-scale demonstration focused on the issue of SEND to happen as far I am aware.[6] For many years, smaller demonstrations have taken place on local levels, but the advent of social media and the ability for parent carers to connect across the country, and many social media groups being active since the reforms of 2014 eased the ability to coordinate and organise such an event. Several local authorities had been taken to judicial review[7] following cuts to SEND budgets, and the teachers unions too were demonstrating and vocal about the cuts to school budgets; hence, the conditions for a mass demonstration were ripe.

The objective was to have many voices heard including children, young people and siblings. In Leeds, I set up a banner and hearts for demonstrators of all ages to add their voices and messages as to why they were demonstrating as a participatory engagement piece. I sat back as they populated the banner with hearts and words (see Figure 20.2). Following the march, I took the artwork produced by the demonstrators to a gallery and included it in an exhibition for visitors to add their voices, but taking these out of the context of the march and the time specific, elicited a different reaction, with the general public seeing it as a protest against cuts in art education while those responding to the work in its intended form in the gallery setting, later identified themselves as parents or professionals who worked within SEND.

Enframing activism within a gallery in this instance failed to draw the same attention it did within the context of the rally. The political conditions had not entered the psyche of the general public. The demonstration received airplay on local and national television, and there were several radio interviews across each region highlighting the march and the purpose behind it. However, unless the population have experience and are affected by the issues being raised as part of their being in the world, then the understanding is lost and they try to make sense of what they see in relation to their everyday context.

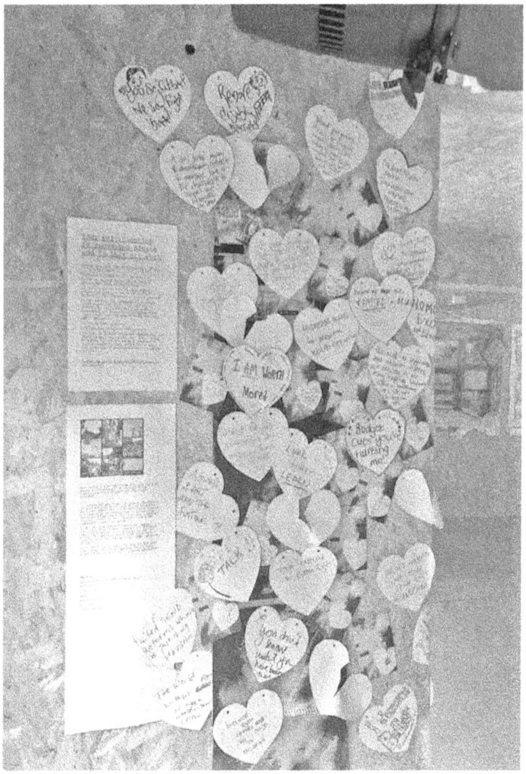

Figure 20.2 Yorkshire and Humber SEND crisis hearts. Photograph credit, Kerry Fox (2019)

SEND Action

SEND Action followed the SEND Crisis March with a Judicial Review in July 2019 and drew upon the work of Ernest Withers (1968) documenting the civil rights movement of the 1960s in America and the sanitation workers demonstration with the exclamation of "I AM" for their demonstration outside the High Court (see Figure 20.3).

Being part of SEND Action, SEND Crisis and a year of campaigns and demonstrations informed my final artwork for my master's degree (York St John University, 2019). Taking the bureaucracy of the officious documents with ruptures, twisting and inks bleeding through, adding the "I AM" representations of the loud hailers from the SEND Crisis March, and including the narratives from mother carers were all part of the process of making this project with a variety of materials (see Figures 20.3a,b,c).

Asking mother carers to sum up their experiences of navigating the bureaucracy they faced when seeking provision for their child/young person read like a litany of despair, despondency, gaslighting, with words that have not changed during decade upon decade for parents challenging the SEND system, including the labels attributed to them such as agitator, warrior, difficult parent, words that both valorise and vilify them (Runswick-Cole & Ryan, 2019). The use of "agitator", "difficult parent" and "warrior mum" started as derogatory statements referring to the mother carers who fought against the system. Edward Timpson (It Must Be Mum,

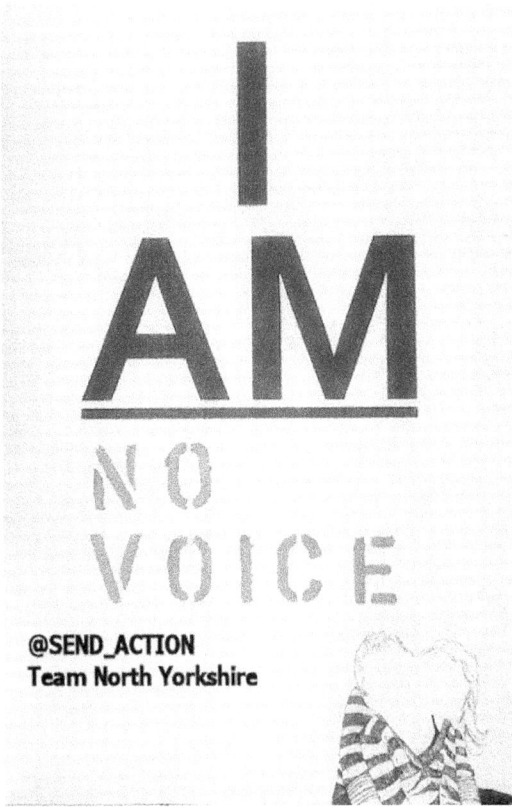

Figure 20.3 "I AM" SEND Action (2019)

2017). the then-children's and families minister, referred to mother carers, in his address to a national conference, as agitators. This was soon taken up by mother carers who then began to use his words to describe themselves as agitators and began to use "I am the difficult parent" hashtags and social media pseudonyms as a symbol that they were battling for their children's rights. I asked for mother carers to submit keywords that expressed the impressions they had of functioning within the bureaucracy that is the special educational needs and disabilities system. In order to collate which words fell into the "I am" category (Mother Carer) and those that fell into the "you are" (officious bureaucracy) category, for example: "I am defeated". "You are complicit". Was there an assumption about which words fell into which category? The answer is yes, they came from the viewpoint of my experiences and wit(H)ness in the same position with inside knowledge of the discourses engaged in by mother carers, parent carers and parent-led organisations. The words collected had several repetitions, and common themes were identified, almost forming a rhythm that lent itself to poetry. (Faulkner, 2009) The use of words woven into poetry as a tool to say what may not otherwise be said, poetry as methodology, allows a magnification of experiences and a means where the researcher and the researched can interweave their experiences; therefore, the use of poetry as methodology and as material brings the voice of the mother carer into an arena that allows for a stronger platform (see Figures 20.4a,b,c).

An ode

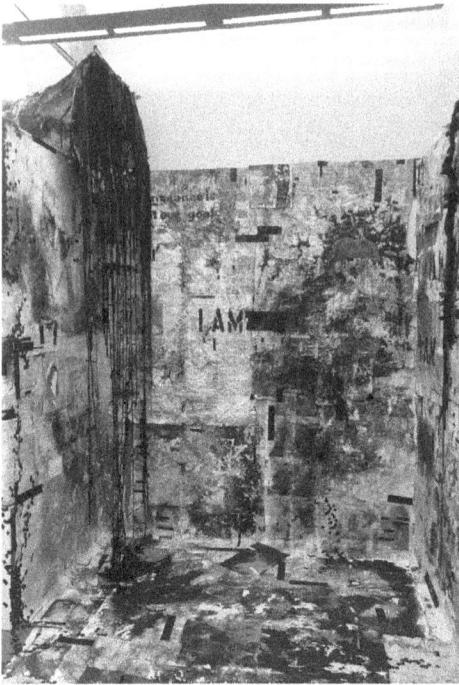

Figure 20.4a   Photograph credit Kerry Fox (2019)

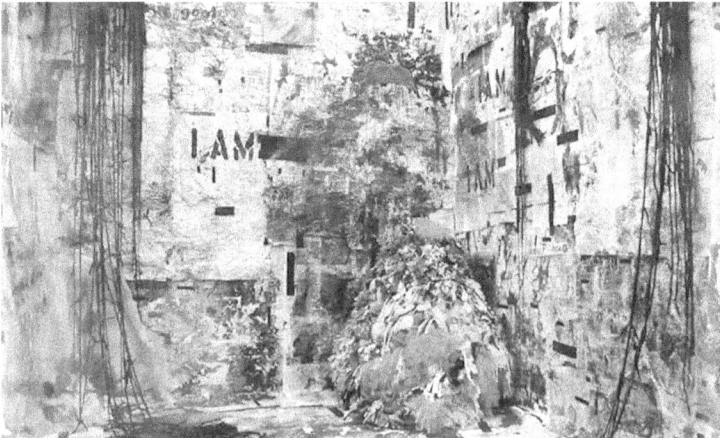

Figure 20.4b   Photograph credit Kerry Fox (2019)

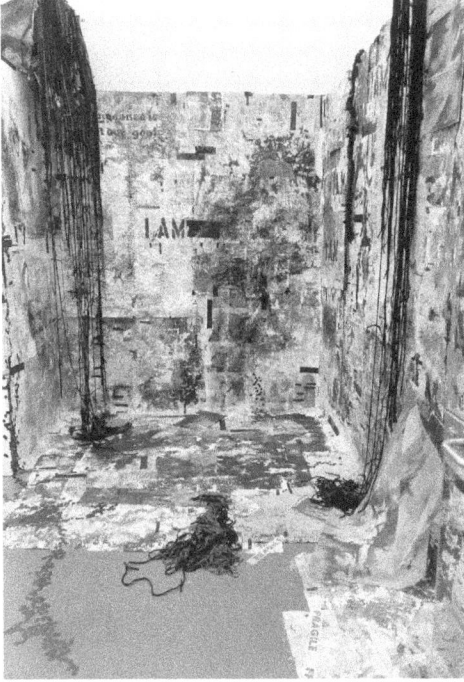

Figure 20.4c   Photograph credit Kerry Fox (2019)

"Ode To Bureaucracy"

I am the exhausted
I am lost
Disheartened, despondent, dejected
Battle hardened and weary
I am the mother
I am the carer
I am the other
The wind that blows in the in between
A mother
An other
The silenced
The charity case

I am the outspoken
You redact me
I outrage you
I am gagged
You gaslight
I am silent
I am the whisper
I roar

I am agitator
I am tiger
I am the warrior
The difficult parent
Mother blame

You are indifferent

You are silent
The twists
The barbs
You are tension
I am adversarial
I am ignored
I have no voice
You are complicit

I am the complainer

I am waiting
The deferred
The referred
The censored
You are assessment
The Censor
The Faceless
I am No one

I am broken

I am reduced
Exhausted
Tired
I battle on
You are relentless

You are Indifferent

You are bureaucracy
The officious
The policies
The cuts
You keep your silence
I am the petition

The re petition

The repetition
The silent
Never heard
Never seen
The loaded gun
The trigger
Silence
You pull
BANG BANG

Case study two: Justice for LB – Sara Ryan

The preventable death of Sara's 18-year-old son, Connor Sparrowhawk (see Figure 20.5), also known as Laughing Boy or LB, in July 2013, and the campaign that followed, #JusticeforLB, is an example of the blurring of scholarship and activism. Connor, diagnosed with autism, learning disabilities and epilepsy, was left to bathe unsupervised in an assessment and treatment unit and drowned. The NHS Trust responsible initially claimed Connor died from natural causes. His devastated family began a five-year battle to gain answers and accountability.

Since 2010, Sara had been documenting everyday family life on her blog: https://mydaftlife.com

The blog included a series of observations filled with joy and humour. When Connor became unwell and was admitted to the unit where he subsequently died, the blog became a bleak diary of the 107 days he spent there. Following Connor's death, the Trust and local authority focused their attention on blaming Sara, including circulating a briefing document about the blog the day after Connor died. Through the response on social media to Connor's death, the responsibility for gaining answers and accountability gradually became a collective endeavour among a diverse range of people, the majority of whom had never met Connor or his family and who campaigned under the #JusticeforLB.

In 2014, a celebration of the 107 days Connor spent in the unit before his death involved people adopting days between 19 March and 4 July to fundraise for the family's inquest legal fees or raise awareness more broadly about the issues people with learning disabilities face. There was an explosion of brilliant contributions from people as far away as Canada, the US, France, Spain

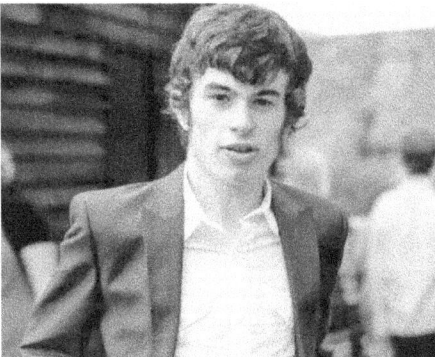

Figure 20.5　Photo of Connor

and New Zealand. Sporting events, artwork, cake sales, films and animations, musical events, academic talks, workshops, the creation of a #JusticeforLB quilt, bus rides and a #JusticeForLB flag which travelled to the Glastonbury music festival were carried out in Connor's memory and to raise awareness of the discrimination people with learning disabilities face. The full details of these activities can be seen here: https://107daysofaction.wordpress.com/

For four years, each attempt, by the Trust and local authority, to blame Sara for Connor's death was met with a lively resistance by the #JusticeForLB collective (Ryan, 2017). Social media played a crucial role in ensuring transparency and scrutiny, and Connor's inquest was the first inquest to be tweeted live, allowing a large audience to follow the proceedings online. Live tweeting was crucial as it made visible what is typically invisible in court proceedings, which included attempts to censor and silence (Ryan, 2017).

Eventually, the chief executive of NHS England agreed to commission a review into deaths in the NHS trust's learning disability and mental health services across a five-year period. This review (Mazars 2015) revealed scandalous dismissal and disregard of the lives of patients with learning disabilities and/or mental health issues and led to an urgent debate in both Houses of Parliament.

A prosecution of the trust by the Health and Safety Executive led to the biggest fine of a trust in the history of the NHS. The judge, in his closing remarks, pointedly referred to the mother-blame Sara experienced; "it is clear on the evidence that Dr Ryan, in particular, faced not merely resistance but entirely unjustified criticism as she pursued her Justice for LB campaign".

The campaign produced two further key documents; the LB Manifesto and a Private Members Bill, the #LBBill in the UK Parliament. The LB Manifesto clearly laid out the aims of the campaign in relation to accountability for what happened to Connor and other young people. The LB Bill[8] aimed to change the law for disabled people so that they have more control over what happens in their lives (Ryan, 2017). Although the LB Bill did not become law, the then-secretary of state for social care, Norman Lamb, drew on sections of the bill and worked with campaigners when producing the Green Paper *No Voice Unheard, No Right Ignored* (Department of Health, 2015).

The Justice for LB Campaign was awarded a Liberty Human Rights award and Sara was recognised with an honorary doctorate of science by Oxford Brookes University in June 2019. And yet, despite all these changes, as we suggested above, what counts as impact in academic circles is highly contested, so much so that the university Sara works for chose not to engage with her scholar activism to the extent the university-wide staff magazine refused to include a piece about #JusticeforLB. Sara was, however, asked to be interviewed about a four-day exchange trip to Japan around learning disability provision in both countries. Sara was left wondering why her scholar activism didn't count in the same way.

Case study three: A broken social contract: coronavirus and disabled people – Katherine Runswick-Cole

In March 2020, as the coronavirus began to tighten its grip in the UK, the government passed a range of legislation giving it extraordinary powers to manage the pandemic. The Coronavirus Act effectively broke the social contract between disabled people and government that had persisted for the previous 30 years by:

- Giving local government the authority to "ease" their responsibilities to deliver social care under the Care Act, 2014;

- Giving the secretary of state for education the power to disapply the law in relation to pro-vision for disabled children and young people;
- Making it easier for people to be detained under the Mental Health Act (MHA) 1983 (Runswick-Cole et al., 2020)

In March 2020, Derbyshire County Council was one of nine local authorities that made the decision to introduce "easements" under the Coronavirus Act that would allow them to downgrade their duties under the Care Act (2014). This decision had a potentially devastating impact on Katherine's son William. Twenty-four-year-old William relies on direct payments for social care to deliver the support he needs to live an ordinary life as part of his community. Derbyshire's "easing" of Care Act duties put this support at risk, and it appeared to Katherine that William was facing the prospect of potentially reduced, or even no, support.

Through her involvement with #JusticeforLB and as part of her work on a research project, "Big society? Disabled people with learning disabilities and civil society",[9] Katherine already knew Steve Broach, a barrister at 39 Essex Chambers. Steve put Katherine in touch with Alex Rook, at the public law firm Rook, Irwin, Sweeney (RIS Law). With support from RIS Law's Education, Health and Care Social Justice Fund,[10] pre-action steps were taken towards potential judicial review proceedings in relation to the Council's triggering of the easements. In an exchange of legal letters, the team discovered that Derbyshire triggered the easements on March 30, 2020, but did not communicate this decision, even as they were required to, to the secretary of state, and then only published the decision squirrelled away in a 210-page Cabinet Report document.

Derbyshire said that the council "has learned lessons from having to react swiftly to a situation never encountered before and will certainly respond differently in the future, should the need arise, in a number of respects, but certainly in relation to publicity and communication" (Samuel, 2020).

The Law Society (2020, p. 37) commented that:

> a failure to comply with the required processes undermines the already reduced protections for vulnerable individuals who may be reliant on care services. In the case of Derbyshire Council, the legal approach prompted it to reconsider and rectify its actions. This demonstrates the value of legal advice for challenging improper imple-mentation of emergency measures and providing redress when necessary, especially in the face of reduced scrutiny from alternative mechanisms.

The legal challenge had the potential to benefit all disabled residents of Derbyshire; nonethe-less, we feel that it is important to acknowledge that activism by academics can reinforce their position of privilege. Access to justice was made possible through Katherine's scholar-activist networks. We need to be aware of such privilege and to share knowledge and resources within and beyond our networks wherever possible.

Conclusion

We began with the promise of a reflection on what we have learned through our work. For us, scholar activism is a contested term, but it should remain so – always in contention and always the subject of debate. Sitting with the uncertainty and the blurring of the boundaries between scholarship and activism is an important part of the work we do. Global crises, like the COVID-19 pandemic, have shone a spotlight on the bankruptcy of models of scholarship that seek to maintain a "respectable" distance between scholarship and activism. And yet, it is important to recognise the activism of marginalised and minoritised groups remains under-recognised as sites for the emergence of radical social movements.

In our case study examples, we see the power of community, the emergence of online activism and the importance of the arts for bringing together communities of practice. Embracing the arts can build connections and much-needed collective strength and solidarity when times are tough, and this inevitably means engaging the imagination to explore injustice and to address power imbalances. We also saw the power of alliances with lawyers and the need for greater access to justice, particularly in times of crisis.

Finally, theoretical perspectives matter. They guide our work, but, at the same time, we know that theorisation does not only take place inside the academy. As Ahmed (2000) has noted, radical (feminist) theorising often takes place in activist spaces. Mothers of disabled children are engaged in everyday theorising about the lives of their children as they navigate the often hostile waters of education, health and social care. And while some philosophers become mothers of disabled children (Kittay, 2019), all mothers of disabled children become philosophers.

Notes

1 A statement of special educational needs is the document in which children's additional learning difficulties and the provision intended to address these is set out in the education system in England. In 2015, following a review, this was replaced with an Education, Health and Care Plan to reflect the health and social care needs of children in addition to their learning needs

2 SENDIST (The Special Educational Needs and Disability Tribunal) is the court where challenges can be made by young people and their parents/carers to decisions about support for their education set out in the statement or Education, Health and Care Plan. Parents/carers report accessing the tribunal as extremely stressful (Runswick-Cole, 2007)

3 SEND is the acronym used in the English education system to describe children with special educational needs and/or disabilities.

4 The SEND National Crisis campaign wants the government to better meet the needs of SEND pupils, and bridge the estimated £1.2 billion shortfall in high needs funding in England that has opened up since 2015 (Oscroft, 2019).

5 SEND Action is a UK network of families, individuals and organisations committed to upholding the rights of disabled children and young people

6 Mass protests took place in the 1990s which led to the Disability Discrimination Act (DDA) (HMSO, 1995). The DDA made it illegal for employers and service providers to discriminate against disabled people, which included schools, but, in contrast to the SEND Crisis March, education was not the only focus of the protests.

7 Judicial Review is a court case where the claimant challenges the lawfulness of the government's decision.

8 See: https://lbbill.wordpress.com/

9 Details of the project can be found here: https://bigsocietydis.wordpress.com

10 Details of the Education, Health, Care (EHC) Social Justice Fund can be found here: https://rookirwinsweeney.co.uk/social-justice-fund/

References

Ahmed, S. (2000). *Strange encounters: Embodied others in post-coloniality*. Routledge.

Altermark, N. (2020). The function of risk groups in Sweden, disability and Covid: The global impacts. iHuman. University of Sheffield. http://ihuman.group.shef.ac.uk/global-impacts-of-covid/

Andermahr, S. (2015). Decolonizing trauma studies: trauma and postcolonialism – introduction. *Humanities, 4*, 500–5.

Bolt, B. (2011). *Heidegger reframed*. I. B. Tauris.

Bruce, E., & Schultz, C. (2002). Non-finite loss and challenges to communication between parents and professionals. *British Journal of Special Education, 29*, (1), 9–13.

Bruguera, T. (2017. *Art + activism = artivism.* TED Archive. [Video]. YouTube. www.bing.com/videos/search?q=tania+bruguera&&view=detail&mid=D2D97DA7F614538B3F9ED2D97DA7F614538B3F9E&&FORM=VDRVRV&ajf=10, 2017

Campbell, J., & Oliver, M. (1996). *Disability politics: Understanding our past, changing our future.* Routledge.

Chomsky, N. (2010). Intellectuals and the responsibilities of public life. In J. Sandlin, B. Schultz, & J. Burdick (Eds.), *Handbook of public pedagogy* (pp. 576–83). Routledge.

Crow, L. (1996). Including all of our lives: Renewing the social model of disability. In J. Morris (Ed.). *Encounters with strangers: Feminism and disability* (pp. 206–26). Women's Press.

Curran, T.,& Runswick-Cole, K. (2014). Disabled children's childhood studies: An emerging domain of inquiry? *Disability & Society, 29*(10), 1617–30.

Darder, A. (2009). Imagining justice in a culture of terror. In S. Macrine (Ed.), *Critical pedagogy in uncertain times* (pp. 151–66). Palgrave.

Darling, R.B. (1979). *Families against society: A study of reactions to children with birth defects.* Sage.

Department of Health. (2015). *No voice unheard, no rights ignored.* https://assets.publishing.service.gov.uk/government/uploads/system/uploads/attachment_data/file/409816/Document.pdf

Douglas, P. (2014). Refrigerator mothers. *Journal of the Motherhood Initiative, 5*(1), 94–114.

Douglas, P., Runswick-Cole, K., Ryan, S., & Fogg, P. (2021). Mad mothering: Learning from the intersections of madness, mothering and disability. *Journal of Cultural and Literary Disability Studies, 15*(1), 39–56.

Fanon, F. (1986). *Black skins, white masks.* Pluto.

Farnum, R. (2016, June 3). Scholar activism – a growing movement of scholar activists. *University World News.* www.universityworldnews.com/article.php?story=20160530142606345

Faulkner, S. (2009). *Poetry as methodology* (1st ed.).Routledge.

Goffman, E. (1963). *Stigma: Notes on the management of a spoiled identity.* Simon & Schuster.

Goodley, D. (2013). Dis/entangling critical disability studies. *Disability & Society, 28*(5), 631–44. https://doi.org/10.1080/09687599.2012.717884

Goodley, D., & Lawthom, R. (2005). *Disability and psychology: Critical introductions and reflections.* Palgrave MacMillan.

Goodley, D., & Runswick-Cole, K. (2014). Big society? Disabled people with the label of learning disabilities and the queer(y)ing of civil society. *Scandinavian Journal of Disability Research, 17*(1), 1–13.

Goodley, D., Miller, M., & Runswick-Cole, K. (2017). Teaching critical disability studies. In C. Newness (Ed.), *Teaching critical psychology* (pp. 64–81). Routledge.

Goodley, D., Runswick-Cole, K., & Liddiard, K. (2015). The dishuman child. In *Discourse: The cultural politics of education*, 37(5), 770–784.

Green, S. E. (2002). Mothering Amanda: Musings on the experience of raising a child with cerebral palsy. *Journal of Loss and Trauma*, 7, 21–34.

Hanisch, C. (1970)."The personal is political." In S. Firestone & A. Koedt (Eds.), *Notes from the second year: Women's liberation* (pp. 76–8). Radical Feminism.

Heidegger, M. (1962). *Being and time.* (Trans. J. Maquarrie & E. Robinson). Blackwell.

Her Majesty's Stationary Office (HMSO) (1995). The Disability Discrimination Act. HMSO.

It Must Be Mum. (2017). SEND Parent = Agitator? https://itmustbemum.wordpress.com/2017/02/24/send-parent-agitator/comment-page-1/.

Jensen, T. (2012). Tough love in tough times. *Studies in the Maternal, 4*(2), 1–26.

Kagan, C., Burton, M., Duckett, P., Lawthom, R., & Siddiquee, A. (2011). *Critical community psychology* (1st ed.). Wiley-Blackwell.

Kitchin, R.M., & Hubbard P.J. (1999). Research, action and "critical" geographies. *Area, 31*, 195–8.

Kittay, E.F. (2019). *Learning from my daughter: The value and care of disabled minds.* Oxford University Press.

Ktenidis, A. (2020). Covid and the implications of its ontologically violent message. iHuman. University of Sheffield. http://ihuman.group.shef.ac.uk/global-impacts-of-covid/

The Law Society. (2020). Law under lockdown: The impact of COVID-19 measures on impact to justice for vulnerable people. www.lawsociety.org.uk/topics/research/law-under-lockdown-the-impact-of-covid-19-measures-on-access-to-justice-and-vulnerable-people

Lazarus, R.S., & Folkman, S. (1984). *Stress, appraisal and coping.* Springer.

Lloyd, M. (2001). The politics of disability and feminism: Discord or synthesis? *Sociology, 35*(3), 715–28.

Mazars. (2015, December). *Independent review of deaths of people with a Disability or Mental Health problem in contact with Southern Health NHS Foundation Trust April 2011 to March 2015.* www.england.nhs.uk/south/wp-content/uploads/sites/6/2015/12/mazars-rep.pdf

McRuer, R. (2006). *Crip theory: Cultural signs of queerness and disability.* NYU Press.

Michalko, R. (2002). *The difference that disability makes.* Temple University Press.

Morris, J. (1992). Personal and political: a feminist perspective on researching physical disability. *Disability, Handicap & Society, 7*(2), 157–66.

Nguyen, T.X. (2018). Critical disability studies at the edge of global development: Why do we need to engage with southern theory? *Canadian Journal of Disability Studies, 7*(1), 1–25.

Office for National Statistics. (2020). *Coronavirus (COVID-19) related deaths by disability status, England and Wales: 2 March to 14 July 2020.* www.ons.gov.uk/peoplepopulationandcommunity/birthsdeathsandmarriages/deaths/articles/coronaviruscovid19relateddeathsbydisabilitystatusenglandandwales/2marchto14july2020 - main-points

Oliver, M. (1990). *The politics of disablement.* Macmillan.

O'Reilly, A. (2016). *Matricentric feminism: Theory, activism & practice.* Demeter Press.

Oscroft, A. (2019). Campaigners to march on Downing Street over SEND funding crisis. *Schools Week.* https://schoolsweek.co.uk/campaigners-to-march-on-downing-street-over-send-funding-crisis/

Prilleltensky, I., & Nelson, G. (1997). Community psychology: Reclaiming social justice. In D. Fox & I. Prilleltensky (Eds.), *Critical psychology: An introduction* (pp. 166–84). Sage.

Research Excellence Framework. (2018, January). *Draft guidance on submissions.* www.ref.ac.uk/publications/draft-guidance-on-submissions-201801/

Roberts, A.L., Koenen, K.C., Lyall, K., Ascherio, A., & Weisskopf, M.G. (2014). Women's post traumatic stress symptoms and autism spectrum disorder in their children. *Research in Autism Spectrum Disorders, 8*(6), 608–16.

Routledge, P., & Driscoll Derickson, K. (2015). Situated solidarities and the practice of scholar-activism. *Environment and Planning D: Society and Space, 33*(3), 391–407.

Runswick-Cole, K. (2007). "The tribunal was the most stressful thing: more stressful than my son's diagnosis or behaviour": The experiences of families who go to the Special Educational Needs and Disability Tribunal (SENDIST). *Disability and Society, 22*(3), 315–28.

Runswick-Cole, K.&Ryan, S. (2019.) Liminal still? Unmothering disabled children. *Disability & Society,* 1125–39. https://doi.org/10.1080/09687599.2019.1602509

Runswick-Cole, K., Goodley, D., & Liddiard, K. (2020). Human disposability in England. iHuman. University of Sheffield. http://ihuman.group.shef.ac.uk/global-impacts-of-covid/.

Ryan, S. (2017). *Justice for Laughing Boy.* Kingsley.

Ryan, S.,&Runswick-Cole, K. (2008a). From advocate to activist? Mapping the experiences of mothers of children on the autism spectrum. *Journal of Applied Research in Intellectual Disabilities, 22*(1), 43–53.

Ryan, S., & Runswick-Cole, K. (2008b). Repositioning mothers: Mothers, disabled children and Disability Studies. *Disability & Society, 23*(3), 199–210.

Said, E.W. (1993). *Culture and imperialism.* Vintage.

Samuel, M. (2020, June 5). Council says it has learned lessons after care act legal challenge dropped. *Community Care Magazine.* www.communitycare.co.uk/2020/06/05/council-says-learned-lessons-care-act-legal-challenge-dropped/

Taylor, M. (2014). "Being useful" after the Ivory Tower: Combining research and activism with the Brixton Pound. *Arena, 46*(3), 305–12.

Thomas, C. (1999). *Female forms: Experiencing and understanding disability.* Open University Press.

Thomas, C. (2007). *Sociologies of illness and disability: Contested ideas in disability studies and medical sociology.* Palgrave MacMillan.

Wark, M. (2011). This shit is fucked up and bullshit. *Theory and Event, 14*(4). https://muse.jhu.edu/issue/24512

Webb, D. (2019). Prefigurative politics, utopian desire and social movement learning: reflections on the pedagogical lacunae in Occupy Wall Street. *Journal for Critical Education Policy Studies, 17*(2), 204–45.

Withers, E. (1968). *Iamaman.* Prezi. https://prezi.com/-vbynwzph4io/i-am-a-man-photography-by-ernest-c-withers-1968/

21

BUILDING PARTNERSHIPS FOR COMMUNITY-BASED SERVICE-LEARNING IN POVERTY-STRICKEN AND SYSTEMICALLY DISADVANTAGED COMMUNITIES

Jacqueline Akhurst and Nqobile Msomi

Abstract

Post-apartheid resource constraints in South Africa demand responses beyond individually focused psychology. People's health and well-being are impacted by contextual challenges such as: family dislocation and disruption, widespread unemployment and poverty, and the high incidence of violence and crime (given the violent past of the apartheid state). Increased access to psychological assistance may offer support and promote mental health.

Recently in universities, community engagement has been emphasised alongside teaching and research, to promote knowledge exchange with community partners. Given imperatives to decolonise knowledge in psychology, community-based service-learning (CBSL) provides a mechanism. We explore CBSL for trainee psychologists, within a Community Psychology master's module, focusing upon the often-neglected perspectives of community partners. Through three case examples from organisations working with children and youth, accounts of collaborative work illustrate trainees' contributions and the impacts of contextual factors. We make recommendations, to support more sustainable CBSL partnerships, aimed towards civic empowerment and social change.

Resumen

Las limitaciones de recursos posteriores al apartheid en Sudáfrica exigen respuestas que van más allá de la psicología centrada en el individuo. La salud y el bienestar de las personas se ven afectados por desafíos contextuales tales como: dislocación y ruptura familiar, desempleo y pobreza generalizados, y la alta incidencia de violencia de género y otras formas de violencia

DOI: 10.4324/9780429325663-26

(dado el pasado violento del país). Un mayor acceso a la asistencia psicológica puede ofrecer apoyo social y promover la salud mental.

Recientemente, en las universidades, se ha enfatizado la participación de la comunidad junto con la enseñanza y la investigación, para promover el intercambio de conocimientos con socios comunitarios. Dados los imperativos para descolonizar el conocimiento en Psicología, el aprendizaje en servicio basado en la comunidad (CBSL en inglés) proporciona un mecanismo para dicha transformación. Exploramos CBSL para psicólogos en formación, dentro de un módulo de Maestría en Psicología Comunitaria; centrándose en las perspectivas frecuentemente descuidadas de nuestros socios de la comunidad. A través de tres ejemplos de casos de organizaciones que trabajan con niños y jóvenes, los relatos del trabajo colaborativo evidenciaremos las contribuciones de los alumnos y los impactos de los factores contextuales. Hacemos recomendaciones, para apoyar alianzas para CBSL más sostenibles, dirigidas hacia el empoderamiento cívico y el cambio social.

Context

In South Africa (SA), post-apartheid resource constraints demand responses that are wide-reaching, since people's needs cannot be met through individually focused traditional psycho-logical interventions. The number of psychologists per capita is relatively low (Sodi, 2017), and to seek individual assistance, people need medical insurance (available to less than 20% of the population). Many of the problems causing widespread mental distress relate to the structural and systemic inequalities in a country with a GINI coefficient amongst the highest in the world (World Bank, 2019). Such inequalities result in elevations in a number of indices of mental distress, for example teenage pregnancy rates, levels of illiteracy, numbers of prisoners and sub-stance dependencies (Wilkinson & Pickett, 2009).

As a consequence of contextual issues, many people struggle with multiple challenges, including very limited income opportunities leading to widespread poverty, and family dis-location and disruption due to migrations into metropolitan areas (Mlambo, 2018), often for poorly paid work opportunities. Associated issues are inadequate housing (often in informal settlements), under-resourced schools and limited infrastructure, due to local authorities not keeping pace with service delivery demands. Additionally, a high incidence of gender-based and other forms of violence exist (much of this a legacy of the violent apartheid past); thus, people experience high levels of crime. All of the above have concomitant effects on health (Flisher et al., 2012).

When faced with such systems-related issues, psychologists need to work with community-based partners, to multiply the effectiveness of potential interventions and to collaborate with other agencies. Some community-based organisations (often constituted as non-profit organisations, NPOs) work to advocate for structural social change, and there is potential to work in solidarity with them. A social action model of Community Psychology (Ahmed & Pretorius-Heuchert, 2001) seems best suited to the context, to prompt greater responsiveness from local and regional governmental structures.

Although very locally based in a small city in the Eastern Cape, SA, our chapter refers to challenges common in marginal settlements of the major cities in SA and in other low- and middle-income countries. Many of the issues above could be tackled with increased access to psychological assistance, to promote mental health and increase support. This chapter explores community-based service-learning (CBSL) as a means of providing assistance, as incorporated into the Community Psychology coursework of trainee psychologists, in their final year of studies before completing a year-long practicum (internship). Since service-learning is often managed by central university units, it has infrequently overlapped with Community Psychology. We hope this chapter will illustrate the synergies between the two.

We are writing this chapter at a time of change. Jacqueline (the first author) recently retired from her full-time position, in which she managed and supervised the work of trainees that we reflect upon. Nqobile was appointed as an early-career lecturer to take on this work, contributing in a number of ways: during 2019, she had worked in one of the NPOs who hosted CBSL, so has a sense of the partner experience; then, she conducted the interviews that form the basis of the case accounts in this chapter; finally during 2020, she became coordinator of the CBSL module and has implemented changed (and more systemic) activities, during the COVID-19 crisis.

Community Psychology and community-based service-learning

In recent years, our university has emphasised community engagement (CE) alongside teaching and research, in order to promote knowledge exchange through building stronger social compacts with community partners. This derives from post-apartheid national imperatives for greater contributions from universities to societal reconstruction (Department of Education, 1997), with service-learning as a key mechanism. Some universities might have approached these requirements through centralised units that have had limited influence: thus seeming to pay "lip-service" to CE. This has not been the case in our university, where the number and quality of CE programmes has grown and made valuable contributions. In psychology, given the need to decolonise knowledge construction (Barnes & Siswana, 2018), CBSL has the potential to contribute towards transformation. In postgraduate psychology we have actively developed modules with embedded CBSL, planning activities that resonate with many students' desires to assist communities. Being committed to the values, principles and theoretical underpinnings of Community Psychology, we consider how we might translate these into "real world" practice through CBSL.

For this chapter, we will focus on CBSL within a compulsory Community Psychology module, completed by master's-level (the final academic exit point for practitioners) trainee clinical and counselling psychologists. Table 21.1 provides a snapshot of the overall structure of training for SA counselling or clinical psychologists.

During the first year (M1) of many programmes in SA, Community Psychology is part of professional training, to equip trainees with skills that are broader in scope than those focused on individual interventions (Carolissen, 2006), enabling work in community settings. Trainees will have had various levels of prior exposure, depending on their earlier studies, though some may never have studied Community Psychology. The M1 module is partially intended to equip trainees for a governmental innovation that expands services provided by the state health system, in which clinical psychologists are mandated to complete an additional paid "community service" year (Ahmed & Pillay, 2004), after completing their degree and second-year internship (M2, within psychiatric settings). Counselling psychology trainees do not complete an equivalent third year, though the field's scope in SA has strong leanings towards Community Psychology-related work (Bantjes et al., 2016).

Table 21.1 Master's degree studies for counselling and clinical psychologists in South Africa

Year of master's study	Short-name	Cohort of students
Year 1 (theory / practice)	M1	Counselling/clinical
Year 2 (practicum)	M2	Counselling/clinical
Year 3	Community service	Clinical only

Table 21.2 Basic outline of module activities

1. Introductory weeks of Community Psychology module – March		
2. M2 presentations of previous year's projects – April		
Project 1 with partner A	Students 1 & 2	3. CBSL activities
Project 2 with partner B	Students 3 & 4	May–November
Project 3 with partner C	Students 5 & 6	
Project 4 with partner D	Students 7 & 8	
Project 5 with partner E	Students 9 & 10	
Project 6 with partner F	Students 11 & 12	

In M1, the Community Psychology module (with design and facilitation influenced by Vygotskian and humanistic influences, see Lawthom, 2011) prepares trainees for and then supports their CBSL. Reflexive elements encourage trainees to make links between theory and practice (Gilbert & Sliep, 2009), with an emphasis on balancing societal and partners' needs. Trainees critically reflect upon the ways in which values: social justice, stewardship and building community or solidarity (Kagan et al., 2020), underpin their approaches to partnership working and activities.

Practically, after the introductory weeks of the module, trainees from the previous year present information on possible continuing projects. Potential new projects are also outlined, where community-based organisations have requested assistance. This allows for some evolution in projects from one year to the next, with some partnerships ending naturally, others continuing and there being new opportunities. Table 21.2 provides an overview of the module structure over one calendar year.

The cohort of 12 M1 trainees select those CBSL projects in which they are interested, with discussions if necessary to negotiate final placements. Six projects (one per pair) are facilitated between May and November. After preliminary briefings by us as tutors, trainees then contact their partners, meet up and discuss the intended work. Some projects may require a needs analysis, for example through asset-based community development (ABCD, Kagan et al., 2020). The work is planned and further negotiated with partners to set realistic goals and activities. The trainees actively engage for up to six months, with many paying weekly visits to their respective settings during coursework time. The tutors are allocated approximately two hours supervision for each pair over the period, and trainees attend weekly peer group supervision (Akhurst & Kelly, 2006).

Building partnerships

This study draws from the often-neglected voices of our community partners (Akhurst, 2016), reporting their perspectives of working in partnership with M1s. It is useful to introduce literature that highlights partnership-working and development in CBSL, before presenting the case examples.

As in the evolution of Community Psychology towards more critique, literature in CBSL mirrors practitioners' deepening insights, through reflexivity about their roles and key elements for partnership-building and maintenance. Whereas earlier CBSL illustrates partnerships in which academics lead in "knowledge exchange", with students seeming to benefit more from the partnership than members of the target community, in the past two decades, more critical lenses have been applied to CBSL. This has led to debates about power and the motives of participants, and questions around resources and who benefits. Preece (2012) emphasises the role of stronger social compacts with community partners for meaningful student engagement, recommending that partnerships evolve in socially accountable ways. It is therefore important to examine the basis for partnership-building, the nature of the relationships established, the expectations and goals of the collaboration and the exchanges of knowledge and other resources that occur.

Earlier partnerships in CBSL relied on an "exchange": altruistic intentions enabled community access to the labour and knowledge of trainees, who in their turn needed "real world" experiences, in order to gain skills and apply their theoretical learning. NPOs in SA often feel frustration at the lack of delivery of services and funding from the various governmental education, social care or health sectors, and staff time limitations may also inhibit the achieving of goals. They thus appreciate offers of assistance from other sources. The proliferation of NPOs in Africa in recent years has been noted (Matthews & Nqaba, 2017). In SA's early post-apartheid transitionary years, the funding of NPOs was redirected to government. However, the increasing failure of government provision of services represents a part of the current political crisis.

To avoid a deficit approach, it is important to discuss the assets that each partner brings to the collaboration, perhaps through an inclusive ABCD assessment (Kagan et al., 2020). Community partners often want access to what they perceive as the resources of the university (e.g. Cox, 2000), but the establishment of such partnerships might also enable the leverage of further funding and status for the NPOs.

Trainees often speak of making a difference or "giving back" to communities (Akhurst & Mitchell, 2012), which are viewed as groups with deficits or needing access to resources. Such approaches risk being "charitable" giving of time and sharing of resources (Lewis, 2004), leading to unequal relationships and the potential for patronising approaches, rather than transformative work towards social change (du Plessis & Van Dyk, 2013). It is therefore important to think carefully about the basis of the partnership: who has initiated it, what is the nature of the "exchanges", and how will negotiations enable open dialogue about needs and expectations, as well as resources desired and to be provided, for equity?

The process of partnership-building begins with communication and relationship-building between the tutor managing the course and the "gatekeeper(s)" of the organisations, providing access to the setting (du Plessis & Van Dyk, 2013). Then, relationships will need to be built between the trainees who will provide the "services" and workers in the setting, who may also be gatekeepers or managers. There are also relationships to be built with other community members, perhaps "service users" who may benefit from the trainees' work. Relationships are thus multiple, bidirectional and need careful attention, built upon mutual respect and open dialogue (Holland, 2005).Furthermore, the boundaries and the sustainability of the relationships need clarification, in relation to the continuation of the partnership and any associations beyond the time limits of CBSL. Finally, given the legacies of SA's apartheid past, establishing relationships that feel more equal may be more difficult for people of different ethnic origins (Netshandama, 2010). People have varied valuable experiences and their collective contributions are important.

Mitchell (2008) reminds us of systems of power that need to be considered when working in participatory ways towards greater equality. CBSL partnerships may be defined as "a set of relationships between people and/or systems where power is derived from Actor A's control of resources that Actor B needs or strongly desires" (Donaldson & Daughtery, 2011, p. 84).The "exchange" of resources, including knowledge and skills, thus needs attention. This includes negotiating expectations and goals, both at the beginning and at various times. What degree of sharing occurs in the planning of trainees' learning outcomes, the activities planned and the vision for what is achievable in the timeframe? And what is the nature of the capacity-building that is desired?

These considerations are therefore embedded in all of the above: the nature of power differentials; access to people and resources; perceptions and attitudes that need exploration and clarification; the influences of sociocultural factors and languages used; and then systemic issues related to the contexts of both the NPO and the university. Some of these may be summarised as "upstream" and "downstream" influences (Riemer et al., 2020) that impact on both the creation and the sustaining of the partnership. What are potential synergies between the differing demands and needs of the two contexts, between the community-based partners and the academic staff and trainees? Both careful negotiation and continued opportunities to think things through have an influence on the success of the activities.

Case examples of partnerships

In what follows, we will describe aspects of collaborative partnerships, through a selection of three case examples. Approval for the study was granted by the Rhodes University Ethical Standards Sub-committee (RUESC no. 2020-1427-3434), after gaining gatekeeper permissions. We are both qualified adult lecturers, with training in research and the methodologies of teaching and learning. The trainees involved in CBSL are adult M1s, thus likely to be in the age range of 24–45, from diverse backgrounds and ethnic groups.

The data were generated from interviews with some of our community partners between 2016 and 2019, with whom our M1s worked. The interviews followed a template of questions, to probe experiences and perceptions of the value and challenges of the work, with examples. We explored the experiences of four partners from three different settings: gaining their perspectives, both to illustrate aspects of partnership-building and also to highlight the limitations encountered. We describe the initial negotiations and trainees' briefing, actual student activities and their facilitation, and reflective opportunities. We hope to illustrate partners' understandings of CBSL, establishing what is needed to improve partnership-working, both in the setting up and the delivery of such projects.

This multiple case study approach was analysed and conceptualised on two levels: firstly, within-case analyses of the three cases, as they were summarised to form examples; secondly, a cross-case analysis, to identify emergent themes. Through these examples, we provide evidence from partners' accounts of the impacts of their work with the trainees, with participants' words shown in italics. These case examples illustrate work in settings where the focus is on young people.

Case example 1

The setting is an NPO childcare shelter for boys, known by the pseudonym EX. There is capacity for 15–30 males (ages 5–18) to live there at any time. Some are housed temporarily, whereas others stay for longer periods (as negotiated by the Department of Social Services), depending on their circumstances, the level of parental involvement and the need for, and the availability of, foster placements. The negotiating partner, with whom the trainees liaised, was a social worker based at EX and she was happy to be interviewed. She describes the residents with:

All these social problems [...] some of them they have been neglected from childhood [...] and some of them have been exposed to abuse [...] They've been on the streets living under bridges for such a long time and now they come to a structured space, where now we have to change their living and [...] their systems; so now we have to unwind [...] what has been happening throughout the years.

This displacement of young boys, vulnerable to social ills, is a remnant of our sociopolitical history and the disruptions of family systems. The description above outlines the challenges faced by the staff members, as they encourage the residents to adapt to structured routines and to ameliorate some of the emotional impacts of their previous circumstances. A former chair-person had initially requested our assistance because there were changes in staffing of the centre, and the social worker noted that she "*got excited when you guys reached out to me [.] it was really assisting [...] because we had a crisis of the staff*". After initial discussions, in 2016 the first pair of trainees ran workshops and team-building exercises for staff members over a period of months, which she describes as "*teamwork and communication and anger management*" along with assertive ways of speaking, such as: "*I feel*" statements. She noted:

I still have a clear picture of the programme [...] I still remember everything [...] from the staff, a better way of working and understanding each other without all these feelings and fights [...] and a way of [...] presenting the challenge rather than looking at the problem and making <u>more</u> problems.

This excerpt suggests that the planned activities with the staff were experienced as helpful.

Then in 2017, the subsequent pair of trainees negotiated a programme to work in more focused ways through workshops with the residents (the boys' expressed needs influenced the topics covered). The partner reported the following about those initial discussions:

I'm sitting with this challenge then they said do I have any ideas of how I want them to do it [.] so I said I don't have any problem they can draw up a plan then I will have a look at it [...] so they drew us a plan then they presented it and I was comfortable with it.

When asked about her experiences of working with the two successive pairs of trainees, she remarked: "*they were very humble, they were very sweet [...] they were very professional [...] because they were here for the staff, but they would engage with the boys as well [...] so they went beyond my expectations*". She also commented that the trainees had taken note of "*the struggles of the staff [...] while they deal directly with the angers of these boys*".

When further probed about her experiences of the trainees' activities, she responded:

they were thrown in the deep end [...] there's a crisis, now deal with this crisis [...] so for them it was a reality because there was no sugar coating of things [.] they experienced those things first-hand [...] they came up with the results [.] they didn't give up, they were not scared to face up [...] they executed everything [...]

This illustrates the trainees' capacities to utilise their skills in the situation, and to provide professional assistance where needed. Finally, when asked about any limitations or suggestions for future working, she noted that to start with, she would like:

firstly to make a presentation, what is the status quo now [...] I wanna be part of the plan so that we're not off tune [...] I wouldn't change anything but I would appreciate if I'm part of the plan. At the end of any CBSL, she suggested: can we have a session whether it's a day session

> *[…] when EX is closed […] whatever the activities, so that we do the debriefing so that in the following year when we start […] we start afresh […]*

This highlights the need for key staff members to be briefed and consulted beforehand (in this case the initial negotiations had been done with the chairperson), and for an evaluative workshop to close the engagements for the year. Subsequently, due to further staff changes at EX, the partnership did not continue into 2018–2020; however, the original social worker has now returned to EX, and through participating in these interviews, expressed hopes that the partnership might resume from 2021.

This case example occurs in the context of displacements of people as a remnant of our apartheid history. It exemplifies collaboration with an NPO in the welfare sector. The psychosocial support provided for childcare staff was reported to be valuable and helped strengthen the team, providing care and support to the boys. The case illustrates collaboration, with the partner site offering opportunities for the trainees to utilise workshopping skills, and the staff and residents seemingly gaining from the relationships built and the content presented. Whilst the facilitation of the work depended mostly on the trainees' professional capabilities, they had outlined their plans and gained prior approval from the partner for their suggestions. It seemed as if they were then given autonomy to present their material in an engaging way. In her reflections, the partner suggested a way to promote continuity from one year to the next, which might provide some challenges for us, given that the requests for input from trainees might exceed the number available for CBSL.

Case example 2

WS is the pseudonym for an initiative by an education-focused NPO. The partner, the head teacher of this programme, describes WS as "*a pull-out programme*" at two schools.

> *We pull children out of their normal classrooms during their normal school hours in small groups and focus mainly on literacy support […] but a lot of our work is also around social and emotional issues as well […] simply because of the nature of the situation in the context that we're working in […] we're part of the schools that are no-fee paying schools […] that serve […] children coming from a very low socio-economic background […] and the schools themselves being classed as dysfunctional.*

Although the two settings are geographically close to one another, with similar sociocultural and contextual challenges: "*you could run the same programme at both of the two schools but talking to very different children actually from quite different backgrounds*". The partner described school A as located

> *in our most deprived socio-economic area […] most of the children are either in child-led homes or they're being raised by granny or are kind of raising themselves a lot of the time […] so very, very difficult circumstances […] very, very poor […] it's very seldom that children […] actually move outside of that area.*

The partner described school B's

> *socio-economic status, while still not great, is a little bit better […] there is more likely to be […] working-class employed parents, whereas at [school A] a lot of children are coming from homes where their parents are unemployed and surviving on benefits and pensions.*

In the context of grave disadvantage and resultant educational outcome inequalities, the NPO partners with local schools to advocate for structural change in the public schooling sector, designing supplementary educational programmes to contribute to improved educational outcomes. However, the presence of multiple sociocultural and contextual stressors impedes children's learning and their development in the school setting. These stressors result from the economic and demographic crises highlighted by the partner. She notes relative socio-economic disparities in the context of poverty, unemployment, child-led homes and ageing people taking care of children. In addition, levels of literacy and numeracy development are particularly poor. When the prospect of a collaborative project was mentioned in 2019, by one of the NPO's staff members, the partner reported feeling

> quite excited about the idea of getting involved [...] I had felt for a long time that through our work that we had been doing with the children at WS that the children are generally in desperate need of some sort of psychological support.

The trainees responded to the challenges identified by the partners by developing a series of conflict-resolution workshops. The partners noted the "*physical bullying [...] that happens in the classroom because children don't have the language or the skills to deal with frustration or [...] heavy emotions in any other way [...] also because of what's modelled before them in their context*". This partner also mentioned the remnants of interpersonal violence from the country's apartheid past (characterised by state-sponsored violence against the oppressed majority).

Reflecting on the nature of the partnership established, the partner noted that the "consultative approach" taken by the trainees was very useful:

> they came in [...] with a "we want to do something. We want to work with you. We're keen to work with children but we don't know what your needs are". And that was our first meeting and it was very much kind of brainstorming together specific needs that we [...] identified.

This highlights the participatory approach taken by the trainees, which contributed to the value of the project for the NPO and the children. Not only was the approach employed by the trainees in the initial stages of the project, but it was sustained throughout the project. The partner highlights that the trainees "*were quite happy for me to chip in and [...] help clarify points [...]*". In addition,

> the content that they developed was really lovely [...] we gave them sort of broad guidelines [and] they really ran with those and you could see that they put a lot of effort and time into thinking about how they were going to approach the topics and what they were going to cover and that was great.

When asked to reflect on the limitations of the project as well as to suggest areas of future development, the partner expressed a desire to extend the scope of the project to include the educators, due to the contextual stressors facing them too. The partner noted that educators sometimes "*become demoralised and realise that 'well I can't really do anything to change these circumstances. Every child has a terrible story.'*" In addition, the partner highlighted the need for evaluation and perhaps revision of the material after a period of time had lapsed:

> [...] So let's say you do three consecutive weeks and then a month later go back and visit the children again and see how much of it is stuck [...] because I come from an NGO background so monitoring and evaluation is like very central.

This case example illustrates the challenges faced in poverty-stricken and systemically disadvantaged schooling communities. It demonstrates the value of CBSL activities by trainees, which focused more on the children's behavioural and emotional responses, alongside efforts that focus on literacy and numeracy development. The participatory approach taken by the trainees in negotiating entry and the way the project unfolded was particularly valuable to the partners. The case demonstrates the value of CBSL activities supporting organisations in their intervention efforts, focusing on the psychosocial challenges that result from systemic injustice and multiple interdependent crises. However, the case also highlights the systemic crises that constrain the efforts of multiple role players to enable social change. NPOs working in the context of structural injustices underscore the relative deprivation within which they work, the remnants of interpersonal violence, disrupted family systems and constrained social mobility. Educators feel overwhelmed and demoralised at the magnitude of multiple and intersecting crises. Efforts by practitioners-in-training, via CBSL activities, although supportive are constrained in contributing to systemic-level change.

Case example 3

This secondary school (NB) became a site for CBSL through negotiation with the former head teacher. It is a non-fee-paying state school, situated in an area where many families live in poverty, and the head teacher described that before she began working there (about five years ago), it had "*fallen into disrepair*", having previously been well run. She believed that the run-down "*tangible and visible*" physical infrastructure was a manifestation of "*a psyche*" of people around the school feeling neglected by the government system. She explained that when one is working in a

> *poverty dominated kind of environment, [...] even keen teachers, even enthusiastic teachers [...] become overwhelmed by all that needs to be done and by the [...] lack of discipline and enthusiasm of other teachers [...] it weighs you down.*

A peer support initiative (run by volunteer psychology postgraduates) had previously been started at a nearby youth centre, but there had been limited recruitment of youth, even though there were identified needs. As the head teacher of NB, she responded to the request to assist with: "*yes please come we've got space and that's the one thing [...] one asset we really had, space and we have needs*". At NB school, she noted that class sizes are large and "*teachers are stretched*"; and "*almost every child has a special case*". When we approached her initially, she could envisage the possibilities of trainees offering forms of psychosocial support to some learners, because there were:

> *not enough teachers to go around [...] to do all the pastoral stuff as well as the academic stuff [...] and so I was really just hoping that we would have a soft-landing space [...] for some of the kids who really, really needed additional support [...] sometimes some of your psychological issues are to do with [...] your school environment and it's [...] so it's hard to find help within the school [...]*

The M1s thus negotiated to run group psychoeducational sessions within the school day (since afterschool sessions were not possible). Whilst the head teacher was initially unsure, the sessions were better received than she expected: "*I had a query as to how much kids would open up in front of each other [...] but they did so and it seemed to be well structured in terms of following*

334

up on certain topics". She emphasised that the CBSL activities of support matched up with learners' needs:

> *one of the great tragedies [...] at the moment is that failure [...] possibly in our country [...] to meet the need and [...] the support sometimes isn't available [...] accessing it and getting those two things to come together [...] is a challenge.*

Here the head teacher highlights the gap between the access to mental health support services and the needs of youth. Initially, she had attempted to facilitate the trainees' work in the school, but given the demands of her role, this became unworkable. She then handed over responsibility to the learner support agent staff member, and that worked better. In her evaluation of the CBSL, she noted: "*I have to stress how really grateful I was [...] and how really grateful the school was to have the service*". When asked to suggest improvements, she noted: (1) that a tutor be more involved with the trainees in planning and talking through the proposed material, to enable it to be as relevant to the setting as possible, promoting trainees' confidence; and (2) the need for an evaluation meeting after each term, including learner representatives and the responsible teacher, to

> *really probe for what are the problems ... you kind of almost have to really dig for them, because otherwise ... you don't look a gift horse in the mouth, there's a problem with information sharing, partner to academic.*

The above comment highlights the importance of enabling frank communication about difficulties that were encountered, because partner organisations might be reluctant to be critical, not wanting to risk losing the assistance provided. The influence of environmental stressors on learners is evident in this case, in particular the levels of poverty in the context, highlighting both the potential value of support to some learners, but also the limitations of only being able to reach a few of the many who face difficulties. Overall, this case illustrates the lack of provision of psychosocial support for many needy learners by the formal system, with no time or opportunity for such support within an educational curriculum. Trainees were thus a resource to assist.

Discussion

The three case examples originated from interviews with four community partners (with two different sites for WS). In each case, the strong influence of contextual factors is clearly evident, produced by intersecting economic, political and social crises, as well as the crisis of violence. In each case, the trainees planned group activities to support the young people. It became clear that all the partners valued the assistance provided by the trainees, because they were intervening in ways not provided by other resources (Hlalele, 2012), thus complementing the partners' work.

Trainees' competence in planning, time investment in the work, and professionalism was evident. These reports resonate with trainees' accounts of their developing competencies, built upon relational foundations, evolution of activities and self-management (Akhurst, 2020). In each case, the trainees approached the partners in a consultative way, developing customised materials following initial suggestions by the partners. The partners thus seemed to value the relationships built in their settings, a key element identified by other authors (e.g. Preece, 2012; du Plessis & Van Dyk, 2013). The partners seemed satisfied with the amounts of consultation; however, each would have liked a stronger evaluative element. This highlights the need for evaluations to be built in from the start, rather than being an "add-on" at the end, when feedback may be overlooked, due to other demands upon people's time. This was also a function of the lack of work time allocated to tutors to manage relationships and evaluations with partners. From a professional training perspective, the module coordinator needed to keep a watch on what community partners hoped for and expected, to see that these aligned with what students could offer, in terms of their skills as trainee psychologists.

The consultative partnership approach seemed to diffuse potential power differentials between the partners and the trainees, moving beyond community–university bifurcation (Srinivasan & Collman, 2005) towards collaboration, underpinned by mutual values (du Plessis & Van Dyk, 2013). The partners planned together with the trainees to identify needs and appropriate intervention strategies, while the trainees were committed to collaborating, in order to meet the psychological needs of people in resource-deprived communities.

All three case examples show the violence of poverty (Rylko-Bauer & Farmer, 2016) that results from the persistent systemic injustices and crises in our context. With regards to case example 1, the challenges that face care workers at youth care centres have received attention (Goelman & Guo, 1998), when working with young residents (Seti, 2008). At EX, staff members also faced interpersonal tensions, so, in this setting work was done with both staff members and young people.

The effects of socio-economic crises are evidenced in the school settings. Sustained inequality has resulted in poor educational outcomes in the city's public schools, as well as affecting children's development (Spaull, 2013). WS works in this context to remediate educational outcomes and advocate for change, and the head teacher at NB highlighted the infrastructural challenges in that setting. Crumbling infrastructure and overcrowded classrooms are reported across multiple provinces in SA (Amnesty International, 2020). The headteacher also noted low teacher morale and lack of psychosocial support for learners, also reported elsewhere (e.g. Matoti, 2010; Hlalele, 2012).

Partners and trainees collaborated to address the influences of systemic crises on well-being, notably related to poverty and inequality. In these contexts, the trainees were able to work at microlevels of the systems, often with groups. However, they were constrained in their aspirations to work from the perspective of a social action model (Ahmed & Pretorius-Heuchert, 2001), being unable to influence systemic change. The limitations of this CBSL relate to their status as trainees, the nature of the work negotiated, their lack of formal role or representation within the systems, as well as limited time periods for the work. These highlight the limits of this work to become more oriented towards promoting social justice, since it would require another staff member in a longer-term oversight role. Such a person needs to work together with partners to build capacity, solidarity and team support, to enable them to make their voices as stakeholders heard within governmental and district structures.

From an academic staff perspective, a challenge of CBSL is its time-consuming nature. Two of the partners' comments suggested that they would have liked more focused tutor support of trainees and evaluation activities that would provide feedback. This resonates with research that has emphasised the staff-intensive nature of CBSL (e.g. Ziegert & McGoldrick, 2008). As the module coordinator, Jacqueline relied on the trainees to act as a "bridge" linking and communicating between the university and the settings since her role only permitted time for trainees' supervision. The partners' suggestions and the point above about a dedicated coordinator highlight the need for more staff resources, to better enable development and capacity-building. In addition, this may lead to improved partner input into the planning of the academic aspects of the module. However, given the economic models dominant in many universities, there is little likelihood of extra staff resourcing.

From the perspective of intervention models, whilst the trainees were attracted to the potential of the social action model (Ahmed & Pretorius-Heuchert, 2001), their limitations to influence systemic factors have become clear, due to lower status and loose association with the organisations. CBSL is thus constrained as a means to challenge broader contextual factors, and more attention needs to be given to further capacity-building amongst community partners, to enable them to be more assertive about their needs from formal structures. This requires further attention from universities' CE, to contribute to societal reconstruction. In the interim, working in sustained ways in conjunction with NPOs who are already lobbying for change, may contribute to improved social justice.

Conclusion

There is no doubt that CBSL provided much-needed assistance in our resource-constrained settings, but this work is limited by the small number of trainees involved. Ways of expanding CBSL in Community Psychology modules should be considered, to develop more partnerships and find ways of working towards greater social change. In modest ways this could enable the social capital of universities to play a greater role in tackling "real world" societal issues. However, since this work relies on the "human capital" of partners and trainees, who in the latter case are themselves in transition spaces, it is time limited, and the academic staff member plays a pivotal role in sustaining relationships over time.

Given these reflections, engendered through experiences and the evaluation of the case studies, Nqobile was aware of the need to redesign the CBSL to strive towards greater impact on social change. A number of serendipitous events occurred in 2020: (1) due to the COVID-19 crisis, she needed to repurpose the CBSL for online delivery; (2) the realisation of the greater potential impact of working with educators as service providers, meant she was open to other possibilities; and (3) she was approached by a national NPO to contribute to online materials and workshop development for educators and associated staff. This led to the CBSL taking on a different form: online work meant that a greater number of participants could benefit from the trainees' work, and they were able to reach educators distributed across national centres, enabled by the NPO's web platform. Hence, the work described in this chapter has evolved, and the 2020 developments will be evaluated, to report on changes in the nature and provision of CBSL. However, one unfortunate limitation of these developments is that they could exclude the more "in-person" local partnerships that were developed with the participants of the case studies.

This chapter illustrates the potential synergies between CBSL and Community Psychology (two fields that have not necessarily previously been considered as mutually supportive). CBSL emphasises the reciprocity of partnerships (Donaldson & Daughtery, 2011) and appears to be a useful transition space for trainees towards community-based practice. The reflections by partners of their experiences of CBSL activities underpinned by careful collaboration, highlight the possibilities to move beyond "resource exchange" towards greater participatory parity (Fraser, 2009) in relationships, to achieve common goals in our context of persistent systemic injustice.

References

Ahmed, R., & Pretorius-Heuchert, J.W. (2001). Notions of social change in Community Psychology: Issues and challenges. In M. Seedat, N. Duncan, & S. Lazarus (Eds.), *Community psychology: Theory, method, and practice* (pp. 67–86). Oxford University Press.

Ahmed, R., & Pillay, A.L. (2004) Reviewing clinical psychology training in the post-apartheid period: Have we made any progress? *South African Journal of Psychology, 34*(4), 630–656.

Akhurst, J. (2020). A South African perspective on community psychology practice competencies. *Journal of Community Psychology, 48*(6), 2108–23.

Akhurst, J.E. (2016). International community-based service learning: Two comparative case studies of benefits and tensions. *Psychology Teaching Review, 22*(2), 18–29.

Akhurst, J.E., & Kelly, K. (2006). Peer group supervision as an adjunct to individual supervision: Optimising learning processes during psychologists' training. *Psychology Teaching Review, 12*(1), 3–15.

Akhurst, J. E., & Mitchell, C.J. (2012). International community-based work placements for UK psychology undergraduates: An evaluation of three cohorts' experiences. *Psychology Learning and Teaching, 11*(3), 401–5.

Amnesty International. (2020). *Broken and unequal: The state of education in South Africa.* Amnesty International Ltd.

Bantjes, J., Kagee, A., & Young, C. (2016). Counselling psychology in South Africa. *Counselling Psychology Quarterly, 29*(2), 171–83.

Barnes, B., & Siswana, A. (2018). Psychology and decolonisation: Introduction to the special issue. *South African Journal of Psychology, 48*(3), 297–8.

Carolissen, R. (2006). Teaching community psychology into obscurity: A reflection on community psychology in South Africa. *Journal of Psychology in Africa, 16*, 177–82.

Cox, D.N. (2000). Developing a framework for understanding university-community partnerships. *Citiscape: A Journal of Policy Development and Research, 5*(1), 9–26.

Department of Education (DoE). (1997). *Education White Paper 3. A Programme for the Transformation of Higher Education.* DoE.

Donaldson, L.P., & Daughtery, L. (2011). Introducing asset-based models of social justice into service learning: a social work approach. *Journal of Community Practice, 19*(1), 80–99.

Du Plessis, C., & Van Dyk, A. (2013). Integrating the community voice into service learning: Engaging with communities. In N. Petersen, & R. Osman (Eds.), *Service learning in South Africa* (pp. 2–32). Oxford University Press.

Flisher, A.J., Dawes, A., Kafaar, Z., Lund, C., Sorsdahl, K., Myers, B., … Seedat, S. (2012). Child and adolescent mental health in South Africa. *Journal of Child and Adolescent Mental Health, 24*(2), 149–61.

Fraser, N. (2009). *Scales of justice: Reimagining political space in a globalizing world.* Columbia University Press.

Gilbert, A., & Sliep, Y. (2009). Reflexivity in the practice of social action: From self- to inter- relational reflexivity. *South African Journal of Psychology, 39*(4), 468–79.

Goelman, H., & Guo, H. (1998). What we know and what we don't know about burnout among early childhood care providers. *Child & Youth Care Forum, 27*(3), 175–99.

Hlalele, D. (2012). Psychosocial support for vulnerable rural school learners: in search of social justice! *Journal for New Generation Sciences, 10*(2), 67–73.

Holland, B. (2005). Reflections on community-campus partnerships: What has been learned? What are the next challenges? In P.A. Pasque, R.E. Smerek, B. Dwyer, N. Bowman, & B.L. Mallory (Eds.), *Higher education collaboratives for community engagement and improvement* (pp. 10–17). National Forum on Higher Education for the Public Good.

Kagan, C., Burton, M., Duckett, P., Lawthom, R. & Siddiquee, A. (2020). *Critical community psychology: Critical action and social change* (2nd ed.). Routledge.

Lawthom, R. (2011). Developing learning communities: using communities of practice within community psychology. *International Journal of Inclusive Education, 15*(1), pp. 153–64.

Lewis, T.L. (2004). Service learning for social change? Lessons from a liberal arts college. *Teaching Sociology, 32*(1), 94–108.

Matoti, S.N. (2010). The unheard voices of educators: Perceptions of educators about the state of education in South Africa. *South African Journal of Higher Education, 24*(4), 568–84.

Matthews, S., & Nqaba, P. (2017). Introduction: Rethinking the role of NGOs in struggles for social justice. In S. Matthews (Ed.), *NGOs and social justice in South Africa and beyond* (pp. 1–16) (Thinking Africa Series). University of Kwa-Zulu Natal Press.

Mitchell, T.D. (2008). Traditional vs. critical service-learning: engaging the literature to differentiate two models. *Michigan Journal of Community Service Learning, 14*(2), 50–65.

Mlambo, V. (2018). An overview of rural-urban migration in South Africa: its causes and implications. *Archives of Business Research, 6*(4), 63–70.

Netshandama, V.O. (2010). Community development as an approach to community engagement in rural-based higher education institutions in South Africa. *South African Journal of Higher Education, 24*(3), 342–56.

Preece, J. (2012). Community engagement in Africa: Common themes, challenges and prospects. In J. Preece, P.G. Nteane, O.M. Modise, & M. Osborne (Eds.), *Community engagement in African universities: Perspectives, prospects and challenges* (pp. 215–29). NIACE.

Riemer, M., Reich, S., Evans, S., Nelson, G., & Prilleltensky, I. (Eds.) (2020). *Community psychology: In pursuit of liberation and well-being* (3rd ed.). Macmillan.

Rylko-Bauer, B., & Farmer, P. (2016). Structural violence, poverty, and social suffering. In D. Brady and L.M. Burton (Eds.), *The Oxford handbook of the social science of poverty* (pp. 47–74). Oxford University Press.

Seti, C.L. (2008). Causes and treatment of burnout in residential child care workers: A review of the research. *Residential Treatment for Children & Youth, 24*(3), 197–229.

Sodi, T. (2017, September 14). *Shortage of psychologists hits SA.* PsySSA. www.psyssa.com/shortage-of-psychologists-hits-sa/

Spaull, N. (2013). *South Africa's education crisis: The quality of education in South Africa 1994–2011.* Centre for Development & Enterprise.

Srinivasan, S. & Collman, G.W. (2005). Evolving partnerships in community. *Environmental Health Perspectives, 113*(12), 1814–16.

Wilkinson, R., & Pickett, K. (2009). *The spirit level: Why more equal societies almost always do better.* Allen Lane.

World Bank. (2019). *South Africa: Overview.* www.worldbank.org/en/country/southafrica/overview

Ziegert, A.L., & McGoldrick, K. (2008). When service is good for economics: Linking the classroom and community through service-learning. *International Review of Economics Education, 7*(2), 39–56.

22

MOBILISING CRITICAL CONSCIOUSNESS IN EDUCATIONAL CONTEXTS

A Community Psychology approach

Bruna Zani, Cinzia Albanesi, Elvira Cicognani,
Antonella Guarino and Iana Tzankova

Abstract

This chapter addresses critical consciousness (CC) in educational and Community Psychology interventions with young people.

We first introduce the conceptualisation of CC and its components, the main research findings on the links between CC and some individual and contextual variables, and its association with positive developmental outcomes. Then, we focus on interventions aimed to foster CC development in adolescents and young adults, presenting two case studies.

The first case study is based on Youth-led Participatory Action Research (Y-PAR). The main goal was to promote critical active European citizenship, involving students at an Italian high school in a practical experience of PAR on social issues at local and European level. The second case study is based on the implementation of the service-learning (SL) methodology to promote CC and civic and cultural competences in Italian university students. Here the focus is on analysing the reflexive process in SL as a "tool" to critically understand and address social and cultural issues.

Finally, the implications of CC for a future Community Psychology praxis are discussed.

Resumen

El capítulo aborda el tema de la conciencia crítica (CC), por lo que concierne las intervenciones basadas en psicología educativa y comunitaria entre la población joven.

En principio presentamos la conceptualización de CC y sus componentes, los principales resultados sobre los vínculos entre CC y algunas variables individuales y contextuales, y su asociación con resultados de desarrollo positivo. Posteriormente, nos enfocamos en el análisis de intervenciones destinadas a promover el desarrollo de CC en adolescentes y jóvenes.

El primer estudio de caso fue basado en la Investigación Acción Participativa dirigida por jóvenes (IAP). El objetivo principal era promover la ciudadanía europea crítica activa, involucrando a los estudiantes de una escuela secundaria italiana en una experiencia práctica

DOI: 10.4324/9780429325663-27

de IAP sobre temas sociales a nivel local y europeo. El segundo estudio de caso fue basado en la implementación de la metodología de Aprendizaje-Servicio (ApS) para promover CC y competencias cívicas y culturales en los estudiantes universitarios italianos. El enfoque era analizar el proceso reflexivo en ApS como "herramienta" para comprender y abordar críticamente los problemas sociales y culturales.

Finalmente, las implicaciones para una futura praxis de Psicología Comunitaria fueran discutidas.

Introduction

This chapter addresses critical consciousness (CC), an issue that has been the object of increasing attention and interest by researchers in recent years and is now an established and fast-growing field, particularly in educational and Community Psychology (CP) interventions with young people. Heberle et al. (2020) in their systematic review have identified 67 studies of CC development in adolescents and young adults, published between 1998 and 2019, 60% of which appeared in 2016 or later. This exponential growth of research suggests that CC is a crucial issue, particularly in the current historical period, more than it has ever been (Rapa & Geldhof, 2020). On the one hand, CC is increasingly considered an important skill to be promoted through educational and empowerment-oriented interventions; on the other hand, evaluation research has confirmed the positive association between CC and positive developmental outcomes.

We will first introduce the conceptualisation of CC and its components; then, a short presentation of the main research findings on the links between CC and some individual and contextual variables will be provided (e.g. parent and peer socialisation, school climate, social emotional functioning, community engagement). We will conclude by focusing on interventions aimed to foster CC development in adolescents and young adults.

The conceptualisation of CC

The conceptualisation of CC is traced back to the foundational critical pedagogy theory developed by Paulo Freire (1973, 1968/2000), as well as to more contemporary theorisation on sociopolitical and CC development (Watts et al., 2011). Based on Freire's pedagogy that is rooted in the link between theory and praxis to develop CC, Jemal's (2017) recent review of the literature provides an in-depth analysis of the inconsistencies in the divergent scholarship within CC theory and practice, and suggests ideas to support the need for a new, CC-based construct, *transformative potential*. In particular, the author underlines the different conceptualisations of CC regarding the number of components considered, from just one (critical reflection, a purely cognitive state that derives from the critical analysis of sociopolitical inequity; Diemer & Li, 2011); to two (the capacity to critically reflect but also to act upon one's oppressive environment; Campbell & MacPhail, 2002); to three (cognitive – critical reflection or critical social analysis, attitudinal or political efficacy – the perceived capacity to realise sociopolitical change, and behavioural – civic or political action; Watts et al., 2011). Another critical point is that some definitions formulate CC as a continuous *process* of growth and development rather than an *outcome* derived from the process of *conscientisation* (i.e. consciousness-raising). Finally, a further issue of confusion in the literature is that some scholars include the tools, strategies and methods for conscientisation within the definition of CC, whereas for Jemal (2017), it is important to distinguish between CC and the tools used to develop CC.

The list of tools to promote CC development at school, which can be embedded in formal education curricula, includes: dialogue or open discussions regarding inequity; reflective questioning; psychosocial support; establishment of co-learning; non-hierarchical, respectful relationships between students and teachers engaged in a process of co-constructing knowledge; small-group discussions and interactions. Despite these distinctions, which sometimes appear "artificial" and linked to the different operationalisations for research purposes, it seems that all scholars rely on Freire's position on CC:

> Within the word we find two dimensions, reflection, and action, in such a radical interaction that if one is sacrificed – even in part – the other immediately suffers. There is no true word that is not at the same time a praxis.
>
> *(Freire, 1968/2000, p. 87)*

More recently, two contributions have been published: firstly, a special issue of the *Journal of Applied Developmental Psychology* edited by Rapa and Geldhof (2020), on new directions for understanding the development of CC during adolescence, which addresses key issues related to its measurement, mechanisms, precursors and outcomes. The second, a systematic review by Heberle et al. (2020) also provides a critical assessment and recommendations for future research. There is consistency across the existing literature in acknowledging as key components of CC critical reflection, critical motivation and critical action. *Critical reflection* occurs when people identify structural inequalities, perceive those inequalities as unjust and connect them to discriminatory systems (Diemer et al., 2017). *Critical motivation* is people's sense of sociopolitical efficacy (i.e. beliefs about their ability to impact sociopolitical conditions) and their commitment to enacting change (Diemer et al., 2016). *Critical action* is the behavioural component of CC and refers to how people go about engaging in activities intended to effect change and address inequalities. Critical action can occur at both individual and group levels (Tyler et al., 2020).

In CP work, promoting all the above dimensions of CC among young people is crucial to foster sociopolitical development and reduce the negative impact of structural inequalities and conditions of oppression on young people's well-being and psychosocial health (Watts et al., 2011). Community psychologists can use tools for *conscientisation* in the context of education to address oppressive conditions and educational disparities, as well as to facilitate youths' agency in challenging the status quo (Jemal, 2017).

Link between CC and variables of adolescent development

We now have a substantial body of literature that provides robust findings on links between CC and some individual and contextual factors impacting on adolescent development (e.g. parent and peer socialisation, school climate, social emotional functioning, community engagement). There is evidence of the positive relation between **parent and peer socialisation and CC**, particularly the reflection and motivation dimensions of CC: CC increases when parents and peers engage adolescents in discussions over social issues and support critical analysis of conditions of injustice. The findings are mixed for critical action, depending on how the variable of socialisation has been operationalised (Heberle et al., 2020).

Some studies have analysed the association between critical action and **school climate**, operationalised as levels of teacher encouragement of open discussion of challenging social and political issues at school: this climate favours adolescents' awareness about conditions of injustice and oppression, stimulating "critical curiosity" and supporting CC development in marginalised youth (Clark & Seider, 2017). For marginalised youth (such as high-school-aged girls of colour in the USA, in the research of Clonan-Roy et al., 2016), there is evidence that CC is related to **social-emotional functioning**, including positive sense of self, leadership skills, positive youth development competencies and also resistance and resilience. Nevertheless, not all the studies show the expected positive relations between social-emotional functioning and the dimensions of CC. The same mixed results emerged in the studies on relations between CC and academic functioning or achievement outcomes.

A further relevant issue in this context is the link between the development of CC and **community engagement**, defined as participation in community-based activities. Some studies provide evidence of such a link, that is, that community engagement can promote critical reflection and critical action, but many questions remain unanswered, such as the characteristics of community-engaged experiences or activities, and the potential reciprocal relations between various dimensions of CC and community engagement (Heberle et al., 2020).

Interventions: how to promote CC in young people?

Community psychologists are increasingly required to act as CC mobilisers when working with youth and local communities, by fostering young people's competences, promoting empowering processes in and out of school, or reducing the intergenerational gap with elders. How can the new generation of community psychologists learn knowledge and skills to develop and mobilise CC among youth and community members? Heberle et al.'s (2020) review summarised the extensive literature on curricular interventions used by teachers to support the development of CC, within different school subjects (literature, arts, social sciences, civic education, ethnic studies) and using a range of methods to discuss issues of unfairness, injustice, power, privileges and oppression, stereotypes and bias, to relate the content of the texts to their lived experience and to critically reflect on such content. Findings of these studies showed an increase in critical awareness, political efficacy and critical action among participants (Kozan et al., 2017). As to extracurricular interventions, it is worth mentioning some out-of-school programmes that used Y-PAR (Sánchez Carmen et al., 2015) or service-learning activities (Winans-Solis, 2014): these were designed specifically to promote critical reflection and critical action among marginalised youth, through consciousness-raising about discrimination, oppression and socio-economic inequity.

In the following sections we illustrate two examples of how we used reflexivity and experiential engaged learning as "tools" to address social and cultural challenges and promote CC in Italian high school students and university students. The first intervention utilised Y-PAR, the second is based upon service-learning.

Promoting critical consciousness through Y-PAR

Y-PAR is a theoretical-methodological approach used to enhance young people's empowerment and civic engagement as well as positive development (Anyon et al., 2018). Young people are trained and involved in all phases of a research process in order to identify and analyse issues relevant to their lives, report to relevant stakeholders and advocate for solutions or influence policies and decisions (Ozer et al., 2010).

How might Y-PAR promote critical consciousness?

Ozer and Douglas (2015) identified the following core processes of Y-PAR: youth–adult partnerships and research with the aim of identifying and investigating social issues; iterative integration of research and action; the practice of critical reflection and discussing strategies for social change; and building supportive networks with stakeholders. For Cammarota and Fine (2008), "Y-PAR teaches young people that conditions of injustice are produced, not natural; are designed to privilege and oppress; but are ultimately challengeable and thus changeable" (p. 2). Several research studies have highlighted that Y-PAR can foster critical thinking in discussions about the root causes of social issues (Foster-Fishman et al., 2010) or when discussing contrasting interpretations of data (Scott et al., 2015). Y-PAR promotes new, systemic, ecological views of a problem and skills in research inquiry, considering evidence, communication, teamwork and advocacy.

Y-PAR in the school context

A critical approach to teaching and learning, as in Y-PAR, might contribute to youth empowerment through the development of critical reflection (Anyon et al., 2018). However, its implementation in the school context requires that several challenges be addressed: moving teacher–student relationships towards greater horizontality; adapting activities to existing structure, timing and the competing demands of school curriculum; enabling different capacities of schools to network with external stakeholders; and establishing youth-adult partnerships (Ozer et al., 2010). The potential of Y-PAR to foster critical awareness and sociopolitical development (SPD) may also be offset by teachers' reluctance to address politically sensitive or controversial topics (Kornbluh et al., 2015).

There is also the risk of "schoolification" of Y-PAR as in: "the transformation of the inquiry and action process from internally motivated and holistic to a series of graded assignments" (Rubin et al., 2017, p. 183). This danger is related to the inherent tensions resulting from applying Y-PAR in a compulsory setting, which pose fundamental constraints to the voice and power of students. To avoid the depoliticisation of Y-PAR and maintain its focus on critical and transformational analysis, interventions in schools should be explicit and balance carefully decision-making dynamics and power-sharing between adults and students.

Case study 1: A Y-PAR intervention targeting the development of active citizenship

To exemplify the use of Y-PAR to promote CC at school, we present an intervention with the main goal of promoting critical active European citizenship as part of the H2020 European Project CATCH-EyoU. The intervention was rooted in the theories of SPD and empowerment (Wallerstein et al., 2005; Zimmerman, 2000) as well as the theory of Freire (1968/2000) about the banking and problem-posing concepts of education. Moreover, we applied the principles of youth-adult partnerships (Anyon et al., 2018).

The aim of this intervention was to involve students in a practical experience of Y-PAR focusing on concrete social issues that they identified as relevant in their own lives and for other people in their local communities, with a European dimension. The goal was to involve young people in elaborating strategies to address the selected issues, either individually or collectively, by eliciting solutions from political institutions.

The Y-PAR intervention, which lasted two school years, was offered to students (16- and 17-year-olds) attending the third year of an Italian high school within a specific mandatory curricular schedule, in which students must learn job-related skills. This allowed at least 100 hours per year, good flexibility in adjusting it, as well as the collaboration of researchers and teachers as tutors.

Students decided on the topic, the methods to collect data and how to share it with the local community. The collaborating adults were teachers and community psychologists. Teachers received training and guidelines on the Y-PAR method and principles in international workshops. The adults supported the participants throughout the process, but the responsibility for the students' work at each stage was in their own hands.

We adopted a two-step participatory approach, in which participants were involved in the cycle of research (analysis of social issues) and intervention (elaborating proposals to address the social issues) at a local level and subsequently at an international European level. In the first year (2016–17), students were involved in the phases of identifying social issues located in their community, mapping and understanding the issues by collecting data, and sharing findings with stakeholders in their local communities and with students and researchers at an international level (at the H2020 project's conference).

After the first year, a phase of reflection allowed students to understand how the social issues identified at a local level could be addressed on a European level. In the second year (2017–18), students: (1) were provided information on the structure and the functioning of the European Union (EU); (2) collected data by contacting representatives of EU institutions, shared research material and had discussions between students from different countries through an online platform; (3) contacted EU organisations and representatives to explore how to address the issue at the EU level; (4) provided ideas for intervention/solution for the EU institutions; (5) attended as main protagonists the H2020 project final conference in Brussels, to discuss and share their proposals with representatives of the EU institutions, public officials and peers from other European countries.

The impact evaluation of the intervention was conducted using a mixed-method approach, including questionnaires and focus groups, both at the beginning and at the end. The quantitative quasi-experimental evaluation revealed that, compared to a control group, Y-PAR participants reported higher scores on social well-being, institutional trust and participation, and lower scores on political alienation (Prati et al., 2020). These improvements in active citizenship were consistent with previous research documenting the effect of Y-PAR in terms of developmental benefits and civic engagement (Anyon et al., 2018).

Examining further the perspectives of participants on the experience, using thematic content analysis of focus groups, we found that students also developed a more nuanced and sophisticated representation of active citizenship, by incorporating critical awareness into the notion (Albanesi et al., 2021). They moved from a "concrete" factual view (e.g. demonstrating, volunteering, voting) towards a more complex view where critical awareness played a key role, both at an individual and at the community level. On a transnational level, the intervention allowed participants to increase their critical awareness of the role the EU plays or potentially could play, in addressing social issues located in their communities (e.g. immigration). The intervention seemed to impact variables that had to do more with the practical experience of being citizens in Europe, while variables related to an abstract support for the EU did not seem to be influenced (Prati et al., 2020). The students involved in the intervention may become less supportive of EU policies and identify less with the EU, but this does not mean that they will be less engaged or committed to changing those policies. This finding may be the result of the practice of critical reflection on the current EU policies and political agenda, including both supportive and critical views on national and EU political institutions.

Overall, in applying Y-PAR, we stress the importance of enhancing students' involvement in the process of research on social issues relevant to them (ownership), requiring critical analysis of information sources (including direct access to reliable sources of information), to better understand their nature and their root causes and reflect on measures that could be adopted to address them.

Y-PAR in school can offer concrete opportunities to develop a critical understanding of societal issues, supporting the notion that participation can change the way of approaching the teaching and learning process. Some challenges also emerged during the different phases of the project implementation. One of the main challenges in implementing Y-PAR in educational settings is the risk of considering inquiry and the research action process as traditional school tasks that require evaluation for grades. Based on this case study, we underline the importance of successful partnerships with teachers and school administrations to ensure the transformative capacity of Y-PAR and promote empowering processes in educational settings. We were very attentive to requiring the school to fulfil some conditions that in our perspective, and coherently with the literature, are needed to translate Y-PAR principles into practice. Indeed, teachers were asked to let students develop the different phases of Y-PAR autonomously in methods and content, with their support when needed. Moreover, teachers were trained on Y-PAR principles and methodology at the beginning of the project, accepted the risk of horizontality and collaboration, and were not afraid to share part of their power and lose their traditional authoritative role.

Service-learning to promote critical consciousness in higher education

Service-learning methodology: the role of reflexivity

Service-learning (SL), sometimes referred to as community-based or community-engaged learning, integrates service for the community and learning with the aim of enhancing the civic responsibility of the students and strengthening the community resources through work on a real-world problem (Aramburuzabala et al., 2019). On the one hand, SL is designed to offer students the opportunity to acquire new competencies and skills, through direct experience in the community that is relevant to their learning, and to be involved in an organisation located in a specific context. On the other hand, SL is designed to meet the organisation's needs identified by the community through university–community partnerships, which offer community organisations different ways (e.g. providing mentoring activities and direct service, and spending time with community members, expanding their networks) to advance their mission, while having a direct impact on community members (McIlrath et al., 2012).

For students, learning and civic development "do not necessarily occur as a result of experience itself but as a result of a reflection process" (Jacoby & Associates, 2003, p. 4). Indeed, SL is not just about doing; it is about reflecting on what is done (e.g. activity, service), how it is done (process and methods of implementation), and where it is done (organisation and community context). The reflective process refers to regular and ongoing activities, where students analyse and think critically about emotional responses to service activities in the context of a particular course or curriculum. The process is guided by academics or community partners, and allows for the understanding of the diverse perspectives inherent in the community challenges that students are experiencing. The goal is to help students acquire and use complex information and develop abilities to identify, frame and address social problems.

The cycle of reflection that occurs within a SL project develops through: making links with the learning objectives; scheduling activities regularly to expand the service experience; offering guidance for the activities; allowing feedback and assessment; engaging in clarification of values (Hatcher & Bringle, 1997). Reflection needs to be situated within the political and ethical contexts of teaching and learning, by directly addressing questions pertaining to equity, accessibility and social justice; these concepts should shape the learning experience for students.

Promoting civic and cultural competences through SL

SL reflective experiences contribute to a deeper understanding of social problems that make it possible for students to identify, frame and address them as engaged citizens, having the opportunity to combine active engagement in communities, and civic and democratic competencies development (Eyler, 2002). As such, SL fits with the educational priorities of EU policy statements that emphasise "active citizenship" and the development of "civic competences" at all levels of education. The Council of Europe developed the Competences for Democratic Culture and Intercultural Dialogue (CDC) model to identify the skills and knowledge that students at different levels of formal education should develop, in order to respond appropriately and effectively to the demands, challenges and opportunities of contemporary heterogeneous complex societies, thus being able to perform democratic, active and responsible citizenship (Barrett, 2016). Openness to cultural otherness and to other beliefs, respect, civic mindedness, responsibility and critical thinking are included in the CDC model and are often reported as the main outcomes of SL for students, besides disciplinary and academic achievements (Celio et al., 2011; Salam et al., 2019).

Special attention has been devoted recently to cultural competence in SL, as its development is becoming more and more important to engage effectively in a culturally diverse society. Vargas and Erba (2017) proposed a conceptualisation of cultural competence as a multidimensional process that involves three dimensions: cultural awareness, cultural knowledge and cultural skills. A fourth dimension was introduced by Súarez-Balcazar et al. (2011), namely cultural practice.

Vargas and Erba (2017) developed a programme of SL based on their conceptualisation, that used creative activities to foster a sense of citizenship by promoting undergraduate students' awareness of the social issues faced by Latino/a youth, a feeling of personal responsibility regarding cultural issues, and a desire to contribute to solve social problems. They reported that students learned to make the connection between the theory around public issues studied in the classroom, and the personal experience they had through their SL. Indeed, the midterm impact evaluation showed an enhanced awareness and sense of citizenship of undergraduate students. Overall, the development of cultural competence requires students' and academics' engagement in a process of (critical) cultural reflection, which involves thoroughly analysing and monitoring beliefs, attitudes and behaviours towards the value of cultural diversity, exploring best practices for teaching culturally diverse students, and being inclusive to incorporate more positive views of culturally diverse students (Gay & Kirkland, 2003).

Case study 2: Reflexive process in SL experiences. How does reflexivity develop? Evidence from the experiences developed in Bologna

As we have seen in the previous paragraphs, the reflexive process is a vital component of SL experiences. As mentioned in the Erasmus Plus project Europe Engage (Aramburuzabala et al., 2019), reflection leads students to link their experiences to the theoretical and methodological background of the academic disciplines and enhances a mechanism that encourages students to link their service experiences to their academic curricula, offering students structured opportunities to reflect upon the effects of their service. Different tools and methods can be used to support students' reflections on the SL experiences, including group/class discussions, essays and other specific assignments that relate the civic learning with the discipline and the curriculum. The reflective journal is one of the most important tools to encourage students to critically reflect on their personal growth and on the process of collaboration developed within university–community partnerships (de los Ríos & Ochoa, 2012). The journal's main purpose is to help students think more deeply and analytically about concepts and experiences arising from the readings, the lectures, field experiences and seminars (Evans et al., 2013). It allows continuous reflection, as students are invited to write their journals weekly and to register any critical incidents that may have occurred during SL; it supports situated reflection as students are invited to reflect on their own experience as it develops in a specific community organisation (situated) and to relate it to core disciplinary contents.

We have developed SL modules that complement CP courses of two different master's degrees (one in clinical psychology and the other on school and Community Psychology); and a SL module that complements the transversal competences courses offered by the University of Bologna, with a specific focus on civic competences. The modules have been developed in partnership with community organisations active in different fields (e.g. health promotion, social inclusion and diversity, active citizenship). In the modules we use reflective journals to help students articulate their learning and recognise its value for them and the communities. We strongly emphasise rigorous reflective writing, offering guiding questions for students, based on specific reflection models (e.g. Description, Examination, Articulation of Learning, DEAL; Ash & Clayton, 2009) and challenging them with provocative questions during class discussions (see Table 22.1). The reflexive journal contains: sections on analysis of personal, organisational and other problems faced in the communities; on the relation between SL, academic learning and curricular contents; and reflections on connections between academic achievement, civic engagement and personal growth.

Some quotes from the reflexive journals give a brief overview of the types of reflection developed during the experiences, and competences acquired during the SL projects:

> *My experience as collaborator in this context [organisation] was useful. It helped to develop my competencies in teamwork, and collaboration with peers and other people. I also discovered [that I have] good communication skills with adolescents, which will be helpful for a future job. I "touched with my hands" what it means to work in a team in a structured organisation, knowing its strengths and weaknesses.*
>
> *(Clinical Psychology student, Post-school service)*

> *Thinking about the need for a change of perspective and networking, I think that the "community" can be the answer [...] the community that has to be educated to take care, to have a wide perspective, to networking and partnership; to unify citizens, to look at resources and not at problems.*
>
> *(Clinical Psychology student, Migrants and refugees centre)*

> *This is another place where a psychologist – above all a community psychologist – could be supportive: none of the people involved in the project knew how to draw up an evaluation plan of a social project and the only ones who were aware of their importance were stakeholders who fund the project. For me, to give an in-depth and sensitive evaluation could make the project valued by all the people interested in and involved.*
>
> *(Community Psychology student, Post-school service)*

Table 22.1 DEAL model guidelines adapted for students' reflection on service learning

DEAL *model of reflection (adapted from Ash and Clayton, 2009)*	
Sequential steps	*Guiding questions*
1. **D**escription of experiences in an objective and detailed manner.	• When did you get the experience? • Where did it take place? • Who was with you? Who wasn't there? • What did you do/say? What did the others do/say? • Was there anything powerful about the experience you did? • What emotions did you feel?
2. **E**xamination of those experiences considering specific learning objectives (in the case of SL at least for academic enhancement, civic learning and personal growth).	Referring to some learning objectives: critical awareness, civic skills, principles and methods of Community Psychology • Use key concepts and theoretical perspectives to analyse some aspects of the experience. • Refer specifically to aspects of experience that have been made clearer by applying the theory, models and tools of discipline.
3. **A**rticulation of Learning that concretises specific learning related to the outcomes.	**"I learned that"** ... Illustrate a meaningful learning from your SL experience Explain which concepts/principles/values you have learned best, as a result of reflection on experience. • How what you have learned can/could be generalised/ applied in a broader sense (contexts/situations)? **"I learned it when"** ... Explain how learning is linked to specific moments/ activities/situations **"What I learned** is important **because"** ... • What's the value of your learning? (it applies to the specific situation, other contexts, as it concerns your profession, your way of being etc) • How is it linked to the key themes of the discipline and the objectives of the SL?

Critical reflexivity emphasises praxis: students are asked to question assumptions and taken-for-granted actions, thinking about who they are and how their professional and civic competences can be developed through community service (Evans et al., 2013). SL offers the opportunity to experience an agentic role through service, and to consider principles, values and practices of Community Psychology in the making (Dalton & Wolfe, 2012). Reflective practice as it develops in SL offers the opportunity to students to think about their (future) roles as community psychologists, to consider their strengths, their weaknesses and their positions regarding the change they want to make as psychologists.

SL allows students to meet real-world challenges of the community and collaborate for solutions that are meaningful and relevant to community partners and students. Engaging in developing solutions, they learn how complex it may be to address the multiple causes of a specific problem, but they also understand that there are multiple ways of contributing, and that their contribution matters. Confronting multiple perspectives, they understand the risks of orthodoxia, but also the importance of having a solid methodological and theoretical preparation; experiencing diversity (inside and outside community organisations), they develop a "new" understanding of taking positions, of accepting diversity, of being invested with responsibility from the community, recognising that these are not merely cognitive processes but involve the person as a whole (Conway et al., 2009).

Conclusion

The substantial growth of the empirical literature on the development CC in adolescents shows the increasing interest in the topic, due to the associations of CC with several positive developmental outcomes. In the present chapter we have first presented recent conceptualisations of CC as consisting of three components: *critical reflection*, *critical motivation* or political efficacy, and *critical action* or engagement in activities intended to affect change. Then the main research findings on the links between CC and some individual and contextual variables were examined. Drawing on these findings, we addressed the question of how to promote CC in young people: it is our belief that this is a crucial question for the new generation of youth that needs tools to understand and face the social and cultural crises they are experiencing during this pandemic period, but also for the community psychologists who need to learn and use new intervention tools.

Community psychologists are trained in interpersonal relationships, including communication skills, teamwork and group process facilitation, with an emphasis on being able to consider multiple perspectives, adopting multilevel approaches for an ecological understanding of social issues, and bearing witness to oppression (Francescato & Zani, 2017). They are also increasingly required to reveal and address social injustice, being able to recognise how it is maintained at the structural, institutional, interpersonal and individual level. As such, community psychologists are also required to make their values and standpoints explicit, not escaping the moral risk of distance. Since its foundation, CP has dealt with a simple though provocative question: *faced with social challenges (inequalities, injustice, exclusion), what shall we do?* Any effort to provide an answer to such a question, requires the community psychologist to be an agent of change. We have chosen two interventions to promote CC in Italian high school students and university students, as examples of how we used reflexivity and experiential engaged learning as "tools" to address social and cultural challenges.

Lessons learned and limitations.

The Y-PAR intervention showed that it is possible to establish a productive partnership with schools, as well as other community stakeholders, to create a joint "learning journey" capable of supporting and strengthening youths' agency and sociopolitical awareness. By supporting youth in learning a range of skills, community psychologists can collaborate with other adults, contributing their specific expertise (e.g., scientific research approach and methods, group management and organisation). To avoid limitations inherent in applying Y-PAR in a compulsory setting, school–university partnerships should be constructed and maintained from the very beginning through continuous interactions between school and university. In this way Y-PAR can change the approach to teaching and learning at school and may be a strong ally for addressing the new demands of the school curriculum (i.e. equipping students with key competences for life).

The SL experience with senior students addressed CC as a complex process that requires an intentional active role of both academics and community partners: who share the responsibility to offer students opportunities to question their experiences; to develop some awareness of the challenges that they may encounter and engage with as citizens and future professionals. Limitations in SL depend mostly on its implementation: sometimes the SL approach drives the community-based experience only in theory, while in practical terms what is offered is not very different from a traineeship or internship; the capacity of the programmes to stimulate reflexivity can be evaluated only post hoc; thus, there is also the risk of offering inconsistent experiences. Other limitations concern assessment: there is little evidence of long-term impact on students, and on faculty. Despite these limitations, we think that by choosing SL as a method to train students, we make explicit and "real" some CP assumptions: engaging personally with the community is mandatory, learning (and competences development) is a relational co-constructed process, neutrality is not an option, thus contributing to designing a clear pathway for developing critical (aware) CP praxis.

What to do next? Challenges for the years to come

The CC development in young people is an area that needs further research. There are methodological problems and key arguments to be explored in more depth, such as the measurement of the construct (Heberle et al., 2020). Rapa et al. (2020), after discussing the limitations of existing CC measures, present their recently developed instrument, the Short Critical Consciousness Scale (CCS-S), which provides evidence on measurement invariance across respondents of different ethnic, age and gender identity groups. Moreover, it is important to: integrate rigorous quantitative methods using control groups or quasi-experimental methods when assessing the impact of existing interventions; use longitudinal research to analyse the developmental pathway to build CC in children and adolescents with varying identities; understand how the relations among the three CC components vary across development in different contexts. At the theoretical level, there are still some unanswered questions and new directions to be explored (Rapa & Geldhof, 2020): the relationship among the components of CC across the developmental periods and over time, both within individuals and across groups; the conditions under which CC can be fostered; the precursors and the outcomes of the interventions aimed at developing CC in children and adolescents.

At the time of writing this chapter (February 2021), the situation in our country and many others is again becoming critical, due to the second wave of the coronavirus: the implications not only for the social and economic system but also for the day-to-day activities of our lives and the psychological consequences are enormous, and in some aspects still unpredictable and unknown. But we want to conclude with a note of hope, underlining the importance of CC right now: CC may contribute to an adaptive development and foster well-being, especially among those experiencing marginalisation and oppression (Rapa & Geldhof, 2020). There are many ongoing experiences that illustrate the capacity of marginalised communities to use CC to deal with actual change supporting a process of adaptive development despite the pandemic. These experiences are precious, and worth being known, understood and shared as they can be used to build different narratives about power, capacity and strength. For this reason, an informal international network of community psychologists (supported by ECPA, European Community Psychology Association; SCRA, Society for Community Research and Action; and the Community Toolbox) has created the New Bank for Community Ideas and Solutions (www.ecpa-online.com/new-bank), a place where anyone can deposit (and even download) stories that can inspire (new generations of) community psychologists. CC may also be a means by which individuals, groups and communities, marginalised or not (that includes more privileged counterparts), try to promote social change for a more equitable world. Our hope is that practitioners, and especially community psychologists, will be able to develop targeted approaches to support young people in their pathways to acquiring CC.

Notes on authorship

The authors are both senior researchers (Bruna Zani, Elvira Cicognani and Cinzia Albanesi) and early career researchers (Antonella Guarino and Iana Tzankova), who have been involved in research and evaluation of educational and community interventions centred on youth socio-political development. All authors were involved in the Catch-EyoU research project, within which a Y-PAR intervention for youth active citizenship was implemented (case study 1). Cinzia Albanesi and Antonella Guarino are currently involved in SL programmes offered at the University of Bologna (case study 2).

References

Albanesi, C., Prati, G., Guarino, A., & Cicognani, E. (2021). School citizenship education through YPAR: What works? A mixed-methods study in Italy. *Journal of Adolescent Research*. Advance online publication. https://doi.org/10.1177/07435584211035564

Anyon, Y., Bender, K., Kennedy, H., & Dechants, J. (2018). A systematic review of youth participatory action research (YPAR) in the United States: Methodologies, youth outcomes, and future directions. *Health Education & Behavior, 45*(6), 865–78. https://doi.org/10.1177/1090198118769357

Aramburuzabala, P., McIlrath, L., & Opazo, H. (2019). *Embedding service learning in European higher education: Developing a culture of civic engagement*. Routledge.

Ash, S.L., & Clayton, P.H. (2009). Generating, deepening, and documenting learning: The power of critical reflection in applied learning. *Journal of Applied Learning in Higher Education, 1*(1), 25–48.

Barrett, M. (2016). *Competencies for democratic culture: Living together as equals in culturally diverse democratic societies*. Council of Europe. https://rm.coe.int/16806ccc07

Cammarota, J., & Fine, M. (2008). *Revolutionizing education: Youth participatory action research in motion*. Routledge.

Campbell, C., & MacPhail, C. (2002). Peer education, gender and the development of critical consciousness: Participatory HIV prevention by South African youth. *Social Science &Medicine, 55*(2), 331–45. https://doi.org/10.1016/S0277-9536(01)00289-1

Celio, C.I., Durlak, J., & Dymnicki, A. (2011). A meta-analysis of the impact of service-learning on students. *Journal of Experiential Education, 34*(2), 164–81. https://doi.org/10.1177/105382591103400205

Clark, S., & Seider, S. (2017). Developing critical curiosity in adolescents. *Equity & Excellence in Education, 50*(2), 125–41. https://doi.org/10.1080/10665684.2017.1301835

Clonan-Roy, K., Jacobs, C.E., & Nakkula, M.J. (2016). Towards a model of positive youth development specific to girls of color: Perspectives on development, resilience, and empowerment. *Gender Issues, 33*(2), 96–121. https://doi.org/10.1007/s12147-016-9156-7

Conway, J.M., Amel, E.L., & Gerwien, D.P. (2009). Teaching and learning in the social context: A meta-analysis of service learning's effects on academic, personal, social, and citizenship outcomes. *Teaching of Psychology, 36*(4), 233–45. https://doi.org/10.1080/00986280903172969

Dalton, J., & Wolfe, S. (2012). Education connection and the community practitioner. *The Community Psychologist, 45*(4), 7–14.

de los Ríos, C.V., & Ochoa, G.L. (2012). The people united shall never be divided: Reflections on community, collaboration, and change. *Journal of Latinos and Education, 11*(4), 271–79. https://doi.org/10.1080/15348431.2012.715507

Diemer, M.A., & Li, C.-H. (2011). Critical consciousness development and political participation among marginalised youth: Critical consciousness and political engagement. *Child Development, 82*(6), 1815–33. https://doi.org/10.1111/j.1467-8624.2011.01650.x

Diemer, M.A., Rapa, L.J., Park, C.J., & Perry, J.C. (2017). Development and validation of the Critical Consciousness Scale. *Youth &Society, 49*(4), 461–83. https://doi.org/10.1177/0044118X14538289

Diemer, M.A., Rapa, L.J., Voight, A.M., & McWhirter, E.H. (2016). Critical consciousness: A developmental approach to addressing marginalisation and oppression. *Child Development Perspectives, 10*(4), 216–21. https://doi.org/10.1111/cdep.12193

Evans, S.D., Malhotra, K., & Headley, A.M. (2013). Promoting learning and critical reflexivity through an organisational case study project. *Journal of Prevention &Intervention in the Community, 41*(2), 105–12. https://doi.org/10.1080/10852352.2013.757986

Eyler, J. (2002). Reflection: Linking service and learning-linking students and communities. *Journal of Social Issues, 58*(3), 517–34. https://doi.org/10.1111/1540-4560.00274

Foster-Fishman, P.G., Law, K.M., Lichty, L.F., & Aoun, C. (2010). Youth ReACT for social change: A method for youth participatory action research. *American Journal of Community Psychology, 46*(1–2), 67–83. https://doi.org/10.1007/s10464-010-9316-y

Francescato, D., & Zani, B. (2017). Strengthening community psychology in Europe through increasing professional competencies for the new Territorial Community Psychologists. *Global Journal of Community Psychology Practice, 8*(1). https://doi.org/10.7728/0801201703

Freire, P. (1968/2000). *Pedagogy of the oppressed*. Continuum.

Freire, P. (1973). *Education for critical consciousness*. Continuum.

Gay, G., & Kirkland, K. (2003). Developing cultural critical consciousness and self-reflection in preservice teacher education. *Theory into Practice, 42*(3), 181–87. https://doi.org/10.1207/s15430421tip4203_3

Hatcher, J.A., & Bringle, R.G. (1997). Reflection: Bridging the gap between service and learning. *College Teaching, 45*(4), 153–8. https://doi.org/10.1080/87567559709596221

Heberle, A.E., Rapa, L.J., & Farago, F. (2020). Critical consciousness in children and adolescents: A systematic review, critical assessment, and recommendations for future research. *Psychological Bulletin, 146*(6), 525–51. https://doi.org/10.1037/bul0000230

Jacoby, B. & Associates. (2003). *Building partnerships for service-learning*. John Wiley.

Jemal, A. (2017). Critical consciousness: A critique and critical analysis of the literature. *The Urban Review, 49*(4), 602–26. https://doi.org/10.1007/s11256-017-0411-3

Kornbluh, M., Ozer, E.J., Allen, C.D., & Kirshner, B. (2015). Youth participatory action research as an approach to socio-political development and the new academic standards: Considerations for educators. *The Urban Review, 47*(5), 868–92. https://doi.org/10.1007/s11256-015-0337-6

Kozan, S., Blustein, D.L., Barnett, M., Wong, C., Connors-Kellgren, A., Haley, J., Patchen, A., Olle, C., Diemer, M.A., Floyd, A., Tan, R.P.B., & Wan, D. (2017). Awakening, efficacy, and action: A qualitative inquiry of a social justice infused, science education program. *Analyses of Social Issues and Public Policy,17*(1), 205–34. https://doi.org/10.1111/asap.12136

McIlrath, L., Lyons, A., & Munck, R. (Eds.) (2012). *Higher education and civic engagement: Comparative perspectives*. Palgrave Macmillan.

Ozer, E.J., & Douglas, L. (2015). Assessing the key processes of youth-led participatory research: Psychometric analysis and application of an observational rating scale. *Youth &Society, 47*(1), 29–50. https://doi.org/10.1177/0044118X12468011

Ozer, E.J., Ritterman, M.L., & Wanis, M.G. (2010). Participatory action research (PAR) in middle school: Opportunities, constraints, and key processes. *American Journal of Community Psychology, 46*(1–2), 152–66. https://doi.org/10.1007/s10464-010-9335-8

Prati, G., Mazzoni, D., Guarino, A., Albanesi, C., & Cicognani, E. (2020). Evaluation of an active citizenship intervention based on youth-led participatory action research. *Health Education &Behavior, 47*(6), 894–904. https://doi.org/10.1177/1090198120948788

Rapa, L.J., & Geldhof, G.J. (2020). Critical consciousness: New directions for understanding its development during adolescence. *Journal of Applied Developmental Psychology, 70*, 101187. https://doi.org/10.1016/j.appdev.2020.101187

Rapa, L.J., Bolding, C.W., & Jamil, F.M. (2020). Development and initial validation of the short critical consciousness scale (CCS-S). *Journal of Applied Developmental Psychology, 70*, 101164. https://doi.org/10.1016/j.appdev.2020.101164

Rubin, B.C., Ayala, J., & Zaal, M. (2017). Authenticity aims and authority: Navigating youth participatory action research in the classroom. *Curriculum Inquiry, 47*(2), 175–94.

Salam, M., Iskandar, D.N.A., Ibrahim, D.H.A., & Farooq, M.S. (2019). Service learning in higher education: A systematic literature review. *Asia Pacific Education Review, 20*(4), 573–93. https://doi.org/10.1007/s12564-019-09580-6

Sánchez Carmen, S.A., Domínguez, M., Greene, A.C., Mendoza, E., Fine, M., Neville, H.A., & Gutiérrez, K.D. (2015). Revisiting the collective in critical consciousness: Diverse socio-political wisdoms and ontological healing in socio-political development. *The Urban Review, 47*(5), 824–46. https://doi.org/10.1007/s11256-015-0338-5

Scott, M.A., Pyne, K.B., & Means, D.R. (2015). Approaching praxis: YPAR as critical pedagogical process in a college access program. *The High School Journal, 98*(2), 138–57. https://doi.org/10.1353/hsj.2015.0003

Suarez-Balcazar, Y., Balcazar, F., Taylor-Ritzler, T., Portillo, N., Rodakowsk, J., Garcia-Ramirez, M., & Willis, C. (2011). Development and validation of the cultural competence assessment instrument: A factorial analysis. *Journal of Rehabilitation, 77*(1), 4–13.

Tyler, C.P., Olsen, S.G., Geldhof, G.J., & Bowers, E.P. (2020). Critical consciousness in late adolescence: Understanding if, how, and why youth act. *Journal of Applied Developmental Psychology, 70*, 101165. https://doi.org/10.1016/j.appdev.2020.101165

Vargas, L.C., & Erba, J. (2017). Cultural competence development, critical service learning, and Latino/a youth empowerment: A qualitative case study. *Journal of Latinos and Education, 16*(3), 203–16. https://doi.org/10.1080/15348431.2016.1229614

Wallerstein, N., Sanchez, V., & Velarde, L. (2005). Freirian praxis in health education and community organising: A case study of an adolescent prevention program. In M. Minkler (Ed.), *Community organising and community building for health* (2nd ed.) (pp. 218–36). Rutgers University Press.

Watts, R.J., Diemer, M.A., &Voight, A.M. (2011). Critical consciousness: Current status and future directions. *New Directions for Child and Adolescent Development, 2011*(134), 43–57. https://doi.org/10.1002/cd.310

Winans-Solis, J. (2014). Reclaiming power and identity: Marginalised students' experiences of service-learning. *Equity & Excellence in Education, 47*(4), 604–21. https://doi.org/10.1080/10665684.2014.959267

Zimmerman, M.A. (2000). Empowerment theory: Psychological, organisational and community levels of analysis. In J. Rappaport & E. Seidman (Eds.), *Handbook of community psychology* (pp. 43–63). Kluwer Academic Publishers. https://doi.org/10.1007/978-1-4615-4193-6_2

23

WORKING WITH LIFE STORIES FOR TRANSFORMATIONAL LEARNING

Tracking our positionality in an educational dialogical space during COVID-19

Yvonne Sliep, Nosipho Faith Makhakhe, Sipho Ngcongo and Bernice Calmes

Abstract

For the past 15 years, a six-month core module, "The Personal Is the Professional", formed part of the Health Promotion Master's degree at the University of KwaZulu-Natal, South Africa. This module facilitates interactive and dialogic transformative learning spaces for learners to share and deconstruct their personal life stories collectively, to increase insight and the ability to respond to their own and others' contexts. In 2020, we started working online because of COVID-19 and wondered how to manage internet-mediated transformation learning. To apply their insights, knowledge and skills, the students facilitated a six-week workshop with the title "The Personal Is the Professional" with an organisation which has diversity and inclusivity as their core business. This chapter includes the voice of the facilitators, the learners and the organisation. We describe the process and examine our positionality doing this transformational learning. Collectively, we deconstructed what happened in the dialogic space which added to transparency and transferability.

Resumen

Durante los últimos quince años, un módulo denominado «lo personal es también lo profesional» ha sido desarrollado como parte del currículo del Master de Promoción de la Saluden la Universidad de KwaZulu Natal (Sudáfrica). Este modulo facilita espacios de aprendizaje y de dialogo interactivos para que los estudiantes puedan compartir y de construir sus propias historias de vida, para así incrementar la visión colectiva y la capacidad de respuesta ante contextos propios y ajenos. En el año 2020 se inició un ciclo de aprendizaje en línea a cause de la pandemia del COVID 19, con la duda de como manejar la enseñanza transformacional a través de las redes informáticas. Con el fin de aplicar sus observaciones, conocimientos y habilidades, los estudiantes facilitaron un taller de seis semanas baja el título de «lo personal es

DOI: 10.4324/9780429325663-28

también lo profesional» para una organización que se especializa en temas relacionados con la diversidad y la inclusión. En este capítulo se unen las voces de los facilitadores, los estudiantes y la propia organización. Se describen los procesos y se examinan los posicionamientos experimentados durante el proceso de aprendizaje transformacional. De forma colectiva, se de construyeron las experiencias adquiridas en el espacio de dialogo. Este proceso tuvo un valor añadido desde el punto de vista de la transparencia y la transferencia de conocimientos.

Introduction

At the University of KwaZulu-Natal (UKZN), we do a module on working with life stories, "The Personal Is the Professional", which forms part of the master's in Health Promotion, offered by the School of Psychology. Working in health promotion, as in Community Psychology, means enabling people to increase control over, and to improve, their health by reducing the risks and increasing skills, strengths and competencies of individuals and settings (Miller & Shinn, 2005). In these disciplines attention is given to the relationship between broader social forces and social distress seen in vulnerable communities, like low socio-economic status, stressful life events, racial and other kinds of injustices. According to the Ottawa Charter for Health Promotion (World Health Organization, 1986), health promotion is seen as a political act addressing the inequality of access to better health outcomes. An empowerment model, like that of Rappaport (1991), argues for a transformative perspective to change personal and social problems. The theory is translated into community projects to anchor understanding in praxis.

This chapter is co-authored by Nosipho Makhakhe and Sipho Ngcongo, who experienced the module themselves and will track how their stories are shaped according to different retellings. The first telling is at the onset of the course, followed by a telling at the end of the module and a further telling when the module is facilitated by the learners for an organisation that deals with diversity and inclusivity as their core business. The director of the organisation, Bernice Calmes, the fourth author, will include the positionality of the organisation which formed part of the multilevel approach.

The master's programme consists of postgraduate students from different generations, race and ethnic groups and various professional disciplines, resulting in a learner community of great diversity. The intention of the module is to develop critical reflexivity in a way that ultimately promotes social justice. In South Africa, health promoters are dealing with the historical legacy of inequality, structural violence and communicable and non-communicable health challenges, including HIV/AIDS and the recent coronavirus disease (COVID-19), which has the biggest impact on the most vulnerable communities. Often people feel it is their fault that they are trapped in poverty. The participants share their life stories and collectively we explore dominant discourses and name the root causes of poverty. Although it does not change the reality, the students get an additional sense of pride that they have made it this far against all odds. By embracing an African worldview, the notion that knowledge is developed only in the Global North, is challenged. Knowledge is dynamic and must be applicable to the context in which it is created – in keeping with the decolonial discourse.

Theoretical model and dialogic space

The foundation of the work is critical reflexivity. Reflexivity is a term used in social science literature, to understand how one's actions are influenced by how one perceives and assesses the actions of others (Gilbert & Sliep, 2009; Sliep, 2010). The critical reflexivity model has been

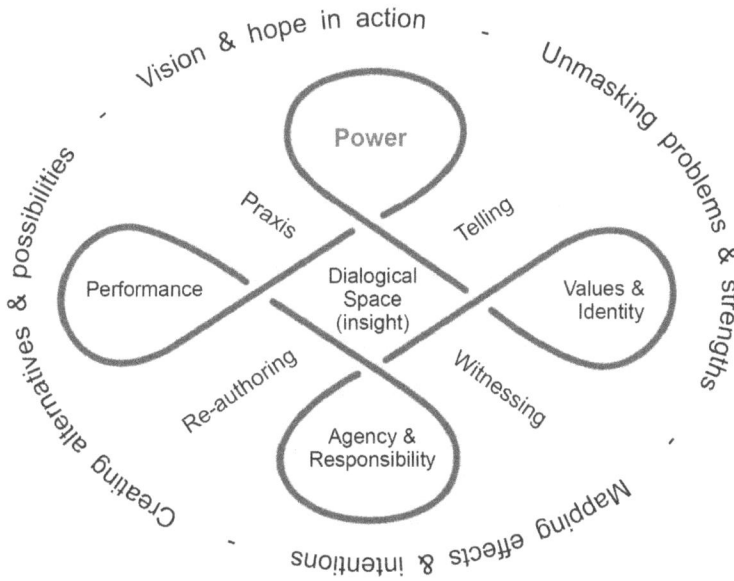

Figure 23.1   Critical relational reflexivity (Sliep, 2020)

useful in various contexts such as higher education (Norton & Sliep, 2020), qualitative research (Naidu et al., 2012), and school and community projects (Norton & Sliep, 2019; Sliep & Kotze, 2008; Sliep, 2016).

The model is embedded in dialogue and narratives. The narrative approach is vital for developing critical reflexivity, because stories help us find meaning in our lives. Narratives are relational between self, others and context. The process of sharing life stories helps us understand how culture and context shapes the person, and it is in the process of understanding the self that we can understand others. At the beginning of the course students develop a tree of life, which is a metaphor that helps them to write and narrate their life stories. The roots represent students' formative years and background. The branches and the leaves represent their personal and educational journeys, and the blossoms and fruits represent their dreams, including personal and professional achievements. The broken branches represent personal failures and hardships.

It is in the process of sharing their life stories, coupled with their learning of the theories that underpin the different loops within the critical reflexivity framework, that the process of developing reflexivity starts. Students are encouraged to reflect on their past and present life course according to the critical reflexivity lens. They analyse the role of power in their lives and how they can reposition themselves in the social world. They engage with the different modes of agency, articulate their values and commit to a course of action informed by their newfound consciousness (performativity), which is termed "walking the talk". The framework comprises four interlinking loops: power, values and identity, agency and responsibility, and performativity. Figure 23.1 provides a visual summary of the loops and the concepts that inform the mechanisms of each loop, each interacting to inform the process of critical reflexivity.

Dialogical space

Reflexivity is anchored and takes place through dialogue. *Dialogos* is a Greek word meaning "conversation" or "discourse". Thus, the term signifies a particular kind of speech that happens between two or more people and is associated with the pursuit of knowledge (reason, argument and discourse). The dialogical space is a social site that enables critical dialogue through different means of communication like spoken words, body language, written and visual means (Rule, 2004). Dialogue occurs at several related levels in this social space, between the members of a group or community that forms the dialogic space, and between outside agents, in this case among the learners, organisations and academics. Actively creating a safe dialogic space provides an opportunity to engage with different perspectives that address complex social problems (Rober, 2005). The created space is a physical or virtual location or place where people meet to interact. It is associated with freedom and mobility, and it is produced by social relations which reproduce, mediate and transform (Bourdieu, 1989).

A culture of "critical acceptance" is considered essential in the creation of a climate of respect where it is safe to question old viewpoints and to try new ideas (Fook et al., 2006). A fruitful online collaboration requires an emphasis on confidentiality and group-generated rules such as showing respect, being non-judgemental and giving place to different ways of being in the dialogue (Salmon, 2009.For an honest discussion to take place, people need to feel safe enough to narrate their stories. Trust was mindfully fostered and nurtured over a period of time to enable dialogue in the virtual space.

Power

Power is unpacked in the Foucauldian sense where it is ever present (Foucault, 1982), and how it is used on both a micro and macro level by others and yourself. We start with the self but take it through to social action, not power *over* but power *with*; not power *for* self but for the collective through social activism in a troubled world. Power affects all interactions, so it is crucial to understand how it works and how it impacts each person's world. According to Laverack (2004) power exists in four different forms authority, force, manipulation, and persuasion. The purpose is to create awareness of the use of power and its effects, starting with the individual right up to the collective use of power for social action (Norton & Sliep, 2018). Reflexivity is aimed at understanding the operations of power rather than its dismantling. A person's positioning in relation to these webs of power will influence their actions.

Values and identity

According to Schwartz and Bilsky (1987), values are concepts or beliefs that guide behaviours and events: they have relative importance based on biological needs, social interactions and the influence of social institutions, for survival. Values are norms reinforced by culture and language and influence identities. We begin by identifying self-values, where they come from and how they help us develop a moral compass for decision-making. Values are dynamic and are established collectively through negotiation and communal participation (Sliep & Norton, 2016). In order to act on the world intentionally, we have to know who we are, where we come from and how we want to live.

Agency and responsibility

Bandura (2001) understands agency as the ability for people to make their own choices and take accountable actions. Reflexivity increases one's sense of awareness about responding to the reality of others. Agency in this context is understood as individual, collective or by proxy.

Responsibility is viewed as the ability to respond (response-ability). Agency needs to be enacted to step fully into responsibility (Gilbert & Sliep, 2009).

Performativity

Performance, according to the critical reflexivity model, requires putting words into accountable action, or walking the talk (Sliep & Norton, 2016). When an action is driven by ethics and values, it becomes an accountable performance. We do this through pulling together all the loops, taking context, language and the positioning of ourselves and others into account, and through the overall reflexive process. Walking the talk is encouraged by dealing with arising issues in terms of moral and collective responsibility. It develops a moral compass to deal with dilemmas and contradictions in beliefs and actions.

Returning to Figure 23.1, we see how the loops are interlinked and that awareness is cultivated through the dialogical space. All the loops are integrated to clarify the overall picture:
- an understanding of context and culture;
- an awareness of power - personal, social and political - in respect of all stakeholders;
- consideration of own and others' values influences identity;
- moral agency for positive performativity; and
- a commitment to dialogue, negotiated positions and actions.

It is important that this is not merely an academic exercise but is internalised so that it becomes anchored into subsequent practice. For the students, this happens during their community practice module (Norton & Sliep, 2018).

Online teaching

Because of COVID-19 that swept across the world in 2020, we had to do our modules online. The academic year in South Africa runs from February to November. We never met the learners face to face in 2020. In February, our campus was rife with protests that meant that people were unsafe, and classes were forbidden. This was followed by a lockdown in the country, which prohibited entry onto campus. The rest of the 2020 academic year was therefore conducted online.

These circumstances left us apprehensive as course facilitators. We did not know how we were going to move this highly interactive, experiential module, based on deep dialogue and trust, to an online module. It was hard to visualise how the sharing of life stories and the co-creation of knowledge would happen remotely. Online learning meant that learners were mostly working in isolation, separate from friends and the campus community. Throughout the modules, we deconstructed what COVID-19 and lockdown meant; how it influenced our lives personally and in our educational setting. Loss of lives among family, friends and colleagues was a hard reality of 2020, for most of the learners and the teaching staff. The result of this online engagement and learning, to our surprise and in contrast with many other university courses, was that we obtained the best results in the past 15 years, despite the extreme hardships that our learners experienced.

Reflexivity embedded in action

Teaching the course online revealed an unexpected challenge and opportunity in relation to the module on community practice. During the lockdown, the students could not enter the community or hold group meetings, including workshops, or work with clinics or schools. The option was either lengthening the course with a whole year or doing an online intervention. If the intervention could not happen in real space, it did not matter how big the physical distance was going to be. On request from an organisation based in the Netherlands, it was decided that "The Personal Is the Professional" module could be provided by the learners to selected members of that organisation.

A series of six workshops was offered covering the theoretical model systematically. The contextual and geographical difference was used to deepen the dialogue in the reflexive loops of power, identity and values, individual and collective agency, and finally, the challenges of walking the talk. Assumptions were revealed, blind spots highlighted, and differences under-stood on a deeper level by participants who were already experienced critical thinkers. The meaningful reflective dialogue provided a space for individual agency and a sense of creating a difference collectively.

Positionality means that one is positioned in relation to others, and therefore reflexivity necessitates an interrogation of that positionality and how it affects the personal as well as the professional aspects of the individual. Positionality in academic writing allows for a reflection of one's position in relation to the social political context of the institution, group or setting. It influenced personal experience and perception of issues (Barrow, 2011). This necessitates that you pause and examine implicit biases and challenge singularities and binaries that influence your view of the world. You may have power and privilege ascribed to you. How can it be dealt with in a way that capacitates and does not hinder transformational learning? Understanding one's positionality, particularly when seeking to create a space for honest dialogue between the academic and the learners, is important because the academic is able to deconstruct their power and privilege within the institution, which has the potential to stifle the voices of learners in the dialogic space (Alexander, 2004).

Coordinator positionality: Yvonne

I brought myself into this work as an educator and researcher in post-apartheid South Africa, which asks for particular action. As a white, middle-aged, middle-class, woman, I have the privilege, responsibility and a heightened sense of accountability to contribute to a more just and inclusive society. My professional identity was very much formed during the apartheid era when, as activists, we were dreaming and working towards a possible post-apartheid future and health system. Nelson Mandela was a symbol, and we never thought he would be released or that he was able to remain the extraordinary human being he was despite 27 years of incarcer-ation. It is what I still bring into my education practices today, providing its own lens. As with any lens, it has a tint that influences how I perceive things. I offer the following example: Over the years, I have witnessed the challenging and often violent context from which the learners come. I have learnt that I must take nothing for granted, especially not how I myself can still be a barrier despite all good intentions. Most learners come from what we call the "born free" generation, referring to being born after the end of apartheid. However, this era brings many other challenges with it. An example is the expectation from parents that their children will become highly qualified and earn well in order to support the extended family. In addition, violence has taken on different forms, with rapes and attacks happening regularly in student residences. It has become vital for me to stay in a position of learning from the students and the realities they face. Living in South Africa is very complex and new pathways may be co-created with the participants.

During 2020, the health theme for the year was COVID-19 —a pandemic that did not differentiate between race and place, but which highlighted inequalities. Many losses were shared during our meetings, and challenges had to be mindfully balanced with support and containment. Despair and helplessness had often been an undercurrent, but in 2020 it was much more palpable. I learnt the importance of "doing hope" as a verb from one of the co-authors who was also a student at the time, breathing week to week through spaces of loss and increasing levels of uncertainty. We used the tree of life as metaphor for sharing life stories:

pollinating possibility
in the breeze that connects the trees
the shape of reflexivity

The online learning space had become a space for vital connectivity. Students used phrases like

I would not have survived if it was not for this space;
My sanity depends on our sessions;
Listening to my classmates' stories. I got to know them on a deeper level. Considering that we haven't met in person. We were able to break many barriers and show our vulnerable side to each other without being judged;
Sharing my story made me feel like I am actively participating in my learning process other than being a sort of a spectator;
The words "you do not know what you do not know" are what I have adopted very earlier on, kept me humble, intrigued and interested;
I began to take responsibility for my own life again that I need to be held accountable for how I feel and how I want to be treated and how I want to live. Thus, little by little, it gave me back my own personal power.

During the past year we needed to play a more containing role than usual. I have a natural nurturing disposition and had to be very mindful that I stayed in a professional learning space. We created more time for individual follow-up. Everyone took the learning journey very seriously. Would we have achieved the same results if our course was online and not during a pandemic that affects us all? I leave this as a question.

I would like to name an ongoing dilemma regarding working with life stories as a tool. For all the time that I have offered the course, I asked myself if it would create a more equal terrain if I shared my own tree of life. Somehow, I found it an even more pressing question during the online course. It felt like I had to make myself more visible, and I missed the face-to-face contact where I could facilitate much more intuitively. I decided against it, like I have every other year. I have lived a long intense life. The state of apartheid had an impact on me and my family on many levels. I have been married to a woman for 30 years. I have Black and white children. I lived and worked in many places and contexts internationally. I have my own sense of ecofeminist spirituality.

Some of the questions I asked were: How will the learners respond to this kind of sharing? Will there be a sense of feeling unsafe as I do not present the norm of society? Will there be a sense of their story being less if there are fewer events to reflect on? Of course, I include examples from my lived experience during our sessions but that is different. I do it to illustrate a particular theoretical point through an example from my own experience. When we come to the end of the course, there is a very different sense of critical reflexivity and it could be the right moment to share. But the sharing of life stories happens at the onset, and then students track and change their stories, which demonstrates their growing sense of reflexivity. It also felt like taking up that space would not contribute to decolonising the teaching space. Both process and content have to be attended to very mindfully. I always thought that if any of the students asked for my story, I would have to stop and rethink. To date that has not happened. At the moment I still think it is better to not share my story in full, but it is a position I will continue to revisit.

I conclude with a co-created pantoum, a structured poem. Everyone involved contributed one sentence of what stood out most for them during the course. These lines are written up in a way that duplicates every sentence twice in the poem, which adds to the rhythm and form.

walking the talk is a lifelong process

prepare to learn, relearn and unlearn

to stand even if standing is uncomfortable
unpack my blind spots, see the privileges I did not earn
what do I do, when am I culpable?

to stand even if standing is uncomfortable

breathing through the discomfort
what do I do, when am I culpable?
our accountability must become overt

breathing through the discomfort

being intentional about our voices and actions
our accountability must become overt
some will follow in the footsteps of those that went ahead

being intentional about our voices and actions

I'm navigating how to be true to myself
some will follow in the footsteps of those that went ahead
walking the talk is a lifelong process

I'm navigating how to be true to myself

unpack my blind spots, see the privileges I did not earn
walking the talk is a lifelong process
prepare to learn, relearn, and unlearn

Co-facilitator positionality: Nosipho

In 2016, I enrolled for the master's in health promotion and had the opportunity to learn about critical reflexivity in "The Personal Is the Professional" module. Through the life story work

I got to narrate my life story, firstly, from a place of naivete and description, oblivious to the social constructs that have shaped me. Prior to this course, during my undergraduate studies in sociology, I did learn about socialisation and agency; however, my understanding of these terms was conceptual, and I did not relate them to my experiences.

This course gave me an opportunity to critically reflect on my life story and to analyse my relationships and how they have shaped me. I got to see the insidious and beneficial uses of power. I also learned that through self-reflection and introspection, I personally have a responsibility to challenge the way I was socialised to engage with societal structures. Through the lenses of agency and critical thinking, I got to learn that power is not static, but it is fluid in nature. This meant that I would find myself in both states of power and powerless depending on my interactions in the social world, that the world was complex and non-binary. By virtue of being a university student, this meant that I had a level of privilege and power over others that I needed to be aware of. This course also helped me understand the realities of others and show more empathy to the things that separate us as well as embrace the things that unite us. At the end of the course, I wrote this poem to show how I had gained my voice and ability to speak out:

Face to face with my inner self

The woman in me has been awakened
The woman in me is no longer afraid
The woman in me is no longer silent
The woman in me wants us to talk
She wants us to meet
Wants us to make peace
Wants us to be introduced to the world
The woman in me is tired of hiding
Tired of struggling
The woman in me wants to fight for all women out there
The woman in me is ready
The woman in me is unstoppable

The shift from being a student to a teaching assistant meant that I was now in a position to teach others about critical reflexivity. It was important for me to engage critically with theories of power, agency and responsibility, values and identity, and performativity through social action. I had to treat the students' narratives with the utmost sensitivity. Being in this position showed me the importance of bringing to life the abstract notion of reflexivity through using examples and making references to current events. Examples are: demonstrating to students what the current dominant discourses are, and the importance of including marginalised voices. The process of transitioning also meant that self-reflexivity had to expand beyond my personal life and into my professional life. I had to contend with the multiple realities of the students and engage with their narratives as they developed their own critical reflexivity. The use of narratives in developing critical reflexivity can cause learners to question their lives and their long-held beliefs. It is important that I make this process explicit at the onset of the course, to prepare students for possible interruptions caused by the questioning and the transitioning they experienced.

The facilitation of an online dialogical space was challenging, particularly because I had not met the group in person and therefore trust was built over a much longer period. As the facilitator I had to allow myself to be vulnerable and share some of my challenges that I was experiencing because of the COVID-19 pandemic. Teaching a course in the midst of such rampant death and grief was one of the most difficult things I have had to do. Each class session began with a check-in: everyone in the group was given the space to express themselves and also to break down if they felt emotionally tender. The group became a safe space where emotions were allowed, and in doing so the co-creation of knowledge occurred.

In my capacity as a researcher, I work with youth from poor communities and sex workers. Both of these groups of people are on the lower spectrum of society. They are marginalised and rendered voiceless by dominant discourses. Working with these groups of people through community interventions, critical reflexivity has helped me be aware of the power dynamic and the importance of trust-building and power-sharing. As a reflexive professional this means that I have the responsibility to engage with these groups in a way that gives them the freedom and a platform to express themselves and to give voice to their struggles. It is also crucial for me to remember that my presence is not one of a saviour or a deliverer of empowerment, but I am merely a catalyst for them to tap into their own internal power as well as join forces and develop into a critical mass that recognises their collective agency so as to engage with and challenge systems of oppression.

Learner positionality: Sipho

I am a Black Zulu man at the age of 28 living in rural South Africa. A typical homestead includes various dwellings that also creates space for our ancestors who came before us. Creating the dialogue poem with my course co-ordinator helped share my life story in a few poetic stanzas. I live in rural Kwa-Zulu Natal with a big extended family. It is not a comfortable place for me as it feels unsafe and there are too many of us living in a small space.

> *lots of bodies moving around chaotically*
> *bad blood amongst all of us*
> *and nowhere at all to go to*
> *violence sparks grudges and jealousy*
> *and nowhere at all to go to*
>
> *first my father was stabbed*
>
> *six times in the chest*
> *the day six cows were slaughtered*
> *to change the wrath*
> *of the ancestors*
>
> *then my brother was stabbed*
>
> *five times in the back*
> *all in the name of envy*
> *punished because he dared*
> *to go to varsity*

I know
I am next in line
I know
it is coming
I too go to varsity

I do not know

who I am
I do not know
where I want to go to
I know it has to be away from here

Many of my fellow students also come from challenging circumstances. The online master's course felt like a lifeline during a time of darkness. It became the most meaningful space of connectivity for me.

My positionality shifts between the different contexts I find myself in. I respond and get responded to as a Black Zulu man in South Africa. My positionality in relation to the system is influenced by low socio-economic status and living within a violent society. The lessons I learned from examining my positionality include the understanding of how my position influenced the decisions, ideas, values, beliefs and issues I had previously prioritised. The shift from such positionalities in relation to gender, culture and race came when I learned about power dynamics and the dominant discourses of patriarchy, the culture of misogyny, and intersectionality through my female colleagues, as well as the people affected by such discourses around me. As a result, I became aware of the privilege my positionality provides. For this, I have learned that through shared struggles, intersectional vulnerabilities can be blurred if not traced or acknowledged.

When we were linked to an international organisation in the Netherlands for our practical, I came to a deeper understanding of how I am situated in a global context. I have understood not only the self-positionality but also the positionality in relation to others in a global context. Before the module I felt that South Africa was inferior to countries in the Global North, that the Northern hemisphere is somehow more civil. I doubted my ability to make a useful contribution. However, during the series of the workshops I became aware of positions we take for granted, like nationality. Being in a country where I was born and raised, not as immigrant or foreigner: how being in this position shielded me from xenophobia and displacement. Knowing where I come from, my tribe, my story and my people became more apparent to me during the international exchange. I understood the power that comes with just knowing how to trace your lineage, which is not the case, for instance, when your ancestors were slaves or when you are an immigrant in a foreign land.

Education offered a bridge from where I come, to the dreams I aspire to reach. The shift from such positionality was to change how I communicate my ideas and beliefs with others, to not use my education and knowledge as power *over others*. I had to understand different views and to accommodate people's values, beliefs and knowledge, even when they are different from mine. Over time, we developed the trust that allowed me to show my vulnerability. Entering an academic world, like writing this chapter, requires an examination of the changes in my thinking, awareness, and curiosity as I gradually enter a new system of privilege.

I end with the following poem:

I found strength in dialogue
speaking of and not into my circumstances
I develop skills to navigate a complex and diverse terrain
Confidently and flexible I take on challenges
knowing we don't know all the answers

I reclaimed my space and became visible

from airborne roots and broken branches
to power kindling from within
I no longer dream about agency
I have self-efficacy and will generate more

so here I am

I bring my truest self with me
re-authoring my identity
doing hope in an unknown landscape
with positive uncertainty

Organisation positionality: Bernice

The organisation called Article 1 Midden Nederland (Central Netherlands) is the provincial registry for discrimination complaints originating in local communities in the Dutch Province of Utrecht. There are more than 25 regional discrimination registry offices in The which form a National Platform called *Discriminatie* (Discrimination). The name of the organisation refers to the first amendment of the *Nederlandse Grondwet* (Dutch Constitution), which states that all citizens are equal before the law. The regional registries were constituted as a result of a national law from 2009, which enables local governments to create and finance a registration facility for discrimination complaints as near as possible to the residence of its citizens and provide information about the service. Article 1 Central Netherlands, in its current form, has existed since 2009. Based on more than ten years of work experience and assistance to survivors of discrimination, Article 1 Central Netherlands also provides policy advice to local governments and training options for professionals and education facilities throughout the Province of Utrecht. We serve 26 municipalities (1.34 million inhabitants).

As the COVID-19 pandemic broke out in early 2020, we saw increased incidences of microaggression and discrimination against citizens with non-traditional Dutch facial features and skin colour. For the first time we had an unusually high number of complaints from the Southeast and East Asian communities who were initially blamed in a "satirical" carnival song for the COVID-19 outbreak in the Netherlands. Subsequent lockdowns had detrimental effects on the relationships between social services and customers, especially the vulnerable and groups at risk of social exclusion and discrimination. The riots and protests in The Netherlands during the month of May 2020, as a result of the police violence and the increased activism of Black Lives Matter, exposed a bulk of marginalised communities denouncing many forms of exclusion.

The sheer number of registered complaints during the COVID-19 pandemic forced an internal reflexivity about the nature of our work and the way we see and provide services to survivors of discrimination. The main challenge resided in understanding why, despite a sound legal framework, many groups expressed their unease with Dutch society and a sense of exclusion. As an organisation we were compliant with regulations and procedures, but were we truly impartial? In the face of the official discourse, were we seen by our customers as independent arbiters between survivors of violence and local governments (our main funders)? Is it possible for an organisation such as Article 1 Central Netherlands to be impartial in the face of cases involving proved racism implicating official bodies and institutions?

These fundamental questions prompted many discussions, both internally between colleagues, and externally with partners and shareholders. The conclusion reached after many sessions was that in order to maintain credibility, we had to stay close to our mandate, which is registry and information. The matching and possibly most consistent action besides publishing about facts and figures derived from the registration process, was to build case studies in order to raise awareness and increase the visibility of target groups at risk of exclusion and discrimination, including broad constituencies, for example, the disabled and chronically ill, seniors, LGBT+ (lesbian, gay, bisexual and transgender) communities, Asians, Blacks, Muslims, young people, workers, and all the intersections within these groups. We achieved this by designing online campaigns targeting the above-mentioned groups through shared stories, movies, poems and songs with the hashtag #youcount and increased our online visibility on social media platforms– our work continued despite the lockdown.

Already in the first half of 2020, we reached out to the University of KwaZulu-Natal in order to explore the possibility of attending parts of the critical reflexivity master's programme, *The Personal Is the Professional*. This resulted in a six-week course attended by three members of the Article 1 Central Netherlands team at a time when, in light of the COVID-19 pandemic and corresponding social transformation processes in the Netherlands, it was necessary to reflect on the course of action that had to be taken.

Referring to the critical reflexivity loops, the course reminded us of the necessity to organise dialogical spaces of trust for team members in the middle of the ordinary dynamics of a regional registry. This is needed because the stories that lie at the core of the discrimination complaints are sometimes heavy, intense and touch the lives of the professionals involved. Adherence to procedures requires consultation and careful reflexivity with self and team to preserve acceptable levels of objectivity and customer care.

During the reflections in the power loop, we affirmed that as an independent organisation relying on municipal subventions, we had to navigate policy priorities, customer interests, organisational interests and stakeholder interests. In navigating with care, we have to remain unblemished and unquestionably a regional body accessible to all: perpetrators of discrimination, survivors of discrimination, sister organisations and government bodies.

Discussing values and identities, we learned to separate layers of compromise and intersectionality. In the end, our organisation is stronger if we can learn to build bridges with the value and identity variables of those who seem at the peripheral spectrum of our work. Sticking to natural partners is not as pivotal for change as reaching out to the unusual suspects.

Analysing agency and responsibility gave perspective to our actions as professionals (sometimes with personal lives as activists or former activists), linked to a clear regulatory framework and mandate. This is at times difficult because the law is based on contextual standards, while in dealing with discrimination survivors you may also need instruments to heal broken souls. The question then is to distil the spirit of the law without breaking away from the regulatory framework, in a way that makes sense to the partner organisations, without alienating customers and survivors.

When we reached the performativity loop, "walking the talk" referred to a balanced and negotiated act in which we can give visibility to the unique set of data and experiences that we collect at the registry, and give visibility to the plea of survivors of discrimination. All of this occurs while maintaining dialogues with communities with opposing views, partner organisations and regional governments.

In conclusion, we offered a pantoum, which captured our experience, to UKZN students and facilitators:

To see yourself as a source of light
Listening attentively without judging
Navigating the personal and the professional
Enriching the soil we root in

Listening attentively without judging

Negotiating through layers of interest and privilege
Enriching the soil we root in
To believe in inevitable growth

Negotiating through layers of interest and privilege

Social and personal responsibilities
To believe in inevitable growth
Attentive to the hearing, careful in the speech

Social and personal responsibilities

The blessing of paying it forward
Attentive to the hearing, careful in the speech
Tracking dynamics and webs of power

The blessing of paying it forward

Every progress is a win
Tracking dynamics and webs of power
To see yourself as a source of light
  Bernice Calmes, Niki Eleveld, Mustapha Bah

Implications for future Critical Community Psychology

We have to continuously critically reflect on what the results of our teaching are, deconstruct the reasons for these results and adapt accordingly (Zawada, 2020). In our situation, having a co-facilitator that bridged the age and race gap made a big difference. Students often stayed online after the session of the day to further discuss with her.

Transformative learning through life story work is a process that is both challenging and uncomfortable. It is in this space of being out of your comfort zone that deeper critical reflexivity takes place. By creating a space of witnessing in deep dialogue, we also create a space of shared meaning-making. It promotes self-awareness and also other-awareness and leads to new ideas and relational possibilities.

When critical consciousness is "embedded in action" through a reflexive process, it signifies a shift or movement, a change in the status quo. In this way, reflexivity becomes a tool for interrogation, change and transformation. The critical reflexivity model includes all the main concepts, and for logical structure these have been described in loops in Figure 23.1. When others apply it in their own work, the context is filled differently but the framework provides the guideline. The important part of it is to continuously reflect on your own positionality and performativity. To use critical reflexivity is anchored and becomes evident in practice and should not stop at exploring the theory.

The knowledge we create comes not only from an intellectual base but also from an experiential and experienced space, opening imagined future possibilities as part of lifelong learning. Our intellectual landscape becomes influenced by creative forces and gives rise to different shapes and contours. We do the work with the belief that we can make a meaningful contribution to our own lives as well as the lives of others. In South Africa, where the learning landscape is embedded with so many structural and contextual challenges, creating an enabling and reflexive environment, based on a future vision of a more equal and inclusive society, makes all the difference.

Conclusion

At the end of the academic year, students reported an increasing sense of agency as well as an ability to tolerate uncertainty. Despite many ongoing technical and uncertainty challenges, there was a heightened sense of understanding of how the personal links to the professional. There was a broader ability to read the complexity of context and adjust responses accordingly. A strong sense of reframing power from a social constructivist perspective resulted in a greater sense of agency. There was also referral to a sense of social responsibility which was enhanced by the international practice exposure.

What happened during the online teaching of class 2020 can best be described as creating a bittersweet symphony. Every participant came to see and express themselves more fully and clearly. Over time, a harmony among all was created. There was a sense of learning together and making a difference together. We know that in order to stay in tune, we have to continue to practice our individual and collective reflexive selves mindfully. To hear the symphony, we have to continue to practice and perform it.

References

Alexander, R.J. (2004). *Towards dialogic teaching: Rethinking classroom talk*. Dialogos.

Bandura, A. (2001). Social cognitive theory: An agentic perspective. *Annual Review of Psychology, 52*, 1–6. https://doi.org/10.1146/annurev.psych.52.1.1

Barrow, G. (2011). Educator as cultivator. *Transactional Analysis Journal, 41*(4), 308–14. https://doi.org/10.1177/036215371104100407

Bourdieu, P. (1989). Social space and symbolic power. *Sociological Theory, 7*(1), 14–25. https://doi.org/10.2307/202060

Fook, J., White, S., & Gardner, F.(2006). Critical reflection: A review of contemporary literature and understandings. In S. White, J. Fook, & F. Gardner (Eds.), *Critical reflections in health and social care* (pp. 3-20). Open University Press.

Foucault, M. (1982). The subject and power. *Critical Inquiry, 8*(4), 777–95. www.jstor.org/stable/1343197

Gilbert, A., & Sliep, Y. (2009). Reflexivity in the practice of social action: From self-to inter-relational reflexivity. *South African Journal of Psychology, 39*(4), 468–79. https://doi.org/10.1177%2F008124630903900408

Laverack, G. (2004). Chapter 3: Power transformation and health promotion practice. In *Health promotion practice: Power and empowerment* (pp. 33–42). Sage.

Miller, R.L., & Shinn, M. (2005). Learning from communities: Overcoming difficulties in dissemination of prevention and promotion efforts. *American Journal of Community Psychology, 35*(3–4), 169–83.

Naidu, T., Sliep, Y., & Dageid, W. (2012). The social construction of identity in HIV/AIDS home-based care volunteers in rural KwaZulu-Natal, South Africa. *Journal of the Social Aspects of HIV/AIDS Research Alliance, 9*(2), 113–26. www.tandfonline.com/doi/full/10.1080/17290376.2012.683585

Norton, L., & Sliep, Y. (2018). A critical reflexive model: Working with life stories in health promotion education. *South African Journal of Higher Education, 32*(3). https://doi.org/10.20853/32-3-2523

Norton, L., & Sliep, Y. (2019). #WE SPEAK: exploring the experience of refugee youth through participatory research and poetry. *Journal of Youth Studies, 22*(7), 873–90.

Norton, L.M. (2016). Pathways of reflection: Creating voice through life story and dialogical poetry. *Forum Qualitative Sozialforschung/Forum: Qualitative Social Research* 18(1). https://doi.org/10.17169/fqs-18.1.2516

Rappaport, J. (1981). In praise of paradox: A social policy of empowerment over prevention. *American Journal of Community Psychology, 9*(1), 1–25.

Rober, P. (2005). The therapist's self in dialogical family therapy: Some ideas about not-knowing and the therapist's inner conversation. *Family Process, 44*(4), 477–95. https://doi.org/10.1111/j.1545-5300.2005.00073.x

Rule, P. (2004). Dialogic spaces: Adult education projects and social engagements. *International Journal of Lifelong Education, 23*(4), 319–34. https://doi.org/10.1080/026037042000233476

Salmon, G. (2009). E-moderating. In *Encyclopedia of Distance Learning* (2nd ed.) (pp. 890–7). IGI Global. www.igi-global.com/chapter/moderating/11852

Schwartz, S.H., & Bilsky, W. (1987). Toward a universal psychological structure of human values. *Journal of Personality and Social Psychology, 53*(3), 550–62.

Sliep, Y. (2010). Teaching for transformation: The use of narrative metaphor to develop reflexive professionals. *Acta Academica, 2010*(2), 109–32. https://journals.ufs.ac.za/index.php/aa/article/view/1292/1275

Sliep, Y. (2016) Poetry as dialogue – Navigating the storms of life. The violent contexts of tertiary education students in South Africa. In Laura Formenti & Linden West (Eds.), *Stories that make a difference. Exploring the collective, social and political potential of narratives in adult education research* (pp. 172–80). Pensa MultiMedia.

Sliep, Y. (2020). The shape of hope: troubling activism in an academic setting. Paper presented in February 2020 at the Annual Conference of ESREA – European Society for Research on the Education of Adults – Life History and Biography Network.

Sliep, Y., & Kotze, E. (2011). Weaving a learning community by the telling, deconstructing and re-telling of life stories. In K. Maree (Ed.), *Shaping the story: A guide to facilitating narrative career counselling* (pp. 138–51). Brill. https://doi.org/10.1163/9789004406162_013

World Health Organization. (1986). Ottawa charter for health promotion. The 1st International Conference on Health Promotion, Ottawa. www.who.int/publications-detail-redirect/ottawa-charter-for-health-promotion

Zawada, B. (2020). Invisible statues of colonisation: Regulatory curriculum requirements in South African higher education. *Africa Education Review, 17*(3), 142–57. https://doi.org/10.1080/18146627.2019.1683457

PART V

Community Psychology through the lens of hope

24

HOPE

Carolyn Kagan, Jacqueline Akhurst, Jaime Alfaro,
Rebecca Lawthom, Michael Richards and Alba Zambrano

Abstract

In this end note we will revisit the primacy of the ecological crisis as a lens through which to view changing social structures, alliances and possibilities for change. We will then go on to consider ways in which critical community psychological thought and praxis can work with others to recognise the realities of people's lives and engender hope for the future. We recognise the playfulness of the end note. Here we utilise it as a commentary on what has gone before but recognise it is not the end but another opening into future praxis.

Resumen

En esta nota final revisaremos la primacía de la crisis ecológica como una lente a través de la cual ver las estructuras sociales cambiantes, las alianzas y las posibilidades de cambio. Consideraremos formas en las que el pensamiento y la praxis psicológica comunitaria crítica pueden trabajar con otros para reconocer las realidades de la vida de las personas y generar esperanza para el futuro. Utilizamos el capitulo final como un comentario de lo que ha sucedido antes, pero reconocemos que no es el final sino otra apertura a la praxis futura.

The primacy of the ecological crisis

This handbook did not set out to cover all the basics of the discipline of Community Psychology, nor did it set out to cover all approaches: instead it focuses on contemporary issues and debates, through which to view critical thinking and practice. We framed the writing of this handbook in terms of addressing those systemic challenges that arise from intersecting and multiple crises affecting the lives of people around the world. We outlined those crises as (i) an economic crisis; (ii) a sociocultural crisis; (iii) the crisis of conflict and violence; (iv) a political crisis; and (v) an ecological, environmental and energy crisis. Rather than present the chapters in terms of the crises, because of their overlapping nature we viewed theory and praxis through different lenses, each of which embraced the systemic crises in different ways. However, one of the lenses was the ecological lens, which is the only one that directly coincided with a systemic crisis. This

DOI: 10.4324/9780429325663-30

needs some explanation: it is not to assert a hierarchy of importance of the crises, but rather to use the ecological lens as a vehicle for revealing new possibilities for change.

We are at a particular moment in history when the ecological crisis, after a long gestation period, has caught the public imagination – if not yet sufficient government attention. Furthermore, some of the work presented here, in solidarity and partnership with indigenous peoples or First Nations, requires us to think, and reflect differently about humans as just one part of the natural world. It is no accident that several chapters address climate change, environmental protection, biodiversity loss and associated action in one form or another. These issues are deeply enmeshed in and cannot be separated from their economic, political and social contexts, and viewing praxis through an ecological lens throws light on inequalities and power arrangements, but also on possibilities for change in new ways. The ecological crisis is so pervasive, so entwined with capitalism and its attendant inequalities, so threatening to human well-being, so tied in with political priorities and so influenced by cultural beliefs and practices that it warrants a lens of its own. It is not just the public imagination that the ecological crisis has influenced – it is also spawning new alliances and actions (as, indeed did the pandemic, as we saw in the Introduction).

This is a view elaborated by Beck (2016, p. 38), who suggests that

> climate change alters society in fundamental ways, entailing new forms of power, inequality and security, as well as new forms of cooperation, certainty and solidarity across borders.

He argues that traditional boundaries of inequalities are changing; new social norms, laws, industries, technologies and understanding of the nation state are emerging; and public discourse now recognises that principles of national sovereignty, independence and autonomy are obstacles to the survival of humans and other species. Beyond this, however, Beck argues that climate change is a force with the potential to redistribute radical social inequalities and is therefore a matter of justice. Old and new social inequalities are produced and reproduced through the political responses to climate change, but also through the physical processes themselves. Thus, poor coastal communities in the majority world have commonality with rich riverside dwellers in the Global North, as both risk losing homes and livelihoods through climate change-induced flooding (although clearly only one of these groups has the means to provide alternative living). Almost certainly the political response to each scenario will differ and the rich communities are likely to be protected, but the poor will not. However, the possibilities for shared solidarities remain, and the challenge for Community Psychology is to understand how the distribution of assets and systems of power will place some communities at greater risk than others – climate change being just one lens through which to view this challenge.

Thus, Beck argues that climate change is best seen as a device for viewing the metamorphosis of the world. For him, metamorphosis implies a much more radical transformation than "change" – a transformation in which the old certainties of modern society are falling away and something quite new is emerging. To grasp this metamorphosis of the world, he argues, it is necessary to explore the new beginnings, to focus on what is emerging from the old and seek to grasp future structures and norms in the turmoil of the present. Metamorphosis, by definition, is unfinished, unfinishable, open-ended and – this is important to notice – irreversible, but there is still a real danger that it may be harnessed by, and used for imperialistic purposes.

Similarly recognising the planetary interconnectedness of systems, the United Nations Sustainable Development Goals (SDGs) were adopted by all member states in 2015 to widespread acclaim. The 17 SDGs aim to protect the planet, to end poverty and to ensure that everyone achieves peace and prosperity; pledging to "Leave No One Behind". Whilst achieving any of the SDGs by 2030 is increasingly becoming less and less likely, they have been a useful mechanism to promote more targeted planning, giving more focus to specifying attainable goals. The SDGs recognise that progress in any one area may affect other outcomes; and the intersectoral nature aims for more balanced development that also considers future sustainability.

So, this handbook has offered a diverse snapshot of some of the ways in which Critical Community Psychology is incorporating some of the new structures and methods amongst the turmoil – or metamorphosis – of the 2010–2020 decade. This is reflected not so much in issues under discussion, but more in the processes at work and their implications for work beyond the specific issue at hand.

Facing the future with hope

Community Psychology is evolving – perhaps not quickly enough, but nevertheless, as we have seen, part of the critical fringes have gained ground and are being better incorporated into the mainstream. The chapters in this handbook offer practical ways of thinking and working in solidarity with others for change – mostly small scale and local, but tapping into wider social movements. This practice is underpinned by critical theoretical ideas, taking seriously "other" worldviews, and a thorough understanding of the complex networked systems in which we all live, beyond conceptualisations of relatively simple nested systems. The scale and scope of the projects differ but have a shared set of values guiding the work and a sense of hope.

As we have seen, some Critical Community Psychologies are embracing participative ways of identifying priorities and actions, even seeing Community Psychology as a resource to be used by others. They are challenging the privilege of highly educated professionals, recognising the grip of colonialism on people's lives and the damage it still wreaks on social institutions, and on professional education and practice. They are putting into practice "seeing with two eyes" – the sharing of different kinds of knowledge, whilst at the same time, questioning the very nature of those knowledges in perpetuating and strengthening inequalities. We can see a slowing down, a pause, a praxis that seeks to understand the situation of people's lives, not theoretically but practically through processes of deep understanding including, for example, anti-colonial recovery of historical memories, accompaniment and collaborative arts practices. We see a slowing down of the rush to intervene, to design programmes from afar and collect copious amounts of statistical data that tell us what we already know about the impact of inequality, wealth inequalities, violence and the separation of many lives from the natural world. Through this kind of work we can see, not assume, ways in which "participatory parity" (Fraser, 2003) or "mattering" is achieved (see Prilleltensky, 2019). The work represented here reflects value-based, participatory, constructivist and liberatory paradigms of thought and of praxis: alternative paradigms are for another project.

It would be relatively easy to draw a dystopian picture of the crises affecting us all; as we have seen (and know) there are momentous changes afoot, not least because of the pandemic. What this has done is to enable us to

> see with new clarity the systems – political, economic, social, ecological – in which we are immersed as they change around us. We see what's strong, what's weak, what's corrupt, what matters and what doesn't.
>
> *(Solnit 2020)*

These insights might motivate wider struggles for liberation and for change even though, at the same time, we surely know they will lead to a closing down of the interests of capital, power and prestige. We are well placed to continue to work with others in the struggles for equality, livelihoods, peace and recognition. As Freire noted, in his reworking of *Pedagogy of the Oppressed*:

> Without a minimum of hope, we cannot so much as start the struggle. But without the struggle, hope, as an ontological need, dissipates, loses its bearings and turns into hopelessness.
>
> *(Freire with Freire, 1992/1999, p. 9)*

It is not enough, in Freire's view, to simply hold on to hope for better things to come. Hope needs practice, he argues, for it to become historical concreteness (i.e. contribute to real, lasting social change). It is through action that we can emerge from the dystopian black hole into which our struggles can lead us; it is through action that we can maintain hope and through hopefulness that we are prompted to action. Conversely, hopelessness and despair are both the consequence and the cause of inaction or immobilism (Freire with Freire, 1992/1999, p. 9).

Hope does not mean denying the material realities of people's lives or the very real challenges we are faced with, but it does mean also recognising the movements, actions and shifts in consciousness and understanding that have been, and are occurring, whilst simultaneously recognising the need for constant action. Solnit (2016; foreword) cites Patrisse Cullors, one of the founders of Black Lives Matter, who recognised that grief and rage at injustices can coexist with hope, when early on in the movement's history she described the mission as to:

> Provide hope and inspiration for collective action to build collective power to achieve collective transformation, rooted in grief and rage but pointed towards vision and dreams.

We hope that the chapters in this book have, in some small way, inspired continued collective action, moving away from the singular disciplinary straitjacket to action that is cross-disciplinary and with a stronger cross-national focus.

There are, maybe, two ways to envisage the role of Community Psychology's offer, as but one community practice: they are not mutually exclusive. The first is to find ways of ensuring all the locally transformative, but small-scale, changes join up – to become something greater than the sum of the parts. This will involve constant dialogue, not only within Community Psychology but with diverse social movements, for the boundary between community action and academic or professional Community Psychology to be permeated. Community-led action, with community psychologists and Community Psychology as allies and resources to be harnessed, is one way forward.

The second is to solidly engage with our values, to harness some of those Community Psychologies that occur at local and community levels, and politicise them, in order to enable people to play their part in social transformation. In the face of the crises we face and the metamorphosis of change we are undergoing, that will mean at least and at most, to weaken the grip of capital, promote climate and environmental action and to reduce inequalities. What will this take? Kagan (2020) offered a shortlist:

Abandoning a simplistic hierarchical systems model of understanding human experience and the possibilities for change, in favour of more complex, soft systems thinking, drawing ideas and models from different fields, and unpicking ideology-action-structure complexes (Kagan and Burton, 2014).

Employing methods of critical and political consciousness-raising in order to harness local networks and energies for transformational change.

Taking seriously anti- and decoloniality, and the search for epistemic justice and finding ways of recognising different cultural and knowledge bases.

Unpacking the concept of solidarity so as to move beyond the boundaries of Community Psychology thinking, understanding and practice.

Organising internationally, across discipline and professional boundaries and working as part of wider social movements, not confining ourselves to our Community Psychology.

This politicisation is not to confine us to the realm of protest, although of course that has a place, for as the great cultural analyst Raymond Williams (1980/1989, p. 209) said:

> unless protest can be connected with and surpassed by significant practical construction, our strength will remain insufficient, It is then in making hope practical rather than despair convincing, that we must resume and change and extend our campaigns.

Whilst the pandemic continues to leave unprecedented changes, the human need for a responsive and nourishing community lives on. The chapters in this book have illustrated some of the ways in which we, as community psychologists, can contribute to making hope practical and to a positive metamorphosis of the world.

We leave you with some food for thought about the links between the COVID-19 pandemic, which has framed all of our lives throughout the production of the book, and the concerns of Community Psychology.

Reflexiones en tiempos de pandemia (Alba Zambrano, 2021)

Me pregunto: ¿Esta pandemia es nueva para quienes viven en los márgenes?
Aquellos que no tienen agua, ni alimento garantizados cada día,
Aquellos que viven en la calle, como único refugio.
Aquellas, que despiertan y experimentan el miedo profundo de la violencia,
de quienes por ser hombres se han establecido como sus opresores.
Aquellos pueblos, que ya sin tierra, deben someterse a la brutalidad del que se cree superior,
y por ello, dueño de la geografía y de la dignidad.
De aquellas comunidades que por ser definidas como "menos desarrolladas",
han debido silenciar la fuerza y riqueza de su origen e identidad.

¿Es nueva la pandemia, para las otras especies?
Aquellas, que sin ninguna tregua debieron saciar el apetito desmedido de la civilización "moderna".
Con ello, rompimos una y otra vez el patrón que sostenía la vida,
olvidando que la vida solo es posible si cuidamos la compleja red de relaciones
que involucran una comunidad, incluida la humana.
Cada uno de nosotros, a su modo, también es parte de otras pandemias;

Cuando hemos ido matando uno a uno los sueños, esos de justicia, de vida respetuosa de las vidas otras.

Cuando nos hemos ido ajustando sin voz a las fórmulas del mercado.

Cuando hemos exterminado: naturaleza, vida, culturas, otros modos de vida, otras cosmovisiones.

De variados modos, somos pandemia, viviendo una nueva pandemia.

Pero también somos vida conectada con la vida;

Con sueños pausados, y con una mayor conciencia acerca de que la vida tiene el riesgo de la muerte.

Reflections in times of pandemic (Alba Zambrano, 2021)

I wonder: Is this pandemic new to those who live on the margins?

Those who don't have water or food guaranteed every day

Those who live on the streets – their only shelter.

Those women who on waking feel the deep fear of violence

from those men who have become their oppressors.

Those peoples without land who must submit to the brutality of those who consider themselves superior

and thereby control both place and dignity.

Those communities, that by being defined as "less developed"

Have had to silence the strength and wealth of their heritage and identity.

Is the pandemic new to the other species?

Those that, without relief, have had to satisfy the insatiable appetite of "modern" civilisation.

We have broken, over and over again, the patterns that sustain life,

forgetting that life is only possible if we care for the complex web of relations

that are involved in a community, including the human one.

Every one of us is, in our own way, part of other pandemics

When we've been killing, one by one, those dreams of justice, of respect for the lives of others

When we've been silently adjusting ourselves to the laws of the market

When we've been destroying nature, life, cultures, other ways of life, other worldviews

In different ways, we are a pandemic, living a new pandemic.

But we are also life connected to life

With our dreams on hold, and with greater awareness of the fact that to live is to risk death

References

Beck, U. (2016). *The metamorphosis of the world.* Polity.

Fraser, N. (2003). Social justice in the age of identity politics: Redistribution, recognition, and participation. In N. Fraser & A. Honneth (Eds.), *Redistribution or recognition? A political-philosophical exchange.* Verso.

Freire, P., with Freire, A.M.A. (1992/1999). *Pedagogy of hope: Reliving pedagogy of the oppressed* (R.R. Barr, Trans.). Continuum.

Kagan, C. (2020). *Values and the metamorphosis of change.* European Community Psychology Association Conference, December, 2020. Bratislava (moved online).

Kagan, C.M., & Burton, M.H. (2014) Culture, identity and alternatives to the consumer culture. *Educarem Revista*, Curitiba, Brasil, n. 53, 75–89 (Dossier: Educação, Cotidiano e Participação: desafios e contribuições para a formação). http://ojs.c3sl.ufpr.br/ojs/index.php/educar/article/view/36583

Prilleltensky, I. (2019). Mattering at the intersection of psychology philosophy and politics. *American Journal of Community Psychology, 65*(1–2), 16–34.

Solnit, R. (2016). *Hope in the dark: Untold histories, wild possibilities.* Canongate.

Solnit, R.(2020, April 7). "The impossible has already happened": What coronavirus can teach us about hope. *The Guardian.* www.theguardian.com/world/2020/apr/07/what-coronavirus-can-teach-us-about-hope-rebecca-solnit

Williams, R. (1980/1989). The politics of nuclear disarmament. In *Resources of hope* (pp. 189–209). Verso.

INDEX

For Product Safety Concerns and Information please contact our EU
representative GPSR@taylorandfrancis.com
Taylor & Francis Verlag GmbH, Kaufingerstraße 24, 80331 München, Germany

boilerplate
www.ingramcontent.com/pod-product-compliance
Lightning Source LLC
Chambersburg PA
CBHW081040220326
41598CB00038B/6942

```
9 781032 160917
```